MW00837431

VisualDx: Essential Dermatology in Pigmented Skin

VisualDx: Essential Dermatology in Pigmented Skin

SENIOR EDITORS:

Aída Lugo-Somolinos, MD
Associate Professor of Dermatology
Department of Dermatology
University of North Carolina-Chapel Hill
Chapel Hill, North Carolina

Lynn McKinley-Grant, MD
Associate Professor
Division of Dermatology/Dermatology Residency Program
Georgetown University Hospital/Washington Hospital Center
Washington, District of Columbia

ASSOCIATE EDITORS:

Lowell A. Goldsmith, MD, MPH
Emeritus Professor of Dermatology
Department of Dermatology
University of North Carolina-Chapel Hill
Chapel Hill, North Carolina

Art Papier, MD
Associate Professor of Dermatology and Medical Informatics
Department of Dermatology
University of Rochester School of Medicine and Dentistry
Rochester, New York

ASSISTANT EDITORS:

Chris G. Adigun, MD
Resident in Dermatology
University of North Carolina-Chapel Hill
Chapel Hill, North Carolina

Stephanie Diamantis, MD
Resident in Dermatology
University of North Carolina-Chapel Hill
Chapel Hill, North Carolina

Donna Culton, MD, PhD
Assistant Professor of Dermatology
Department of Dermatology
University of North Carolina-Chapel Hill
Chapel Hill, North Carolina

Arden Fredeking, MD
Resident in Dermatology and Internal Medicine
Georgetown University Hospital/Washington Hospital Center
Washington, District of Columbia

Ivy Lee, MD
Resident in Dermatology
Georgetown University Hospital/Washington Hospital Center
Washington, District of Columbia

Mat Davey, MD
Resident in Dermatology
University of North Carolina-Chapel Hill
Chapel Hill, North Carolina

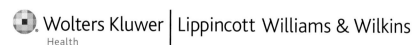
Wolters Kluwer | Lippincott Williams & Wilkins
Health

Philadelphia · Baltimore · New York · London
Buenos Aires · Hong Kong · Sydney · Tokyo

Acquisitions Editor: Sonya Seigafuse
Product Manager: Kerry Barrett
Production Manager: Alicia Jackson
Senior Manufacturing Manager: Benjamin Rivera
Marketing Manager: Kim Schonberger
Design Coordinator: Terry Mallon
Production Service: SPi Global

© 2011 by LIPPINCOTT WILLIAMS & WILKINS, a WOLTERS KLUWER business
Two Commerce Square
2001 Market Street
Philadelphia, PA 19103 USA
LWW.com

All rights reserved. This book is protected by copyright. No part of this book may be reproduced in any form by any means, including photocopying, or utilized by any information storage and retrieval system without written permission from the copyright owner, except for brief quotations embodied in critical articles and reviews. Materials appearing in this book prepared by individuals as part of their official duties as U.S. government employees are not covered by the above-mentioned copyright.

Printed in China

Library of Congress Cataloging-in-Publication Data
  VisualDx. Essential dermatology in pigmented skin / senior editors, Aída Lugo-Somolinos, Lynn McKinley-Grant ; associate editors, Lowell A. Goldsmith, Art Papier ; assistant editors, Chris G. Adigun ...[et al.].
    p. ; cm. — (VisualDx essential dermatology series)
  Essential dermatology in pigmented skin
  Includes bibliographical references and index.
  ISBN-13: 978-1-4511-1605-2
  ISBN-10: 1-4511-1605-5
  1. Skin—Diseases—Diagnosis. 2. Skin—Diseases—Treatment. 3. Pigmentation disorders. I. Lugo-Somolinos, Aída.
II. McKinley-Grant, Lynn. III. Title: Essential dermatology in pigmented skin. IV. Series: VisualDx essential dermatology series.
  [DNLM: 1. Skin Diseases—diagnosis. 2. Skin Manifestations. 3. Skin Pigmentation—physiology. WR 141]
  RL105.V57   2012
  616.5—dc22

                                                                                                    2010054172

Care has been taken to confirm the accuracy of the information presented and to describe generally accepted practices. However, the authors, editors, and publisher are not responsible for errors or omissions or for any consequences from application of the information in this book and make no warranty, expressed or implied, with respect to the currency, completeness, or accuracy of the contents of the publication. Application of the information in a particular situation remains the professional responsibility of the practitioner.

The authors, editors, and publisher have exerted every effort to ensure that drug selection and dosage set forth in this text are in accordance with current recommendations and practice at the time of publication. However, in view of ongoing research, changes in government regulations, and the constant flow of information relating to drug therapy and drug reactions, the reader is urged to check the package insert for each drug for any change in indications and dosage and for added warnings and precautions. This is particularly important when the recommended agent is a new or infrequently employed drug.

Some drugs and medical devices presented in the publication have Food and Drug Administration (FDA) clearance for limited use in restricted research settings. It is the responsibility of the health care provider to ascertain the FDA status of each drug or device planned for use in their clinical practice.

To purchase additional copies of this book, call our customer service department at (800) 638-3030 or fax orders to (301) 223-2320. International customers should call (301) 223-2300.

Visit Lippincott Williams & Wilkins on the Internet: at LWW.com. Lippincott Williams & Wilkins customer service representatives are available from 8:30 am to 6 pm, EST.

                                                                                    10 9 8 7 6 5 4 3 2 1

Contributors

Chris G. Adigun, MD
Resident in Dermatology
University of North Carolina-Chapel Hill
Chapel Hill, North Carolina

Naurin Ahmad, MD
Resident in Dermatology and Internal Medicine
Georgetown University Hospital/Washington Hospital Center
Washington, District of Columbia

Kimberly Capers Arrington, MD
Resident in Dermatology and Internal Medicine
Georgetown University Hospital/Washington Hospital Center
Washington, District of Columbia

Nasir Aziz, MD
Resident in Dermatology
Georgetown University Hospital/Washington Hospital Center
Washington, District of Columbia

Suzanne Berkman, MD
Resident in Dermatology
Georgetown University Hospital/Washington Hospital Center
Washington, District of Columbia

Rodolfo E. Chirinos, MD, MSc
Resident in Dermatology
Georgetown University Hospital/Washington Hospital Center
Washington, District of Columbia

Morgana Colombo, MD
Resident in Dermatology and Internal Medicine
Georgetown University Hospital/Washington Hospital Center
Washington, District of Columbia

Donna Culton, MD, PhD
Assistant Professor of Dermatology
Department of Dermatology
University of North Carolina-Chapel Hill
Chapel Hill, North Carolina

Mat Davey, MD
Resident in Dermatology
University of North Carolina-Chapel Hill
Chapel Hill, North Carolina

Cynthia Marie Carver DeKlotz, MD
Resident in Dermatology and Internal Medicine
Georgetown University Hospital/Washington Hospital Center
Washington, District of Columbia

Kristina L. Demas
Medical Student
George Washington University
Washington, District of Columbia

Jennifer Alston DeSimone, MD
DermAssociates
Silver Spring, Maryland

Stephanie Diamantis, MD
Resident in Dermatology
University of North Carolina-Chapel Hill
Chapel Hill, North Carolina

Kamilah Dixon
Medical Student
Georgetown University
Washington, District of Columbia

Sridhar Dronavalli, MD
Resident in Dermatology and Internal Medicine
Georgetown University Hospital/Washington Hospital Center
Washington, District of Columbia

Meaghan Canton Feder, NP
Division of Dermatology
Georgetown University Hospital
Washington, District of Columbia

Arden Fredeking, MD
Resident in Dermatology and Internal Medicine
Georgetown University Hospital/Washington Hospital Center
Washington, District of Columbia

Lowell A. Goldsmith, MD, MPH
Emeritus Professor of Dermatology
Department of Dermatology
University of North Carolina-Chapel Hill
Chapel Hill, North Carolina

Laurie Good, MD
Internal Medicine Preliminary Intern
Saint Joseph Hospital
Denver, Colorado

Jennifer Hensley, MD
Melanoma Fellow
Division of Dermatology
Georgetown University Hospital/Washington Hospital Center
Washington, District of Columbia

Randa Khoury, MD
Melanoma Fellow
Division of Dermatology
Georgetown University Hospital/Washington Hospital Center
Washington, District of Columbia

Ivy Lee, MD
Resident in Dermatology
Georgetown University Hospital/Washington Hospital Center
Washington, District of Columbia

Aída Lugo-Somolinos, MD
Associate Professor of Dermatology
Department of Dermatology
University of North Carolina-Chapel Hill
Chapel Hill, North Carolina

Erin Luxenberg, MD
Resident in Internal Medicine and Dermatology
University of Minnesota
Minneapolis, Minnesota

Lynn McKinley-Grant, MD
Associate Professor
Division of Dermatology/Dermatology Residency Program
Georgetown University Hospital/Washington Hospital Center
Washington, District of Columbia

Mary Gail Mercurio, MD
Associate Professor
Department of Dermatology
University of Rochester School of Medicine and Dentistry
Rochester, New York

Tess Nasabzadeh, MD
Resident in Dermatology and Internal Medicine
Georgetown University Hospital/Washington Hospital Center
Washington, District of Columbia

Sabrina Newman, MD
Resident in Dermatology and Internal Medicine
Georgetown University Hospital/Washington Hospital Center
Washington, District of Columbia

Alicia Ogram, MD
Resident in Dermatology
Georgetown University Hospital/Washington Hospital Center
Washington, District of Columbia

Katie L. Osley, MD
Resident in Internal Medicine
Thomas Jefferson University Hospital
Philadelphia, Pennsylvania

Saurabh Singh, MD
Resident in Dermatology
Georgetown University Hospital/Washington Hospital Center
Washington, District of Columbia

Pooja Sodha
Medical Student
Georgetown University
Washington, District of Columbia

Adam Tinklepaugh
Medical Student
George Washington University
Washington, District of Columbia

Suraj Venna, MD
Director of the Melanoma Center
Washington Cancer Institute of Washington Hospital Center
Assistant Professor, Division of Dermatology/Dermatology
    Residency Program
Georgetown University Hospital/Washington Hospital Center
Washington, District of Columbia

Table of Contents

Preface

For the past decade, Logical Images has had an explicit goal to capture the rich variations of skin diseases, including those variations related to skin pigmentation and ethnicity. Early in 2001, we incorporated two modules into the VisualDx system—"Rashes in Dark Skin, and Lesions and Growths in Dark Skin"—edited by Paul Kelly, MD, one of the world's experts in skin disease in pigmented skin, and Lowell A. Goldsmith, MD, MPH. Those modules began to fill the gap that existed, because almost all textbooks and atlases are deficient in illustrations of cutaneous diseases in darkly pigmented skin (for an overview of this deficiency, see *J Am Acad Dermatol.* 2006 Oct;55:687–690). Even in the Logical Images' database of nearly 70,000 images, we find that there are insufficient images of some diseases in pigmented skin.

VisualDx: Essential Dermatology in Pigmented Skin is a monograph edited by Aída Lugo-Somolinos, MD, from the University of North Carolina (and previously on the faculty of the University of Puerto Rico) and Lynn McKinley-Grant, MD, of the faculty of Georgetown University, two clinicians who have extensive experience caring for patients with pigmented skin, including Hispanics, African Americans, and diverse patients from many countries. This volume has over 700 pictures of skin diseases in adults and children with darkly pigmented skin. This text and its illustrations are important not only for the health professionals who are using the book for diagnosis and treatment but also for their patients—whom they will be able to show images of "their disease" as it presents in a skin type resembling their pigmentation. Using pictures to more effectively connect the patient and the physician is an essential part of exemplary medicine.

This volume complements two books in our *VisualDx: Essential Dermatology* monograph series: one addressing skin disease in children (edited by Craig N. Burkhart, MD, and Dean Morrell, MD) and a volume on skin disease in adults (edited by Noah Craft, MD, and Lindy Fox, MD). The monograph series is a combined book/online product blending the strengths of a traditional book format with the innovative online VisualDx diagnostic system. The online VisualDx diagnostic database has extensive disease- and therapy-related data, which were used by contributing authors to develop the *VisualDx: Essential Dermatology* texts. Only a small percentage of the images in this volume have appeared in the other *VisualDx: Essential Dermatology* books.

The books are stand-alone publications addressing the tasks of diagnosis and therapy and are immeasurably strengthened and enriched when used by those accessing the online and other electronically sourced materials.

These books and the VisualDx electronic media are developing synergistic interactions to lead to outstanding patient care, and Wolters Kluwer/Lippincott Williams & Wilkins is our talented and enthusiastic partner in developing this pacesetting set of critically needed texts.

Aída Lugo-Somolinos, MD
Lynn McKinley-Grant, MD
Art Papier, MD
Lowell A. Goldsmith, MD, MPH

Acknowledgments

Many of the photographs in this book are from the collections of many contributors including the slide collections of the senior and associate editors and the institutional collections at New York University, the University of Rochester School of Medicine and Dentistry, and the Washington Hospital Center. Special thanks to Drs. Charles Crutchfield III, Jeffrey Callen, Thomas Nigra, and Nancy Esterly whose slides of skin diseases in those with pigmented skin were especially valuable for this project. Other contributors include Victor D. Newcomer, MD; Karen Wiss, MD; Tor Shwayder, MD; Stephen Estes, MD; Shahbaz A. Janjua, MD; Steven Oberlender, MD, PhD; David Foster, MD, MPH; Noah Craft, MD, PhD; David Elpern, MD; Bernardo Gontijo, MD, PhD; Lawrence Parish, MD; Mary Gail Mercurio, MD; Frances J. Storrs, MD; Robert Baran, MD; Robert Brodell, MD; Robert Chalmers, MD; Flavio Ciferri, MD; Sethuraman Gomathy, MD; Elaine Siegfried, MD; Mary J. Spencer, MD; William Bonnez, MD; Robert A. Briggaman, MD; Walter Brooks, MD; E. Dale Everett, MD; Benjamin Fisher, MD; Kenneth G. Gross, MD; Alan Gruber, MD; Robert Kalb, MD; Edith Lederman, MD; Jason Maguire, MD; Karen McKoy, MD; and Larry E. Millikan, MD.

Illustrations of morphologic lesion types in pigmented skin were created by Glen Hintz, MS, Professor of Medical Illustration at the Rochester Institute of Technology.

Portions of therapy tables in Chapter 5 were first developed by Drs. Craig N. Burkhart and Dean S. Morrell for *VisualDx: Essential Pediatric Dermatology* and Drs. Noah Craft and Lindy P. Fox for *VisualDx: Essential Adult Dermatology*.

The VisualDx database at Logical Images has been developed for over ten years by dozens of contributors and is the source of portions of this book.

Special thanks to Layla Heimlich at the William B. Glew, MD, Health Sciences Library of Washington Hospital Center for help in finding published materials related to skin diseases in pigmented skin.

All the authors and editors are grateful for the extraordinary care and diligence that Angela Delacenserie and Frances Reed gave to the preparation and redaction of the text and for the professional skill with which Stephanie Piro prepared the large number of clinical images for this book. Sonya Seigafuse, Kim Schonberger, and Kerry Barrett at Lippincott Williams & Wilkins helped make this complex project a reality.

Introduction to the VisualDx: Essential Dermatology Series

Welcome to the *VisualDx: Essential Dermatology* series. The goal of this series is to assist you in making the diagnosis and planning for the treatment of the most common skin disorders you will encounter in your daily clinical practice. *VisualDx: Essential Dermatology in Pigmented Skin* addresses the common and some serious skin disorders in patients with darkly pigmented skin.

You have purchased two stand-alone but synergistic products: a book and a digital database that can be accessed on your desktop computer, laptop, tablet, or smartphone device.

1. Book: This book has a unique approach to the diagnosis and treatment of skin diseases in adults and children with dark skin pigmentation. The book is organized by skin lesion morphology to assist the differential diagnostic process. The diseases in the book can also be accessed using a traditional index. Individual diseases are summarized in clinically oriented, concise texts providing an overview of the disease and visual signs and symptoms, diagnostic pearls, best laboratory tests, differential diagnosis, therapy, and key literature references. Each diagnosis is extensively illustrated with the highest quality color photographs. The book can be rapidly used during the patient encounter or as a study aid away from the patient visit.

2. Electronic Access—Online and Mobile Platforms: The online version of *VisualDx: Essential Dermatology in Pigmented Skin* is one component of the VisualDx visual diagnostic decision support system. VisualDx is more than an online atlas or textbook; the system is used at the point of care to develop visually rich differential diagnoses. The online system includes thousands of images and expert-written and -edited text. It can be accessed on the Internet or mobile device by signing in at www.essentialdermatology.com/pigmented if you are a first-time user or www.visualdx.com/visualdx if you have already set up your password and by accessing the VisualDx application for your mobile source (iPad, iPhone, iTouch, and Android devices).

Whether on the desktop or mobile device, VisualDx is typically used to read about a diagnosis and view images, or build a differential diagnosis based on patient factors.

- Individual diseases can be accessed from the home page, or a complete differential diagnosis can be developed in seconds.
- Novices unfamiliar with morphologic terminology are assisted by interactive icons; searches can be conducted through these icons or by typing in the patient findings.
- Users can search signs and symptoms, medications, medical history, travel history, laboratory findings, and more.
- In addition to building a custom differential diagnosis with patient findings, users who choose to look up a specific diagnosis can quickly see a "textbook" differential diagnosis and access diagnoses within the differential by hyperlink.
- Disease information and images can be printed and shared with patients or coworkers.

We certainly hope that this product will be useful to you and the patients you care for.

Please look for other titles in the *VisualDx: Essential Dermatology* series.

Introduction to VisualDx: Essential Dermatology in Pigmented Skin Online

To access your personal-use online subscription, go to www.essentialdermatology.com/pigmented and register using the code found in the front of this book.

VisualDx is a diagnostic clinical decision support system that integrates search, imagery, and text in an easy-to-use Web browser-based system. VisualDx allows you to "look up" information by multiple parameters simultaneously rather than by a single index term, as found in print-based resources. It is important to know that online VisualDx does not only work by a simple search of this textbook or a search of text in an online database. Our authors and editors have reviewed the medical literature and created a search technology that allows you, the user, to search by patient findings. Through organization by patient characteristics such as symptoms, signs, visual clues, laboratory, and so forth, you will receive highly relevant information results. This distinction is important: when using a search engine such as Google or Yahoo, one is searching millions of pages of text. In decision support systems such as VisualDx, you do not experience the randomness of millions of pages of search and results; you are searching purposefully designed medical relationships derived from the medical literature. The search results are more accurate, easier to read, and more comprehensive from the point of view of clinical differential diagnosis. And the process takes much less time than it took to read this paragraph!

Investigate this distinction, and prove it for yourself. Start by registering your VisualDx online account. Visit www.essentialdermatology.com/pigmented and enter the code as instructed on the inside cover of this book. If you have already registered, login at www.visualdx.com/visualdx. With your user ID and password, you can also download a VisualDx application for your mobile device (iPad, iPhone, iTouch, and Android devices).

Look Up a Diagnosis

If you have a presumptive diagnosis and are looking for more images of the disease, or you are interested in delving deeper into the "textbook" differential diagnoses, simply type the diagnosis name into the search box on the VisualDx home page; you may choose from the type-ahead menu. Click on the diagnosis name to access the disease summary, organized by disease synopsis, visual signs and symptoms, diagnostic pearls, differential diagnosis, best laboratory tests, management and therapy, and key literature references. Disease summaries for conditions listed in the differential diagnosis may be accessed via hyperlink, as can PubMed abstract pages for journal articles in the key references.

Differential Builder

To build a custom differential based on your patient's findings, click the Differential Builder button on the VisualDx home page. You will see a series of problem-oriented choices. Choose the clinical scenario (content area) that is most clinically relevant for your patient. Once within a particular clinical scenario (e.g., Differential Builder: Dark Skin Rash), click the Quick Start button to guide your process, or bypass the quick start option and enter findings directly by typing them into the Type to Add Findings text box and selecting from the type-ahead menu. The Quick Start button guides the user through the entry points on the left side of the screen: lesion type (morphology), body location or distribution, and key questions. Browse All Findings allows the user to view findings by category (e.g., appearance of the patient).

Note: For a review of morphology and distribution terms, use the free interactive tutorial LearnDerm at www.logical-images.com/educationalTools/learnDerm.htm.

Searching by a single characteristic such as distribution or lesion type can often give dozens of results. You can narrow your search by entering multiple characteristics, including lesion distribution (Fig. 1), lesion type (Fig. 2), timing of onset and duration of lesions, and other signs and symptoms. Figure 2 shows the vesicular/pustular lesion types in pigmented skin, and Figure 3 depicts the visual differential diagnosis of pustule (lesion type) and widespread (distribution) with thumbnail clinical images.

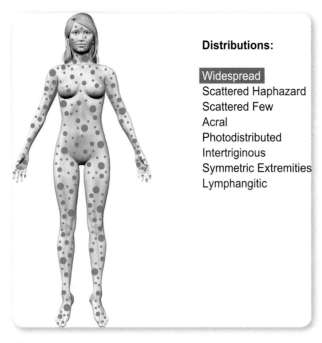

Distributions:

Widespread
Scattered Haphazard
Scattered Few
Acral
Photodistributed
Intertriginous
Symmetric Extremities
Lymphangitic

Figure 1 A widespread distribution selected for adult.

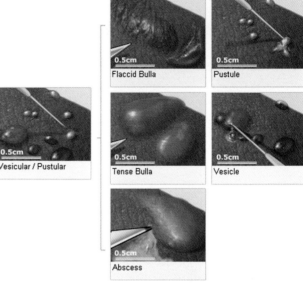

Figure 2 Vesicular/pustular lesion morphology and its subtypes, including pustule.

4 diagnoses match all 2 current findings

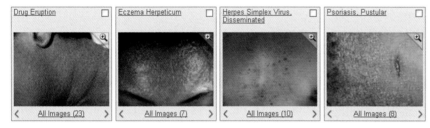

56 diagnoses match 1 of 2 current findings

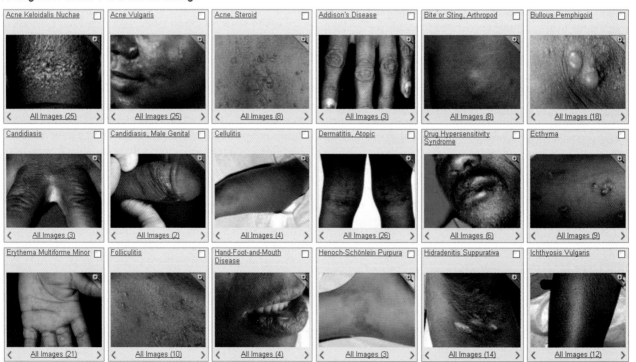

Figure 3 As findings are entered, VisualDx returns a visual differential diagnosis organized by the diagnoses with most matched findings.

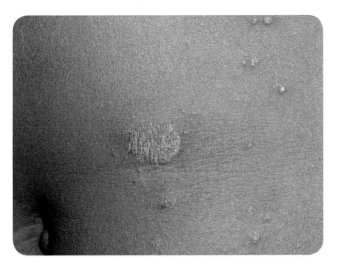

Figure 4 In dark skin, small papules are common as well as the more typical scaly plaques in pityriasis rosea.

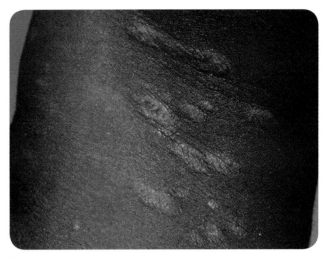

Figure 5 Typical oval plaques of pityriasis rosea following lines of cleavage in the neck.

Further, you can view multiple images of a single disease appearing in the visual differential diagnosis to see disease variation, as for pityriasis rosea (Figs. 4 and 5), a common disorder in pigmented and lightly pigmented skin. The online system has many examples of the classical and non-classical morphologies and distributions, and the system interface will re-sort the thumbnail results depending on lesion type, thus accounting for the variation possible with each disease.

We have planned this book and computer resource to be useful to you and your patients.

Please look for other titles in the *VisualDx Essential Dermatology* series: *VisualDx: Essential Adult Dermatology* and *VisualDx: Essential Pediatric Dermatology*.

CHAPTER 1

Approach to the Dermatologic Patient

In all successful patient-doctor visits, the needs of both parties are satisfied. In all patient-doctor visits that are less than successful, the differences between the two participants are not addressed appropriately. As the amount of time available for doctors and patients to get to know each other diminishes, encounters between physicians and patients, who are frequently of different cultural backgrounds, are particularly complex.

In this chapter, we discuss the implicit and explicit challenges that can arise in approaching and communicating with patients who are from different ethnic or cultural backgrounds than their physician and may have pigmented skin. We offer some practical advice about how to ensure that the dermatology visit is successful and meaningful.

Importance of Cultural Competency

What does the approach to patients have to do with the color of their skin? In one sense, the answer to this question is "nothing." All patients, regardless of skin color, should be treated with courtesy and respect. But in another sense, the answer to the question is that the approach to patients with pigmented skin is different because physicians must take into account the patients' unique cultural backgrounds, attitudes toward diagnoses and treatments, and unique susceptibility toward certain dermatologic conditions.

The ethnic composition of the U.S. population has changed in recent decades and is likely to change even more in the future. For example, between 2000 and 2010, the proportion of whites in the United States decreased from 81.0% to 79.3%, while the proportion of blacks increased from 12.7% to 13.1% and of Hispanics from 12.6% to 15.5%.[1] The U.S. Census Bureau predicts that in 2050, 72.1% of Americans will be white, 14.6% will be black, and 24.4% will be Hispanic. As a result of these changes, a larger proportion of the dermatology patient population will consist of people with pigmented skin.

The racial and ethnic backgrounds of physicians do not currently match those of their patients, and this is unlikely to change drastically in the near future. Although the proportion of white physicians, 76.8% in 2009, is similar to the proportion of whites in the general population, the proportions of black (5.7%) and Hispanic (11.1%) physicians are lower than in the general population.[2]

Before approaching any patient, today's physicians must be aware that many of their patients will probably have a different racial and ethnic background than the physician. This is important because it could have a major impact on the type of approach to the patient that will be most successful. Physicians must also be prepared to tailor their approach to the patient based on whether the patient and physician are of the same gender and whether the patient is a member of one of several hundred ethnic minority groups in the United States.

Because of the high likelihood that physicians and patients will come from different ethnic and cultural backgrounds, physicians must be culturally competent. For example, physicians need to be aware of their patients' cultural background whenever they prescribe a treatment that will change the patient's skin color. In some cultures, making skin darker is taboo, and patients from these cultures are unlikely to adhere to a medication that has this effect. In this situation, the physician needs to be honest about the medication's potential effects and explain why the treatment is important. If the patient still refuses the treatment, the physician needs to consider alternative treatment approaches.

Cultural competency requires an understanding of the different ways in which people from different cultures interpret body language, including hand movements and touching by others, as well as eye contact. In some cultures, physical contact between unrelated men and women is prohibited. Culturally competent physicians also understand that certain dermatologic features, such as moles or scars, have different implications for people from different cultures. An awareness of how patients with pigmented skin might respond to different dermatology diagnoses or terms can help the physician customize his or her communication approach to meet the patients' needs.

The Patient History

All patients approach cosmetically obvious skin lesions with apprehension. However, patients with pigmented skin are more likely to have particular concerns about certain dermatology conditions. For example, a vitiligo diagnosis in people from certain areas of Asia might raise fears of Hansen disease. Similarly, hyperpigmentation, which is common in people with pigmented skin, in a young person might result in decreased self esteem and increase the risk of being a victim of bullying at school. Patients might not raise these issues spontaneously, so physicians must be ready to discuss them at the proper moment.

Taking the patient history in dermatology serves as the basis for the relationship between the physician and the patient. In fact, this first interaction portends the rapport between the patient and physician. During this process, the physician asks general questions and chooses which additional questions to ask based on the patient's responses, as well as the physician's observations.

Taking a good history from a patient who has a dermatology problem requires using virtually all of the physician's senses. For example, the physician uses his or her ears to hear what the patient is saying and how he or she is saying it (such as whether the patient hesitates or refuses to answer certain questions); eyes to observe the patient's skin, clothing, and body language, as well as other members of the patient's family if any are present; touch to feel the hydration and morphology of any lesions; and smell to gather clues about a patient's skin disorder.

Information that might seem extraneous to the patient can be very valuable to the physician. The physician uses this information to assess the patient's mindset and his or her likely response to any therapeutic plan the physician proposes. The best histories involve consideration of a variety of conditions and insightful questions.

Obtaining a history may be especially challenging when the patient's native language is not one that the physician can speak or when ethnic or religious traditions prevent frank discussion. When the patient and physician do not speak the same language, the physician can ask a family member to interpret for the patient or arrange for an on-site or telephone interpreter to assist. If the patient's cultural or ethnic background makes discussing certain topics difficult, asking others in the examination room to step out of the room can sometimes help.

Social (including where the patient comes from and where and when the patient has recently traveled), occupational, family, and noncutaneous medical histories are vital for establishing the full and rich substrate for the physician–patient relationship. For the time-challenged physician, these histories remain essential because many dermatologic diseases are influenced by environmental, genetic, and occupational factors. By the end of the history, the physician's approach should have established in the patient's mind that the medical encounter is proceeding successfully, the physician is a very competent professional, and the patient will be part of the short- and long-term solution to the problem. The patient needs to feel that he or she has come to the right place and that the doctor understands what the patient is experiencing.

Communicating with the Patient

Throughout the visit, the physician should explain to the patient what the physician is observing. This will make the patient a participant in the process and will ultimately enlist him or her in the diagnostic, prevention, and treatment plans.

Most patients are uncomfortable with the uncertainty that is intrinsic to many facets of medicine. Clear communication about the diagnostic and therapeutic processes may allay some of the patient's anxiety. The physician must be careful not to demonstrate any anxiety because this could exacerbate the patient's anxiety.

The physician should try to build rapport with the patient throughout the visit by discussing conditions using terms that are common in the patient's community and demonstrating knowledge about the home and folk remedies that the patient might have used before consulting the physician. The physician should not make any assumptions or judgmental comments about home remedies that the patient has used or might be considering; some of these home remedies could be effective, although the physician should warn the patient not to use any remedies known to be harmful.

If the physician prescribes a medication, he or she needs to ensure that the patient understands how to take the medication properly and is aware of any potential side effects. This is another instance where cultural sensitivity is important because, when choosing which treatment to prescribe, the physician should be aware that people in some cultures are not comfortable taking pills, whereas others will only take medicine in the form of pills or injections.

The physician should determine the patient's literacy level because a patient who cannot read will not be able to follow instructions for taking a medication, for example, if these instructions are only delivered in writing. If a patient cannot read or cannot read English, the physician should determine whether another member of the patient's household might be able to read the information to the patient. The physician should also consider whether the patient might have a hearing or visual impairment that might require a more tailored communications approach. Finally, if the patient does not speak English well or at all, the physician should not simply speak English more loudly—finding a family member or professional interpreter is a much more appropriate, culturally competent, and effective approach.

If the physician needs to disclose bad news (such as the need for further treatment based on lab test results) to the patient, this should be done in person and not over the phone.[3] If the news might be very upsetting, the physician should suggest that the patient brings a family member or friend to provide support. The physician should demonstrate a caring and compassionate sense of connection with the patient and pace the discussion according to the patient's emotional state. The physician should avoid using jargon and, if the patient or a household member can read English, should write out the name of the condition for the patient or give the patient a pamphlet or handout with details on the disease. The physician should make sure that the patient does not blame himself or herself for the problem. The physician should confirm that the patient has understood the information by asking the patient to explain the information using his or her own words. The visit should include time for the patient to integrate the information and ask questions, and the physician should be prepared to refer the patient to a dermatologist or community-based resources where appropriate.

Approach to Dealing with Potential Abuse

If the physician suspects that the patient might have experienced sexual or physical abuse, the physician should report these suspicions to the appropriate local social service agency.[4] If the physician is not sure whether to report the case, he or she should discuss the situation with local adult or elder abuse consultants.[5]

During the dermatology visit, the physician should keep in mind that certain cultural practices, such as cupping and coining, lead to ecchymosis formation in distinctive patterns. Proper evaluation is necessary because the use of cultural practices does not exclude the possibility that the patient has experienced physical abuse.

When the physician suspects sexual or physical abuse, he or she should complete a full physical examination to identify signs of abuse. If the patient has symptoms suggesting a sexually transmissible infection, the physician should test the patient for common sexually transmitted infections before initiating treatments that could interfere with the diagnosis of such infections.

Approach to HIV/AIDS

If the physician suspects that a patient with pigmented skin might have HIV/AIDS or a sexually transmitted disease, the physician must explain his or her suspicion in a way that will not make the patient feel guilty or think that the physician is basing this suspicion on the patient's social or ethnic background.

If the physician suspects that the patient has HIV/AIDS, in particular, the physician must determine whether the patient has any of the risk factors for this condition. The physician can ask questions about HIV/AIDS risk factors as part of the past medical history. Specifically, when collecting the patient's vaccine history, the physician should ask whether the patient has been tested for HIV. For example, the physician might ask, "Have you had the hepatitis vaccine? Have you ever been tested for HIV? If so, what were the results? If not, would you like to be tested?"

Other questions should address previous blood transfusions, intravenous drug use, sexual contact, and sexual orientation. Questions about sexual contact and sexual orientation, in particular, must be asked with cultural sensitivity. To be able to discuss HIV/AIDS in a culturally sensitive way, physicians should become familiar with the meanings of HIV in different cultures.

References

1. U.S. Census Bureau. Projected Population of the United States by Race and Hispanic Origin: 2000 to 2050, Table 1a. http://www.census.gov/population/www/projections/usinterimproj/natprojtab01a.pdf.

2. U.S. Department of Labor, U.S. Bureau of Labor Statistics. Labor Force Characteristics by Race and Ethnicity, 2009. Report 1026. http://www.bls.gov/cps/cpsrace2009.pdf

3. Levetown M; American Academy of Pediatrics Committee on Bioethics. Communicating with children and families: from everyday interactions to skill in conveying distressing information. *Pediatrics*. 2008;121(5): e1441–e1460.

4. Centers for Disease Control and Prevention; Workowski KA, Berman SM. Sexually transmitted diseases treatment guidelines, 2006. *MMWR Recomm Rep*. 2006;55(RR-11):83–86.

5. Kellogg N; American Academy of Pediatrics Committee on Child Abuse and Neglect. The evaluation of sexual abuse in children. *Pediatrics*. 2005;116(2):506–512.

CHAPTER 2

Examination of Pigmented Skin

What does the color of the skin have to do with prevention, diagnosis, and treatment of skin disease? From a visual perspective, the background color of the skin has *everything* to do with making the correct diagnosis. What is considered pigmented skin? It is a term that has been used along with terms such as dark skin, ethnic skin, brown skin, and skin of color to describe patients with Fitzpatrick skin Types III–VI.[1] Ethnic groups more commonly referred to include Hispanic or Latino, black or African American, Native American, Asian, Pacific Islander, South East Asian, Indian, and Middle Eastern.

With projections from the Census indicating that, by the year 2056, more than 50% of the US population will be nonwhite, the study and recognition of the different dermatologic conditions presenting in these populations is even more important. For example, lesions commonly presenting as macules and patches in white skin (Fitzpatrick Types I and II) may present as papules or nodules in darker skin, and pigmented skin is more likely to develop postinflammatory hyperpigmentation or hypopigmentation than white skin.

The physical exam is where the special skills of the physician come to the fore. Thoroughness establishes the physician as the consummate professional and expert. Looking in the mouth and between the toes, carefully parting the hair to examine the scalp, and inspecting all of the nails may never have been done before in an exam, and the patient will be impressed by the assiduous search for disease and etiology. Pigmented lesions are more common on the hands, feet, and oral mucosa of people with pigmented skin. Explaining this to the patient will make him or her feel that the physician is familiar with pigmented skin.

The health care provider must be sensitive as to how to examine each area of the body in people of different ethnic and religious backgrounds. The physician must ask who can be present in the room, how much of the body can be exposed, and what parts are not to be examined. It is best to take the lead from the patient.

The Patient

The examination of the patient starts when you walk into the room and introduce yourself to the patient and to anyone else in the room who is part of the patient's support team. It is best to first interact with the patient, including pediatric patients, and then quickly acknowledge and identify the support team. We prefer to have patients identify the relationship with others in the room because complications may ensue when you assume who the spouse, parents, grandparents, or other friends or family members are. Also it is very important to identify who will be the interpreter in cases where the physician does not speak the language of the patient.

The examination requires the health care provider to use multiple senses—including sight, smell, hearing, and touch—to help make the diagnosis. Using sight, you may be able to see the distribution of a rash, and you can observe family members present to see if the condition may be hereditary or congenital or to identify the culture of the patient. Certain bacteria and fungi have an odor; the smell of cigarette smoke is distinct; and using smell, you may be able to assess level of hygiene. You can hear the patients speak and identify whether English is their second language and determine their literacy level and level of education. With touch, you can feel the hands to see if there is involvement of the rash on the hands.

When patients ask the physician to examine a particular lesion or area of involved skin, the physician often focuses on the patient complaint without looking elsewhere. Looking at an isolated lesion without examining the patient completely, however, may lead to misdiagnosis or nondiagnosis of potentially serious lesions. There are many cutaneous clues that will assist the physician in diagnosing systemic diseases. For example, not only will patients who smoke smell like smoke, but their skin color will be darker and grey, they will have fine wrinkles around the lips, and the teeth will be brown—in these patients, you may want to look for weight loss and other signs of lung cancer or bladder cancer.

Encourage your patient to completely disrobe and wear a gown, explaining how other clues or problems might be hidden on skin covered by clothing. We must be aware particularly of the cultural implications of what nakedness represents. For example, Hispanic and Middle Eastern patients are more comfortable when examined by a physician of the same sex, and female patients should always be examined in the presence of a chaperone. We recommend chaperones for physician and patient interactions of opposite sex and total body skin exam or genitalia exam. Some religious beliefs may also prevent the physician from performing a complete skin examination.

Once the patient is prepared for the examination, it is more acceptable and less invasive to start with the fingers, nails, and upper extremities. After establishing comfort and observing for nail-related findings, the examiner can work his or her way to the rest of the body, verbalizing where he or she is going in advance and what is being seen. Verbalizing your findings will allow for patient input, provide reassurance and instill confidence in the clinical interaction, and distract the patient from potential fear.

When performing a skin examination, the entire skin surface should be examined, including the scalp, oral cavity, genitals, and nails. Gloves are worn for examination of the genitals, feet, scalp, intraoral palpation, and palpation of potentially infectious lesions that are moist, hemorrhagic, or crusted. Gloves are not necessary for examination elsewhere unless there is a concern about infection; some patients may feel more at ease if the provider does wear gloves, but sometimes wearing gloves for the complete examination may cause the patient to feel embarrassed or self-conscious. Further, in a patient with a common, easily diagnosed, and noninfectious condition such as psoriasis, touching the patient's psoriatic plaques or shaking his or her hands without gloves can make him or her feel normal and comfortable. This can be reassuring to the patient as well as to family members, illustrating that he or she is not contagious. The use of gloves is thus part of the art of dermatology, and patients can participate in the gloves decision for the general body epidermis examination.

Hospitalized Patient

It is important to examine the entire skin surface of a hospitalized patient to look for critical clues to systemic disease, infections, and inflammatory processes. The physician should try to understand the cultural meaning of being in the hospital. The examination may require nursing assistance to turn the patient, remove bandages, etc. The lighting can be poor in hospitals, so in pigmented skin the physician will need all of the tools included below. In most life-threatening diagnoses, the key to early detection is recognition of erythema, which is the earliest sign of infection and inflammation in drug reactions, toxic epidermal necrolysis, and sepsis from line infections.

Signs, Symptoms, and Physical Findings

Lighting

Good lighting, either artificial or natural, is essential for a good skin examination, especially in darker-skinned patients where the color of the lesions may be more difficult to visualize. Fixed or standing lighting frees both hands for examination and manipulation of lesions. Oblique illumination (side lighting)

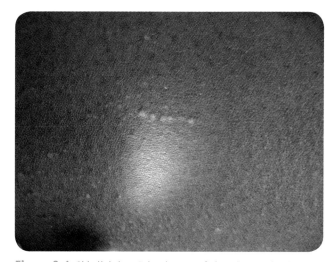

Figure 2-1 Side lighting. Faint degrees of elevation can be detected by side lighting, as seen in this side lighting of the tiny linear papules of lichen nitidus.

of a slightly elevated papule confirms its raised character by the shadow it casts (Fig. 2-1). This should be done in a dimly lit or dark room. Intense light (e.g., the head of an ophthalmologic penlight) is used to transilluminate cystic lesions and reveal the homogeneity of the structure. Focused, intense light should not be used for the complete examination because it can wash out important details. Polarized light can aid in seeing erythema in pigmented skin—both on the skin and in images.[2]

Wood Light

The Wood lamp ("black light") produces long-wave ultraviolet rays (365 nm peak UVA range) with relatively low energy. No special precautions are required for its routine use, except that the room should be as dark as possible. Melanin absorbs strongly at 365 nm, so that minor losses of melanin are accentuated. Hypopigmented areas are paler than normal skin, and depigmented areas are stark or milk white under Wood light (Fig. 2-2). The Wood lamp is especially useful in the

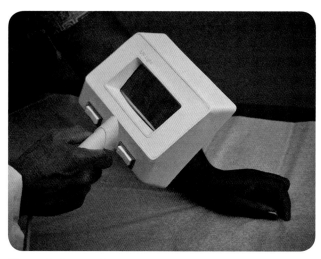

Figure 2-2 A Wood lamp uses a 365-nm-long wavelength of ultraviolet light, causing the skin over the lower arm to look darker. With the Wood lamp, areas of hypopigmentation or hyperpigmentation are accentuated compared with the background skin color.

TABLE 2-1	**Fluorescent Characteristics of Certain Conditions**
Characteristics	**Conditions**
Yellow-green fluorescence of hair	*Microsporum canis*
Yellow-green fluorescence of skin	*Pseudomonas* infection
Pink fluorescence of urine	Uroporphyrins of porphyria cutanea tarda
Coral fluorescence of toes, axillae, groin	Erythrasma infection

diagnosis of vitiligo or in seeing the hypopigmentation of tinea versicolor in early stages. Certain conditions have characteristic fluorescent patterns (Table 2-1). The Wood lamp is also useful for checking urine specimens for uroporphyrins (pink fluorescence), which are characteristic of porphyria cutanea tarda. Multiple exogenous substances, including markers, lint, dyes, and lipstick, can fluoresce on the skin.

Magnification

Magnifying lenses (5× to 10×) should be strong enough to allow the physician to easily observe lesions. Episcopes or dermatoscopes allow the examination of skin lesions under magnification with excellent illumination and permit resolution of fine detail and size (Fig. 2-3). They are especially useful for viewing complex pigmented lesions and melanomas. They can be used to view erythema in all skin types.

Lenses are especially useful for detecting altered skin markings and contours in tumors, and especially melanoma. Lenses are also used to observe nail fold telangiectasia in connective tissue diseases and to detect the subtle surface changes (Wickham striae) in lichen planus. When mineral oil, immersion oil, or alcohol is placed on the skin, the stratum corneum becomes more transparent, revealing deeper structures

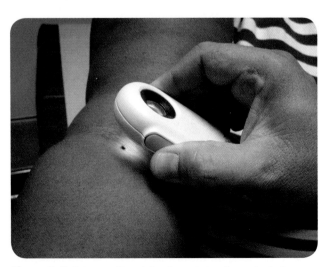

Figure 2-3 Episcope. Especially pigmented and vascular lesions can be examined in more detail by use of bright optics and polarization.

in more detail. This technique allows easier visualization of telangiectases, Wickham striae, and similar findings.

Normal Anatomical Findings (Futcher Lines)

Normal anatomical lines of demarcation, Futcher lines are easily visible on pigmented skin (Figs. 2-4 and 2-5). They represent a normal variation and are not signs of any disease.

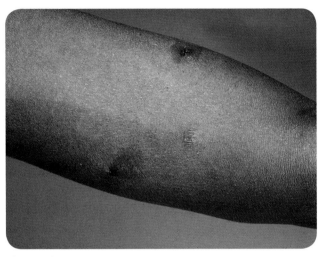

Figure 2-4 Futcher line with plaques of eczematous dermatitis.

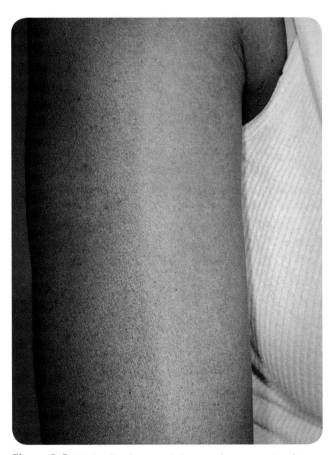

Figure 2-5 Futcher line is more obvious on the upper extremity and is a linear line of demarcation in pigmentation.

Purpura and Erythema

A well-known sign of life-threatening disease, purpura appears as purple-red discoloration in lighter skin tones but can appear brown or almost gray in skin with more pigmentation. Likewise, many inflammatory and infectious diseases present with erythema, or redness of the skin, and the change in appearance can be very subtle in darker skin. On exam, erythema in pigmented skin will be red to purple to black, and the temperature of the area is increased. In Figure 2-6A–F, similar "red" papular drug eruptions are shown in patients with varying degrees of skin pigmentation ([A] shows the least intrinsic pigmentation, [F] the most). Although the basic reaction has prominent erythema, the degree of perceived redness varies based on the underlying skin pigmentation.

Detection of early erythema can save lives and decrease health care costs, and in pigmented skin it depends on the clinician's ability to recognize shades of red as well as distinguish subtle color variations across the skin. High-tech solutions for measuring skin redness are being developed, but on the front lines, close visual observation—and excellent lighting—are still very important. So, too, is listening: often, the best aid comes from the patient who says, "My skin is now red." Listen to that patient!

Palpation of Skin Lesions

Palpation reveals the lesion's depth, extension, texture, firmness, and fixation to underlying structures of skin. Light pressure can reveal a thrill in a vascular lesion, implying an arteriovenous malformation. Lateral compression of dermatofibromas causes them to become depressed and to indent the overlying skin (Fitzpatrick sign). Firm stroking of apparently normal skin can induce histamine release, redness, and edema; this phenomenon, known as dermographism, is accentuated in urticaria (Fig. 2-7). Stroking of individual papules leading to local erythema and edema (and, rarely, vesiculation) is diagnostic of urticaria pigmentosa. This phenomenon is named Darier sign. Stroking the skin of atopic patients produces a white line without a red phase (white dermographism), which in dark brown skin is a light-tan color. In nevus anemicus, firm rubbing makes the surrounding normal skin bright red but does not induce erythema in the hypopigmented skin. In blistering diseases, rubbing apparently normal skin may induce new blisters; this occurs in patients with pemphigus vulgaris and toxic epidermal necrolysis. Extension of an intact blister by application of pressure to the lesion (Asboe-Hansen sign) indicates an intraepidermal blister.

Diascopy

Observing the changes in a skin lesion with compression (diascopy) is often useful in the diagnosis of skin diseases. Compression may be performed with a magnifying glass, microscope slide, or clear plastic plate. These instruments are all considered *diascopes*. Blue to red lesions that blanch when compressed are vascular lesions, and their gradual refilling is observed by seeing the red color return. Purpuric lesions do not blanch completely with pressure; raised, purpuric, non-blanchable lesions indicate cutaneous small-vessel vasculitis. In Type IV–VI skin types, these changes occur, but the blue, red, and purpuric lesions are more of a dark purple. Compression of brown to yellow-brown papules may reveal the apple-jelly nodules of granulomatous diseases (e.g., sarcoidosis, tuberculosis).

Itching with No or Minimal Skin Lesions

The description of the itching becomes most important when there are no lesions present. A sensation of biting described with the itching can be a sign of xerosis. A deep itching, not on the surface, is more consistent with systemic disease. A burning itching may be a neuropathy or sign of systemic disease.

It is important to know that itching has many causes, ranging from skin diseases (such as eczema, psoriasis, and scabies) to internal conditions (such as hyperthyroidism, kidney or liver disease) to some blood-related diseases. In addition, itch can be caused by water contact in the bath or shower, or it may be plain, garden-variety winter itch.

Physicians and patients are very troubled by severe and persistent itching with no or minimal skin lesions. The anguish of these patients and the possibility that the pruritus indicates an underlying systemic disease often leads to extensive laboratory testing and the use of multiple medications within a short period of time. There is often no lesion to biopsy.

These patients are best approached by having a diagnostic scheme of the causes of itching in these circumstances, some basic laboratory testing, and a therapeutic approach to provide some relief.

A useful approach has been outlined by Yosipovitch et al.[3] Involving the patient's primary physician is useful to avoid unnecessary testing.

- Chronic renal disease—basic renal chemistries and serum calcium
- Hyperthyroidism—TSH for screening
- Cholestasis—often due to bile salts, especially during pregnancy; screening with routine liver chemistries and bile salt levels if evidence is suggestive
- Hematologic disease and lymphomas—careful node exam, routine hematology studies
- HIV-associated pruritus
- Paraneoplastic syndrome with solid tumors—careful history and physicals before extensive screening
- Itching related to psychiatric disease—early psychiatry consultation very helpful; often delusions of parasitosis and itch with obsessive-compulsive disorder, and itching associated with anorexia nervosa
- Aquagenic pruritus—water-induced itching with polycythemia and lymphoma relationships

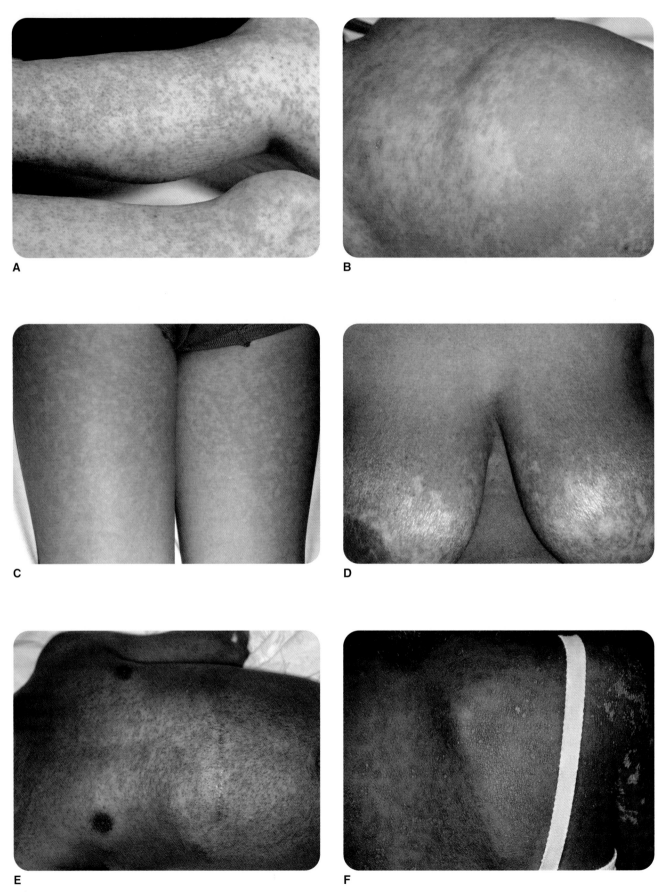

Figure 2-6 A–F: Similar "red" papular drug eruptions are shown in patients with varying degrees of skin pigmentation ([**A**] shows the least intrinsic pigmentation, [**F**] the most). Although the basic reaction has prominent erythema, the degree of perceived redness varies based on the underlying skin pigmentation.

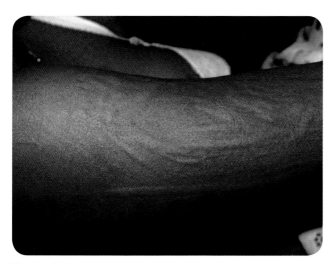

Figure 2-7 Dermographism. Histamine release is accentuated in patients with reactive vasculature in hypersensitivity reactions.

- Itching in the elderly—very disturbing to the patient, especially as multiple negative tests are found
- Neuropathic itching associated with stroke, diabetes, and Creutzfeldt-Jakob disease; postherpetic neuralgia, notalgia paresthetica, and brachioradial pruritus (the latter usually due to cervical disc disease)
- Drug-associated pruritus
- Opiates and their analogues
- Hydroxyethyl starch

Treatment will depend on the cause, but emollients, cooling agents, reduction in bathing, and antihistamines will help these patients.

Cultural Practices, Cosmetic Customs, and Tribal or Social Markings

Many cultures use folk health remedies to treat various illnesses. Some common cultural methods used include cupping, coining, spooning, moxibustion, caida de mollera, salting, herbal rubs, and acupuncture. (See Cultural Practices at VisualDx online for a more detailed discussion.) These widely practiced alternative forms of medicine create marks on the skin—such as petechiae, purpura, and hyperpigmentation—and may cause contact dermatitis. Cupping often produces 4- to 6-cm circular burns from the heat and central ecchymosis and petechiae from the suction effect. In coining or spooning, the edge of a smooth object, such as a coin or spoon, rubbed against the skin (typically on the back) produces linear erythematous patches, petechiae, or purpura. Ecchymotic streaks, often in a parallel and in symmetrical distribution, are characteristic. The lesions of moxibustion appear as a pattern of small discrete, circular, targetlike burns that may be confused with cigarette burns. The practice can lead to second-degree burns, with bullae progressing to scar formation.

It is very important to understand the cultural background of the patient and family and consider cultural practices when assessing skin conditions. It is necessary to specifically ask about cultural practices because families may not volunteer information. Although the therapies may be well-intentioned, they can cause damage to the skin and underlying tissue. Treatment for burns or for secondary infection of lesions as well as pain control should be considered.

Many cultures—both inside and outside of the United States—employ methods of body modification (piercings, tattoos, scarification, hair styles) for decoration; for religious, ethnic, or tribal identification; or to show allegiance to or membership in a social or professional group such as a college fraternity, a branch of the armed forces, or even a criminal gang. Trauma to the skin can result in the development of keloids, which occur most frequently in black patients and those of Mediterranean ancestry but are possible in any skin type.

Special Diagnostic Procedures

These tests are described for education purposes. Before they are performed in the actual care and management of patients, the professionals involved should become familiar with the current state of the Clinical Laboratory Improvement Amendments (CLIA) regulations.

Organism Detection and Presumptive Identification

Organism identification is essential for the rational treatment of skin infections and infestations. Procedures important for dermatology are outlined in this section; standard infectious disease and microbiology texts should be consulted for further details. Superficial crusts, exudate, and topical medications should be swabbed with alcohol to remove saprophytes and secondary contaminating bacteria.

Potassium Hydroxide Preparation for Fungus

1. With an alcohol swab, cleanse the skin of any ointment.
2. With the edge of a microscope slide or scalpel, vigorously scrape the skin onto a second microscope slide. The best areas for scraping are the following:
   - Inner surface of a blister roof or the blister base
   - Moist, macerated areas, such as between toes, at the edge of the lesion, away from potential secondary infections that may interfere with fungal growth
   - Rim or leading edge of lesions
   - Under nail or under paronychial fold
   - Base of a plucked hair
3. Place a drop of 10% to 20% KOH on the scale-covered slide and apply a coverslip.
4. Warm gently. Avoid actual boiling, as this causes the KOH to crystallize (Fig. 2-8).
5. Examine with a microscope by scanning at 10× and then confirming hyphae with the 40× objective at low illumination. This is achieved by setting a low level of light and racking the condenser all the way down (Fig. 2-9).

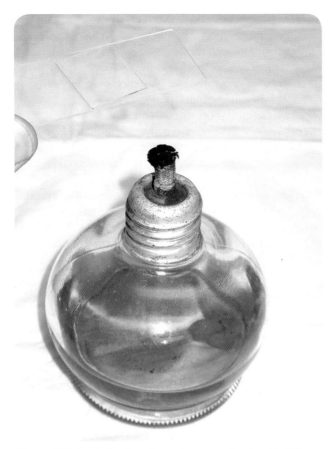

Figure 2-8 Gentle heating of a small amount of scale with KOH over an alcohol lamp is the key for a useful fungal preparation.

Small amounts of scrapings on a slide frequently yield the best results because the coverslip rests on the slide, producing the best optical properties. Potassium hydroxide (KOH) hydrolyzes the epidermal proteins but not the fungal elements. The cell envelopes of the stratum corneum remain and should not be confused with fungi.

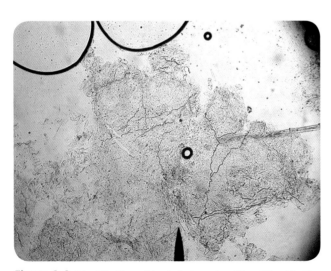

Figure 2-9 Identification of hyphal elements with a 10× objective and low illumination allows hyphae to show up as dark objects against the background. Using a 40× objective confirms the diagnosis.

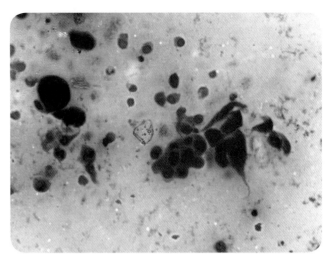

Figure 2-10 Multinucleated cells or giant nuclei characterize herpes simplex or herpes zoster infections of the skin.

Tzanck Smear for Giant Cells

A Tzanck smear is very important for the rapid diagnosis of patients with vesicles and does not require special techniques such as PCR or fluorescent microscopy. The demonstration of multinucleated giant cells indicates that the causative agent is either herpes simplex virus or varicella-zoster virus. The procedure is as follows:

1. Select a fresh umbilicated vesicle.
2. Unroof the vesicle with a scalpel blade.
3. Gently scrape the base of the vesicle with the scalpel, and smear scrapings onto a microscope slide.
4. Fix with 95% alcohol.
5. Stain with Wright or Giemsa stain, using the technique that is used for routine white cell differential counts.
6. Examine under the microscope using the 10× or 40× objective. A positive preparation demonstrates very large multinucleated giant cells with a high nuclear-cytoplasmic ratio. Examination with the oil immersion objective is often required in equivocal cases (Fig. 2-10).

Examination for Lice

Nits (eggs of lice) on pubic, axillary, scalp, or other hairs may be directly examined with the microscope. Organisms and empty, highly refractile egg cases are easily observed with the 10× objective (Fig. 2-11). Adult lice can be seen with the naked eye and are dramatic under the lower objective (Fig. 2-12).

Examination for Scabies

Scabietic mites may be removed from burrows with a scalpel after applying 10% KOH or mineral oil to the suspected burrow. The oil optically clears the stratum corneum, enhancing visualization of the mite. Application of a tetracycline solution (500 mg tetracycline in 20 mL glycerin and 80 mL absolute ethanol), followed 1 minute later by shining a Wood lamp on the skin, accentuates the burrow. Burrows fluoresce a brilliant green, allowing easy removal of a suspected organism. Alternatively, a small drop of ink placed on the opening of the

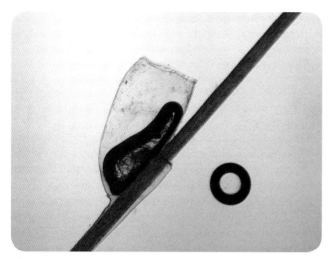

Figure 2-11 Hair with a louse egg case (nit). 10× objective.

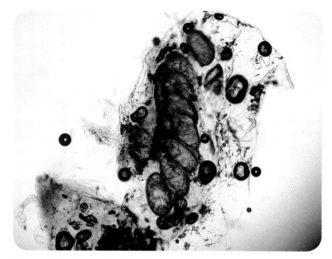

Figure 2-13 Scraping from burrow with an adult *Sarcoptes* mite, in lower-left corner, and a string of eggs containing organisms.

TEST [Allerderm, Phoenix, AZ]). The patches are applied for 48 hours under occlusion and then examined for a delayed hypersensitivity that may vary from mild erythema to actual vesiculation (Fig. 2-16). False-negative tests are frequent, and many positives (e.g., to nickel) may not be clinically relevant to the condition at hand. For that reason, this testing should be done by a trained specialist in patch testing, usually a dermatologist.

Culture Techniques

Sabouraud medium is useful for the isolation of most fungi. It is commercially available, stored cool, and then incubated with specimens at room temperature. Sabouraud medium with cycloheximide (Actidione) and chloramphenicol suppresses bacterial and saprophytic fungi. It is very important to avoid use of this medium if *Cryptococcus* is suspected because cycloheximide suppresses the growth of *Cryptococcus*.

India Ink Stain for *Cryptococcus*

A smear of an exudate is mixed with one small drop of commercial India ink, and a coverslip is applied. If the preparation

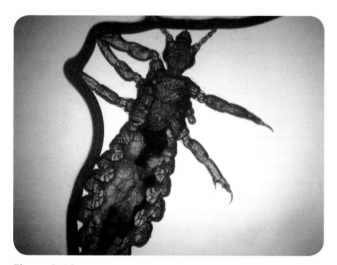

Figure 2-12 Adult louse from scalp. 10× objective.

burrow that is then rapidly wiped away with a tissue may also reveal tracks (Figs. 2-13–2-15).

Gram stain for bacteria and *Candida*

1. Air-dry the slide.
2. Cover with 1% crystal violet for 15 seconds. Wash with water.
3. Cover with Gram iodine for 15 seconds. Wash with water.
4. Decolorize for 15 seconds with acetone alcohol. Wash with water.
5. Cover with 2.5% safranin for 15 seconds. Wash with water and air-dry.
6. Examine with 10×, 40×, and oil immersion lenses.

Special Techniques

Patch Testing

Patch testing is done to determine delayed hypersensitivity to exogenous substances. The materials are specially prepared or may be available in the form of kits (e.g., T.R.U.E.

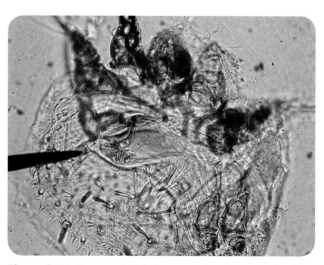

Figure 2-14 Close-up of adult *Sarcoptes* mite, the cause of scabies.

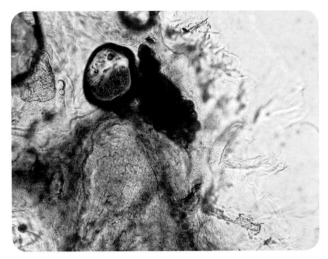

Figure 2-15 Clump of scabies feces. The presence of this alone is diagnostic of scabies.

is too dark, water may be added to dilute the ink. The large, translucent capsules of *Cryptococcus*, with a small central nucleus that may contain a nucleolus, can be seen. The buds have a narrow base; blastomycosis and other fungi have a broad base.

Acid-Fast Stain

In suspected lepromatous leprosy and orificial tuberculosis, direct stains may be positive. In other forms of cutaneous leprosy and cutaneous tuberculosis, the chance of a positive smear is so small that a direct smear is not indicated. *Nocardia* in mycetomas will also stain with the acid-fast stain.

Punch Biopsy

The punch biopsy is a common biopsy used by dermatologists. When properly performed, the procedure can be done rapidly with a very low incidence of adverse events or significant

scarring. In the patient with pigmented skin, the site selection is important. Avoid the chest, back, upper arms, and jaw line. Always advise all patients that the procedure will result in a mark or a scar.

1. Prepare a punch biopsy tray: Include alcohol pads, local anesthetic, gloves, punch instrument, forceps, scissors, gauze, needle driver, and suture.
2. Prepare the patient: Explain the procedure to the patient step by step in a gentle, reassuring manner. Ideally, the patient should be reclining or supine during the procedure to avoid an accident if he/she loses consciousness.
3. Anesthetize the patient: Topical anesthetics, such as topical lidocaine or EMLA, under occlusion, may be used to reduce the discomfort caused by needle sticks, but they are not usually necessary. If using a topical anesthetic, once the cutaneous surface is appropriately anesthetized, wipe the area clean with an alcohol pad and use a syringe with a 30-gauge needle to inject local anesthetic into the deep dermis **(Fig. 2-17)**.
4. Punch biopsy: Apply gentle lateral traction around the area of skin to be biopsied. The punch biopsy is then performed by applying slight downward pressure on the skin while rotating the punch instrument clockwise and counterclockwise **(Fig. 2-18)**. One will feel a gentle pop as the instrument penetrates the dermis into the subcutaneous tissue.
5. Remove the biopsy tissue: Gently grasp the sample with forceps, lift until resistance is felt, and cut the tissue free at the subcutaneous level **(Fig. 2-19)**.
6. Close the defect with one to three simple interrupted sutures **(Fig. 2-20)**: Choose the appropriate suture based on the patient's age, anatomic site, and size of the biopsy. In general, nonabsorbable (nylon or polypropylene) 4-0 suture is appropriate for superficial suturing of lesions on the trunk and extremities, and 5-0 suture is preferred for the face and genitalia.

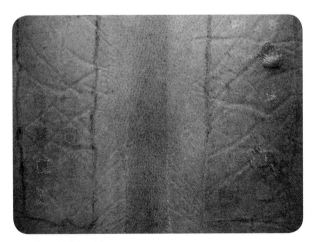

Figure 2-16 Vesicular patch test reaction. Patch test material is often applied on a small disc under occlusion.

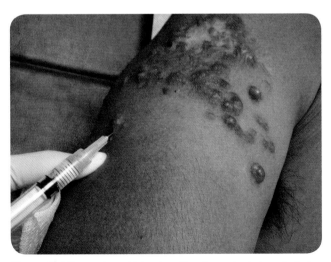

Figure 2-17 Intradermal injection of local anesthesia into the lesion using a 30-gauge needle. Biopsy usually does not need to include normal skin for its interpretation.

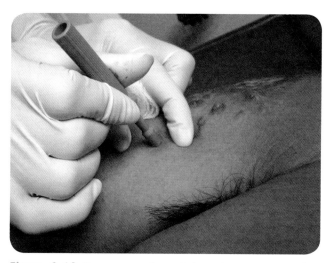

Figure 2-18 Firm pressure is applied to the cutaneous surface while rotating the punch biopsy instrument between the thumb and forefinger.

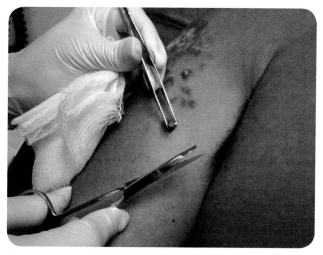

Figure 2-19 Remove the tissue gently using forceps with teeth, removing deep dermis when indicated. Very superficial biopsies often have to be repeated.

7. Dress the wound: Apply a thin layer of white petrolatum or antibiotic ointment, cover the area with a nonadherent pad (e.g., Telfa [Kendall, Mansfield, MA]), and secure the pad with adhesive tape.
8. Provide the patient with written postoperative instructions explaining proper wound care, activity restrictions, and a number to call in case an adverse event occurs.
9. Remove sutures: The patient should return in 5 to 7 days for removal of facial sutures and 10 to 14 days for removal of sutures on the torso and extremities.

Shave Biopsy

The shave biopsy is another common biopsy technique used by dermatologists. When properly performed, the procedure can be done rapidly with a very low incidence of adverse events or significant scarring. Shave biopsy is most commonly performed when ruling out skin cancer in an exophytic lesion.

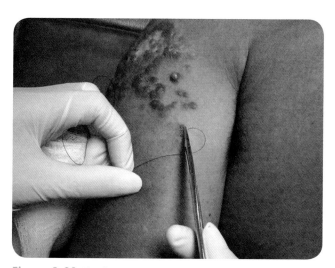

Figure 2-20 The best wound closure can be obtained if wound edges are approximated with simple interrupted sutures.

1. Prepare a shave biopsy tray: Include alcohol pads, local anesthetic, gloves, flexible or rigid scalpel, forceps, gauze, an agent for hemostasis (20% aluminum chloride solution), and bandage.
2. Prepare the patient: Explain the procedure to the patient step by step in a gentle, reassuring manner. Ideally, the patient should be reclining or supine during the procedure to avoid an accident if he/she loses consciousness.
3. Anesthetize the patient: Topical anesthetics, such as topical lidocaine or EMLA, under occlusion, may be used to reduce the discomfort caused by needle sticks, but they are not usually necessary. If using a topical anesthetic, once the cutaneous surface is appropriately anesthetized, wipe the area clean with an alcohol pad and use a syringe with a 30-gauge needle to inject local anesthetic into the deep dermis.
4. Shave biopsy: Apply gentle lateral traction around the area of skin to be biopsied. The shave biopsy is then performed using the scalpel to gently cut through the base of the lesion using a side-to-side sawing motion. If needed, use the back of a cotton swab to cut against when the final attachment of tissue is reached. Alternatively, forceps can be used to grab the specimen.
5. Remove the biopsy tissue.
6. Hemostasis: Using a cotton swab, apply aluminum chloride solution to the area as an agent of hemostasis. Vigorous rubbing can help stop bleeding more quickly. This technique should not be used near the eyes. If bleeding is persistent, continued pressure or electrocautery may be required to achieve hemostasis.
7. Dress the wound: Apply a thin layer of white petrolatum or antibiotic ointment, cover with a nonadherent pad (e.g., Telfa), and secure the pad with adhesive tape.
8. Provide the patient with written postoperative instructions explaining proper wound care, activity restrictions, and a number to call in case an adverse event occurs.

References

1. Fitzpatrick TB. The validity and practicality of sun-reactive skin types I through VI. *Arch Dermatol.* 1988;124(6):869–871.

2. Anderson RR. Polarized light examination and photography of the skin. *Arch Dermatol.* 1991;127(7):1000–1005.

3. Yosipovitch G, Dawn AG, Greaves MW. Pathophysiology and clinical aspects of pruritus. In: Wolff K, et al., eds. *Fitzpatrick's Dermatology in General Medicine.* New York, NY: McGraw-Hill; 2008:902–911; chap 102.

CHAPTER 3

Morphology and Distribution

Learning to describe skin findings is the fundamental and essential skill of dermatologic diagnosis. Learn to describe what you see with the words defined in this chapter and online at www.essentialdermatology.com/pigmented (if you are a first-time user) or www.visualdx.com/visualdx (if you already have your password set up). See also the LearnDerm interactive tutorial at www.logicalimages.com/educationalTools/learnDerm.htm. In this chapter, there are precise definitions of the key morphologic terms with illustrative examples. Online, there are additional images; an interactive self-assessment; and further training in configurations, distributions, and variants of disease presentation. Master these definitions in this chapter and online, as they lead to more efficient and precise diagnoses.

Morphology

The ability to use the standard morphologic descriptive terminology of dermatology has been the key to developing accurate skin-based differential diagnoses for over a century. The characterization of visual skin findings requires both careful observation and the use of universally accepted terminology. Once you know these terms, you will be able to use the differential diagnosis index in Chapter 4 and use the online differential diagnosis engine of VisualDx more effectively. In this section, as in VisualDx, the primary morphologic terms are grouped into logical categories. For example, vesicles, bullae, and pustules are grouped because these are terms that represent fluid-filled lesions. The grouping is purposeful. As you examine the patient, ask yourself questions such as, Are these lesions raised? Are these lesions solid or fluid-filled? Do these lesions blanch, or are they nonblanching as in the purpuras? The categories match the skin exam method. In addition to identifying the main categories, you can further describe papules and plaques by checking for surface change such as scale or crust. Visit www.logicalimages.com/educationalTools/learnDerm.htm for access to the Learn-Derm interactive tutorial. The tutorial includes more images, image descriptions, and an interactive self-study test with virtual examination tools.

Group	Lesion Type	Definition
FLAT 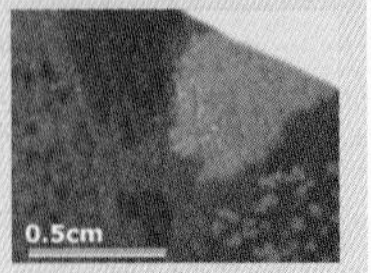	Macule 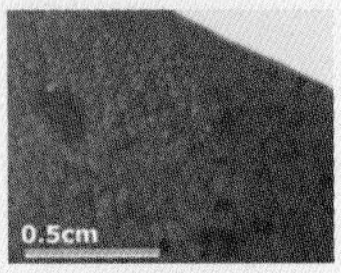	A flat, generally <0.5 cm area of skin or mucous membranes with different color from surrounding tissue. Macules may have nonpalpable, fine scale (see Fig. 3-1).
	Patch 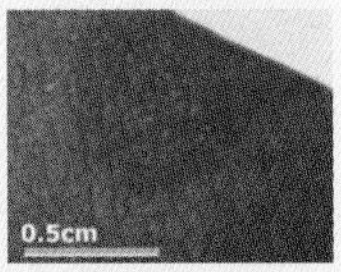	A flat, generally >0.5 cm area of skin or mucous membranes with different color from surrounding tissue. Patches may have nonpalpable, fine scale. When used to describe an early clinical stage of cutaneous T-cell lymphoma (mycosis fungoides), the term patch may include fine textural change such as "cigarette paper" thinning, poikilodermatous atrophy, or slickness secondary to follicular loss (see Fig. 3-2).
RAISED AND SMOOTH 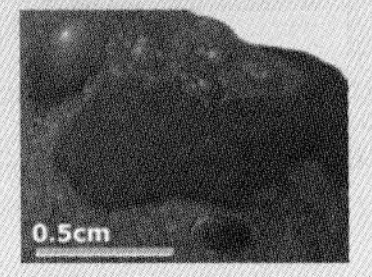	Papule 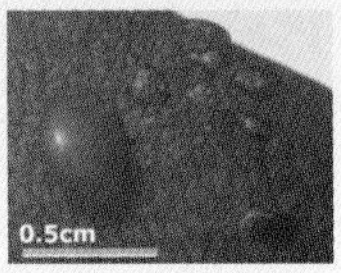	A discrete, solid, elevated body usually <0.5 cm in diameter. Papules are further classified by shape, size, color, and surface change (see Fig. 3-3).
	Plaque 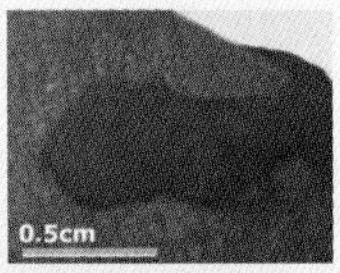	A discrete, solid, elevated body usually broader than it is thick measuring more than 0.5 cm in diameter. Plaques may be further classified by shape, size, color, and surface change (see Fig. 3-4).
	Nodule 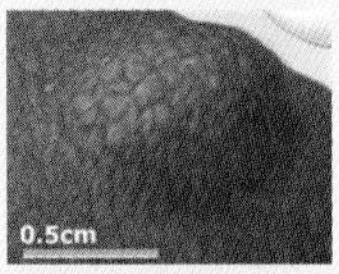	A dermal or subcutaneous firm, well-defined lesion usually >0.5 cm in diameter (see Fig. 3-5).
	Cyst 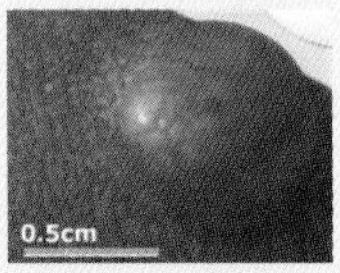	A closed cavity or sac containing fluid or semisolid material. A cyst may have an epithelial, endothelial, or membranous lining (see Fig. 3-6).
SURFACE CHANGE 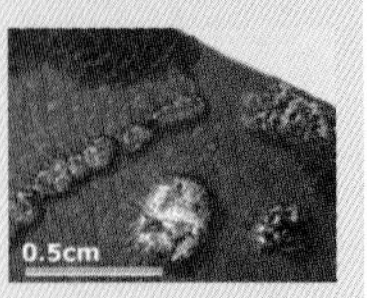	Crust 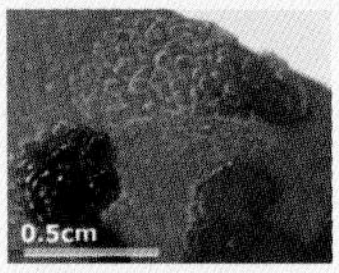	A hardened layer that results when serum, blood, or purulent exudate dries on the skin surface. Crusts may be thin or thick and can have varying color. Crusts are yellow-brown when formed from dried serum, green or yellow-green when formed from purulent exudate, and red-black when formed by blood (see Fig. 3-7).
	Scale 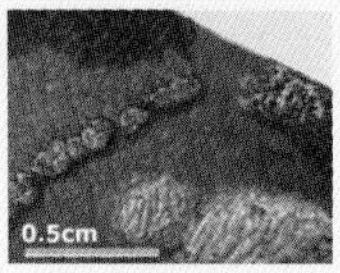	Excess stratum corneum accumulated in flakes or plates. Scale usually has a white or gray color (see Fig. 3-8).

(Continued)

(*Continued*)

Group	Lesion Type	Definition
FLUID-FILLED 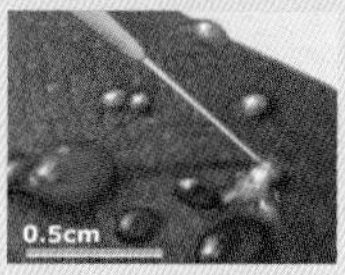	Abscess 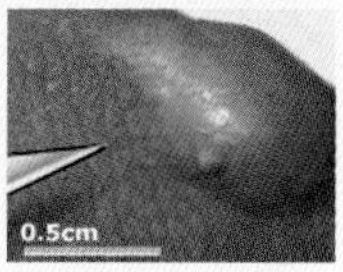	A localized accumulation of pus in the dermis or subcutaneous tissue. Frequently red, warm, and tender (see Fig. 3-9).
	Bulla 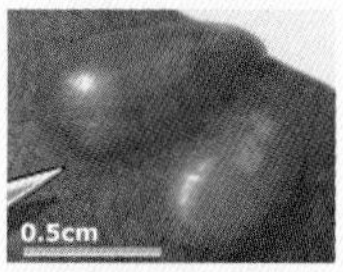	A fluid-filled blister >0.5 cm in diameter. Fluid can be clear, serous, hemorrhagic, or pus-filled (see Fig. 3-10).
	Pustule 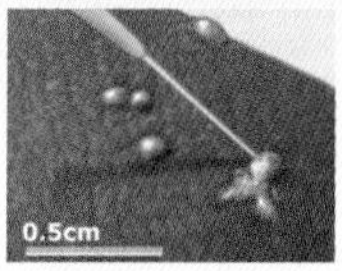	A circumscribed elevation that contains pus. Pustules are usually <0.5 cm in diameter (see Fig. 3-11).
	Vesicle 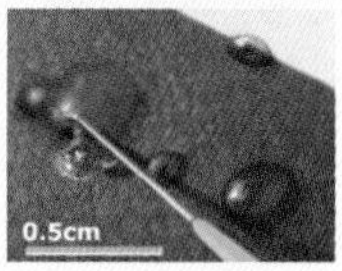	Fluid-filled cavity or elevation <0.5 cm in diameter. Fluid may be clear, serous, hemorrhagic, or pus filled (see Fig. 3-12).
RED BLANCHABLE 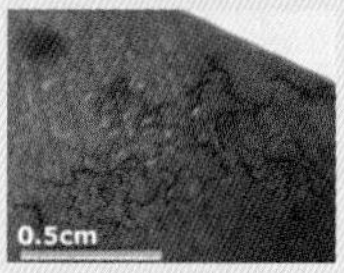	Erythema 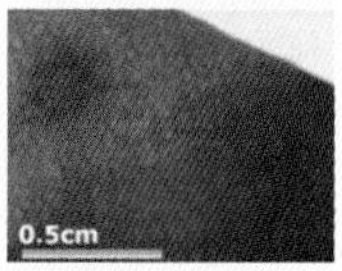	Localized, blanchable redness of the skin or mucous membranes (see Fig. 3-13).
	Erythroderma 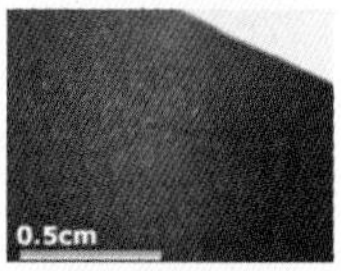	Generalized, blanchable redness of the skin that may be associated with desquamation (see Fig. 3-14).
	Telangiectasia 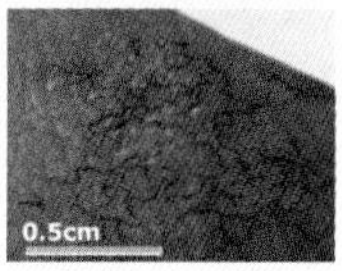	Visible, persistent dilation of small, superficial cutaneous blood vessels. Telangiectases will blanch (see Fig. 3-15).

(*Continued*)

(Continued)

Group	Lesion Type	Definition
PURPURIC	Ecchymosis	Extravasation of blood into the skin or mucous membranes. Area of flat color change may progress over time from blue-black to brown-yellow or green (see Fig. 3-16).
	Petechiae	Tiny 1–2 mm, initially purpuric, nonblanchable macules resulting from tiny hemorrhages (see Fig. 3-17).
	Palpable Purpura	Raised and palpable, nonblanchable, red or violaceous discoloration of skin or mucous membranes due to vascular inflammation in the skin and extravasation of red blood cells (see Fig. 3-18).
SUNKEN	Atrophy	A thinning of tissue defined by its location, such as epidermal atrophy, dermal atrophy, or subcutaneous atrophy (see Fig. 3-19).
	Erosion	A localized loss of the epidermal or mucosal epithelium (see Fig. 3-20).
	Ulcer	A circumscribed loss of the epidermis and at least upper dermis. Ulcers are further classified by their depth, border/shape, edge, and tissue at their base (see Fig. 3-21).
GANGRENE	Gangrene	Necrotic, usually black, tissue due to obstruction, diminution, or loss of blood supply. Gangrene may be wet or dry (see Fig. 3-22).
ESCHAR	Eschar	An adherent thick, dry, black crust (see Fig. 3-23).

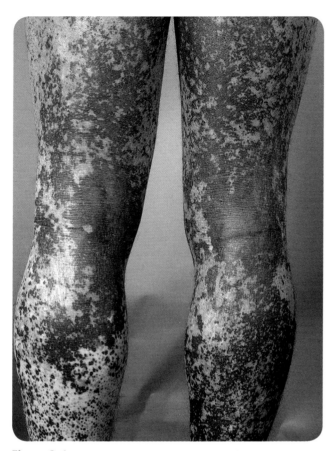

Figure 3-1 Drug-induced hyperpigmentation and hypopigmentation related to azidothymidine.

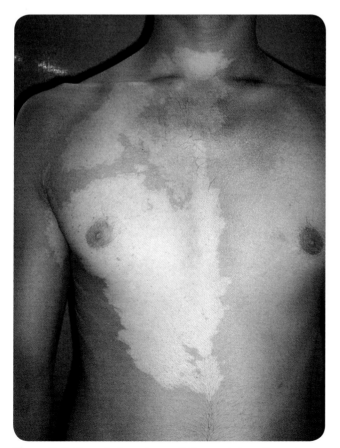

Figure 3-2 Nevus depigmentosus with large patches of hypopigmentation and depigmentation on the right side of the body.

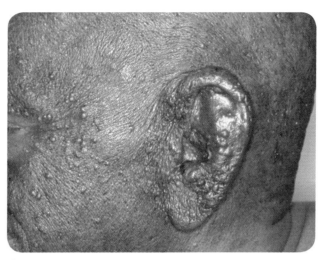

Figure 3-3 Mycosis fungoides (cutaneous T-cell lymphoma) with follicular papules and plaques.

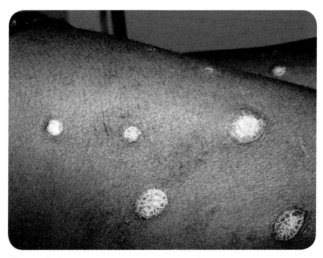

Figure 3-4 Psoriasis with several plaques with white scale.

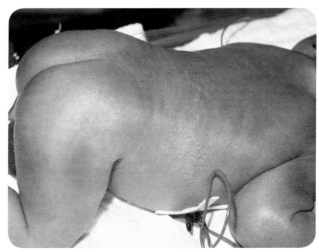

Figure 3-5 Superficial red nodules of varying size due to subcutaneous fat necrosis.

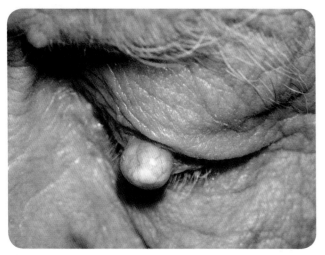

Figure 3-6 Pedunculated epidermoid cyst of the upper eyelid.

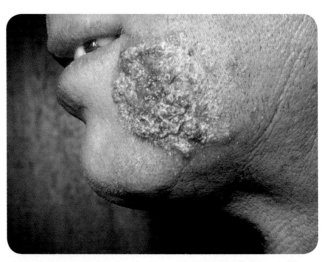

Figure 3-7 Large crusted lesion of superficial dermatophyte (tinea faciale) on the lower face.

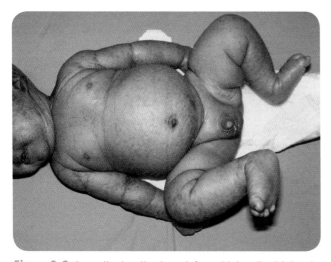

Figure 3-8 Generalized scaling in an infant with lamellar ichthyosis.

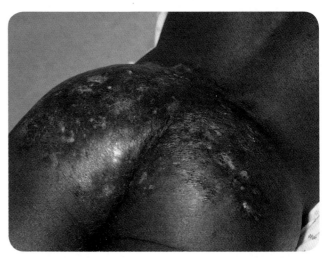

Figure 3-9 Multiple buttock abscesses.

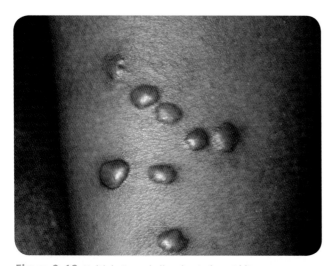

Figure 3-10 Multiple tense bullae due to insect bites.

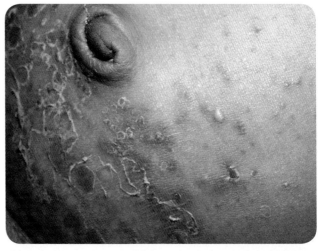

Figure 3-11 Bullous impetigo with pustules of varying size and eroded pustules with annular scale.

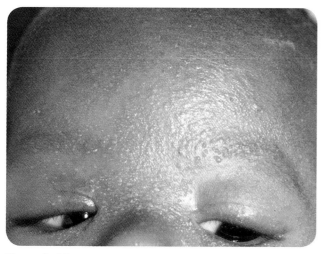

Figure 3-12 Multitudes of tiny clear vesicles in miliaria crystallina.

Figure 3-13 Scarlet fever with blanching erythema and fine papules (sandpaper skin).

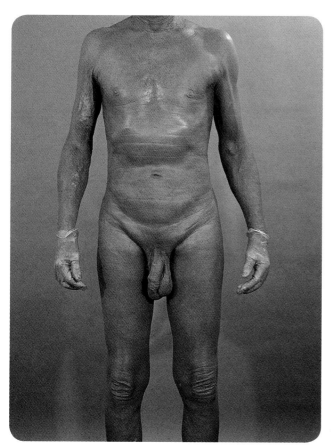

Figure 3-14 Erythroderma being treated with corticosteroids and occlusion, hence the gloves. A "skip area" of normal skin on the right upper arm is suggestive of the diagnosis of pityriasis rubra pilaris.

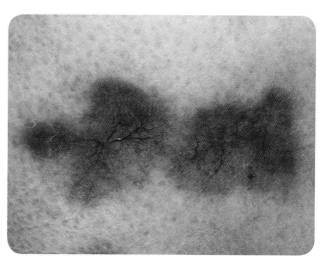

Figure 3-15 Telangiectatic blood vessels, hyperpigmentation, and depressed skin in necrobiosis lipoidica.

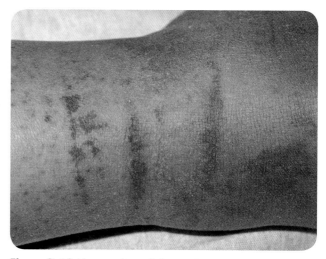

Figure 3-16 Linear ecchymosis in a patient with mixed connective tissue disease.

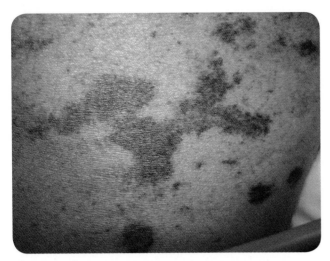

Figure 3-17 Purpura and petechiae in a patient with cutaneous strongyloidiasis with dermatomyositis and immunosuppression.

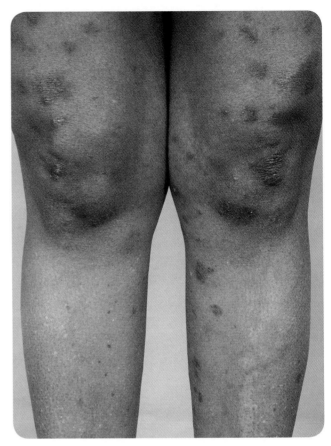

Figure 3-18 Leukocytoclastic vasculitis with bilateral palpable lesions on both legs.

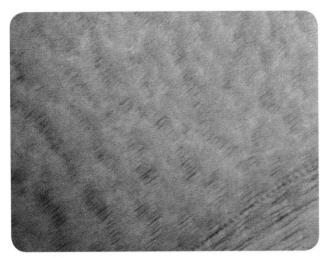

Figure 3-19 Atrophic abdominal striae with wrinkled (cigarette paper) appearance.

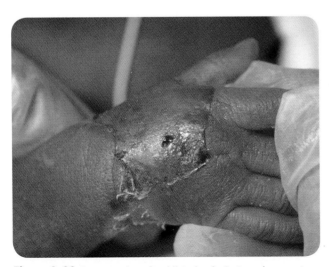

Figure 3-20 Large erosion after blistering in Bart syndrome, a type of epidermolysis bullosa.

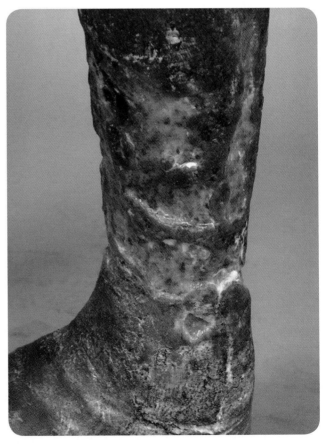

Figure 3-21 Full-thickness skin ulcers in lepromatous leprosy (Hansen disease).

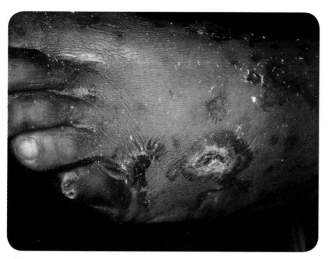

Figure 3-22 Gangrene of toe, ulcers, and purpura in acute meningococcemia.

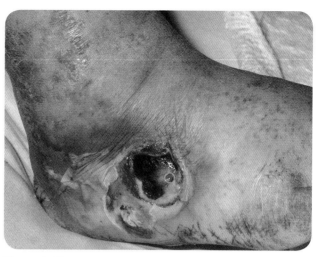

Figure 3-23 Eschar, a hemorrhagic crust, on a lesion of leukocytoclastic vasculitis.

Distributions

Skin lesions can occur at a discrete body location or form a distribution pattern by involving multiple body surfaces. Distribution refers to the pattern in which multiple lesions are arranged. Both location and distribution can be powerful clues in the process of developing a differential diagnosis. Learn the most important distributions in this section and visit www.logicalimages.com/educationalTools/learnDerm.htm for additional definitions and an interactive self-study quiz.

Distribution	Definition
Acral 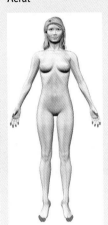	An acral pattern of skin lesions involves the distal aspects of the head (ears and nose) and the extremities (hands, fingers, feet, toes).
Dermatomal 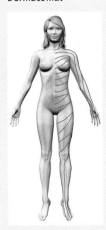	Dermatomal distribution includes an area of skin following the sensory skin innervation of a particular nerve root. Dermatomal distributions do not cross the midline of the body.
Intertriginous 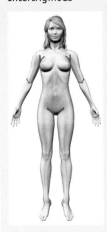	Intertriginous distribution involves skin creases and folds. An intertriginous pattern includes involvement of the axillae, crural fold, gluteal crease, and possibly the inframammary fold.

(Continued)

(*Continued*)	
Distribution	**Definition**
Lymphangitic 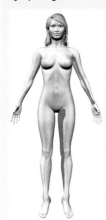	A lymphangitic pattern of skin lesions or subcutaneous lesions appears along the path of the lymph channels of the leg or arm. Sporotrichosis, a deep fungal infection, typically presents with a lymphangitic pattern.
Photodistributed 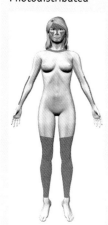	A photodistributed pattern follows the sun-exposed skin. Typical areas of involvement are the forehead, chest, upper back, upper ears, nose, cheeks, upper lip, neck, forearms, and dorsum of the hands.
Scattered 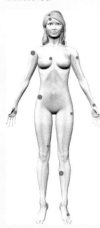	Skin lesions occurring across many body locations can appear to be distributed randomly or haphazardly. A severe case of poison ivy dermatitis could appear widely scattered.

(*Continued*)

(Continued)

Distribution	Definition
Symmetric 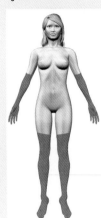	Skin lesions that are found symmetrically on the extremities can be indicative of diagnoses of many etiologies, including infectious, metabolic, genetic, and inflammatory causes.
Widespread 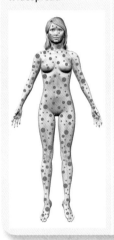	A widespread distribution involves the entire—or almost the entire—body.

CHAPTER 4

Essential Skin Diseases

The purpose of this chapter is to aid clinicians in the diagnosis and management of skin and mucosal conditions in patients with darker skin types (Fitzpatrick Types IV-VI). We recognize this represents a heterogenous multi-ethnic, multi-cultural group. Wherever possible we have tried to be precise in describing populations with reference to skin type, country or geographic area of origin, and/or ancestry. In some studies, race/ethnicity is self-reported by participants selecting from categories such as white, Hispanic, and African American or black. Thus in many instances, we have replicated this terminology for lack of more specific information. This chapter contains over 250 diseases and disorders and their variants organized according to their common presentations. These clinical presentations are divided by morphology and are in the order as shown: Morphology Indexes 4-1 and 4-2 for red skin lesions with and without serious fever and illness; Morphology Indexes 4-3 and 4-4 for skin lesions with prominent pigmentary change and skin lesions with prominent vasculature or purpura; Morphology Indexes 4-5 and 4-6 for smooth skin lesions, few and many;

Morphology Indexes 4-7 and 4-8 for scaly or crusted skin lesions, few and many; Morphology Indexes 4-9, 4-10, and 4-11 for fluid-filled skin lesions, atrophy/sclerosis, and limited number of lesions or growths, respectively; and Morphology Index 4-12 for special body locations (face/neck, mouth, nails, palms and soles, genital region, and scalp). One major challenge of clinical diagnosis is disease variability, for example, the variability of presentation of disease in different age groups and skin tones. These lists are guides for those using this textbook alone. The complexity and number of diseases should encourage the user to refer to the VisualDx online diagnostic resource that accompanies this book. Using the online system is a powerful way to assist with building a differential diagnosis. Start by going to www.essentialdermatology.com/pigmented to activate your free 1-year subscription. Further instructions and your activation product code are detailed on the inside front cover of this book.

Alphabetical Index 4-13 contains all of the discrete diseases in an alphabetical list with the appropriate page number for the disorder.

ALPHABETICAL INDEX 4-13   Alphabetical List

(Continued)

ALPHABETICAL INDEX 4-13   *(Continued)*

Scarlet Fever

Laurie Good

Diagnosis Synopsis

Scarlet fever is an acute erythrogenic toxin-mediated disease caused by infection with Group A beta-hemolytic streptococci (*Streptococcus pyogenes*, or GAS). Most cases follow a streptococcal pharyngitis or tonsillitis. However, streptococcal sepsis, cellulitis, puerperal infection, or surgical infection can initiate scarlet fever. Scarlet fever is most common in children aged younger than 10, but it can affect adults as well. There is no gender or racial predisposition. A 2- to 5-day incubation period precedes the onset of rash. Associated prodromal symptoms include fever, nausea, vomiting, myalgias, headache, and malaise. The characteristic rash begins within 12 to 48 hours of fever onset. Generalized lymphadenopathy is common.

Though scarlet fever was once a fatal disease in the pre-antibiotic era, its associated complications are now fortunately rare with the existence of effective antibiotic therapy. However, meningitis, otitis, sinusitis, pneumonia, arthritis, rheumatic fever, hepatitis, and glomerulonephritis can still rarely occur as complications.

Pediatric Patient Considerations

Scarlet fever is most common in children aged 2 to 10 years old. Hepatitis is a rare complication that occurs more frequently in adults but can occur in children rarely. Meningitis, impetigo, and glomerulonephritis are among the many known complications that can occur in children with untreated GAS infections.

Studies have implicated scarlet fever as a possible immune trigger, as GAS infections are associated with a higher risk of developing Tourette's, tic disorders, attention-deficit hyperactivity disorder, and obsessive-compulsive disorder in children.

Look For

Scarlet fever is characterized by a "sandpaper-like" exanthem with minute (1 to 2 mm) blanchable papules on an erythematous base, resembling a "sunburn with goose bumps" (Fig. 4-1). The lesions begin on the neck and then spread inferiorly to the trunk and extremities. The redness is accentuated in skin folds and flexural areas but may be difficult to see on heavily pigmented skin. Therefore, check flexural areas, where skin is lighter, for Pastia lines (petechial lesions); rely on tactile feel of sandpaper rash if sunburn appearance is difficult to appreciate on deeply pigmented

skin; check mucous membranes for more obvious signs (white and red strawberry lesions).

When streptococcal pharyngitis or tonsillitis is the evoking infection, the tonsils are beefy red and enlarged with a purulent exudate with associated tender submandibular adenopathy. Initially, the tongue is white with red papilla, giving it a characteristic "white strawberry" appearance. Eventually, the tongue becomes bright red ("red strawberry tongue") (Fig. 4-2).

Flushed cheeks with circumoral pallor are characteristic as well as palatal petechiae.

The rash typically lasts for 4 to 5 days. During resolution, desquamation begins on the head and neck and progresses to the acral regions over a period of 2 to 6 weeks (Figs. 4-3 and 4-4).

Diagnostic Pearls

- Classic sandpaper rash following acute pharyngitis or tonsillitis
- White strawberry or red strawberry tongue
- Pastia lines (linear petechiae in the antecubital, axillary, and inguinal areas) are classic findings in more severe cases.

?? Differential Diagnosis and Pitfalls

- Toxic shock syndrome (TSS) originates from *Staphylococcus aureus* infections arising in the setting of superabsorbent tampons, nasal packing, or surgical site infections. Patients are systemically ill and eventually desquamate.
- Staphylococcal scalded skin syndrome usually occurs in young children following an *S. aureus* infection. Affected skin is notably tender.

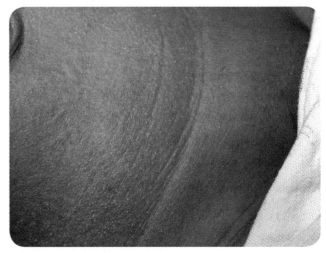

Figure 4-1 Sandpaper skin of scarlet fever.

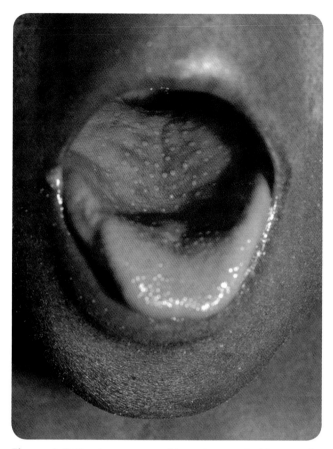

Figure 4-2 Strawberry tongue with erythema and white posterior papillae.

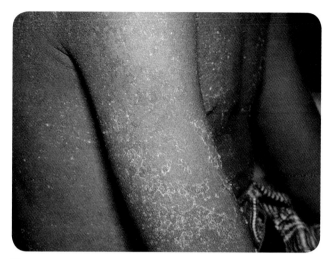

Figure 4-4 Post-scarlet fever desquamation.

- Drug eruptions will have a history of exposure.
- Sunburns occur after sun exposure and are photodistributed.
- Photodrug eruptions are photodistributed.
- Photocontact dermatitis is photodistributed.
- Rubeola has associated cough, coryza, conjunctivitis, and Koplik spots.
- Rubella has occipital and postauricular lymphadenopathy.
- Rat-bite fever
- Infectious mononucleosis has associated lymphadenopathy.
- Primary HIV infection is characterized by lymphadenopathy and rash.
- Lupus erythematosus has associated photosensitivity.

✓ Best Tests

The diagnosis is usually made on clinical grounds and supported by a rising ASO titer and positive throat or wound cultures for *Streptococcus*.

▲▲ Management Pearls

- Because of the potential for complications, do not delay treatment of suspected scarlet fever while waiting for laboratory confirmation.
- Should patients develop complications or if they are found to have a serious source of infection (i.e., osteomyelitis), further workup and treatment are warranted.

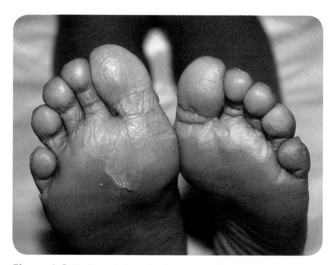

Figure 4-3 Peeling of the soles is common after scarlet fever.

- Kawasaki disease is characterized by "strawberry tongue," conjunctival injection, cervical lymphadenopathy, and rash. This is also more common in children.

Therapy

GAS remain sensitive to penicillin, making it the drug of choice:

- Penicillin G benzathine—1.2 million U IM single dose or penicillin VK 250 mg p.o. three to four times daily for 10 days

Alternatives include the following:

- Erythromycin 333 mg p.o. every 8 hours for 10 days for penicillin-allergic patients
- Amoxicillin 250 to 500 mg p.o. three times daily for 10 days
- Cephalexin 250 to 500 mg p.o. four times daily for 10 days

Pediatric Patient Considerations

Intravenous penicillin (Pen G four divided doses) or erythromycin 1 g IV every 6 hours is the therapy of choice and results in rapid improvement of constitutional symptoms and avoidance of suppurative and nonsuppurative sequelae.

Suggested Readings

Mell LK, Davis RL, Owens D. Association between streptococcal infection and obsessive-compulsive disorder, Tourette's syndrome, and tic disorder. *Pediatrics.* 2005;116(1):56–60.

O'Loughlin RE, Roberson A, Cieslak PR, et al. The Epidemiology of Invasive Group A Streptococcal Infection and Potential Vaccine Implications: United States, 2000–2004. *Clin Infect Dis.* 2007;45:853–862.

Human Immunodeficiency Virus Primary Infection

Laurie Good

▪▪ Diagnosis Synopsis

Primary human immunodeficiency virus (HIV) infection syndrome, also called acute retroviral syndrome, is an acute flulike illness that develops anywhere from 1 to 6 weeks following exposure to HIV. Primary HIV infection is believed to occur in 40% to 80% of newly infected individuals. Symptoms are variable: fever, headache, lymphadenopathy, nausea, diarrhea, rash, and pharyngitis are usually present. Other symptoms include vomiting, arthralgias, and photophobia.

The cutaneous eruption is characteristically a morbilliform exanthem resembling a simple drug or viral exanthem. The palms and soles are usually spared, and lymphadenopathy is usually present. It may last for a few days to several weeks, with most cases resolving within 4 to 5 days. The eruption is self-limited.

Primary HIV infection occurs prior to the development of sufficient HIV antibodies for an individual to test positive on enzyme-linked immunosorbent assay (ELISA, an antibody test) or Western blot. These antibodies can take 2 to 4 months to develop. Primary HIV infection is important to recognize from a public health perspective. Patients with primary HIV infection are ten times more likely to transmit HIV compared to patients in the chronic phase of HIV infection. Patients with primary HIV infection are most likely to present to primary care physicians, emergency rooms, urgent care and walk-in centers, or general medicine clinics. Approximately 90% of cases are not diagnosed at the primary encounter.

The vertical transmission of HIV from breast-feeding mothers to infants is a significant problem, especially in resource-poor settings such as Africa, where rates of HIV infections are high. One study examined the signs of primary HIV infection in breast-fed babies in Africa and found that 95%, compared to 61% of uninfected breast-fed babies, showed at least one of the following clinical signs: mononucleosislike syndrome, dermatitis, or generalized lymphadenopathy. Each of these was an independent factor associated with a primary HIV infection. The presence of any of these signs in a breast-fed child whose mother is HIV positive should prompt consideration of HIV RNA or DNA testing.

◉ Look For

A transient, blanching morbilliform eruption, primarily involving the trunk (Fig. 4-5). Lymphadenopathy is usually prominent. Oral and penile ulcers in men are findings that have also been associated with primary HIV infection.

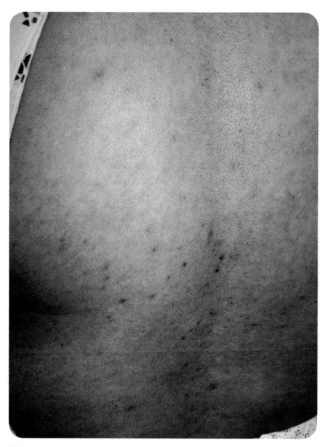

Figure 4-5 HIV (primary infection).

●● Diagnostic Pearls

Diagnosis is based on clinical suspicion in those at risk, such as those who are sexually promiscuous, intravenous drug users, and men who have sex with men. Consider the diagnosis of primary HIV infection in any individual with flulike symptoms and risk factors for HIV. Specifically, fever for >7 days, morbilliform eruption, lymphadenopathy, elevated liver enzymes, and reversal of the CD4:CD8 ratio warrant HIV viral load testing, even if clear risk factors for HIV are not elicited by history.

?? Differential Diagnosis and Pitfalls

- Clinically similar to mononucleosis
- Consider any viral-induced exanthem
- Influenza
- Viral hepatitis (HBV)
- Measles

- Rubella
- Exanthematous drug eruption if there is a history of preceding medication use
- Cytomegalovirus infection
- Secondary syphilis
- Toxoplasmosis
- Brucellosis
- Malaria

Best Tests

- In the acute stage of infection, viral RNA can be detected by polymerase chain reaction (PCR) methods prior to the formation of antibodies. An HIV viral load and CD4+ T-cell count should be performed at initial presentation.
- The diagnosis of primary HIV infection should be confirmed with ELISA in the weeks that follow. Furthermore, Western blot analysis should be used as a confirmatory test on all ELISAs yielding a positive result.
- Skin biopsy is nonspecific and will usually not help to make the diagnosis.

Management Pearls

- Sequential HIV antibody tests are recommended when clinical suspicion is high.
- Immediate partner notification is essential in any patient with primary HIV infection. Have Department of Health notify partners and recommend or obtain HIV testing.

Therapy

When and if therapy is to be instituted is controversial. Points in favor of treatment include decreasing or preventing the seeding of CNS, decreasing HIV transmission, and preserving HIV-directed cytotoxic T lymphocyte. Points against treatment include toxicity, increased risk of resistance, cost of treatment, and the possibility of treating a potential long-term nonprogressor. Consultation with infectious disease specialists may be warranted.

Chinese literature suggests a role for traditional herbal treatments in primary HIV infection as well as HIV prevention, in particular with baicalin.

Suggested Readings

Li BQ, Fu T, Yan YD. Inhibition of HIV infection by baicalin—a flavonoid compound purified from Chinese herbal medicine. *Cell Mol Biol Res.* 1993;39(2):119–124.

Rouet F, Elenga N, Msellati P, et al. Primary HIV-1 infection in African children infected through breastfeeding. *AIDS.* 2002;16(17):2303–2309.

Rickettsiae

Donna Culton

Diagnosis Synopsis

Rickettsiae are a diverse group of diseases caused by obligate, intracellular, Gram-negative bacteria of the genus *Rickettsia*. These diseases are transmitted by arthropod vectors that induce breaks in the skin and allow for transmission of the infectious organism. Proliferation within the endothelial cells of the capillaries, arterioles, and venules leads to a systemic vasculitis and the multitude of clinical findings. The rickettsiae are divided into two major groups: the spotted fever group and the typhus group.

Rocky Mountain spotted fever (RMSF) is the most severe and frequently reported rickettsial infection. It is caused by *Rickettsia rickettsii* and transmitted via the bite of *Dermacentor*, *Rhipicephalus*, or *Amblyomma* ticks. Distribution within the United States ranges from the eastern two thirds of the United States to the Pacific coast, Rocky Mountain states, and southwestern United States. The majority of cases present during the months of April through September. While persons of any sex or ethnicity may be affected, enzyme-linked immunosorbent assay (ELISA) among military personnel has shown higher rates of seropositivity in men and in dark-skinned individuals. When basing diagnosis on clinical findings paired with serology in a more general population, white individuals had a higher incidence. This discrepancy in serological versus clinical incidence among different ethnic groups may be explained by the difficulty in identifying both ticks and the rash of RMSF in more deeply pigmented skin, which can often delay diagnosis in these patients. In fact, the rash of RMSF occurs less frequently in dark-skinned patients; this is felt to be a true variant of disease manifestations and not just a lack of diagnosis by clinicians. Left untreated, the fatality rate is just over 20%. Even with appropriate treatment, the hospitalization rate is over 70% and the fatality rate is 5% to 10%. Fatalities are likely due to delayed diagnosis given the nonspecific clinical findings.

Early clinical manifestations of RMSF include high fever, severe headache, myalgias, nausea, and vomiting. Later manifestations include rash, photophobia, confusion, ataxia, seizures, cough, dyspnea, arrhythmias, jaundice, and severe abdominal pain. Although predominantly a clinical diagnosis, laboratory findings may include thrombocytopenia, hyponatremia, and elevated transaminases.

There are several other tick bite-associated spotted fevers. Mediterranean spotted fever, also known as Boutonneuse fever or Marseilles fever, is caused by *R. conorii* and is transmitted by the brown dog tick, *Rhipicephalus sanguineus*. Disease is endemic throughout Africa, the Middle East, and southern Europe. African tick bite fever is caused by *R. africae* and transmitted by the *Amblyomma* tick. The clinical signs and symptoms are similar to those of RMSF, with the tache noire as the primary distinguishing cutaneous feature. These diseases often have a less aggressive course with a more favorable prognosis compared to RMSF. Travel to an endemic area leads to an increased risk of disease development among nonnatives.

Rickettsialpox is a spotted fever caused by *R. akari* and transmitted by bites from the house mouse mite, *Liponyssoides sanguineus*, with the house mouse as the mammalian reservoir. The bites are painless and often go unnoticed. Rickettsialpox is most common in large urban areas in the northeastern United States, with over half of the reported cases in New York City. This febrile illness is acute and self-limited, often resolving within 2 weeks without treatment. An eschar initially develops at the site of the mite bite within 24 to 48 hours, with fever following in another 1 to 2 days. The clinical findings are otherwise similar to RMSF. The cutaneous findings can resemble varicella infection with poxlike lesions.

Endemic typhus (murine typhus) is caused by *R. typhi* and transmitted by flea bites, with rodents as the mammalian vector. Without treatment, mortality is 1% to 2%, most commonly in the elderly. Risk factors include employment as a sanitation worker in a granary or brewery. Transmission can occur in domestic settings in the developing world.

Epidemic typhus (louse-borne typhus) is caused by infection with *R. prowazekii* and transmitted by the human body louse, which is common in conditions of poor hygiene; wartime, famine, and overcrowding are conditions that favor propagation of the louse vector. In the United States, the southern flying squirrel may serve as the mammalian reservoir. Mortality rate is 20% overall but is higher among the elderly.

Other more geographically limited diseases within the rickettsiae group include the following:

- Queensland tick typhus, caused by *R. australis* and transmitted by the *Ixodes* genus of ticks. This disease is endemic to eastern Australia.
- Japanese spotted fever, or oriental spotted fever, is caused by *R. japonica* and transmitted by ticks. The mammalian reservoir is still undefined. It is limited to the central and southwestern coastal regions of Japan, with about 40 cases reported yearly.
- Scrub typhus is caused by *Orientia tsutsugamushi* and transmitted by the larval stage (chigger) of the trombiculid mite of the *Leptotrombidium* species. Rodents serve as the mammalian reservoir. This disease is endemic to the Indian subcontinent, eastern Asia, and the western Pacific Rim.

Pediatric Patient Considerations

Age-specific incidence of RMSF is highest in children.

⦿ Look For

RMSF

Signs and symptoms typically begin 2 to 14 days after inoculation. Fevers, myalgias, and headaches are the most common manifestations. Rash is present in 90% of cases and begins 2 to 5 days after onset of the fever. Look for multiple 1- to 5-mm erythematous or purpuric papules that begin on the ankles, wrists, and forearms and spread centripetally to the trunk with facial sparing. The palms and soles are commonly affected (Fig. 4-6). Lesions progress from papules to petechiae, which may coalesce to form ecchymoses. Less commonly, the rash may be asymmetric or localized. These subtle findings may be less noticeable in darkly pigmented patients, thereby delaying diagnosis.

Mediterranean Spotted Fever and African Tick Bite Fever

Look for the tache noire (present in 30% to 86% of cases), an erythematous, indurated papule with a black central necrotic eschar. Tache noire may be multiple, especially in African tick bite fever, where these lesions are associated with regional lymphadenopathy. The tache noire is followed by the more generalized cutaneous eruption, which in these diseases may be more diffuse with less petechiae and purpura.

Rickettsialpox

At the site of the mite bite, look for a red papule that quickly evolves into a 1- to 2-cm vesicle with a violaceous or erythematous halo. The vesicle dries and develops into a black eschar (Figs. 4-7 and 4-8). Within 1 day to 1 week, a generalized, scattered papulovesicular eruption develops with eventual crusting of lesions within a few days. Palms and soles are spared.

Endemic Typhus

Look for sudden onset of flulike symptoms. Fifty percent of patients will also develop a widespread maculopapular and/or petechial eruption.

Epidemic Typhus

Look for blanchable pink macules appearing first within the axillae and upper trunk and spreading to the entire body. Within 7 days, exanthema evolves to a more papular appearance. The residual macules may coalesce and become dusky with associated petechiae. There is notable sparing of the palms, soles, and face.

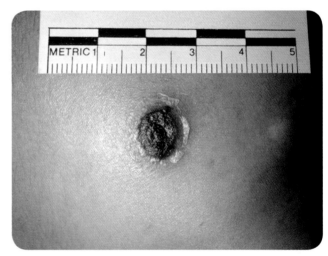

Figure 4-7 Hemorrhagic eschar of rickettsialpox.

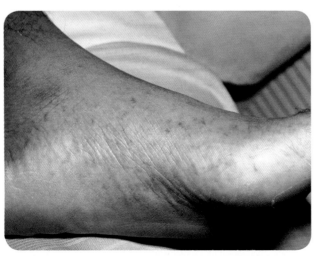

Figure 4-6 Purpura on the feet is characteristic of RMSF.

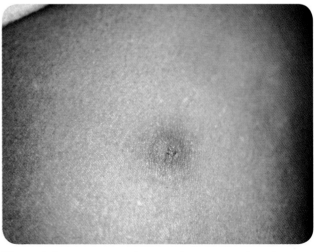

Figure 4-8 Healing stage of rickettsialpox lesion with small crust.

Diagnostic Pearls

- A palm and sole petechial eruption in the setting of high fever, myalgias, and headache is characteristic of RMSF. Involvement of the scrotum or vulva is a clue for RMSF. In areas with high concentrations of disease, consider RMSF as a cause of unexplained fever in spring or summer.
- Rickettsialpox should be considered in patients with a black eschar followed by a more generalized papulovesicular eruption, particularly in metropolitan areas.
- The rash of epidemic typhus begins on the trunk and spreads to the extremities—opposite of the rash of RMSF, which begins on the limbs and spreads centrally.
- A high clinical index of suspicion is necessary for all diseases within this group. A thorough travel history should be obtained, as travelers may contract disease while visiting endemic areas but develop clinical signs and symptoms upon returning home.

Differential Diagnosis and Pitfalls

- Meningococcemia typically occurs in the late winter to early spring with fever and rash appearing within 24 hours of infection. There is also marked lymphadenopathy.
- Measles typically occurs in the winter to spring and has associated symptoms of cough, coryza, conjunctivitis, and Koplik spots.
- Enteroviral infections typically occur in the summer to fall. The fever and rash often appear together. Sick contacts are common.
- Dengue fever, also known as "breakbone fever," has severe arthralgias.
- Vasculitis is marked by palpable purpura rather than petechiae.
- Drug eruptions will have a history of drug exposure.
- Gonococcemia may present with asymmetric monoarticular arthritis and a pustular or petechial rash.
- Meningitis has prominent neurological signs.
- Immune thrombocytopenic purpura presents with a petechial rash.
- Thrombotic thrombocytopenic purpura is characterized by fever, anemia, thrombocytopenia, renal impairment, and neurological deficits.
- Mediterranean spotted fever and African tick bite fever should be considered in persons from endemic areas.

Tache noire

- Brown recluse spider bite (Fig. 4-9)
- Cutaneous anthrax
- Scrub typhus
- Rickettsialpox
- Deep fungal infection

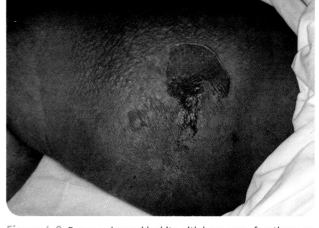

Figure 4-9 Brown recluse spider bite with large area of erythema on thigh, with multiple vesicles and eroded bullae. Sometimes purpura may be present, raising the diagnosis of RMSF.

Rickettsialpox

- Varicella
- Eczema herpeticum
- Eczema vaccinatum
- Echovirus
- Other rickettsial spotted fevers

Best Tests

- Serology
- Indirect immunofluorescence assay (IFA)
- ELISA
- Treatment should be initiated immediately with high clinical suspicion. Early in infection, serologic assays may be unreliable. In the first week of illness, 85% of patients lack diagnostic titers, and up to 50% may lack diagnostic titers 7 to 9 days after onset of illness. It is important to test acute and convalescent samples 2 to 4 weeks apart to confirm infection. A fourfold rise in IFA titers is confirmatory. ELISA is not quantitative.
- Skin biopsy with direct immunofluorescence may help confirm diagnosis in the acute setting with a sensitivity of 70%.
- Immunohistochemical staining, polymerase chain reaction, and electron microscopy may aid in diagnosis.

Management Pearls

- Rapid diagnosis and treatment prevent deaths.
- Removal of the tick within 6 hours of the bite may prevent transmission. However, exposure to a crushed tick or to

tick fecal matter may result in immediate transmission. Antimicrobial prophylaxis following a tick bite is not recommended and may, in fact, delay the onset of disease.

Therapy

Doxycycline is the drug of choice for treatment of all tick-borne rickettsial disease in children and adults. The risks of significant morbidity from RMSF outweigh the low risk of dental staining in children from doxycycline. Therefore, doxycycline is recommended in children of all ages if RMSF is suspected. Clinical response time is typically within 24 to 72 hours. Other broad-spectrum antimicrobials are usually ineffective.

- Adults or children >45 kg (>100 lbs): doxycycline 100 mg twice daily p.o. or IV
- Children <45 kg (<100 lbs): doxycycline 2.2 mg/kg body weight given twice a day p.o. or IV
- Pregnant adult or tetracycline allergic: chloramphenicol 500 mg four times per day IV. Complicated cases in pregnant women should be treated with doxycycline 100 mg daily p.o. or IV.

IV therapy is frequently indicated for hospitalized patients. Oral therapy is acceptable for patients considered to be in early stages of the disease and for those who can be managed as outpatients.

The optimal duration of therapy has not been established, but current recommendations are to treat for at least 3 days after the fever subsides and when evidence of clinical improvement is noted (treatment should be given for 7 to 14 days). Severe or complicated disease might require longer treatment courses.

Although rickettsialpox is self-limited, tetracycline can lead to clinical improvement within 3 to 5 days.

Endemic and epidemic typhus are treated with doxycycline 100 mg p.o. twice daily for 7 days. An alternative option is chloramphenicol 12.5 mg/kg p.o. every 6 hours for 7 days.

Suggested Readings

Dantas-Torres F. Rocky Mountain spotted fever. *Lancet Infect Dis.* 2007;7(11):724–732.

Graf PC, Chretien JP, Ung L, et al. Prevalence of seropositivity to spotted fever group rickettsiae and Anaplasma phagocytophilum in a large, demographically diverse US sample. *Clin Infect Dis.* 2008;46(1):70–77.

Halpern AV, Green JJ, Heymann WR. The Rickettioses, Ehrlichioses, and Anaplasmoses. In: Wolff K, Goldsmith LA, Katz SI, Gilchrest BA, Paller AS, Leffell DJ, eds. *Fitzpatrick's Dermatology in General Medicine.* 7th Ed. New York, NY: McGraw-Hill; 2008:1940–1952.

Rolain JM, Jensenius M, Raoult D. Rickettsial infections—a threat to travelers? *Curr Opin Infect Dis.* 2004;17(5):433–437.

Silber JL. Rocky Mountain spotted fever. *Clin Dermatol.* 1996;14(3):245–258.

Secondary, Tertiary, and Congenital Syphilis

Stephanie Diamantis

▪▪ Diagnosis Synopsis

Syphilis is a sexually transmitted infection (STI) caused by *Treponema pallidum* and is characterized by a chronic intermittent clinical course.

Primary syphilis is characterized by a painless ulceration or chancre that develops 10 to 90 days (average of 3 weeks) after direct inoculation. All patients with primary syphilis develop secondary syphilis if left untreated.

Secondary syphilis usually appears 3 to 10 weeks after the primary chancre and is characterized by papulosquamous eruptions on the body and mucosal involvement.

Latent syphilis occurs after lesions of primary and secondary syphilis have resolved without treatment, and patients are asymptomatic but seropositive. The latent stage may last for years: 60% to 70% of patients remain latently asymptomatic; about 30% will progress.

Tertiary syphilis may appear months to years after secondary syphilis resolves and can involve the central nervous system, heart, bones, and skin. About 16% of untreated patients will develop tertiary lesions.

T. pallidum is transmitted person to person via direct contact, usually genital, and may enter through skin or mucous membranes. It can also cross the placenta and infect an unborn child.

Between 2005 and 2006, the number of primary and secondary syphilis cases increased by 11.8%. Sixty-four percent of syphilis cases were among men who have sex with men. An increased incidence of syphilis in the United States has been observed in African American and Hispanic individuals, sex workers, those exposed to sex workers, and those with a history of other STIs and/or HIV. The incidence rate for non-Hispanic African Americans remains 50 times higher than for non-Hispanic whites. Other concomitant STIs are common, particularly chancroid and herpes simplex virus.

Characteristics

Secondary Syphilis

Skin and mucous membrane lesions of variable morphology are characteristic. Mucocutaneous manifestations and prodromal symptoms last 3 to 12 weeks and resolve spontaneously. If left untreated, up to 25% of patients will relapse within the first 2 years.

Tertiary Syphilis

Tertiary syphilis can occur 3 to 5 years after infection in untreated patients. Both nodular lesions and gummas present on the skin, are destructive, and heal with scarring. Cardiovascular involvement occurs in 10% of untreated patients and most often presents as aortitis. Neurosyphilis occurs in 4% to 9% of untreated patients.

Congenital Syphilis

Congenital syphilis is acquired by the fetus, in utero, from an infected mother. US case report data from 2005 show that the rate of congenital syphilis in African Americans was 19.9 times higher than the rate for whites. Early congenital syphilis is defined as occurring before 2 years of age and is characterized by cutaneous and extracutaneous findings. Half of infected infants are asymptomatic at birth. Historically, infected infants were said to develop a form of rhinitis, snuffles, characterized by excessive blood-stained nasal drainage by the infant's third week of life. Other findings include hepatomegaly, splenomegaly, lymphadenopathy, mucous patches, hemolytic anemia, thrombocytopenia, periostitis, and intrauterine growth retardation. If syphilis remains latent and symptoms occur after 2 years of age, it is considered late congenital syphilis, and findings include tissue malformation at critical growth periods, incisor abnormalities, corneal opacities, and eighth nerve deafness.

◉ Look For

Secondary Syphilis

Skin

- Generalized nonpruritic papulosquamous eruption including the palms and soles, with pink to violaceous scaly papules. Macules are more commonly found in white patients. Papular lesions in dark-skinned patients tend to be more hyperpigmented (Figs. 4-10 and 4-11).

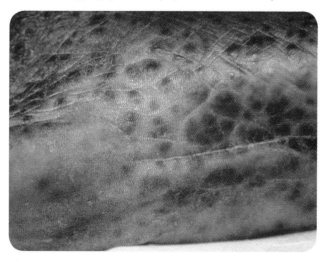

Figure 4-10 Discrete pigmented papules on the sole and foot in secondary syphilis.

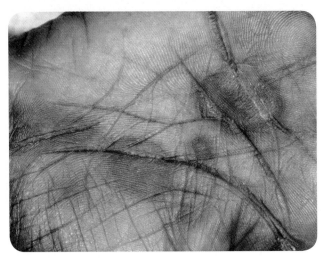

Figure 4-11 Scaling palmar plaques and papules in secondary syphilis.

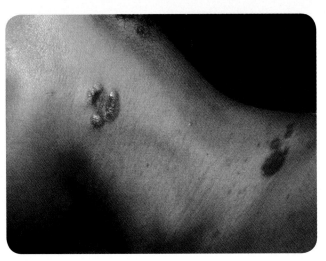

Figure 4-13 Papular and nodular secondary syphilis in a patient with HIV infection.

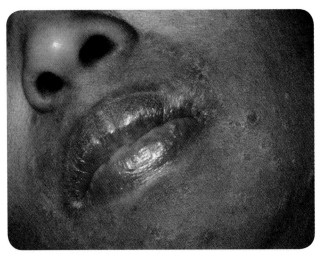

Figure 4-12 Split papules at lip margins characteristic of secondary syphilis; also, scaling papules on the face.

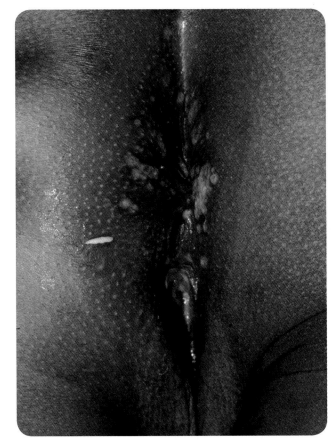

Figure 4-14 Perianal condyloma lata characteristic of secondary syphilis.

- Patchy alopecia with "moth-eaten" scalp and loss of the lateral one-third of the eyebrows
- Presence of a "crownlike" papulosquamous eruption around the frontal scalp line
- Erythematous papules at the angles of the mouth with a central fissure ("split papules") (Fig. 4-12)
- Annular plaques of secondary syphilis are more common in dark-skinned patients and tend to be periorificial in distribution. Follicular lesions are also much more prevalent in dark-skinned patients.
- Palm and sole lesions in Fitzpatrick skin types IV to VI may be scaly or copper colored and resolve with hyperpigmentation.
- Truncal lesions may also leave hyperpigmented macules or, rarely, lead to keloids.
- Lesions may be exuberant with concurrent HIV infection (Fig. 4-13).

Mucosal

- Ulcers/erosions
- Gray-colored plaques (mucous patches) on tonsils, tongue, pharynx, gingiva, genitalia; hoarseness when the oropharynx is involved; highly infectious; split papules on the lips

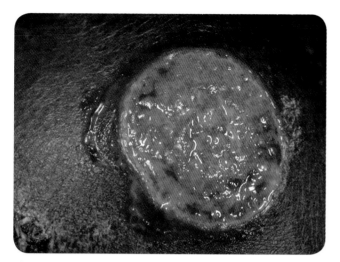

Figure 4-15 Ulcerated tertiary syphilis in a patient with HIV infection.

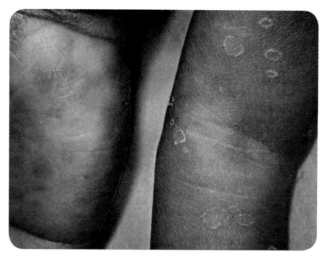

Figure 4-16 Secondary syphilis–like eruption with annular scaling lesions in a newborn due to early prenatal congenital syphilis.

- Condyloma lata—exophytic mucus-covered papules and plaques located in folds of moist skin (i.e., genitalia, anus) (Fig. 4-14); highly infectious

Prodromal Symptoms

- Fever, weight loss, malaise, lymphadenopathy, myalgias, and sore throat

Tertiary Syphilis

Skin/Mucosal

- Nodular—red-brown papules or nodules that may ulcerate and expand while healing in the center, resulting in a serpiginous pattern. They heal with scarring; usually found on the trunk and extensor aspects of the extremities (Fig. 4-15). Ulcers are commonly seen with concurrent HIV.
- Gumma—small papule that enlarges, often with central necrosis; found on lower legs
- Ulceration (especially the tongue), superficial glossitis

Osseous

- Bone pain, especially at night; periostitis, osteomyelitis, gummatous osteoarthritis
- Charcot joints—knees and ankles commonly affected, more common in men

Congenital Syphilis

Early

- Red and purple macules and papules that progress to a copper color over time, usually on the face, arms, buttocks, and legs of the newborn (Fig. 4-16)
- Vesicles and bullae may occur at acral sites, followed by erosion and crusting. Diffuse acral scaling may also herald early congenital syphilis.
- When thrombocytopenia is severe, petechiae may be seen.
- Rhagades are fine, periorificial, linear scars.

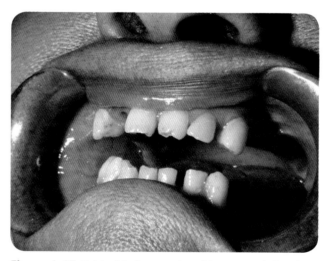

Figure 4-17 Notched incisors, a sign of late congenital syphilis, in a child.

- Condyloma lata are flat-topped papules at mucocutaneous junctions.
- Examine for hepatosplenomegaly.

Late

- Frontal bossing due to periostitis of the parietal and frontal bones; saddle nose; high palatal arch; saber shins
- Hutchinson teeth (cylindrical formation of central upper incisors), mulberry molars (Fig. 4-17)

 ## Diagnostic Pearls

Secondary Syphilis

- Eruption is symmetric and nonpruritic. Involvement of the palms and/or soles with macules and scaly papules is common. Signs of secondary syphilis should prompt serological testing.

- Secondary syphilis is common in a mother of a child born with congenital syphilis.

Tertiary Syphilis

Destructive, scarring, cutaneous lesions.

Congenital Syphilis

Serologic testing of both mother and child (infant's sera, not cord blood) is recommended.

?? Differential Diagnosis and Pitfalls

Secondary Syphilis

Cutaneous Lesions

- Lichen planus—very pruritic, violaceous papules with Wickham striae
- Pityriasis rosea—Look for herald patch, collarette of scale, and orientation of lesions.
- Pityriasis rubra pilaris—Look for orange-red, waxy-like keratoderma of the palms and soles.
- Guttate psoriasis—Systemic signs are absent, and palms and soles are spared.
- Drug eruption—pruritic; appropriate timing after drug use
- Erythema multiforme—also palmar/plantar (usually not truncal); characteristic targetoid morphology
- Active arthritis (Reiter syndrome)
- Tinea—Check KOH.
- Scabies—very pruritic; contacts may be affected; scabies prep useful
- Sarcoidosis
- Mycosis fungoides

Mucous Membrane Lesions

- Herpes simplex virus
- Aphthous ulcers
- Infectious mononucleosis—Check heterophile antibody titer.
- Erythroplakia
- Erosions due to oral candidiasis
- Condyloma acuminata

Patchy Alopecia

- Alopecia areata
- Traction alopecia

Tertiary Syphilis

- Cutaneous malignancy
- Deep fungal infection

- Atypical mycobacterial infection
- Scrofuloderma

Congenital Syphilis

- Congenital rubella, congenital Lyme disease, and congenital cytomegalovirus infection. If blisters are present, consider congenital candidiasis, acropustulosis, and congenital Lyme disease.

✓ Best Tests

The diagnosis of syphilis includes the following strategies:

- Direct visualization of *T. pallidum* via dark-field microscopy in primary—not in secondary
- Direct detection of the bacterial DNA via PCR (useful in genital ulcerations)
- Serologic antibody tests (nonspecific and treponemal specific)

Nontreponemal tests (detection of antibodies to cardiolipin):

- Venereal Disease Research Laboratory (VDRL)
- Rapid plasma reagin (RPR or STS)
- Titers correlate with disease activity; useful in screening and monitoring treatment
- False positives due to pregnancy, lupus erythematosus, lymphoma, antiphospholipid syndrome, cirrhosis, vaccinations, drug abuse, and infectious diseases

Treponemal-specific tests (to be performed when nontreponemal test is reactive):

- Microhemagglutination assay for *T. pallidum*
- Fluorescent treponemal antibody absorption test
- Captia enzyme-linked immunosorbent assay
- Not reactive in early primary syphilis
- Will remain positive forever, so not useful for monitoring response to treatment
- False positives in HIV infection, autoimmune diseases, and additional bacteria from treponeme and spirochete families

Patients with very high antibody titers may have a false-negative test, but serial dilutions will correct for this (prozone phenomenon).

Congenital Syphilis

Diagnosis of congenital syphilis can be made via the following:

- An abnormal physical examination that is consistent with congenital syphilis
- Serum quantitative nontreponemal serologic titer fourfold higher than mother's titer

- A positive dark-field or fluorescent antibody test of body fluid(s)

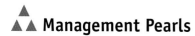

Management Pearls

- Those diagnosed with syphilis should be screened for HIV infection and, if negative, retested 3 months later. Syphilis patients with HIV can be recalcitrant to treatment.
- Management of sex partners—Persons exposed to an infected sexual partner within 90 days preceding the diagnosis may also be infected and should be treated presumptively.
- All infants born to women who have reactive serologic tests for syphilis should be thoroughly examined for evidence of congenital syphilis. Examination of the placenta or umbilical cord by using specific fluorescent antitreponemal antibody staining is suggested.

Therapy

General
Penicillin G (IM or IV) for all stages of syphilis remains the gold standard. Type of preparation, dosage, and length of treatment depend on stage and clinical manifestations with the details obtainable from the CDC.

The Jarisch-Herxheimer reaction is an acute febrile reaction that can occur within the first 24 hours of treatment for syphilis. Headache, myalgias, shaking chills, and malaise can accompany the fever. Early labor and fetal distress may occur in pregnant patients.

Treatment and follow-up for individuals coinfected with HIV differ slightly from the regimens discussed above. Consultation with an infectious disease specialist is recommended.

Suggested Readings

Dourmishev LA, Dourmishev AL. Syphilis: Uncommon presentations in adults. *Clin Dermatol.* 2005;23(6):555–564.

http://www.cdc.gov/STD/treatment/2006/congenital-syphilis.htm

James WD, Berger TG, Elston DM, eds. Syphilis, yaws, bejel, and pinta. In: *Andrews' Diseases of the Skin.* 10th Ed. Philadelphia, PA: Elsevier; 2006:352–364.

Lautenschlager S. Cutaneous manifestations of syphilis: recognition and management. *Am J Clin Dermatol.* 2006;7(5):291–304.

Newman LM, Berman SM. Epidemiology of STD disparities in African American communities. *Sex Transm Dis.* 2008;35(12 Suppl):S4–S12.

Necrotizing Fasciitis

Mat Davey

■■ Diagnosis Synopsis

Necrotizing fasciitis is a deep and often devastating bacterial infection that tracks along fascial planes and expands beyond outward cutaneous signs of infection (i.e., erythema). It most commonly occurs from an extension of an overlying skin and/or soft tissue infection. Inciting events include perforating trauma, surgery, or insect bites. Predisposing factors for necrotizing fasciitis include recent surgery, diabetes mellitus, malignancy, and alcoholism, although most affected patients are healthy individuals.

Classically, group A beta-hemolytic streptococci are associated with necrotizing fasciitis, but many other organisms, including *Staphylococcus aureus*, *Vibrio vulnificus*, *Enterobacteriaceae*, and *Bacteroides* spp., have been reported. Polymicrobial infection is frequent.

Patients with necrotizing fasciitis are acutely ill. They are often thought to have cellulitis that is not responding to standard antibiotic therapy. Pain is out of proportion to physical findings. There is often associated skin necrosis and bullae formation. Signs of systemic illness such as fever, lethargy, hypotension, and tachycardia are present; these may progress to multiorgan failure. When localized to the lower abdominal wall, perineum, or genitals, the condition is known as Fournier gangrene. Diabetic patients are particularly susceptible to Fournier gangrene, which is often polymicrobial with mixed anaerobic organisms.

The mortality of necrotizing fasciitis is high. Treatment includes broad-spectrum intravenous antibiotics and immediate surgical debridement of infected and devitalized tissue.

Look For

Early, there is erythema and edema typical of cellulitis in the setting of a patient who appears severely ill. Despite standard antibiotic therapy, the edema progresses and is often associated with bullae, cyanosis, and eventual gangrene (Figs. 4-18 and 4-19). Crepitus may be present. The subcutaneous tissues will often have a hard, wooden feel.

Diagnostic Pearls

Distinguishing necrotizing fasciitis from a cellulitis that does not require surgical intervention may be challenging. The following clinical features suggest a deep necrotizing infection:

- Constant pain that is often quite severe and is out of proportion with visible skin changes
- Anesthesia to pinprick in affected locations
- Presence of bullae
- Skin necrosis or ecchymosis that precedes necrosis
- Gas in the soft tissues
- Edema extending beyond areas of erythema
- Systemic toxicity (fever, delirium, renal failure, hypotension, tachycardia)
- Cutaneous anesthesia
- Rapid spread despite antibiotic therapy

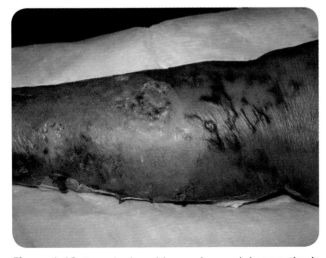

Figure 4-18 Hemorrhagic vesicles, erosions, and desquamation in necrotizing fasciitis.

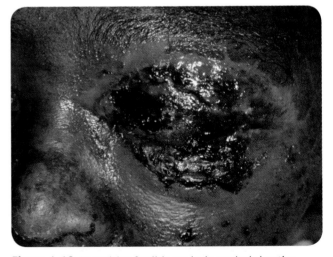

Figure 4-19 Necrotizing fasciitis can be in any body location.

?? Differential Diagnosis and Pitfalls

- Cellulitis
- Erysipelas
- Purpura fulminans complicating varicella
- Vasculitis
- Calciphylaxis
- Ecthyma gangrenosum
- Disseminated intravascular coagulation
- Staphylococcal scalded skin syndrome
- Insect bite (e.g., brown recluse spider)
- Toxic shock syndrome
- Gas gangrene (clostridial myonecrosis)
- Pyoderma gangrenosum

✓ Best Tests

- This diagnosis is made on clinical grounds. Immediate surgical intervention is required. Therefore, if you are considering this diagnosis, contact a surgeon immediately. To confirm suspected necrotizing fasciitis, a small, exploratory incision can be made at the site of maximum suspicion. In cases of necrotizing fasciitis, there will often be a thin, brownish exudate with extensive undermining of the surrounding tissues, which dissect easily with a blunt instrument or gloved finger. The fascia will be swollen and gray, with areas of necrosis.
- CT scan or MRI may demonstrate edema extending along fascial planes, and plain films may demonstrate gas in the tissues. However, definitive treatment of this disease should not be delayed in order to obtain radiologic studies.

▲▲ Management Pearls

- Supportive treatment should be pursued in an intensive care unit setting. In addition to debridement and intravenous antibiotics, patients require wound care and careful attention to fluid and electrolyte balance, nutrition, and temperature regulation. Patients may need ventilatory and/or hemodynamic support.
- Commonly needed consultations (in addition to general surgery) include infectious disease, critical care, and plastic surgery.
- There is an association between nonsteroidal anti-inflammatory drug (NSAID) use and the development of necrotizing fasciitis. Although no studies have been able to show a causative role, it is generally accepted that NSAIDs mask the symptoms and potentially delay

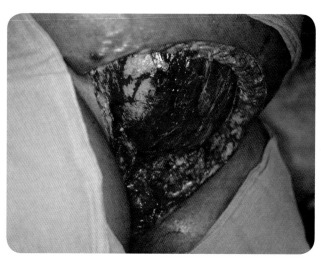

Figure 4-20 Extensive debridement is a necessary therapy for necrotizing fasciitis.

Therapy

Therapy requires immediate surgical intervention in addition to antibiotics. Antibiotics alone are of little benefit because of the ischemia found in these infections. All infected and devitalized tissue must be removed (Fig. 4-20). Often, patients will need multiple (if not daily) trips to the operating room to accomplish this.

Choice of antibiotic therapy can be directed by Gram stain(s) taken at the time of the initial operation. Antibiotics will need to be continued until such time as operative procedures are no longer needed and the patient has been afebrile for 2 to 3 days.

Polymicrobial Infection

- Ampicillin-sulbactam 1.5 to 3.0 g IV every 6 to 8 hours
- Piperacillin-tazobactam 3.375 g IV every 6 to 8 hours plus clindamycin 600 to 900 mg IV every 8 hours plus ciprofloxacin 400 mg IV every 12 hours
- Imipenem/cilastatin 1 g IV every 6 to 8 hours
- Meropenem 1 g IV every 8 hours
- Ertapenem 1 g IV every 24 hours

Streptococcal Infection

- Clindamycin is recommended as additional therapy in cases of group A streptococcal disease to block toxin production

(Continued)

- Penicillin 2 to 4 million units IV every 4 to 6 hours plus clindamycin 600 to 900 mg IV every 8 hours

Staphylococcus aureus Infection

- Nafcillin or oxacillin 1 to 2 g IV every 4 hours
- Cefazolin 1 g IV every 8 hours
- Vancomycin (for methicillin-resistant *S. aureus*) 30 mg/kg/d IV divided in two doses

Clostridial Infection

- Penicillin 2 to 4 million units IV every 4 to 6 hours
- Clindamycin 600 to 900 mg IV every 8 hours

In addition, patients will require aggressive fluid resuscitation.

diagnosis. Thus, NSAIDs should be avoided in patients suspected of having necrotizing fasciitis.

Suggested Readings

Anaya DA, Dellinger EP. Necrotizing soft-tissue infection: Diagnosis and management. *Clin Infect Dis.* 2007;44(5):705–710.

James WD, Berger TG, Elston DM, et al., eds. *Andrews' Diseases of the Skin: Clinical Dermatology.* 10th Ed. Philadelphia, PA: Saunders Elsevier; 2006:261–262.

Saavedra A, Weinberg AN, Swartz MN, et al. Soft tissue infections: Erysipelas, cellulitis, gangrenous cellulitis, and myonecrosis. In: Fitzpatrick TB, Wolff K, eds. *Fitzpatrick's Dermatology in General Medicine.* 7th Ed. New York, NY: McGraw-Hill; 2008:1373–1720.

Souyri C, Olivier P, Grolleau S, et al., French Network of Pharmacovigilance Centres. Severe nectrotizing soft-tissue infections and nonsteroidal anti-inflammatory drugs. *Clin Exp Dermatol.* 2008;33(3):249–255.

Drug Hypersensitivity Syndrome (DRESS Syndrome)

Suzanne Berkman

■■ Diagnosis Synopsis

Drug hypersensitivity syndrome (DHS), or drug reaction with eosinophilia and systemic symptoms (DRESS), is a serious multisystem drug reaction characterized by fever, skin eruptions, eosinophilia, and internal organ involvement, usually hepatitis. The most commonly implicated drugs include anticonvulsants, sulfonamides, and nonsteroidal anti-inflammatory drugs (NSAIDs). Minocycline, allopurinol, metronidazole, dapsone, antiretroviral agents (e.g., nevirapine), clopidogrel, and ticlopidine are other known causes. It typically occurs 1 to 3 weeks after starting a new medication but may develop months later. Sulfonamide-induced DRESS typically has an earlier onset, appearing as early as 7 to 14 days after initiation of therapy.

The specific underlying mechanisms of this condition are unknown, and they likely vary among patients and specific drugs. Defects in the detoxification of anticonvulsants and sulfonamides have been demonstrated in patients with DRESS. Human herpesvirus type 6 (HHV-6) and HHV-7 reactivation have also been demonstrated in many of these patients, although the pathogenic role of this viral reactivation, if any, is yet to be determined.

It is imperative to withdraw the suspect medication(s) as soon as possible when DRESS is suspected, as there is a 10% mortality rate associated with this syndrome. If a patient is rechallenged with the drug, the reaction will occur within 24 hours. Rechallenge is usually *not* performed as a diagnostic procedure.

◉ Look For

The skin is involved in over 80% of cases (Fig. 4-21). A morbilliform, or measles-like, eruption is common, with macules and papules ranging in color from faint pink to dark red and distributed symmetrically and spreading from the face downward. Pustules may also be seen. Lymphadenopathy is another common finding and can be striking, leading to a misdiagnosis of lymphoma or mononucleosis. Facial edema and erythroderma are common (Fig. 4-22).

Some patients will have urticarial plaques that may resemble erythema multiforme. Others will have manifestations of Stevens-Johnson syndrome, with atypical targetoid lesions, vesicles, and mucosal involvement that progress to toxic epidermal necrolysis (TEN). Erythroderma is an additional serious manifestation of this syndrome.

In dark-skinned individuals, the eruption may present with deep red to brown macules and papules that are also distributed in a symmetrical fashion starting on the face and spreading downward.

●● Diagnostic Pearls

The liver, kidneys, and the hematologic system are the most commonly involved internal organ systems, but, rarely, pneumonitis, pericarditis, or myocarditis may be seen.

?? Differential Diagnosis and Pitfalls

- Infectious mononucleosis
- Cytomegalovirus infection
- Roseola
- Measles
- Other viral exanthems
- Leukemia or lymphoma

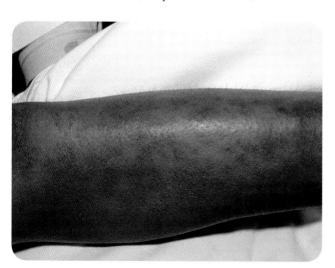

Figure 4-21 DRESS with phenytoin-induced eosinophilia, hepatomegaly, splenomegaly, and lymphadenopathy.

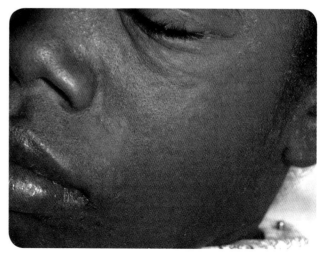

Figure 4-22 Erythroderma with DRESS due to phenytoin.

- Drug eruption not otherwise specified
- Erythema multiforme
- Rocky Mountain spotted fever
- Rickettsialpox
- Secondary syphilis
- Meningococcemia

✓ Best Tests

- It is important to identify any internal organ involvement. Laboratory studies should include the following: liver function tests, CBC with differential to look for the presence of leukocytosis with eosinophilia and atypical lymphocytes, and urinalysis and renal function tests. Chest X-ray and/or ECG can be ordered if symptoms of cough or chest discomfort are present.
- Skin biopsy may show evidence of a common drug eruption but may reveal keratinocyte necrosis indicative of erythema multiforme, Stevens-Johnson syndrome, or TEN.

▲▲ Management Pearls

- The inciting drug must be identified and stopped immediately. Counsel the patient regarding avoidance of the drug and related compounds in the future. Aromatic anticonvulsants cross-react; therefore, all related compounds should be strictly avoided as well. Oral rechallenge tests and skin testing may be harmful and are, therefore, not recommended.
- Conduct a thorough search for signs of systemic involvement. Patients with DRESS warrant hospitalization and may require treatment in an intensive care setting, with meticulous attention paid to wound care, temperature regulation, nutrition, and fluid and electrolyte balance.

Consultations may be needed with dermatology, critical care, gastroenterology, ophthalmology (for patients with TEN), or nephrology.
- Patients who have had DRESS are at an increased risk for becoming hypothyroid. This usually occurs 4 to 12 weeks after the reaction.

Therapy

- Many patients will recover spontaneously, although slowly. Optimize supportive care for any specific organ dysfunction. Monitor for and promptly treat any complicating infections.
- In mild cases, topical high-potency corticosteroids may be helpful for cutaneous manifestations. Systemic corticosteroids are recommended for severe cases of DRESS, particularly when there is involvement of the heart and lung. Intravenous immunoglobulin (IVIG) has been reported to be beneficial in cases of DRESS syndrome secondary to anticonvulsants and nevirapine.

Suggested Readings

Aihara Y, Ito SI, Kobayashi Y, et al. Carbamazepine-induced hypersensitivity syndrome associated with transient hypogammaglobulinaemia and reactivation of human herpesvirus 6 infection demonstrated by real-time quantitative polymerase chain reaction. *Br J Dermatol.* 2003;149: 165–169.

Fields KS, Petersen MF, Chiao E, et al. Case reports: Treatment of nevirapine-associated DRESS syndrome with intravenous immune globulin (IVIG). *J Drugs Dermatol.* 2005;4:510–513.

Shear NH, Spielberg SP. Anticonvulsant hypersensitivity syndrome. In vitro assessment of risk. *J Clin Invest.* 1988;82:1826–1832.

Shiohara T, Lijima M, Ikezawa Z, et al. The diagnosis of a DRESS Syndrome has been sufficiently established on the basis of typical clinical features and viral reactivations. *Br J Dermatol.* 2007;156:1083–1084.

Kawasaki Disease

Laurie Good

■ Diagnosis Synopsis

Kawasaki disease (KD), or mucocutaneous lymph node syndrome, is a multisystem vasculitis that affects infants and children. The exact cause is unknown, though several clinical and epidemiologic features of the disease (such as the temporal, spatial, and seasonal clustering of cases) suggest an infectious, likely viral, etiology that evokes an abnormal immunologic response in genetically susceptible individuals. The disease occurs primarily in children aged younger than 6 years (with about one-fourth of cases occurring before age 1) and affects children of Asian/Pacific Islander descent disproportionately. One study showed rates of KD among white, Hispanic, and Asian/Pacific Islander children <5 years of age to be 15.3, 20.2, and 45.9 of 100,000, respectively. KD is classically characterized by six criteria:

- Fever lasting at least 5 days (usually longer)
- Conjunctival injection without exudate
- Red lesions of the mouth or pharynx
- Acute hand and foot edema followed by peeling
- Polymorphous cutaneous eruption
- Lymphadenopathy

The majority of individuals affected by KD follow a benign course. However, coronary artery aneurysms develop in 20% to 25% of untreated patients. Treatment is aimed at decreasing the risk of developing coronary artery abnormalities and preventing complications from these abnormalities.

Of note, one study identified one predictive factor in the development of coronary artery aneurysm: persistence of fever beyond 5 days. The study examined ethnicity and demonstrated shorter fever duration in African Americans, who also had a significantly reduced risk of developing coronary artery aneurysms as a complication of KD.

As the search for a viral etiologic agent continues, research has also begun looking for susceptibility genes within certain patient populations. On the premise that serum levels of IL-10 are increased in patients with KD, a study in Chinese patients in Taiwan looked at the −592 IL-10 promoter polymorphism as a potential susceptibility or severity marker of the disease. While they found nothing to predict patients who would develop cardiac complications of KD, their findings did suggest involvement of the IL-10−592*A allele in the development of KD in Taiwanese children.

◉ Look For

The classic case definition of KD should be used as a guideline to increase awareness of KD and prevent overdiagnosis. However, one should remember that the principal clinical criteria are typically not all present at a single point of time, and infants will often present with "incomplete" KD, in which criteria are not fulfilled but coronary artery abnormalities do develop. Therefore, all suspected cases should be diagnosed based on (a) ruling out alternative diagnoses, (b) assessment of principal clinical criteria over time, and (c) supportive clinical features and laboratory data.

In the eyes, look for bilateral nonpurulent conjunctivitis. In the mouth, look for strawberry tongue and red, fissured lips. Skin findings are nonspecific and polymorphous. Lesions typically occur on the trunk and extremities with a predilection for the lower abdomen, groin, perineum, and buttocks (Figs. 4-23 and 4-24). Redness and swelling may be seen on the hands and feet (Fig. 4-25). Desquamation occurs during the second week of the illness.

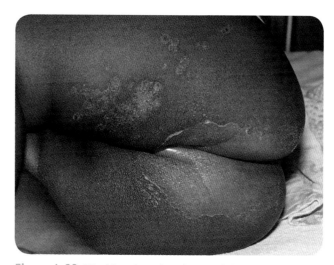

Figure 4-23 KD with perirectal erythema and desquamation.

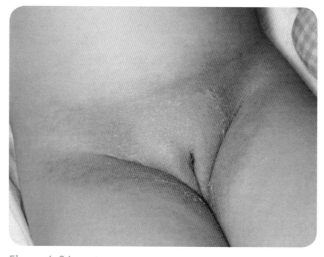

Figure 4-24 Erythema and scaling around the pubic area in KD.

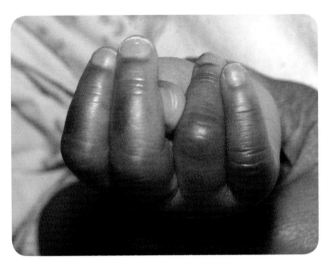

Figure 4-25 KD with diffuse edema of the hand.

Principal Clinical Criteria

- Fever: Remittent and high spiking (>39°C [102.2°F]); fever usually lasts 11 days without treatment or 2 days with appropriate therapy.
- Extremity changes: Erythema or firm induration of the palms and soles that may be painful is typical in the acute phase. Desquamation, usually beginning in the periungual region, occurs 2 to 3 weeks after disease onset.
- Exanthem: Within 5 days of fever onset, an erythematous, diffuse, nonspecific maculopapular eruption occurs, usually with accentuation in the perineal region (Fig. 4-23). Occasionally, the rash is urticarial, scarlatiniform, erythema multiforme-like, or micropustular.
- Bilateral conjunctival injection: Bulbar injection usually begins shortly after fever onset; spares the limbus; and is not associated with pain, exudate, conjunctival edema, or corneal ulceration.
- Oral mucosa changes: Lips may be erythematous, dry, peeling, cracked, and bleeding. The tongue may be erythematous with prominent fungiform papillae ("strawberry tongue"). The oropharyngeal mucosa may be diffusely erythematous.
- Cervical lymphadenopathy: Nodes in the anterior cervical triangle may be unilaterally enlarged (>1.5 cm). Lymph nodes are typically firm, nonfluctuant, and nontender.

Supportive Clinical Findings

- Cardiovascular: Cardiac findings may be prominent in the acute phase and may affect any structure of the heart. Cardiac auscultation of the infant may reveal a hyperdynamic precordium, tachycardia, a gallop rhythm, and an innocent flow murmur. If there is significant mitral regurgitation, auscultation may reveal a pansystolic regurgitant murmur. Other findings may include congestive heart failure, shock, peripheral gangrene, Raynaud phenomenon, or aneurysms of coronary or medium-size noncoronary arteries.

- Musculoskeletal: Arthritis and arthralgias of small and large joints may occur in the first week of illness. Large joints are more often affected after the first week.
- Gastrointestinal: Various manifestations during the acute phase may include diarrhea, vomiting, abdominal pain, hepatic dysfunction, jaundice, hepatic enlargement, and hydrops of the gallbladder.
- Neurologic: Extreme irritability, aseptic meningitis, and transient sensorineural hearing loss may occur during the acute phase.
- Genitourinary: Symptomatic or asymptomatic urethritis may be diagnosed by urinalysis.

Supportive Laboratory Results

- Elevated erythrocyte sedimentation rate (ESR)
- Elevated C-reactive protein (CRP)
- Leukocytosis (>15,000 with granulocyte predominance)
- Thrombocytosis (>500,000 after the first week)
- Anemia
- Abnormal plasma lipids
- Mild to moderate elevation of serum transaminases
- Mild to moderate sterile pyuria
- Pleocytosis of cerebrospinal fluid
- Leukocytosis of synovial fluid

Diagnostic Pearls

- Prolonged fever, conjunctivitis, and extreme irritability are the hallmarks of KD. Perineal erythema, that is, dark red or purple skin, with overlying scale frequently presents early in the disease course and provides a useful clue to the diagnosis.
- "Incomplete" KD should be strongly considered in any infant with unexplained fever for 5 or more days associated with two or more of the principal clinical features and three or more supportive laboratory findings.
- KD is unlikely if platelet counts, ESR, and CRP are normal after 7 days of illness.
- Conjunctival exudates, pharyngeal exudates, discrete intraoral lesions, a bullous eruption, or significant generalized lymphadenopathy weigh strongly against KD.

Differential Diagnosis and Pitfalls

- Patients with toxic shock syndrome most often have focal cutaneous skin infections, abscesses, infections associated with nasal packing, or a history of recent surgical procedures.
- Erythema multiforme presents with symmetrically distributed target lesions. Patients frequently have coexisting herpes orolabialis.
- Viral exanthems such as measles may be difficult to distinguish from KD. However, patients with measles often display an exudative conjunctivitis and Koplik spots within the oral mucosa.

- The cutaneous and mucosal findings in scarlet fever may also easily be confused with KD. However, these patients respond to antistreptococcal antibiotic therapy.
- Staphylococcal scalded skin syndrome presents with erythema and desquamation accentuated within skin folds.
- Distinguishing drug reactions from KD can be difficult. A careful drug history is critical.
- Common pitfalls may include diagnosing an infection in an infant with fever and an enlarged cervical lymph node (bacterial lymphadenitis) or sterile pyuria (partially treated urinary tract infection). The subsequent exanthem and mucosal changes may be misdiagnosed as a drug reaction to the prescribed antibiotics. Viral meningitis may be misdiagnosed in an infant with fever, rash, and cerebrospinal fluid pleocytosis.

Fever and similar mucocutaneous changes may also occur in the following:

- Stevens-Johnson syndrome
- Juvenile rheumatoid arthritis
- Bacterial cervical lymphadenitis
- Behçet disease
- Rocky Mountain spotted fever
- Leptospirosis
- Mercury hypersensitivity reaction

Best Tests

Because KD is idiopathic, no specific tests exist to confirm its diagnosis. Initial investigation should include tests to both support the diagnosis of KD and evaluate for alternative diagnoses. Testing should include a CBC with differential, ESR, CRP, urinalysis for blood and protein, liver function tests, an electrocardiogram, and echocardiogram.

To Support the Diagnosis

- CBC with differential
- ESR
- CRP
- Dip test of urine for blood and protein
- Liver function tests
- Electrocardiogram and echocardiogram

To Suggest Alternative Diagnoses

- Antistreptolysin O titer
- Anti-DNase B
- Nose and throat swab for culture
- Stool sample for culture
- Blood cultures
- Renal function tests
- Coagulation screen
- Autoantibody profile (antinuclear antibodies, extractable nuclear antibodies, rheumatoid factor, antineutrophil cytoplasmic antibodies)

- IgM and IgG serologies for *Mycoplasma pneumoniae*, enterovirus, adenovirus, measles, parvovirus, Epstein-Barr virus, and cytomegalovirus
- Urine microscopy and culture
- Consider serologies for rickettsiae and leptospirosis
- Consider a chest X-ray

Management Pearls

- Echocardiography should be performed at diagnosis, at 2 weeks, and at 6 to 8 weeks after onset. Coronary artery morphology, left ventricular and left valvular function, and the presence of pericardial effusion should be evaluated with each examination. If there is persistent fever or any cardiac abnormalities, echocardiography should be repeated more frequently.
- The diagnosis of KD should be reconsidered if fever persists after giving intravenous immunoglobulin (IVIG).
- Live virus vaccines (measles, mumps, rubella, and varicella) should be deferred for at least 11 months after IVIG administration.
- Patients and parents of patients on long-term aspirin should be warned of the potential for Reye syndrome and should report to the physician any exposures or symptoms consistent with influenza or varicella. Patients should receive an annual influenza vaccine. Consider alternative antiplatelet medications during the first 6 weeks after administration of the varicella vaccine.

Therapy

The acute phase of KD is treated with high-dose IVIG (2 g/kg infused over 10 to 12 hours) and high anti-inflammatory doses of aspirin (80 to 100 mg/kg/d divided into four doses until afebrile for 48 to 72 hours). Patients with persistent or recrudescent fever for 36 or more hours after completion of the first infusion of IVIG should be considered for retreatment with high-dose IVIG or corticosteroids (intravenous pulse methylprednisolone, 30 mg/kg once daily for 1 to 3 days). Low-dose aspirin (3 to 5 mg/kg/d) is continued until no evidence of coronary changes is found on echocardiography at 6 to 8 weeks after illness onset. Aspirin may be continued indefinitely for patients with coronary abnormalities.

Suggested Readings

Hsueh KC, Lin YJ, Chang JS, et al. Association of interleukin-10 A-592C polymorphism in Taiwanese children with Kawasaki disease. *J Korean Med Sci.* 2009;24(3):438–442.

Kao AS, Getis A, Brodine S, et al. Spatial and temporal clustering of Kawasaki syndrome cases. *Pediatr Infect Dis J.* 2008;27(11):981–985.

Porcalla AR, Sable CA, Patel KM, et al. The Epidemiology of Kawasaki Disease in an Urban Hospital: Does African American Race Protect Against Coronary Artery Aneurysms? *Pediatr Cardiol.* 2005;26:775–781.

Systemic Lupus Erythematosus

Aída Lugo-Somolinos

◼◼ Diagnosis Synopsis

Systemic lupus erythematosus (SLE) is a multisystem auto-immune disease that affects the skin and internal organs and is characterized by pathogenic circulating autoantibodies. Sex and ethnicity/race are the strongest risk factors for developing SLE, with a 6:1 female-to-male ratio and with African American women demonstrating a fourfold higher incidence when compared to whites. It is more common and also more severe in African Americans than whites. Women of childbearing potential are most often affected.

The etiology of SLE is poorly understood, but there is a strong association with autoantibodies and SLE. For example, even though the autoantibodies are not organ specific, only certain organs in a given patient demonstrate end-organ damage. It is hypothesized that a complex interplay between genetic proclivity and environmental influences leads to a perpetuated autoimmune response. Autoantibodies play significant roles in the diagnosis, management, and prognosis of SLE. They are as follows:

- Anti-dsDNA—highly specific for SLE. Rising levels correlate with increased SLE activity and an increased risk for SLE nephritis; seen in approximately 55% to 65% of SLE patients.
- Anti-Sm—highly specific for SLE; seen in approximately 25% to 30% of SLE patients; considerable diagnostic value, but levels do not correlate with disease activity.
- Anti-ribonucleoprotein (anti-RNP)—highly specific for SLE; seen in approximately 5% of SLE patients.
- Antinuclear antibody (ANA)—highly sensitive for SLE; seen in approximately 99% of SLE patients. In other words, it is very rare for an SLE individual to have a negative ANA. Considerable screening value, but levels do not correlate with disease activity.
- Antihistones—highly specific for drug-induced SLE.

The organ systems most commonly affected in SLE are skin, renal, pulmonary, CNS, hematologic, and joints. Fever, myalgias, weight loss, and lymphadenopathy are very common nonspecific constitutional findings. Other findings in lupus erythematosus include lymphadenopathy, conjunctivitis, episcleritis, normocytic normochromic anemia (sometimes hemolytic anemia), and leukopenia. Pneumonitis, nephritis, hypocomplementemia, and discoid lesions are more common in African Americans. African American women and Hispanics have an earlier onset of SLE and nephritis. Skin involvement is more common in African Americans.

Of note, SLE patients often require a multidisciplinary team, and, hence, efforts should be made to clarify the level and location of involvement to assist the various disciplines.

There are drug-induced forms of the disease, with a different pattern of autoimmunity and clinical profile.

Pediatric Patient Considerations

In approximately 15% to 20% of patients with SLE, the condition will present during the first 2 decades of life. Constitutional symptoms, fever, fatigue, weight loss, headache, mood disturbances, arthralgias, and skin findings may all be seen. Neurologic and renal involvement is prominent in childhood SLE. The onset of the disease is usually between the ages of 10 and 15; however, it can occur at any age. Girls outnumber boys 8:1 in adolescence, but the incidence nearly equalizes in younger ages.

The disease is more common in nonwhites. It is found worldwide. Genetic factors play a role, and a family history of SLE or lupus erythematosus or an inherited complement deficiency in any form is a risk factor for developing the disease.

◉ Look For

The classic cutaneous finding in SLE is the malar, or "butterfly," blush, which is not as prevalent in African Americans (Figs. 4-26 and 4-27). Photosensitivity is also less common. Erythema covering the nose and medial cheeks can occur after sun exposure and precedes the systemic symptoms by weeks. The erythema often develops into fine, scaling, coalesced papules. The erythema can become intense, and small infarcts and necrosis can develop in fulminant cases. A rash can develop in a photodistribution with prominence on the dorsa of the hands and digits. This rash can involve the

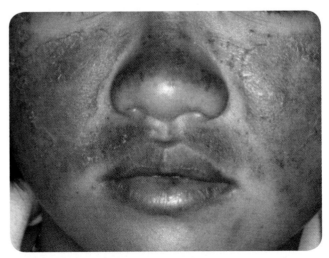

Figure 4-26 SLE in a child with a butterfly rash; note the characteristic sparing of nasolabial folds.

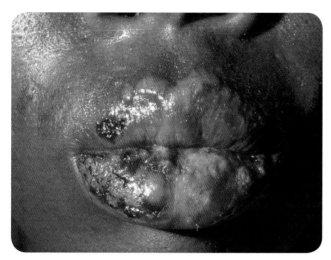

Figure 4-27 SLE with papules, edema, and blistering on the lips.

arms and trunk. Nail fold erythema and even necrosis often occur. Alopecia may also be seen.

Palmar erythema with tenderness is not an uncommon presenting sign in African American women, and when accompanied by tenderness, it signals a worse prognosis. Small mucous membrane ulcers, especially on the palate, can develop but are about two times less common in African Americans compared with whites. Livedo reticularis is common. Discoid lupus lesions can be seen about 2.5 times more frequently in African Americans. If systemic lupus does not start within the first few (often 2) years of the disease, there is a low probability of systemic lupus. Variants also include bullous lupus erythematosus. Purpura can occur secondary to vasculitis and is usually found on the extremities. Lupus profundus is a panniculitis rarely seen in patients with SLE. Some patients with systemic lupus will have psoriasiform or annular lesions in a photodistribution (subacute cutaneous lupus).

Pediatric Patient Considerations

The classic malar, or "butterfly," rash is more common in adolescents.

Diagnostic Pearls

Per the American College of Rheumatology 1982 Revised Criteria for Classification of Systemic Lupus Erythematosus, the criteria for SLE include any four (or more) of the following at any time during a patient's history:

- Malar rash
- Discoid rash
- Photosensitivity
- Oral ulcers
- Arthritis

- Serositis
- Renal disorder
- Neurologic disorder
- Hematologic disorder
- Immune disorder
- Presence of antinuclear antibodies

Sometimes multiple dermatofibromas may be present. Look for periungual telangiectases, erythema, and scaling between the finger joints and temporal hair thinning in addition to the clinical lesions. Alopecia is 1.5 times more common in African Americans than whites.

Pediatric Patient Considerations

Constitutional symptoms are more common than skin findings in children and adolescents. Ulcers, photosensitivity, and alopecia are all less common in children than in adults.

?? Differential Diagnosis and Pitfalls

- Dermatomyositis—Characteristic heliotrope rash (violaceous plaques surrounding eyes), photodistributed cutaneous eruption, and nail fold changes. Look for elevated serum CK levels and proximal symmetric extremity weakness.
- Rosacea—ANA negative
- Antiphospholipid antibody syndrome/lupus anticoagulant—can overlap with SLE; associated with recurrent thromboses and spontaneous abortions, elevated prothrombin time (PT)
- Polymorphous light eruption (PMLE)—Most lesions resolve within several days; skin lesions are located primarily on sun-exposed areas (SLE can occur on sun-exposed and sun-protected areas). Note that previous studies have shown that up to 19% of patients with PMLE can be ANA positive. Hence, an ANA alone may not be sufficient in differentiating PMLE from SLE.
- Phototoxic/photoallergic drug eruptions
- CREST syndrome—can have overlap with dermatomyositis; refers to a subset of patients with limited scleroderma
- Seborrheic dermatitis—no systemic findings; erythema and scale in sebaceous distribution
- Contact dermatitis
- Pityriasis rubra pilaris
- Sarcoidosis
- Scleroderma—Check for anticentromere antibodies and anti-Scl-70 antibodies; typified by sclerotic changes in skin not seen in dermatomyositis.
- Graft versus host disease—occurs after allogeneic stem-cell transplantation
- Mixed connective tissue disease—Check for anti-U1RNP antibody. Most patients are positive for this in mixed connective tissue disease.

- Generalized morphea—asymmetric induration, no Raynaud phenomenon, no systemic involvement
- Polymyositis—without cutaneous findings
- Acute lesions of erythropoietic protoporphyria may have similar locations, especially on the dorsum of the hands, but usually there is no weakness.
- Tinea faciei—Check KOH; will also be ANA negative.

Pediatric Patient Considerations

Same differential diagnosis as for adults except it does not include rosacea, sarcoidosis, or mixed connective tissue disease.

 Best Tests

- Diagnosis is made on clinical and serologic grounds, using the American Rheumatologic Association (ARA) criteria for diagnosis.
- ARA criteria—meet at least four of the following: malar rash, discoid rash, photosensitivity, oral ulcers, arthritis, serositis, renal disorder, neurologic disorder, hematologic disorder, immunologic disorder, and presence of ANA.
- ANA and anti-DNA antibodies are found in a majority of patients.
- Skin biopsy can be diagnostic for lupus, as well as biopsy of uninvolved skin for direct immunofluorescence (DIF—lupus band test). DIF can be very useful when conventional histopathology is not discerning and will demonstrate granular deposition of IgG, IgA, or IgM at the dermal-epidermal junction.
- Check BUN/creatinine (Cr), urinalysis, liver function tests, and serum complement (CH50). Slight elevations in partial thromboplastin time (PTT) and PT might suggest the presence of the lupus anticoagulant. Patients with the lupus anticoagulant are at higher risk for stroke and thrombosis.

Pediatric Patient Considerations

If SLE is suspected, a complete workup should be initiated to include ANA, anti-dsDNA, anti-SSA, anti-SSB, anti-RNP, and anti-Smith antibodies. Diagnosis is made on clinical and serologic grounds, using the ARA criteria for diagnosis. These criteria were revised in 1997. Skin biopsy can be diagnostic for lupus, and biopsy of uninvolved skin for DIF. Check BUN/Cr, urinalysis, liver function tests, and serum complement (CH50). Slight elevations in PTT and PT might suggest the presence of the lupus anticoagulant.

▲▲ Management Pearls

- Consultation with multiple specialists is mandatory for patients with SLE.
- The patient should avoid sunlight (especially at noon and at high altitudes), photosensitive drugs, and exogenous estrogens.

Pediatric Patient Considerations

A multidisciplinary approach is best. Patients should see a pediatric rheumatologist, ophthalmologist, and dermatologist. Prompt diagnosis is important so that early treatment can be initiated.

Therapy

Treatment should be commensurate with the severity of the disease.

Antimalarials
- Hydroxychloroquine: 200 to 400 mg p.o. daily
- Chloroquine: 125 to 250 mg p.o. daily

Glucocorticoids
- Prednisone: 5 to 60 mg p.o. daily or divided two to four times daily; taper over 2 weeks

Immunosuppressives
- Cyclophosphamide: 10 to 20 mg/kg IV every 3 to 4 weeks or 1.5 to 2.5 mg/kg p.o. daily
- Azathioprine: 1.5 to 3 mg/kg p.o. daily, maintenance dose of 1 to 2 mg/kg/d
- Mycophenolate mofetil: 500 mg p.o. twice daily, increase over several weeks to 1,500 mg p.o. twice daily

Arthritis, arthralgias, and myalgias can be managed with nonacetylated salicylates (choline magnesium trisalicylate 500 mg to 1.5 g p.o. two to three times daily) and nonsteroidal anti-inflammatory drugs (NSAIDs) (ibuprofen 400 to 600 mg p.o. every 4 to 6 hours, as needed)

Pediatric Patient Considerations

Oral corticosteroids are the mainstay of treatment. Steroid-sparing agents such as antimalarials, azathioprine, cyclophosphamide, cyclosporine, and mycophenolate mofetil are also used frequently. Anti-B-cell therapy with rituximab has also been successful. Interferon and anti-TNF therapies may also be considered.

Topically, all patients should use sunscreen daily that provides both UVA and UVB blockage. High-potency topical corticosteroids can be used for localized areas of involvement.

Suggested Readings

Cooper GS, Parks CG, Treadwell EL, et al. Differences by race, sex, and age in the clinical and immunologic features of recently diagnosed systemic lupus erythematosus patients in the southeastern United States. *Lupus.* 2002;11:161–167.

Halder RM, Roberts CI, Nootheti PK. Cutaneous diseases in black races. *Dermatol Clin.* 2003;21:679–687.

James WD, Berger TG, Elston DM, eds. Cutaneous vascular diseases. In: *Andrews' Diseases of the Skin Clinical Dermatology.* 10th Ed. Philadelphia, PA: Elsevier; 2006:816–817.

Lau CS, Yin G, Mok MY. Ethnic and geographical differences in systemic lupus erythematosus: An overview. *Lupus.* 2006;15:715–719.

Lee LA. Lupus erythematosus. In: Bolognia JL, Jorizzo JL, Rapini RP, eds. *Dermatology.* 1st Ed. Philadelphia, PA: Elsevier; 2003:601–613.

Alarcón GS, McGwin G Jr, Bartolucci AA, et al. LUMINA Study Group. Systemic lupus erythematosus in three ethnic groups. IX. Differences in damage accrual. *Arthritis Rheum.* 2001;44(12):2797–2806.

Disseminated Purpuras

Sabrina Newman

This is a group of disorders with similar, but not identical, pathophysiologies and often similar clinical presentations. They are all serious, potentially life-threatening conditions and must be approached with urgency. Often, these patients benefit from timely specialized consultations. Acute meningococcemia and purpura fulminans are discussed here. For discussions on disseminated intravascular coagulation (DIC) and gonococcemia, see VisualDx online. (If you are a first-time online user, go to www.essentialdermatology.com/pigmented; if you already have your password set up, go directly to www.visualdx.com/visualdx.)

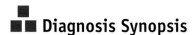 Diagnosis Synopsis

Acute Meningococcemia

Infection with the Gram-negative bacterium *Neisseria meningitidis* is responsible for acute meningococcemia, a severe illness that typically occurs in small epidemics, commonly in military camps or college dormitories. It is transmitted from person to person by respiratory droplets.

Infection begins as a nonspecific viral-like illness that rapidly evolves (within hours) into one of two main presentations: meningitis or septicemia. Most cases are acquired through exposure to asymptomatic carriers. Headache, nausea, vomiting, and myalgias are quickly followed by obtundation and a septic-appearing patient. Altered consciousness and seizures can occur. In asplenic patients, fulminant meningococcemia can occur in hours with sepsis, hypotension, shock, and death. Chronic meningococcemia, often associated with terminal complement deficiencies, is characterized by persistent low fever, rash, and arthralgias and is commonly mistaken for gonococcemia.

Purpura Fulminans

Purpura fulminans is a severe, often fatal condition of intravascular thrombosis and hemorrhagic infection that usually follows a bacterial infection, commonly *N. meningitidis*, resulting in DIC and skin necrosis. Though primarily seen in children, purpura fulminans can occur in patients of all ages. It is also associated with infection with pneumococci, the varicella zoster virus (VZV), the measles virus, staphylococci, and Group A beta-hemolytic streptococci. Acquired deficiencies of proteins C and S may contribute to the pathogenesis. Acute illness is manifest by a septic-appearing patient with high fever and rapid deterioration leading to hypotension and shock. There is progression from acral purpura to widespread ecchymoses and gangrene.

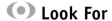 Look For

Acute Meningococcemia

The very early rash is reported to resemble a viral exanthem with erythematous macules and papules, but in most cases, patients present with a petechiae eruption on the trunk and the distal extremities. This may go unnoticed in dark skin. Evaluate areas of lighter pigment such as the palms and nail beds to identify petechiae. Ecchymoses, vesicles, and bullae with central infarcts quickly follow (Figs. 4-28–4-30). In severe cases, the infection will also affect the mucosa of the mouth or the conjunctiva. The petechiae of meningococcemia typically have gray or dusky centers and are slightly vesicular in appearance. Digits and limbs may become gangrenous with well-demarcated gun-metal-gray discoloration. At this stage, patients will have significant central nervous system (CNS) abnormalities and signs of severe sepsis.

Neonatal/Infant Patient Considerations

The typical order of symptoms and signs in meningococcal disease is fever, symptomatic sepsis, then skin involvement, and CNS signs.

Early meningococcal disease usually presents as an acutely febrile child with a viral-like illness (vomiting, malaise, lethargy). Within hours, however, infants will develop signs of septicemia or meningitis.

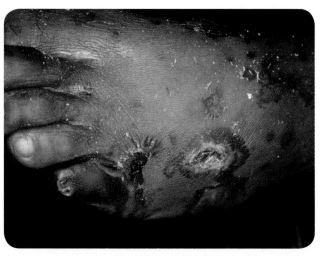

Figure 4-28 Acute meningococcemia with purpura and gangrene.

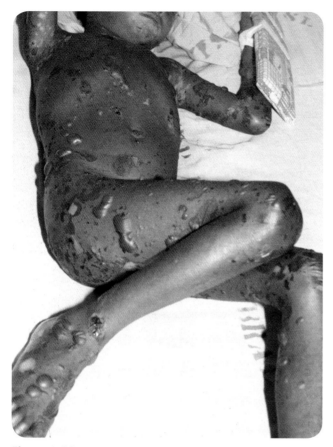

Figure 4-29 Acute meningococcemia with purpura and bullae.

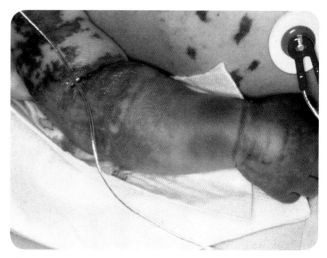

Figure 4-31 Purpura fulminans with disseminated meningococcemia.

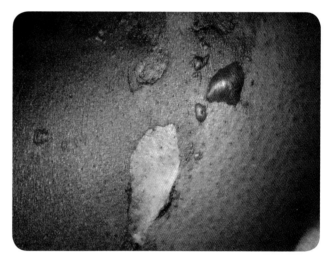

Figure 4-32 Purpura fulminans with vesiculation from meningococcemia.

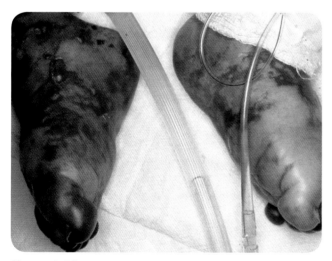

Figure 4-30 Gangrene and skin thrombosis secondary to acute meningococcemia.

moses; however, they evolve rapidly into painful, indurated, well-demarcated, irregularly bordered purpuric papules and plaques that are surrounded by a thin, advancing erythematous border. These areas often then form necrotic areas with vesicles and bullae and, finally, firm eschars that ultimately slough. Purpura and infarctions can involve acral areas and digits. Gangrene and autoamputation can develop.

●● Diagnostic Pearls

Acute Meningococcemia

- Fever and a petechial rash are meningococcal disease until proven otherwise, and treatment is warranted without positive diagnostic testing.

Purpura Fulminans

Sharply demarcated ecchymoses, purpura, and necrosis symmetrically involving the extremities (Figs. 4-31 and 4-32). Sites of involvement may initially appear like ecchy-

- Larger lesions will have complex arcuate and geographic or maplelike borders. Purpura can be subtle on dark skin; be sure to look in the oral mucosa and conjunctiva for petechiae and purpura. Also, evaluate palms, soles, and nail beds where the skin is not as dark.
- Meningococcal disease is less likely if illness lasts longer than 24 hours without progressing.

Purpura Fulminans

- The purpura from Coumadin (warfarin) is more prominent on fatty areas such as breasts, buttocks, and thighs, while purpura fulminans is more extensive.
- Lesions often rapidly progress to purpuric bullae.
- Head, neck, and mucous membrane involvement are uncommon.

?? Differential Diagnosis and Pitfalls

Infection:

- Bacteremia or meningitis (*Streptococcus pneumoniae*, *Haemophilus influenzae* Type b, *Staphylococcus aureus*, group A streptococcus, other Gram-negative cocci or bacilli)
- Viral illness (i.e., hemorrhagic fever group, disseminated herpes simplex virus, VZV, cytomegalovirus, echovirus, coxsackievirus)
- Rickettsiae (Rocky Mountain spotted fever, ehrlichiosis, epidemic typhus)
- Disseminated fungal infection
- Leptospirosis

Vasculitis:

- Henoch-Schönlein purpura
- Acute hemorrhagic edema of infancy
- Kawasaki disease
- Hypersensitivity vasculitis
- Calciphylaxis

Toxin/drug:

- Toxic shock syndrome
- Heparin necrosis

Hematologic diseases

- Hemolytic-uremic syndrome
- Idiopathic thrombocytopenic purpura
- Protein C or S deficiency
- Coumadin necrosis

Physical:

- Petechiae caused by coughing, vomiting, or crying
- Trauma

- Over anticoagulation with heparin or Coumadin
- Bleeding into hemangiomas
- Trauma

✓ Best Tests

Acute Meningococcemia

- Meningococcal disease should be confirmed by isolation of *N. meningitidis* from normally sterile sites (i.e., blood and CSF Gram stain and cultures).
- Meningococcal PCR should also be obtained from whole blood (EDTA specimen) and CSF to increase the sensitivity and specificity and allow rapid diagnosis.
- Histology of skin lesions will show leukocytoclastic vasculitis with hemorrhage and vascular thromboses. Diplococci may be seen in Gram-stained sections.
- Sensitivities should be obtained for all meningococcal isolates.

Neonatal/Infant Patient Considerations

All infants with suspected invasive bacterial infection should have blood drawn for electrolytes, full blood count, aspartate aminotransferase, alanine aminotransferase, coagulation studies (prothrombin time [PT], partial thromboplastin time [PTT], international normalized ratio (INR), fibrin degradation products), arterial blood gas, and blood cultures. Meningococcal disease should be confirmed by isolation of *N. meningitidis* from normally sterile sites (i.e., blood and CSF Gram stain and cultures).

In untreated patients, blood cultures are positive in up to half of patients, and CSF cultures are positive in up to 80% of infants with meningitis. Therefore, meningococcal PCR should also be obtained from whole blood (EDTA specimen) and CSF (if a lumbar puncture is performed) to increase the sensitivity and specificity (>90%) and allow rapid diagnosis (within 4 to 8 hours) of meningococcal disease.

Purpura Fulminans

- Blood cultures
- Gram stain and culture of skin lesions—scrapings, biopsy, or aspirate
- Consider lumbar puncture with Gram stain and culture of CSF.
- Consider throat culture.

- DIC panel (platelet count, PT, fibrinogen, fibrin split products, etc.) and routine blood work—CBC, chemistries
- Hemodynamic monitoring
- MRI may help elucidate the extent of soft tissue involvement.

▲▲ Management Pearls

Acute Meningococcemia

- *If you are thinking of this diagnosis, do not wait for the results of confirmatory tests to initiate therapy, as this can be a life-threatening illness. All children with a petechial eruption and signs of sepsis should be admitted and treated for meningococcal disease without delay.*
- Household contacts should receive prophylactic rifampin, ceftriaxone, or ciprofloxacin (contraindicated in children younger than 2 years and in pregnancy) within 24 hours of diagnosis of the primary case.

Precautions: Standard, droplet. (Isolate patient, wear a mask, and limit patient transport.)

Neonatal/Infant Patient Considerations

- All infants with a nonblanching eruption (purpura) and signs of sepsis should be admitted and treated for meningococcal disease without delay.
- Since early meningococcal disease often presents as a nonspecific febrile illness, if an infant is not hospitalized, parents should be encouraged to seek immediate medical help again if the infant's condition deteriorates or develops a nonblanching eruption.
- Infants with high suspicion for meningococcal disease should be sent to the hospital as soon as possible (often by ambulance).

Purpura Fulminans

The clinical picture should suggest the diagnosis and necessitates immediate implementation of antibiotic and supportive therapy in an intensive care setting. Patients will often require ventilatory and inotropic support in addition to aggressive fluid resuscitation and hemodynamic monitoring. Surgery is frequently needed to débride or amputate devitalized tissue. Several studies have reported that protein C replacement therapy is associated with reduction in mortality and morbidity in patients with purpura fulminans.

Therapy

(See VisualDx online for further details on managing these diseases.)

Acute Meningococcemia

Blood cultures should be taken at the time of intravenous cannula insertion, before giving antibiotics, if possible. However, treatment should not be delayed in order to obtain cultures.

Adults

Intravenous penicillin G is the drug of choice for susceptible isolates:

- 300,000 U/kg IV daily divided every 4 hours. Many adult patients are begun at a dose of 4 million units IV every 4 hours. Continue administration for 5 to 7 additional days after the patient's temperature has returned to normal.

Intravenous chloramphenicol should be used in patients highly allergic to penicillin:

- 1 g IV every 6 hours. Administer for 5 to 7 additional days after the patient's temperature has returned to normal.

Third-generation cephalosporins (cefotaxime, ceftriaxone) may be used as a third alternative and may be considered for initial therapy in areas of the world with penicillin-resistant strains (e.g., the United Kingdom and Spain) or in septic patients while the diagnosis is being confirmed.

- Cefotaxime 2 g IV every 4 hours
- Ceftriaxone 2 g IV/IM every 12 hours
- Administer for 5 to 7 additional days after the patient's temperature has returned to normal.

Prevention: There are vaccines available.

Neonates/Infants and Children

Intravenous benzylpenicillin 300 mg, cefotaxime 50 mg/kg, or ceftriaxone 80 mg/kg should be administered immediately to all suspected cases of meningococcal disease unless there is a history of anaphylaxis to penicillin. If the etiology of sepsis or meningitis is unknown at admission (usual scenario), ceftriaxone or cefotaxime should be given for the first 24 to 48 hours. Chloramphenicol should be administered to those with a history of anaphylaxis to penicillin or cephalosporins.

Purpura Fulminans

Empiric antibiotic coverage should be instituted immediately and directed at the most likely pathogens. For meningococcus,

(Continued)

high-dose penicillin G is the treatment of choice, with chloramphenicol reserved for penicillin-allergic patients:

- Penicillin G 2 to 4 million units every 4 to 6 hours IV
- Chloramphenicol 100 mg/kg/d IV divided every 6 hours

Alternatives include:
- Ceftriaxone 2 g IV every 12 hours initially
- Cefotaxime 2 g IV every 6 hours

Antibiotic therapy should be adjusted once the pathogen and its sensitivities are known.

Patients may benefit from heparin 10 U/kg/h continuous IV infusion. Monitor PTT every 6 hours.

Repletion of proteins C and S with fresh frozen plasma may be important adjunctive therapy in patients with purpura fulminans.

Consider meningococcal vaccination in high-risk patients (college students living in dormitories, military recruits living in barracks, etc.). Chemoprophylaxis for the close contacts of an individual with a meningococcal infection may be with rifampin, ciprofloxacin, ceftriaxone, or azithromycin:

- Rifampin—<1 month of age, 5 mg/kg p.o. every 12 hours for 2 days; >1 month of age, 10 mg/kg p.o. every 12 hours for 2 days; adults, 600 mg p.o. every 12 hours for 2 days
- Ciprofloxacin—adults only, 750 mg p.o. single dose
- Ceftriaxone—younger than 15 years of age, 125 mg IM single dose; adults, 250 mg IM single dose
- Azithromycin—adults, 500 mg p.o. single dose

Pediatric Patient Considerations

Vigorous antibiotic therapy for underlying infection. Heparin can be considered with signs of DIC.

Suggested Readings

Da Ros CT, Schmitt Cda S. Global epidemiology of sexually transmitted diseases. *Asian J Androl.* 2008;10(1):110–114.

Department of Health and Human Services, Centers for Disease Control and Prevention. STD Surveillance 2006: Trends in Reportable Sexually Transmitted Diseases in the United States, National Surveillance Data for Chlamydia, Gonorrhea, and Syphilis.

Hassan Z, Mullins RF, Friedman BC, et al. Purpura fulminans: A case series managed at a regional burn center. *J Burn Care Res.* 2008;29:411–415.

Rosenstein NE, Perkins BA, Stephens DS, et al. Meningococcal disease. *NEJM.* 2001;344:1378–1388.

Taylor FB Jr, Toh CH, Hoots WK, et al. for the Scientific Subcommittee on Disseminated Intravascular Coagulation (DIC) of the ISTH. Towards definition, clinical and laboratory criteria, and a scoring system for disseminated intravascular coagulation. *Thromb Haemost.* 2001;86(5): 1327–1330.

Yung AP, McDonald MI. Early clinical clues to meningococcaemia. *Med J Aust.* 2003;178:134–137.

Erysipelas

Mat Davey

■■ Diagnosis Synopsis

Erysipelas, a bacterial infection of the skin and superficial dermal lymphatics, is caused primarily by group A streptococci (*Streptococcus pyogenes*). It usually occurs in isolation and has a predilection for the extremes of age, debilitated patients, and patients with poor lymphatic drainage. Historically, erysipelas occurred on the face, but at the present time, this infection is more commonly seen on the lower extremities of patients with venous insufficiency and stasis dermatitis. Penile erysipelas starts with erythema, itching, and tingling, followed by swelling and pain. It often results in progressive, chronic lymphedema with permanent swelling of the penis (elephantiasis). Elephantiasis may also develop in the lower extremities from recurring bouts of erysipelas.

As opposed to impetigo, in cellulitis and erysipelas, systemic symptoms of fevers, chills, and malaise often precede or coincide with the appearance of the skin lesions. Complications are not common but can include glomerulonephritis, lymphadenitis, and subacute bacterial endocarditis. If left untreated, both cellulitis and erysipelas can be complicated by bacteremia and death.

Of note, a rising prevalence of community-acquired methicillin-resistant *Staphylococcus aureus* (CA-MRSA) has increasingly been identified as a pathogen of skin and soft tissue infections in otherwise healthy individuals lacking the traditional risk factors for such infections (IV drug use, incarceration, participation in contact sports, etc.). Antibiotic coverage must take into account the risk of MRSA. It is helpful to be aware of patterns of antimicrobial resistance within your local community.

◉ Look For

In erysipelas, look for sharply demarcated, bright red plaques with warmth and tenderness. Borders are elevated, and central clearing may be present. Overlying bullae, vesicles, and purpura (bleeding into the skin) within the lesions can occur (Fig. 4-33). Lymphangitic streaking and regional lymphadenopathy are usually seen. Penile erysipelas may spread to the pubic area. Erysipelas may involve the scrotum and be limited to it.

●● Diagnostic Pearls

Erysipelas is differentiated from angioedema or contact dermatitis of the face by the presence of pain, fever, and an elevated leukocyte count. If infection appears to involve the eyelids and there are signs of proptosis and/or ophthalmoplegia, consider orbital cellulitis rather than erysipelas. Conduct

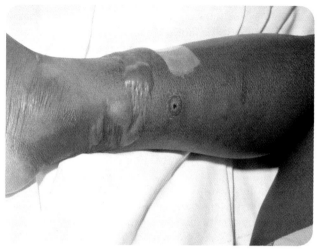

Figure 4-33 The distinction between erysipelas and cellulitis may be difficult to make when there is not a raised border, as in this lesion.

a prompt ophthalmologic exam; orbital cellulitis can lead to vision loss, cavernous sinus thrombosis, abscess formation, and meningitis.

?? Differential Diagnosis and Pitfalls

Impetigo/Cellulitis/Erysipelas

- Stasis dermatitis
- Erythema nodosum (panniculitis)
- Erysipeloid
- Lipodermatosclerosis
- Thrombophlebitis
- Contact dermatitis
- Necrotizing fasciitis
- Deep vein thrombosis
- Herpes zoster
- Erythema chronicum migrans (Lyme disease)
- Vasculitis—polyarteritis nodosa
- Inflammatory carcinoma of the breast
- Eosinophilic cellulitis (Wells syndrome)
- Urticaria
- Sweet syndrome

✓ Best Tests

- Diagnosis is most often made clinically. Mark the leading edge of erythema in patients with cellulitis or erysipelas with pen or marker, and check every 4 to 6 hours. If progressive after 24 hours of therapy, consider more aggressive therapy or other etiologies. Surgical consultation is recommended if necrotizing fasciitis is a possibility. MRI can be performed to evaluate deeper tissue involvement.

- Wound cultures for bacterial identification and antibiotic susceptibility should be obtained. Sensitivities should be performed on any *S. aureus* isolates to determine antibiotic resistance. Consider oropharyngeal, nasal, and conjunctival cultures if there is facial involvement. If diagnosis is in doubt, biopsy can be performed and sent for Gram stain and tissue culture.
- A CBC may show normal or elevated white blood cells. Blood cultures are of very little utility in patients lacking signs of systemic toxicity (tachycardia, hypotension).

▲▲▲ Management Pearls

Given the prevalence of MRSA, maintain a high index of suspicion for this diagnosis and make the initial choice of empiric antibiotic therapy accordingly. It is helpful to be aware of patterns of antimicrobial resistance within your community. In patients with recurrent MRSA infections, eradication of MRSA nasal carriage may be accomplished by application of mupirocin 2% cream (twice daily for 5 days) to the nares. The combination of rifampin (600 mg daily for 10 days) plus TMP-SMX (1 double-strength tab twice daily for 10 days) has also been shown to eradicate colonization.

Therapy

Most of these infections are caused by *S. aureus* or *S. pyogenes*, so the same antibiotic regimen may be used for impetigo, cellulitis, and erysipelas:

- Dicloxacillin 250 to 500 mg p.o. every 6 hours
- Amoxicillin plus clavulanic acid 250 to 500 mg p.o. every 6 hours
- Cephalexin 250 to 500 mg p.o. every 6 hours

- Azithromycin 500 mg p.o. one time, then 250 mg p.o. daily (used for patients with penicillin allergy)

Mild cases can be monitored and treated on an outpatient basis.

Penile erysipelas also requires treatment with steroids (prednisone) to prevent chronic lymphedema and subsequent elephantiasis.

Consider daily prophylaxis with penicillin in patients with multiple recurrent bouts of erysipelas who have poor lymphatic drainage.

Pediatric Patient Considerations

Mild cases can be monitored and treated on an outpatient basis with a 7- to 10-day course of antibiotics covering *S. aureus* or *S. pyogenes*.

Suggested Readings

Bernard P. Management of common bacterial infections in the skin. *Curr Opin Infect Dis.* 2008;21(2):122–128.

Craft NC, Lee PK, Zipoli, MT, et al. Superficial cutaneous infections and pyodermas. In: Fitzpatrick TB, Wolff K, eds. *Fitzpatrick's Dermatology in General Medicine.* 7th Ed. New York, NY: McGraw-Hill; 2008:1694–1703.

Elston DM. Community-acquired methicillin-resistant Staphylococcus aureus. *J Am Acad Dermatol.* 2007;56(1):1–16; quiz 17–20.

James WD, Berger TG, Elston DM, eds. *Andrews' Diseases of the Skin: Clinical Dermatology.* 10th Ed. Philadelphia, PA: Saunders Elsevier; 2006:251–264.

Stevens DL, Bisno AL, Chambers HF, et al. Infectious Diseases Society of America. Practice guidelines for the diagnosis and management of skin and soft-tissue infections. *Clin Infect Dis.* 2005;41(10):1373–1406.

Ecthyma Gangrenosum

Mat Davey

 Diagnosis Synopsis

Less commonly, pyogenic bacterial infections are caused by anaerobic and/or Gram-negative bacteria. Ecthyma gangrenosum (EG) is a cutaneous manifestation of *Pseudomonas aeruginosa* bacteremia, which typically develops in patients with underlying immunosuppression. Clinical manifestations mimic abscesses; however, most patients are systemically ill with associated fever, chills, and hypotension.

 Look For

Initial lesions of EG are painless and present as erythematous or purpuric macules. Within 12 to 24 hours, abscesses, vesicles, or bullae develop (Fig. 4-34). Lesions often rupture, leaving a gangrenous ulcer with a central black eschar.

 Diagnostic Pearls

Pseudomonas sepsis commonly occurs after surgical procedures, especially urologic procedures. Patients present with fever a few days prior to lesion development.

?? Differential Diagnosis and Pitfalls

Infectious:
- Cellulitis or erysipelas
- Cat scratch disease
- Atypical mycobacterial infections (*Mycobacterium marinum*)

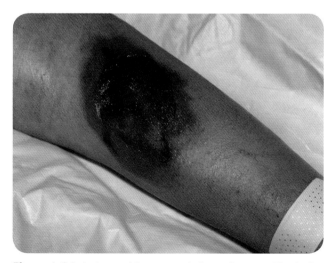

Figure 4-34 A plaque with purpura, dusky erythema, and beginning erosions is typical of the early stages of ecthyma gangrenosum. Later stages may have a tightly adherent hemorrhagic crust.

- Deep fungal infection
- Herpetic whitlow

Noninfectious:
- Ruptured subcutaneous cyst
- Gout
- Large dermal nodules of lymphoma/pseudolymphoma may mimic abscesses
- Eosinophilic cellulitis

 Best Tests

- The diagnosis is usually suggested by the rapid course and systemic toxicity. Needle or incisional aspiration of purulent material allows for rapid diagnosis and specific therapy.
- Gram and fungal stains of exudate or aspirate may yield immediate microbiologic diagnosis. Cultures take a few days (bacterial) to weeks (fungal) to yield results.
- Sensitivities on all cultures should be performed to determine antibiotic resistance.

▲▲ Management Pearls

Pseudomonal sepsis occurs frequently after surgical procedures, especially urologic procedures. Chronic indwelling urinary catheters and long-term intravenous catheters have also been associated with EG. Prolonged use of antibiotic therapy targeting nonpseudomonal organisms may promote overgrowth of *P. aeruginosa*.

Therapy

In patients with known or suggestive EG and/or systemically ill patients with atypical bacterial isolates, inpatient empiric IV antibiotics and supportive care must be pursued.

Initial treatment should be with an aminoglycoside (tobramycin, gentamicin, or amikacin) combined with an antipseudomonal penicillin (carbenicillin, piperacillin, or ticarcillin), a cephalosporin (ceftazidime or cefepime), or carbapenem (meropenem).

Granulocyte-macrophage colony-stimulating factor may adjunctively be used in neutropenic patients and those with myeloid dysplasia.

- Ceftazidime—2 g IV every 8 hours
- Cefepime—2 g IV every 12 hours

(Continued)

- Ticarcillin—3 g IV every 4 hours
- Piperacillin—4 g IV every 4 hours
- Gentamicin and tobramycin—3 to 5 mg/kg in two to three divided doses daily
- Amikacin—7.5 mg/kg IV every 12 hours
- Meropenem—0.5 g every 8 hours or imipenem 0.5 g every 6 hours

For patients with beta-lactam allergies:

- Aztreonam—1.5 g every 6 hours
- Piperacillin-tazobactam—3.375 g every 4 hours

Suggested Readings

Craft NC, Lee PK, Zipoli MT, et al. Superficial cutaneous infections and pyodermas. In: Fitzpatrick TB, Wolff K, eds. *Fitzpatrick's Dermatology in General Medicine*. 7th Ed. New York, NY: McGraw-Hill; 2008:1694–1703.

James WD, Berger TG, Elston DM, eds. *Andrews' Diseases of the Skin: Clinical Dermatology*. 10th Ed. Philadelphia, PA: Saunders Elsevier; 2006:251–264.

Toxic Shock Syndrome

Laurie Good

■■ Diagnosis Synopsis

Toxic shock syndrome (TSS) is a severe exotoxin-mediated bacterial infection that is characterized by high fevers, headache, pharyngitis, vomiting, diarrhea, and hypotension. Two subtypes of TSS exist, based on the bacterial etiology: *Staphylococcus aureus* and group A streptococci. Significantly, the severity of TSS can range from mild disease to rapid progression to shock and end-organ failure. The dermatologic manifestations of TSS include the following:

- Erythema of the palms and soles that desquamates 1 to 3 weeks after the initial onset
- Diffuse scarlatiniform exanthem that begins on the trunk and spreads toward the extremities
- Erythema of the mucous membranes (strawberry tongue and conjunctival hyperemia)

TSS was identified in and most commonly affected menstruating young white women using tampons in the 1980s. Current TSS cases are seen in postsurgical interventions in men, women, and children, as well as in other settings, in addition to cases of menstrual TSS, which have declined with increased public education on tampon usage and TSS. One study in Japanese patients found the highest TSS incidence to occur among children with burns, as staphylococcus colonization is high in this subgroup and antibody titers are not yet sufficient to protect children from the exotoxins causing TSS.

Staphylococcal TSS is caused by *S. aureus* strains that can produce the toxic shock syndrome toxin-1 (TSST-1). TSST-1 is believed to cause disease via direct effects on end organs, impairing clearance of gut flora–derived endotoxins, with TSST-1 acting as a superantigen leading to massive nonspecific activation of T cells and subsequent inflammation and vascular leakage. In this form of TSS, risk factors include lack of an antibody to TSST-1, surgical packing, abscesses, surgical mesh, and tampon use. A late 1980s study showed a lower rate of tampon usage among African American and Mexican American women compared to white women, and while this may help explain the lower incidence of TSS in African American women, the authors did not believe that the findings were sufficient to explain the discrepancy entirely. They hypothesized that perhaps the erythema of TSS is more difficult to see on darker-pigmented skin, thus resulting in clinicians failing to recognize or report TSS because they failed to recognize one of the criteria for diagnosis.

Streptococcal TSS is also caused by exotoxins that cause massive stimulation of T cells via a superantigen mechanism. Clinically, the most common presenting symptom is severe pain in an extremity with or without underlying soft tissue infection. A prodrome of fever, diarrhea, and myalgias is often seen. The macular exanthem seen in staphylococcal TSS is much less commonly found in streptococcal TSS.

Approximately 48 to 72 hours after the initial onset, shock and multiorgan failure follow. In this form of TSS, risk factors include varicella infection, bites, and lacerations.

Epidemiological studies from 2000 to 2004 in the United States show that the incidence of invasive group A streptococcus infections, such as streptococcal TSS, is higher among African Americans than other groups. The case fatality rate, however, was not different between groups.

Interestingly, there is an emerging pathogen, *Streptococcus suis*, which can be transmitted from pigs to humans and has been responsible for several large outbreaks of disease, including TSS, in Asia, specifically Thailand and China. The consumption of raw or undercooked pork is the number one risk factor. In one Thai study, 23% of patients with positive cultures developed TSS, and the mortality rate from infection with certain serotypes of *S. suis* has proven to be exceptionally high. Thus, this new pathogen has been the cause of great concern worldwide.

All forms of TSS can result in confusion and coma, renal impairment, liver impairment, adult respiratory distress syndrome, and disseminated intravascular coagulation. Supportive measures (intravenous fluids, vasopressors, etc.) and appropriate antibiotics are the mainstays of treatment.

Pediatric Patient Considerations

Children are most susceptible to TSS between the ages of 6 months and 2 years. Before 6 months, the mother's antibodies are protective, and after age 2, the child begins producing antibody titers in higher amounts. Beyond age 41, antibodies against TSST-1 are at their highest levels.

Closed environment (hospital, school, military, familial) outbreaks of TSS have occurred, and an outbreak of group A streptococcal TSS was reported in a day care in Spain that led to one child's death and several hospitalizations.

TSS mortality rates are much lower in children than adults at 5% to 10% and 3% to 5%, respectively, for streptococcal versus staphylococcal types.

Immunocompromised Patient Considerations

Although infections with *S. aureus* are common in HIV-infected people, the complication of TSS is rare. This is thought to be related to the immune deficits and T-helper cell dysfunction in HIV-positive people. However, in cases that have been reported, they tend to present with a recurrent and prolonged disease course. Attributed to delayed antibody production against TSST-1 by HIV-positive individuals, a protracted disease course has been reported in HIV-positive teens, adults, and children.

Look For

Early diffuse, macular, or scarlatiniform exanthem. Exanthem may initially appear over the trunk but always spreads to the arms and legs. Also look for palms and soles with erythema and edema, intense erythema of the mucous membranes, and, 1 to 2 weeks after onset of illness, diffuse desquamation with sheetlike peeling (Fig. 4-35). Patchy alopecia (reversible) and fingernail shedding have been described.

Note: The exanthema in these areas—flexural areas, palms, and mucous membranes—may be more appreciable on deeply pigmented skin.

Staphylococcal TSS

- Diffuse macular erythroderma
- Desquamation of palms/soles 1 to 3 weeks after onset of symptoms
- High-grade fever
- Hypotension
- Multiorgan involvement

Streptococcal TSS

- Severe localized pain in an extremity
- Prodromal symptoms
- Desquamation of palms/soles 1 to 3 weeks after onset of symptoms
- Hypotension within 48 to 72 hours of initial onset of symptoms
- Multiorgan involvement

Note that there are significant differences between staphylococcal and streptococcal TSS. They are as follows:

- Diffuse macular erythroderma is commonly seen in staphylococcal but not in streptococcal TSS.
- Soft tissue infections are rare in staphylococcal TSS but common in streptococcal TSS.

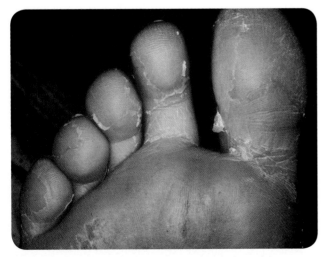

Figure 4-35 Desquamation of the foot after toxic shock.

- Positive blood cultures are seen in <15% of staphylococcal TSS cases but in over 50% of streptococcal TSS.
- Mortality rates are approximately 3% in staphylococcal TSS and 30% to 60% in streptococcal TSS.

Group A streptococci can be isolated from blood, CSF, tissue biopsy, surgical wound, sputum, throat, vagina, and superficial skin lesion.

Diagnostic Pearls

The early exanthem is flexurally accentuated. The underlying infection can be limited and minor in appearance.

Differential Diagnosis and Pitfalls

The CDC diagnostic criteria for TSS are as follows:

- Fever, hypotension, and characteristic rash
- Involvement of three or more organ systems

No serologic evidence of the following: Rocky Mountain spotted fever, measles, leptospirosis, syphilis, Epstein-Barr virus, hepatitis B, or antinuclear antibodies

The differential for TSS includes the following:

- Staphylococcal scalded skin syndrome
- Scarlet fever—1-mm erythematous papules, always elevated WBC with left shift, eosinophilia in up to 20% of patients
- Necrotizing fasciitis—violaceous hue, bullae or necrosis, and severe localized pain
- Drug eruption
- Stevens-Johnson syndrome—drug induced, high fevers, skin tenderness, mucosal erosions, and skin detachment about 1 to 3 weeks after the inciting medication is started
- Toxic epidermal necrolysis—drug induced, high fevers, skin tenderness, mucosal erosions, and skin detachment about 1 to 3 weeks after the inciting medication is started
- Kawasaki disease—fever lasting for more than 5 days with oral mucosal changes, conjunctival injection, and cervical lymphadenopathy
- Meningococcemia—rapid decompensation, characteristic petechial eruption caused by *Neisseria meningitidis*
- Rocky Mountain spotted fever—characteristic retiform purpura; check for serologies

Best Tests

The clinical picture and exam are more important than any test and should prompt initiation of therapy as soon as possible. The following tests and findings support the diagnosis:

- Blood cultures
- Culture of any potentially infected site (e.g., skin lesions, throat)

- CBC—leukocytosis, occasionally thrombocytopenia and/or anemia
- Electrolyte abnormalities, including azotemia
- Liver function tests—Often bilirubin and/or transaminases will be elevated.
- Coagulation studies— Partial thromboplastin time (PTT) and fibrin split products may be elevated.
- Arterial blood gas—metabolic acidosis
- Creatine kinase may be increased.
- Urinalysis may be abnormal, with myoglobulin or casts.
- Serologic testing as mentioned in "Differential Diagnosis and Pitfalls" may be performed to rule out other causes of the clinical findings.

Depending on the clinical scenario, further testing will be needed to investigate or monitor possible complications and may include the following:

- Electrocardiograph/continuous cardiac monitoring
- Invasive hemodynamic monitoring
- Chest radiographs
- Echocardiogram
- Plain films, CT, or MRI of any suspected site of infection
- Lumbar puncture

▲▲▲ Management Pearls

- Excellent supportive care in a tertiary medical center (if possible) is necessary for a successful outcome.

Precautions: Standard and contact (Isolate patient, wear gloves and a gown, limit patient transport, and avoid sharing patient-care equipment.)

Therapy

Immediate intervention for shock and systemic antistaphylococcal/streptococcal antibiotics is essential. Aggressive fluid support will be needed. Cardiovascular, pulmonary, and metabolic intervention/support may be necessary.

Nafcillin or oxacillin 2 g IV every 4 hours OR:

- Cefazolin 1 g IV every 8 hours
- Clindamycin 600 to 900 mg IV every 8 hours (covers streptococci and some MRSA)

Also for MRSA or penicillin-allergic patients:

- Vancomycin 30 mg/kg/d IV divided twice daily
- Linezolid 600 mg IV every 12 hours

Continue antibiotics for a total of 10 to 14 days.

Immune globulin (400 mg/kg over 2 to 3 hours) contains antibody to TSS and may be used for patients with refractory foci of infection.

Pediatric Patient Considerations

Intravenous penicillin (Pen G four divided doses) or erythromycin 1 g IV every 6 hours is the therapy of choice and results in rapid improvement of constitutional symptoms and avoidance of suppurative and nonsuppurative sequelae.

Suggested Readings

Aguero J, Ortega-Mendi M, Eliecer Cano M, et al. Outbreak of invasive group A streptococcal disease among children attending a day-care center. *Pediatr Infect Dis J.* 2008;27(7):602–604.

Chen C, Tang J, Dong W, et al. A glimpse of streptococcal toxic shock syndrome from comparative genomics of *S. suis* 2 Chinese isolates. *PLoS One.* 2007;2(3):e315.

Chuang YY, Huang YC, Lin TY. Toxic shock syndrome in children: Epidemiology, pathogenesis, and management. *Paediatr Drugs.* 2005;7(1):11–25.

Finkelstein JW, von Eye A. Sanitary product use by white, black, and Mexican American women. *Public Health Rep.* 1990;105(5):491–496.

Fongcom A, Pruksakorn S, Netsirisawan P, et al. *Streptococcus suis* infection: A prospective study in northern Thailand. *Southeast Asian J Trop Med Public Health.* 2009;40(3):511–517.

Lun ZR, Wang QP, Chen XG, et al. *Streptococcus suis*: An emerging zoonotic pathogen. *Lancet Infect Dis.* 2007;7(3):201–209.

Shah A, Moss W, Champion S, et al. Nonmenstrual toxic shock syndrome in a young child with human immunodeficiency virus infection. *Pediatr Infect Dis J.* 1996;15(7):639–641.

Tang J, Wang C, Feng Y, et al. Streptococcal toxic shock syndrome caused by *Streptococcus suis* serotype 2. *PLoS Med.* 2006;3(5):e151.

Exfoliative Dermatitis

Donna Culton

◼◼ Diagnosis Synopsis

Exfoliative dermatitis, or erythroderma, is defined as diffuse erythema and scaling involving >90% of the body surface area. This condition typically represents an end-stage process or severe consequence of many distinct disorders, each of which must be considered as the possible underlying etiology. The erythema and scale often begin in localized areas and quickly extend to involve almost the entire body surface area with associated pruritus or allodynia (painful skin). Exfoliative dermatitis is considered to be a medical emergency, as many systemic complications can arise (see below).

Diseases that most often progress to exfoliative dermatitis include psoriasis, atopic dermatitis, drug hypersensitivity, mycosis fungoides (cutaneous T-cell lymphoma), seborrheic dermatitis, generalized contact dermatitis, and pityriasis rubra pilaris, although many others have also been reported. One-half of patients presenting with exfoliative dermatitis already have a known underlying dermatosis. The remaining patients require a thorough history and biopsy to help distinguish among these causative conditions. Even after extensive studies, approximately 20% of patients are eventually labeled as having an idiopathic disease without defined etiology.

When the condition is due to a drug hypersensitivity, the onset is typically 2 to 6 weeks after starting the medication. Onset and resolution are typically more rapid in erythroderma due to drug hypersensitivity compared to other causes. Of note, the erythema can be quite subtle in pigmented skin, thereby delaying diagnosis in these patients.

Immunocompromised Patient Considerations

Drug reactions are the most common cause of exfoliative dermatitis in HIV-infected individuals.

◉ Look For

Look for widespread erythema and scale involving >90% of the total body surface area with, usually, sparing of the mucosa (Figs. 4-36–4-38). With chronic disease, edema, lichenification, scarring alopecia, and nail changes may occur as well. In general, patients often appear ill. Erythema in skin Types V and VI will present as dark red to purple (Fig. 4-39). In darkly pigmented skin, widespread loss of pigmentation can be seen as a sequel.

●● Diagnostic Pearls

If present for prolonged periods of time, the intense pruritus and continuous scratching can lead to lichenification and erosions.

?? Differential Diagnosis and Pitfalls

Differential Diagnosis for Underlying Cause

- Psoriasis
- Atopic dermatitis
- Drug hypersensitivity

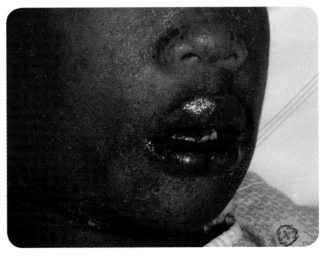

Figure 4-36 Carbimazole-induced exfoliative dermatitis with redness and scaling.

Figure 4-37 Drug-induced exfoliative dermatitis with lip swelling.

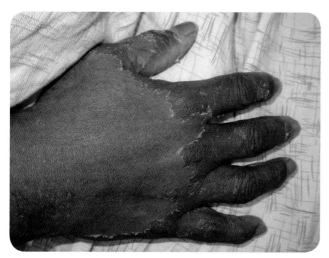

Figure 4-38 Exfoliative dermatitis 4 days after exposure to icodextrin in a patient with lepromatous leprosy.

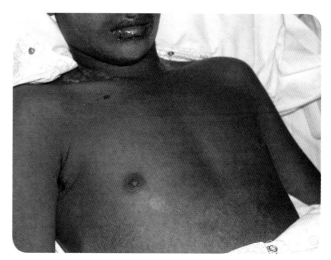

Figure 4-39 Carbimazole-induced exfoliative dermatitis with intensive erythema.

- Mycosis fungoides (cutaneous T-cell lymphoma)
- Contact dermatitis
- Seborrheic dermatitis
- Pityriasis rubra pilaris
- Graft versus host disease
- Lupus erythematosus
- Dermatomyositis
- Staphylococcal scaled skin syndrome
- Toxic shock syndrome
- Bullous disorders
- Malignancy

Pediatric Patient Considerations

As above, but in addition:
Congenital disorders

✓ Best Tests

Biopsy is often indicated to determine the underlying etiology, except in cases where the patient has a well-documented history of a disorder commonly known to progress to exfoliative dermatitis (atopic dermatitis, psoriasis, etc.). Laboratory studies typically show general abnormalities including elevated erythrocyte sedimentation rate, leukocytosis, and eosinophilia. A Sézary prep can be useful when considering mycosis fungoides (cutaneous T-cell lymphoma). When T-cell lymphoma is suggested by the skin biopsy, T-cell receptor gene rearrangements are necessary.

▲▲ Management Pearls

Complications can be severe and include fever, leukocytosis, eosinophilia, edema, lymphadenopathy, organomegaly, and liver and renal dysfunction. More severe complications include electrolyte and fluid imbalance, thermoregulatory disturbance, tachycardia, and high-output cardiac failure. Patients often respond well to hospitalization and topical steroids with wet wraps performed three times daily by a skilled nursing staff. Once improved, identification and optimized treatment of the underlying disorder are critical. Noncompliance with previously prescribed topicals, running out of medications, or worsening of underlying disease often leads to progression to erythrodermic state. If a medication or drug hypersensitivity is felt to be the cause, the causative drug should be avoided. Patients with exfoliative dermatitis should be followed over time with repeat biopsies if necessary to establish a diagnosis, as some patients with idiopathic disease have gone on to develop cutaneous T-cell lymphoma.

Therapy

Treatment of the underlying disease is critical for effective management. If drug-induced, discontinuing the systemic agent is critical. Topical corticosteroids (triamcinolone cream or ointment 0.1% twice daily) under an occlusive sauna suit or wet wraps and topical steroids will greatly aid in relief of erythema, scaling, and itching.

Antihistamines (hydroxyzine 25 to 50 mg four times daily or 2 to 4 mg/kg/d, or cetirizine 10 mg twice daily) may

(Continued)

73

provide some relief of itching. Systemic corticosteroids are often less helpful than expected; however, prednisone 0.75 to 1.0 mg/kg/d tapering over a 2- to 3-week period may help improve symptoms.

When refractory to topical treatment, exfoliative dermatitis may require the use of systemic immunosuppressive agents such as prednisone (which should be avoided when psoriasis is the underlying disorder), methotrexate, cyclosporine, acitretin, and other biologics.

Suggested Readings

Moror N, Slova N, Gupta AK, et al. Erythroderma: A comparison between HIV positive and HIV negative patients. *Int J Dermatol.* 1999;38: 895–900.

Rothe MJ, Bernstein ML, Grant-Kels JM. Life-threatening erythroderma: Diagnosing and treating the "red man." *Clin Dermatol.* 2005;23:206–217.

Seghal VN, Srivastava G. Erythroderma/generalized exfoliative dermatitis in the pediatric practice: An overview. *Int J Dermatol.* 2006;45:831–839.

Sehgal VN, Srivastava G, Sardana K. Erythroderma/exfoliative dermatitis: A synopsis. *Int J Dermat.* 2004;43:39–47.

Calciphylaxis
Arden Fredeking

Diagnosis Synopsis

Calciphylaxis is the diffuse deposition of insoluble calcium salts in the skin resulting from systemic dysregulation of calcium metabolism. Disorders of calcium metabolism can be broadly categorized into four main groups: dystrophic, metastatic, idiopathic, and iatrogenic. Calciphylaxis is the most severe form of metastatic calcification and is most commonly associated with chronic renal failure, patients on hemodialysis, and secondary hyperparathyroidism. The most common causes of chronic kidney disease are diabetic nephropathy, hypertension, and glomerulonephritis. Together these comprise over 75% of all cases of chronic kidney disease. The incidence of calciphylaxis has increased to 5% from 1% in end-stage renal patients receiving hemodialysis over the last 15 years, and 32% to 38% of calciphylaxis cases are kidney transplant recipients. Calciphylaxis affects whites more than dark-skinned individuals, and the female-to-male incidence is 3:1.

While the exact pathogenesis is unclear, characteristic pathologic findings include progressive medial calcification of cutaneous blood vessels and subsequent ischemic necrosis of the skin. In addition, the process is believed to be triggered by chronic hypocalcemia from decreased intestinal absorption of calcium; this leads to increased levels of parathyroid hormone (PTH) and subsequent recruitment of calcium and phosphate from bone. It is believed that disturbances in calcium and phosphorus homeostasis can cause a calcium-phosphorus product, which precipitates out of the serum and lodges within small vessel walls. This then creates intimal fibroplasia and thrombosis of subcutaneous arterioles.

Painful violaceous patches are initially seen clinically, followed by necrosis, ulcers, and/or gangrene (Figs. 4-40–4-42).

Mortality from calciphylaxis is high (60% to 87%) and is secondary to sepsis from large nonhealing ulcers.

Risk factors for calciphylaxis include renal and/or liver disease, elevated calcium level, elevated phosphorus level, elevated calcium-phosphate product over 70 mg^2/dL^2, hypoparathyroidism or hyperparathyroidism, diabetes, female sex, white race, obesity, decreased albumin level, elevated alkaline phosphatase level (most likely indicates increased bone turnover), elevated erythrocyte sedimentation rate (ESR), serum aluminum >25 ng/mL, Coumadin (warfarin) use (inhibition of g-carboxylation of matrix GLA protein, which has an essential role in inhibiting mineralization), systemic corticosteroid use, vitamin D administration, and protein C or S deficiency. The condition has also been observed in patients with breast cancer treated with chemotherapy, systemic lupus erythematosus, end-stage liver disease, and Crohn disease.

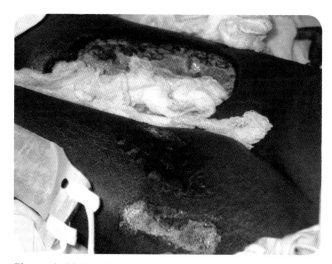

Figure 4-41 Calciphylaxis with superficial and deep ulcerations.

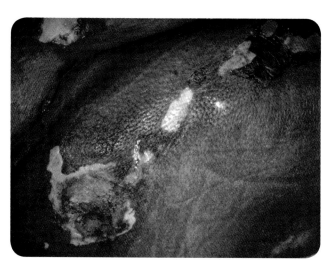

Figure 4-40 A sixty-year-old woman treated with hemodialysis for 8 years, with hemorrhagic crusts and ulcerations characteristic of calciphylaxis.

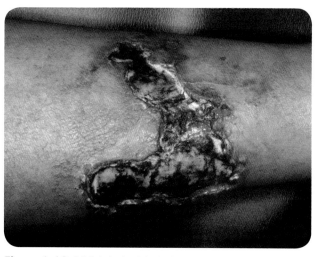

Figure 4-42 Calciphylaxis with thick adherent hemorrhagic crust.

Immunocompromised Patient Considerations

There have been recent reports of calciphylaxis in the immunosuppressed patient with normal renal function. While calcium, phosphorus, and calcium-phosphorus products are within normal limits in these patients, they often have one or more of the above risk factors associated with calciphylaxis. Examples include diseases such as diabetes, markers of illness such as elevated ESR, low albumin levels, and long-term medication usage of prednisone or Coumadin.

⊙ Look For

In darker-skinned individuals, livedo reticularis may appear as dark brown or violaceous reticular patches or net-like erythema. Deep, painful red or purple indurated plaques may be present.

⦁⦁ Diagnostic Pearls

- Calciphylaxis may be classified as proximal (on the trunk, buttocks, face) or distal (extremities). Those patients with distal lesions tend to have a better prognosis. The presence of a painful proximal myopathy may be the first indication of calciphylaxis.
- Scrotal or penile involvement in males is common.

?? Differential Diagnosis and Pitfalls

- Cholesterol emboli
- Cryoglobulinemia
- Cellulitis
- Hypercoagulable state—Check protein C and S and antithrombin III as well as antiphospholipid antibodies.
- Coumadin necrosis—indurated, necrotic areas on the breasts, thighs, and buttocks; usually in the first week of starting Coumadin therapy
- Vasculitis
- Disseminated intravascular necrosis
- Nephrogenic systemic fibrosis
- Lupus profundus lesions may have calcification on X-ray.
- Dermatomyositis and CREST syndrome may have associated calcification.
- Myxoma emboli
- Pancreatic panniculitis
- Peripheral atherosclerotic vascular disease—Check venous and arterial Doppler if ulcerations appear distally.

- Pyoderma gangrenosum
- Wegener granulomatosis

✓ Best Tests

Note that there are no laboratory findings that are specific for calciphylaxis. Some but not all patients demonstrate elevated calcium-phosphate product and/or elevated PTH.

Labs

- Calcium, phosphate, PTH, vitamin D_3 serum levels
- Coagulation factors (prothrombin time [PT], partial thromboplastin time [PTT], protein C and S levels, anticardiolipin antibody, lupus anticoagulant, factor V Leiden)
- Cryoglobulin, cryofibrinogen, hepatitis C antibody
- CBC with differential
- Calculate a calcium-phosphate product (>70 mg/dL has been reported in 33% of cases and is associated with calcification).

Radiologic

- Plain radiographs—may see calcification of small arteries
- High-resolution CT
- Three-phase technetium-99m methylene diphosphonate bone scintigraphy

The gold standard for diagnosis of calciphylaxis is tissue biopsy, but this is subject to sampling error and may initiate ulcer formation. Biopsy should be deep (e.g., wedge excision deep into the subcutaneous tissue). One can see necrosis of the epidermis and superficial dermis with fibrin microthrombi in the dermal and superficial subcutaneous vasculature with minimal inflammation and without vasculitis. One should see intramural calcium deposition in subcutaneous arterioles with associated intimal hyperplasia and ischemic changes of the surrounding panniculus.

▲▲ Management Pearls

- Aggressive wound care
- Pain management
- Surgical consultation is often necessary for wound debridement and/or parathyroidectomy.
- Nutritional consult

Patients often require a multidisciplinary team of specialists including a nephrologist, an internist/critical care expert, a surgeon, a dermatologist, and a pain specialist.

Therapy

Treatment is largely supportive, with aggressive wound care and management of the underlying disease.

First-line Treatments
- Aggressive wound care and pain management
- Normalization of serum calcium and phosphate levels (calcium-phosphate product <55 mg^2/dL^2) via non–calcium-based phosphate binders (sevelamer, lanthanum carbonate)
- Normalization of PTH levels (cinacalcet or parathyroidectomy)

Second-line Treatments
- Intravenous sodium thiosulfate (i.e., 25 g IV over 30 to 60 minutes three times weekly)
- Hyperbaric oxygen therapy
- Low-dose tissue plasminogen activator

Suggested Readings

Fine A, Zacharias J. Calciphylaxis is usually non-ulcerating: Risk factors, outcome and therapy. *Kidney Int.* 2002;61:2210–2217.

Guldbakke KK, Khachemoune A. Calciphylaxis. *Int J Dermatol.* 2007;46: 231–238.

Kalajian AH, Malhotra PS, Callen JP, et al. Calciphylaxis with normal renal function. *Arch Dermatol.* 2009;145(4):451–458.

Mazhar AR, Johnson RJ, Gillen D, et al. Risk factors and mortality associated with calciphylaxis in end-stage renal disease. *Kidney Int.* 2001;60: 324–332.

Raymond CB, Wazny LD. Sodium thiosulfate, bisphosphanates, and cinacalcet for treatment of calciphylaxis. *Am J Health-Syst Pharm.* 2008;65: 1419–1429.

Rogers NM, Coates PT. Calcific uraemic arteriolopathy: An update. *Curr Opin Nephrol Hypertens.* 2008;17:629–634.

Swanson AM, Desai SR, Jackson JD, et al. Calciphylaxis associated with chronic inflammatory conditions, immunosuppression therapy, and normal renal function: A report of 2 cases. *Arch Dermatol.* 2009:145: 723–725.

Weenig RH, Sewell LD, Davis MD, et al. Calciphylaxis: Natural history, risk factor analysis, and outcome. *J Am Acad Dermatol.* 2007;56:569–579.

Leukocytoclastic Vasculitis and Gonococcemia

Naurin Ahmad • Stephanie Diamantis

These are destructive diseases of varying-sized vessels in the skin. For discussions about two disorders with related clinical presentations, polyarteritis nodosa (PAN) and cryoglobulinema, see VisualDx online. (If you are a first-time online user, go to www.essentialdermatology.com/pigmented; if you already have your password set up, go directly to www.visualdx.com/visualdx.) For discussion of Henoch-Schönlein purpura, see page 83.

■■ Diagnosis Synopsis

Leukocytoclastic Vasculitis

Leukocytoclastic vasculitis (LCV) predominantly involves inflammation in the small postcapillary venule. PAN affects medium-sized arterial vessels and is discussed separately, as are Henoch-Schönlein purpura (HSP) and cryoglobulinemia.

LCV, or cutaneous small-vessel vasculitis, is characterized by purpuric or erythematous papules, vesicles, urticarial lesions, or petechiae in small blood vessels due to a complex interplay of immune cells and mediators.

LCV can occur at any age, in all ethnicities/races, and in both sexes. It is more commonly found in adults; 10% of cases are children. Clinical features include a single eruption of palpable purpuric papules or nodules, vesicles, urticarial plaques, or petechiae cropping up in dependent areas approximately 1 week after an inciting factor. Inciting factors include medications (especially antibiotics, nonsteroidal anti-inflammatory drugs [NSAIDs], and diuretics), pathogens (hepatitis viruses, HIV, streptococci), foods or food additives, malignancy, inflammatory bowel disease, and collagen vascular diseases. Up to 50% of cases, however, have no identifiable cause and must be considered idiopathic at this time.

LCV is the most common vasculitis in populations with deeply pigmented skin and is often precipitated by infectious. Noninfectious causes of vasculitis (collagen vascular disease, neoplastic diseases, and paraproteinemias, etc.) are more common in the industrialized nations. In Western Africa, streptococcal infection, *Mycobacterium leprae*, and *Mycobacterium tuberculosis* are common infections associated with vasculitis—especially during the summer. Endemic viral infections such as hepatitis B and C often precipitate vasculitis, despite continuous campaigns to reduce risk of transmission. Vasculitis precipitated by medication use is common in Africa because of a wide range of drugs used and uncontrolled usage. In Sao Paulo, Brazil, the majority of adult vasculitis was classified as Takayasu arteritis, thromboangiitis obliterans, collagen vascular disease–associated vasculitis, and PAN. A study in Kuwait demonstrated that LCV/cutaneous small-vessel vasculitis was the most common type in this population. A study in Thailand demonstrated that possible etiologies of LCV include streptococcal infection, drug hypersensitivity, and systemic lupus erythematosus (SLE).

The highest incidence of hepatitis B–associated vasculitis in world is in Alaskan natives, especially those living in southwest Alaska, an area hyperendemic for hepatitis B.

HIV-associated LCV is a common cause of vasculitis, and is often complicated by low CD4 counts and coinfection with hepatitis viral infections.

While the majority of patients are asymptomatic, LCV can be associated with pruritus, pain, and burning. A skin biopsy confirms the diagnosis. Over 90% of patients with LCV limited to the skin will experience spontaneous resolution over several weeks to months.

Variants or subcategories of LCV include the following:

- HSP—acute onset of palpable purpura, usually seen in children aged younger than 10 years in the lower extremities/buttocks 1 to 2 weeks after a respiratory infection. Fever, arthralgias, and renal and gastrointestinal involvement are common. Renal disease is correlated with spread of purpura above the waist, adult onset, elevated ESR, and fever. While HSP is common in African children and adolescents, in South Africa, the clinical features of HSP do not differ greatly among ethnic populations.
- Urticarial vasculitis—recurrent, painful eruptions of urticarial lesions that last for more than 24 hours (differentiating from chronic urticaria) with or without angioedema (Fig. 4-43). Fever, malaise, myalgias, and arthritis are common. Occurs with SLE, Sjögren syndrome, and viral infections. Complement levels can predict systemic involvement: normal levels are seen in diseases limited to skin, and hypocomplementemic levels are seen with arthritis and with gastrointestinal and pulmonary involvement.

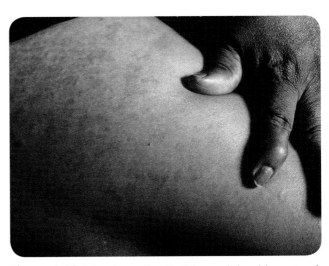

Figure 4-43 Late stage of urticarial vasculitis with scattered, slightly pigmented brown macules.

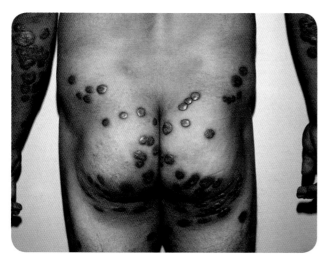

Figure 4-44 Multiple roughly symmetrical hyperpigmented nonscaly plaques characteristic of erythema elevatum diutinum.

A recent study demonstrated that compared to patients in western countries, Thai patients appear to have less severe symptoms and a lower hypocomplementemic, less urticarial vasculitis and SLE.

- Erythema elevatum diutinum—violaceous papules and plaques on extensors symmetrically; chronic with spontaneous resolution after 5 to 10 years (Fig. 4-44)

Gonococcemia

Gonococcemia from *Neisseria gonorrhoeae* in the bloodstream often leads to disseminated gonococcal infection. Gonococcemia occurs in approximately 1% to 3% of patients with gonorrhea. Gonorrhea is the second most commonly reported sexually transmitted infection in the United States, after chlamydia.

Disseminated gonococcal infection is more common in women, due to a higher incidence of occult infection and the increased risk of gonococcemia during menstruation and pregnancy. Other risk factors are HIV, lupus, or complement deficiencies; multiple sexual partners; low socioeconomic status; drug use; being a man who has sex with men; being in an ethnic minority; and a prior history of sexually transmitted infections.

The onset of gonococcemia is often abrupt, with fever (usually 38.33°C to 40°C [101°F to 104°F]), skin lesions, and arthralgias and/or tenosynovitis. Successive crops of hemorrhagic pustules, papules, petechiae, or areas of necrosis may appear during febrile episodes in 40% to 70% of patients. Arthralgias are asymmetric and migratory, involving at first the extensor tendons of wrists, fingers, knees, and ankles. In untreated disseminated disease, septic arthritis with progressive joint destruction may occur. Complications include endocarditis, meningitis, perihepatitis, and pelvic inflammatory disease.

⊙ Look For

Leukocytoclastic Vasculitis

In LCV and small-vessel vasculitis, features include palpable purpura, urticaria, and subcutaneous nodules (Fig. 4-45). Retiform purpura, ulcers and necrosis, and livedo reticularis are often seen in medium- and large-vessel vasculitis. Palpable purpura is the most common skin finding in LCV, with nonblanching 1- to 3-mm violaceous round papules, involving the lower extremities. Lesions enlarge and coalesce into nodules and plaques that may ulcerate (Fig. 4-46). Older lesions may have brownish-red color. In severe cases, vesicles, bullae, and ulcers on the ankles and legs can appear. Facial, palmoplantar, and mucosal lesions are uncommon. Palpable purpura may resolve with atrophic scarring and/ or hyperpigmentation, especially in dark-skinned patients. Urticarial lesions may appear prior to the purpura, last longer than classic urticaria, and resolve with hyperpigmentation.

Gonococcemia

Hemorrhagic pustules, papules, petechiae, and/or areas of necrosis are seen especially during periods of fever and bacteremia (Figs. 4-47–4-50). Hemorrhagic lesions begin as red puncta that enlarge. Vesiculopustules begin as macules and

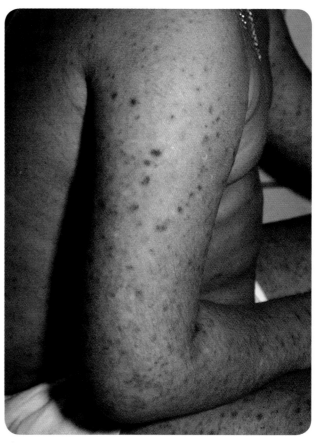

Figure 4-45 Vasculitis with scattered purpuric lesions.

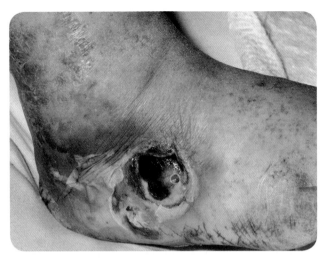

Figure 4-46 Vasculitis on dorsum of foot with hemorrhagic crusts over a large ulcer.

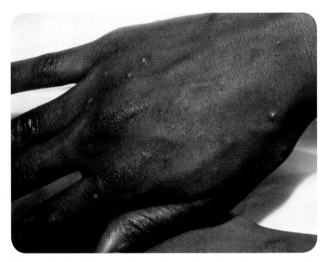

Figure 4-49 Multiple acral pustules in disseminated gonococcemia.

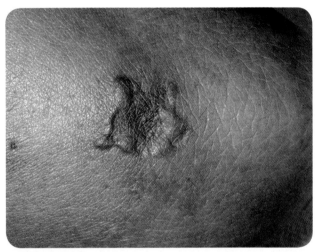

Figure 4-47 Pustules, erythema, and purpura in a 47-year-old HIV-infected Latino man, who presented with a fever, headache, and arthralgias. Blood cultures grew *N. gonorrhoeae*.

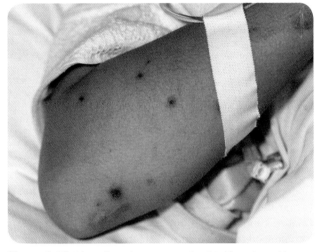

Figure 4-50 Disseminated gonococcemia with disseminated hemorrhagic vesicopustules.

often become necrotic. Palpable purpuric skin lesions may also be seen. Lesions are usually acral. The face, scalp, palms, soles, and trunk are classically spared. There are between 5 and 50 lesions, often in different stages of development.

Diagnostic Pearls

Leukocytoclastic Vasculitis

- Diascopy is a simple and useful maneuver. Pressing a glass slide over a purpuric papule does not blanch the skin.
- Lesions are often in a distinct linear arrangement due to trauma.
- Careful history of medications and other supplements or alternative therapies, preceding infections
- Brownish hyperpigmentation, often faint, distinguishes urticarial vasculitis from urticaria

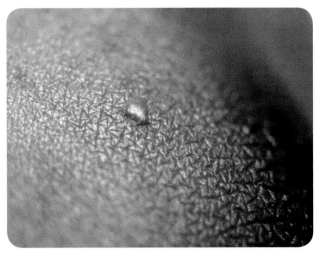

Figure 4-48 Peripheral pustular lesion in gonococcemia.

Gonococcemia

- Women may have minimal genital symptoms but have a positive culture.
- Limited numbers of lesions in an acral distribution (i.e., <20) suggests this diagnosis.

?? Differential Diagnosis and Pitfalls

Leukocytoclastic Vasculitis

Multiple causes must be investigated. The differential diagnosis for vasculitis is extensive. A skin biopsy will largely aid in the diagnosis. Secondary causes of LCV, such as infection, drug exposure, neoplasms, and autoimmune connective tissue disorders, should be sought.

- Bacterial infections
- Viral infections—hepatitis A, B, or C; HIV; varicella-zoster virus; parvovirus B19; cytomegalovirus
- Arthropod bites
- Erythema multiforme—systemic involvement is rare, targetoid lesions
- Still disease—high spiking fevers
- Drug exposure—NSAIDs, penicillins, quinolones, anti-tumor necrosis factor biologics, hydralazine, granulocyte colony-stimulating factor (G-CSF), angiotensin-converting enzyme inhibitors
- Cryoglobulinemia and cryofibrinogenemia—Check for serum IgM and IgG cryoglobulins and cryofibrinogens, hepatitis C virus infection (Fig. 4-51).
- Microscopic polyangiitis—Anti-neutrophilic cytoplasmic antibodies (ANCA) positive, palpable purpura, and constitutional symptoms; look for evidence of pulmonary and renal involvement.
- Wegener granulomatosis—ANCA positive; necrotizing granulomatous inflammation of the upper and lower respiratory tracts; glomerulonephritis (Fig. 4-52) is more common in whites than in African Americans

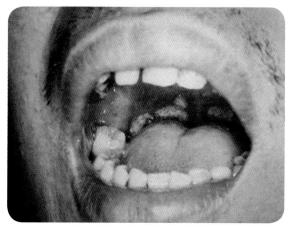

Figure 4-52 Plaques and ulcerations of the soft palate in Wegener granulomatosis.

- Churg-Strauss syndrome—ANCA positive; associated with eosinophilia and asthma; characteristic findings on histology
- PAN—medium-vessel vasculitis with subcutaneous nodules, livedo reticularis, ulcers, and gangrene as cutaneous manifestations.
- Behçet disease—aphthous stomatitis, uveitis, recurrent genital ulcerations
- Immune thrombocytopenic purpura—isolated thrombocytopenia
- Rheumatoid vasculitis—very high rheumatoid factor levels (Fig. 4-53)

Sometimes nonvasculitic purpura on the lower extremities may be palpable, such as those seen in the following:

- Overanticoagulation with warfarin or heparin
- Early disseminated intravascular coagulation
- Pruritic insect bites
- Schamberg disease
- Rocky Mountain spotted fever
- Meningococcemia

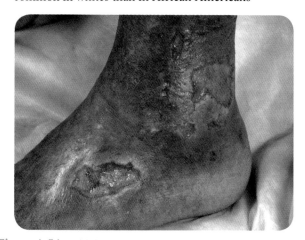

Figure 4-51 Multiple peripheral ulcers due to cryoglobulinemia.

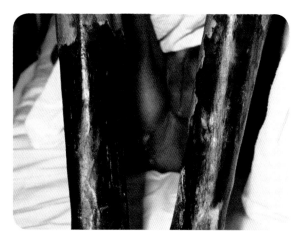

Figure 4-53 Rheumatoid vasculitis with infarctions producing large areas of skin purpura and necrosis.

Immunocompromised Patient Considerations

In the immunosuppressed patient or the patient with low polymorphonuclear leukocytes, the distribution of the lesions may be similar to that in the normal host, but the degree of induration and the purpura may be less or even absent.

Gonococcemia

- Other forms of vasculitis and septic vasculitis have to be considered.
- Bacterial endocarditis
- Meningococcemia
- Ecthyma gangrenosum
- *Vibrio vulnificus* infection
- Rocky Mountain spotted fever
- Emboli
- Disseminated herpes zoster

Best Tests

Skin biopsy is usually necessary for a discrete diagnosis.

Further workup to rule out infectious or rheumatologic etiologies is indicated once vasculitis is confirmed. This is often accomplished with the following tests:

- ANA, ANCA, rheumatoid factor, anti-Ro and anti-La, complement levels, cryoglobulins, HIV and hepatitis B and C serologies

Select patients may require echocardiography, angiography, direct immunofluorescence tests of skin biopsy samples, pulmonary function testing, and screening for malignancy.

Gonococcemia

Gram stain of urethral or cervical exudate showing intracellular Gram-negative diplococci is diagnostic for gonorrhea.

Management Pearls

Leukocytoclastic Vasculitis

Therapy is first directed at any underlying trigger, such as infection or withdrawal of a medication. Defining the nature of the vasculitis and the size of the vessel is important in planning for therapy and should precede, if possible, beginning strong systemic medications. Oral corticosteroids are often required. Consider dietary restriction in patients in whom a food substance may be the inciting agent. Most LCV is self-limited and will resolve in 3 to 4 weeks with postinflammatory hyperpigmentation.

The following supportive/symptomatic measures may be taken:

- Remove offending agent
- Rest with elevation of the legs
- Graduated compression stockings
- NSAIDs for myalgias and arthralgias
- Antihistamines for pruritus, especially in urticarial forms:
  - Diphenhydramine—25, 50 mg tablets or capsules: 25 to 50 mg nightly or every 6 hours as needed
  - Hydroxyzine—10, 25 mg tablets: 12.5 to 25 mg every 6 hours as needed
  - Cetirizine—5, 10 mg tablets: 5 to 10 mg/d
  - Loratadine—10 mg tablets: 10-mg tablet once daily

Depending on the clinical scenario, the speciality consultations may be helpful.

Gonococcemia

- Empiric treatment should be initiated if this diagnosis is suspected, even if supporting microbiological data are pending. Patients with suspected disseminated disease should be hospitalized for initial therapy and screened for signs of meningitis and endocarditis. CDC guidelines for therapy should be followed.

Therapy

Systemic therapies when indicated are discussed online for each disease.

Suggested Readings

Abu-nassar H, Hill N, Fred HL, et al. Cutaneous manifestations of gonococcemia. *Arch Intern Med.* 1963;112:731–737.

Fauci AS. The vasculitis syndromes. In: Wilson JD, Braunwald E, Isselbacher KJ, et al., eds. *Harrison's Principles of Internal Medicine.* 12 Ed. New York, NY: McGraw-Hill; 1991:1456–1463.

Garcia AL, Madkan VK, Tyring SK. Gonorrhea and other venereal diseases. In: Wolff K, Goldsmith LA, Katz SI, Gilchrest BA, Paller AS, Leffell DJ, eds. *Fitzpatrick's Dermatology in General Medicine.* 7th Ed. New York, NY: McGraw Hill; 2008:1993–1996.

http://www.cdc.gov/std/Gonorrhea

Hurlburt KJ, McMahon BJ, Simonetti JP, et al. Hepatitis B associated vasculitis in Alaska Natives: Viral genotype, clinical and serological outcomes. *Liver Int.* 27(5):627–632, 2007.

Kulthnan K, Cheepsomsongsong M, Jiamton S. Urticarial vasculitis: Etiologies and clinical course. *Asian Pac J Allergy Immunol.* 2009;27(203):95–102.

McMahon BJ, Bender TR, Templin DW, et al. Vasculitis in Eskimos living in an area hyperendemic for hepatitis B. *JAMA.* 1980;244(19):2180–2182.

Miller KE. Diagnosis and treatment of *Neisseria gonorrhoeae* infections. *Am Fam Physician.* 2006;73:1779–1784, 1786.

Otedo AE, Oyoo GO, et al. Vasculitis in HIV: Report of eight cases. *East Afr Med J.* 2005;82(12):656–659.

Tapsall JW. *Neisseria gonorrhoeae* and emerging resistance to extended spectrum cephalosporins. *Curr Opin Infect Dis.* 2009;22:87–91.

Zenilman JM. Ethnicity and sexually transmitted infections. *Curr Opin Infect Dis.* 1998;11:47–52.

Henoch-Schönlein Purpura

Stephanie Diamantis

■■ Diagnosis Synopsis

Henoch-Schönlein purpura (HSP) is an idiopathic small vessel vasculitis of uncertain etiology characterized by IgA-immune complexes and C3 deposition in venules, capillaries, and arterioles. The disease occurs mostly in children, with a peak incidence at 5 to 6 years of age, but may also be seen in adults. HSP occurs more often in men and has a seasonal predilection, with most cases occurring during winter. HSP affects all ethnicities but is rare in African American patients.

A history of preceding upper respiratory tract infection is frequently elicited. Patients may experience a 2- to 3-week history of fever, headache, myalgias, arthralgias, and abdominal pain that precedes the skin eruption. The classic tetrad of clinical manifestations includes hematuria, colicky abdominal pain, arthritis, and palpable purpura. Additional symptoms include fever, malaise, headache, vomiting, hematemesis, diarrhea, hematochezia, melena, and scrotal pain. An individual episode may persist for 3 to 6 weeks, and recurrences are frequent.

Extracutaneous manifestations include arthritis, gastrointestinal bleeding, pulmonary hemorrhage, and nephritis. Renal involvement is typically mild and self-limited with transient microscopic hematuria and minimal proteinuria. However, approximately 2% of patients progress to end-stage renal disease (risk factors include older age, purpura extending onto the trunk, or nephritic or nephrotic syndrome at presentation). Occasionally, inflammation of the bowel may lead to appendicitis, ileus, and intussusception. Arthritic complaints most commonly involve the ankles and knees. Neurologic complications include headache, behavioral changes, and rarely convulsions and subarachnoid hemorrhage. Fatalities occur in 1% to 5% of patients.

Consensus criteria for the diagnosis of HSP include palpable purpura plus at least one of the following:

- Diffuse abdominal pain
- Acute arthritis or arthralgias
- Renal involvement
- A skin biopsy showing IgA deposition

◉ Look For

Eruption begins with erythematous macules and papules or urticarial lesions that quickly evolve into purpura within 24 hours. Palpable purpura (violaceous, erythematous, non-blanchable papules) is symmetrically distributed on the legs and buttocks but occasionally involves the upper extremities, face, and trunk (Figs. 4-54–4-57). Vesicles, bullae, and necrotic ulcers may also be seen. Localized soft tissue edema of the hands, feet, scalp, ears, or scrotum may also be present. Individual lesions resolve with hyperpigmentation over 5 to 7 days, but recurrent crops tend to appear over a period of 6 to 16 weeks.

●● Diagnostic Pearls

Look for linear purpura in areas of externally applied pressure: elastic at the top of socks on legs, wrinkles of hospital bed sheets on the back in a recumbent patient, etc. HSP should be considered in a patient with palpable purpura over dependent areas such as the buttocks and legs and over pressure points in the setting of a recent upper respiratory tract infection. The spread of purpura to the upper parts of the trunk portends a higher likelihood of renal involvement. In patients with severe abdominal pain, consider an acute surgical abdomen, intussusception, or paralytic ileus.

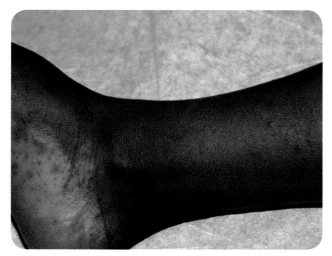

Figure 4-54 Child with various-sized areas of purpura on the sole.

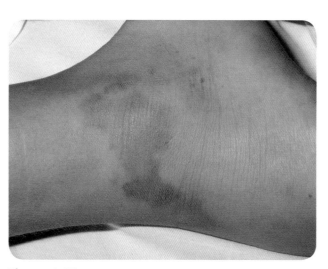

Figure 4-55 Discrete areas of purpura and hyperpigmentation around the ankle.

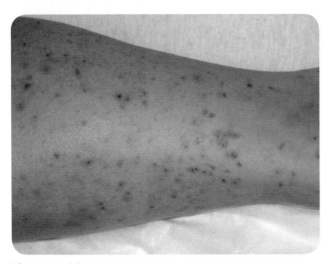

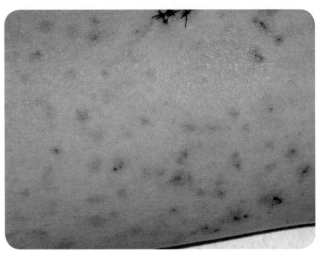

Figure 4-56 A nineteen-year-old Asian man with hematuria, generalized arthralgias, malaise and lower extremity eruption, guaiac-positive stool, and multiple purpuric lesions.

Figure 4-57 Close-up of lesions in patient seen in Figure 4-56.

Pediatric Patient Considerations

In infants, lesions may have purpuric centers and urticarial rims resembling a target.

?? Differential Diagnosis and Pitfalls

- Other small-vessel vasculitides (Kawasaki disease, Wegener granulomatosis, Churg-Strauss syndrome, microscopic polyangiitis, or essential cryoglobulinemia)—also present with palpable purpura and systemic symptoms. Positive direct immunofluorescence and negative basic immunologic investigations (ANA, dsDNA, anti-neutrophilic cytoplasmic antibodies, immunoglobulins, C3 and C4) are helpful in differentiating HSP from other vasculitides.
- Erythema elevatum diutinum—palpable purpura over extensor surfaces that later become fibrotic
- Acute hemorrhagic edema of infancy—children aged 4 months to 2 years; internal involvement is rare
- Urticarial vasculitis—painful urticarial lesions that last longer than 24 hours
- Pigmented purpura—nonblanchable macules with no associated vessel inflammation
- Erythema multiforme—erythematous, targetoid plaques most commonly acrally distributed
- Systemic lupus erythematosus—can have purpuric lesions, arthritis, and nephritis, but photosensitivity is usually present
- Meningococcemia—may result in purpura fulminans characterized by necrotic, nonblanchable palpable purpura on predominantly acral areas

- Disseminated intravascular coagulation (DIC)—Patients are more systemically ill.
- Endocarditis—palpable purpura over acral areas
- Thrombocytopenic purpura—presents like DIC with petechiae
- Rickettsial infections—characteristic purpura on the hands and feet. Patients are systemically ill.
- Leukocytoclastic vasculitis secondary to infections, drugs, connective tissue diseases, and malignancies
- Drug eruption
- Abuse (particularly in children)
- Leukemia

Pediatric Patient Considerations

Children with HSP are usually systemically well, and alternative etiologies should be strongly considered and evaluated for in the systemically unwell child.

✓ Best Tests

- HSP is largely a clinical diagnosis, but commonly ordered laboratory tests to evaluate for systemic involvement include a urinalysis, CBC with differential, ESR, BUN, creatinine, coagulation studies, ASO titers, and fecal occult blood testing.
- Leukocytosis, elevated ESR, hematuria, proteinuria, and a positive stool Hemoccult test are often seen. BUN and creatinine may also be elevated. An elevated serum IgA is suggestive. The Rumpel-Leede tourniquet test (application of tourniquet or blood pressure cuff causes petechiae)

may be positive but difficult to see in darkly pigmented patients.

- Skin biopsy and direct immunofluorescence studies are diagnostic. Histologic exam shows leukocytoclastic vasculitis, and direct immunofluorescence shows IgA deposits within blood vessel walls.
- Abdominal and/or testicular ultrasounds may be conducted to rule out intussusception or testicular torsion.

▲▲ Management Pearls

- Second episodes may be common despite adequate therapy. Recurrences are more common in patients with renal involvement.
- Close follow-up with repeat urinalysis is necessary to exclude associated renal nephritis and renal failure. Studies to exclude streptococcal infection as a precipitating factor should be performed.
- The long-term prognosis in patients with HSP is associated with the presence or absence of renal disease.

Therapy

- HSP is usually benign and self-limited, and treatment is often supportive, including rest and adequate hydration. Recovery is usually expected within 4 weeks.
- Systemic corticosteroids (approximately 1 mg/kg p.o. daily) have been used to treat the associated vasculitis, nephritis, abdominal pain, and subcutaneous edema. However, steroids do not prevent the recurrence of skin lesions.
- Corticosteroids may be effective in treating abdominal pain and arthritis, although reliable data on their effect on purpura, duration of the illness, or in mitigating potential long-term renal disease are lacking. Several reports point to a possible benefit of high-dose corticosteroids alone or in combination with other immunosuppressive agents (e.g., cyclophosphamide, azathioprine) in patients with HSP with progressive renal disease. Early administration of oral prednisone may reduce the intensity of joint or muscle pain but does not prevent renal disease.

Treatment for Skin Lesions
- Bed rest and leg elevation
- Prednisone—low to intermediate doses (30 to 60 mg/d)
- Dapsone 50 to 200 mg/d after glucose-6-phosphate dehydrogenase testing
- Colchicine 0.6 mg/d to 1.2 mg twice daily

Treatment for Abdominal Symptoms
- H2 blockers
- Corticosteroids 1 to 2 mg/kg/d

Renal Disease
- Systemic corticosteroid use is controversial
- Intravenous immunoglobulin

Nonsteroidal anti-inflammatory drugs may be helpful in alleviating arthralgias but should be avoided if renal and gastrointestinal manifestations are present.

Suggested Readings

Chartapisak W, Opastiraku SL, Willis NS, et al. Prevention and treatment of renal disease in Henoch-Schönlein purpura: A systematic review. *Arch Dis Child.* 2009;94:132–137.

Fervenza FC. Henoch-Schönlein purpura nephritis. *Int J Dermatol.* 2003;42:170–177.

James WD, Berger TG, Elston DM, eds. Cutaneous vascular diseases. In: *Andrews' Diseases of the Skin Clinical Dermatology.* 10th Ed. Philadelphia, PA: Elsevier; 2006:833.

Piette WW. What is Schönlein-Henoch purpura, and why should we care? *Arch Dermatol.* 1997;133:515–518.

Reamy BV, Williams PM, Lindsay TJ. Henoch-Schönlein purpura. *Am Fam Physician.* 2009;80(7):697–704.

Weiss PF, Feinstein JA, Luan X, et al. Effects of corticosteroid on Henoch-Schönlein purpura: A systematic review. *Pediatrics.* 2007;120(5):1079–1087.

Frostbite

Kristina L. Demas • Lynn McKinley-Grant

◼◼ Diagnosis Synopsis

Frostbite is a localized cold injury to the skin, soft tissue, and deeper structures in severe cases. This tissue injury is the result of exposure to temperatures below the freezing point 0°C (32°F). Blood vessels near the skin initially respond by vasoconstricting to help preserve core body temperature. Pathogenesis is related to local, cold-induced crystallization of tissue water into ice that causes hypoxia, release of inflammatory mediators, and ultimately tissue damage and cell death. The extremities, chin, nose, ears, and cheeks are most affected. Indirect damage such as thrombosis or vasodilation may also occur. Frostbite typically occurs over extended cold exposure (minutes or hours) but may also result from instantaneous exposure to cold metal.

Early symptoms of frostbite include loss of pain sensation or a burning/tingling sensation. Complete anesthesia may occur with continued exposure. Clinical features of frostbite include cellular tissue effects (e.g., endothelial injury and membrane damage), a thermoregulatory response (e.g., shivering), and a systemic response (e.g., shock, neuromuscular dysfunction). There are two clinical presentations: superficial frostbite and deep frostbite. Deep frostbite involves subcutaneous tissue and most often leads to tissue loss.

Young, elderly, and intoxicated persons are most at risk for frostbite. Research has shown that African American men and women are slightly more prone to develop frostbite than whites. Other people who may be more predisposed to frostbite are those of Arabic descent and those who reside in warmer climates. Men develop frostbite more often than women, but this may reflect a greater participation in sports and outdoor activities and a higher number of men who are homeless; athletes in cold climates and homeless persons without adequate shelter or clothing are at-risk populations for frostbite. Diabetes, the use of beta-blockers, Raynaud phenomenon, and peripheral neuropathy may also predispose to frostbite development.

Pediatric Patient Considerations

Infants and children have an increased susceptibility to frostbite because they lose heat from their skin faster because of their increased surface-to-body mass ratio. Oftentimes, children may not communicate their symptoms at early onset.

◉ Look For

A history of cold exposure that describes pain and burning followed by anesthesia. Look for large clear blisters, gangrene, and ulcerations in extremities, neck, face, and ears.

Superficial frostbite results in bulla and erythema formation. The frozen part is waxy, firm, and resilient below the surface when gently depressed with thumb. Skin may appear white or yellow (Fig. 4-58). Erythema is more orange, and edema has a grey-purple hue.

Deep frostbite manifests as gangrene, anesthesia, hemorrhagic blisters, ulceration, or hyperesthesia (Fig. 4-59).

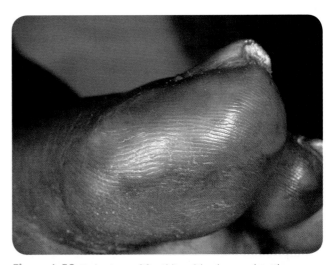

Figure 4-58 Early stage of frostbite with edema and erythema.

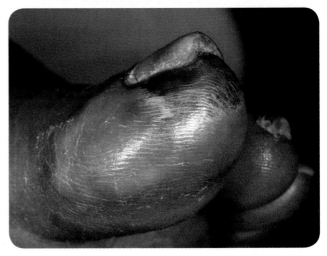

Figure 4-59 Progression of frostbite to bullae and necrosis.

Skin may be hard or wooden without resilience. Gangrene may develop in 3 to 7 days. Pain and pruritus associated with frostbite may last as long as 8 weeks and 6 months, respectively. There also remains an increased sensitivity to cold in the areas of frostbite.

 ## Diagnostic Pearls

- The clinical appearance of frostbite may be deceiving; clinical history is a key to diagnosis. Very few patients arrive with tissue still frozen. Red-yellowish skin that becomes hardened with loss of pain sensation is often indicative of frostbite.
- Frostbitten fingers or toes will often first appear bright red or deep purple. They will then turn gray, and then a stark, icy white over time on the plantar or palmar surfaces. Darker skin will ultimately become an ashy gray color.

 ## Differential Diagnosis and Pitfalls

A diagnosis of frostbite is usually made based on a history of cold exposure and clinical presentation. Make sure to consider the following differential diagnoses:

- Frostnip—a milder form of cold injury that only involves the superficial and subcutaneous tissue. Pain usually resolves in 2 to 4 weeks.
- Pernio—a form of cold injury associated with damp or humid environment. Look for recurrent painful and/or pruritic erythematous, violaceous papules on fingers and/or toes; often seen with poor vascular circulation.
- Trench foot—a condition affecting the feet that is associated with damp and cold environments. Unlike frostbite, it does not require exposure to freezing temperatures.
- Bullous pemphigoid—Look for systemic, tense, and intensely pruritic blisters.

 ## Best Tests

Diagnosis of frostbite relies on clinical history and presentation. Laboratory workup is not indicated unless the patient has signs of systemic hypothermia. Technetium scintigraphy, magnetic resonance imaging and angiography, and triple-phase bone scanning may give some indication of viability of tissue and bone.

 ## Management Pearls

Educate the patient about exposure risks and preventative measures such as the use of layered clothing, staying dry, and protecting the face, head, and neck in cold, windy weather.

Therapy

Rapid rewarming is the objective of treatment.

- Remove wet or constricting clothing.
- Never rub or massage affected area, as this may cause more damage.
- Rapidly rewarm affected tissue in thermometer-controlled running water (37°C to 40°C [98.6°F to 104°F]) for 10 to 45 minutes.
- Warm IV fluids can be given to assist in rewarming.
- Analgesics or narcotics can be given to reduce pain.
- If deep frostbite, affected tissue has a poor prognosis, and debridement or amputation is generally necessary.

Suggested Readings

Biem J, Koehncke N, Classen D, et al. Out of the cold: Management of hypothermia and frostbite. *CMAJ.* 2003;168:305–311.

Burgess JE, Macfarlane F. Retrospective analysis of the ethnic origins of male British army soldiers with peripheral cold weather injury. *J R Army Med Corps.* 2009;155(1):11–15.

Jurkovich GJ. Environmental cold-induced injury. *Surg Clin North Am.* 2007;87:247–267.

Mailler-Savage EA, Adams BB. Skin manifestations of runners. *J Am Acad Dermatol.* 2006;55:290–301.

Patel N, Patel D. Frostbite. *Am J Med.* 2008;121:765–766.

Viral Exanthems (Rubeola [Measles], Cytomegalovirus Infection, and Asymmetric Periflexural Exanthem of Childhood)

Laurie Good

This chapter contains common conditions that are often diagnosed without special diagnostic studies. Measles, cytomegalic infection, and asymmetric periflexural exanthem of childhood (APEC) are discussed in this chapter. Discussions on other viral exanthems such as mononucleosis and neonatal enteroviral infections can be found on VisualDx online. (If you are a first-time online user, go to www.essentialdermatology.com/pigmented; if you already have your password set up, go directly to www.visualdx.com/visualdx.)

■■ Diagnosis Synopsis

Rubeola (Measles)

Rubeola (measles) is caused by a single-stranded RNA virus of the *Paramyxoviridae* family. The disease is worldwide in distribution and primarily occurs in late winter and spring. Cases are more common in developing countries, as the vast majority of individuals in industrialized nations have been vaccinated. The majority of cases of measles in the United States in recent years have been from patients recently living abroad. Classically, the disease is seen more often in children. In an unvaccinated population, children aged younger than 5 years are at highest risk of infection and death.

Measles is transmitted via respiratory droplets, and it is highly infectious. The incubation period after the measles virus infects the upper respiratory tract and nasal passages is typically 10 to 14 days. A prodrome characterized by coryza, cough, and conjunctivitis occurs for about 3 to 4 days followed by the onset of the characteristic morbilliform rash. A characteristic enanthem of grayish, slightly raised papules/bumps on the buccal mucosa, known as Koplik spots, occurs during the prodrome and is pathognomonic. The coryza, cough, and conjunctivitis will increase in severity until the rash reaches its peak. Treatment is supportive.

Encephalitis is a complication in about 1 of 1,000 cases. Others include diarrhea, bronchopneumonia, croup, hepatitis, myocarditis, and otitis media. Subacute sclerosing panencephalitis is a late complication, occurring on average 10 to 11 years after acute infection. This catastrophic sequela is characterized by changes in personality, seizures, and coma and eventuates in death.

Ethnic differences have been demonstrated in the United Kingdom with regard to MMR (measles, mumps, and rubella) vaccine uptake. In an urban UK study comparing vaccination rates among Asians, Caribbean individuals of African descent, non-Caribbean individuals of African descent, Chinese, and whites, only the Asian population was found to have increased the percentage of vaccinated people after the negative public media surrounding the MMR vaccine gained strength in 1998; all other ethnic groups experienced a decline. Caribbean individuals of African descent had the lowest MMR uptake. This is significant, as measles requires a high vaccination rate for herd immunity; thus certain ethnic communities could be at higher risk of measles outbreaks.

In the United States, the measles epidemic of 1989–1991 was found to affect nonwhite children at a four- to sevenfold higher rate than non-Hispanic white children. This led to a public health campaign to eliminate the ethnic/racial gap due to differences in vaccination coverage, and, according to the CDC in 2001, all ethnic/racial groups had achieved an uptake of around 90% (89% for African American, 92% for Hispanic, 92% for white, 94% for American Indian/Alaska Native, and 90% for Asian/Pacific Islander children).

Adverse reactions are a feared consequence of any vaccination, but few if any vaccines have received more hype than the MMR. Although unsubstantiated claims have been made regarding potential reactions to this vaccine, several legitimate reports have led to the conclusion that high-risk children should be tested for metabolic disorders or inherited endocrine disorders prior to receiving vaccinations. One Chinese series reported seven cases of acute metabolic crisis in children with diagnosed and undiagnosed metabolic or endocrine disease following vaccination; two of these cases (one child with glutaric aciduria type 1 and another with Leigh disease) occurred after the measles vaccination. While MMR has been the subject of negative media coverage, it is indisputably the reason for reduced childhood mortality worldwide.

A higher mortality rate due to measles is experienced by malnourished children, in whom vitamin A supplementation is beneficial for reducing mortality and preventing blindness.

Immunosuppression is a risk factor for the development of measles and its complications; immunosuppressed patients frequently lose vaccinated humoral immunity. In one series, 25% of children receiving chemotherapy had absent serum immunity to measles.

Cytomegalovirus Infection

Cytomegalovirus (CMV) is a herpesvirus that causes a wide spectrum of disorders in adults, ranging from an asymptomatic subclinical infection or a mononucleosislike syndrome in healthy individuals to disseminated disease in immunocompromised patients. Adults and occasionally older children may develop the mononucleosis syndrome. The symptoms are identical to traditional mononucleosis caused by the Epstein-Barr virus (EBV) and include sore throat without exudate, fever to 39°C (102.2°F), malaise, and myalgias.

Patients with immunosuppression due to AIDS and/or chemotherapy, transfusion recipients, transplant recipients, and pregnant women are at risk for disseminated disease.

Hepatosplenomegaly, lymphadenopathy, chorioretinitis, gastroenteritis, esophagitis, pneumonia, CNS infection, adrenalitis, and a wasting syndrome have been reported. Like other herpesviruses, CMV establishes a latent infection that may reactivate during periods of relative immunosuppression.

CMV is transmitted by body secretions, including saliva, blood, urine, breast milk, semen, and cervical fluid. The prevalence of seropositivity tends to be higher in people of lower socioeconomic status as well as ethnic/racial minorities, in particular Asian and North African ethnic groups.

The administration of ampicillin to a patient with CMV may precipitate the appearance of an exanthem. A posttransfusion syndrome may appear 3 to 6 weeks after a blood transfusion and is identical to the mononucleosis syndrome.

Meningoencephalitis is common in AIDS patients, in whom disseminated CMV may be a terminal event. Interstitial pneumonia, colitis and toxic megacolon, severe hepatitis, retinitis, and other complications are often seen. Perforated colon has also been reported in AIDS patients. A morbilliform eruption is seen in approximately one-third of patients. CMV infection is seldom a source of morbidity and mortality in immunocompetent patients.

Of note, recurrent and, in particular, primary infections in pregnant women may lead to congenital CMV infection. These infants may have growth retardation, thrombocytopenic purpura, hepatosplenomegaly, jaundice, microcephaly, and chorioretinitis. The prognosis is generally poor.

Asymmetric Periflexural Exanthem of Childhood

APEC, also known as unilateral laterothoracic exanthem of childhood, is a self-limited inflammatory condition of infancy and early childhood. It is typically a mildly pruritic exanthem that usually follows a mild upper respiratory infection (URI) or GI illness. APEC occurs primarily in late winter and early spring and shows a 2:1 female-to-male predominance. Most patients are 2 to 3 years of age, although it has been described in children from 8 months to 10 years.

Fever is found in 40% of cases. Pruritus is noted in two-thirds of patients: mild intensity in one-fourth, moderate in nearly one-half, and severe in another one-third. Very rarely, children have an associated enanthem. Children may have low-grade or more significant fever. Lesions spontaneously resolve in 2 to 6 weeks.

◉ Look For

Rubeola (Measles)

An oral mucosal enanthem, referred to as Koplik spots, will develop prior to the generalized eruption. Koplik spots are minute, grayish-white papules with a central bluish-white speck. They are usually opposite the second molars. Bluish-gray or white spots can also be seen on the tonsils. These spots slough off as the morbilliform rash appears. This eruption is pathognomonic for measles.

The exanthem consists of erythematous macules and papules beginning behind the ears and at the forehead and then spreading down the neck, upper extremities, trunk, and finally the lower extremities (Figs. 4-60–4-62). Confluent lesions can occur on the face. The rash typically peaks for 3 to 4 days and then begins to fade at day 5, in the same cephalocaudad manner in which it appeared. Desquamation may take place after approximately 1 week. Thrombocytopenia, with resultant purpuric lesions, may complicate measles.

Variant: atypical measles (in those with killed vaccine or in whom immunization has failed) will spread from the extremities inward. Petechiae, vesicles, or papules can occur. Cough and conjunctivitis are not as marked as in typical rubeola.

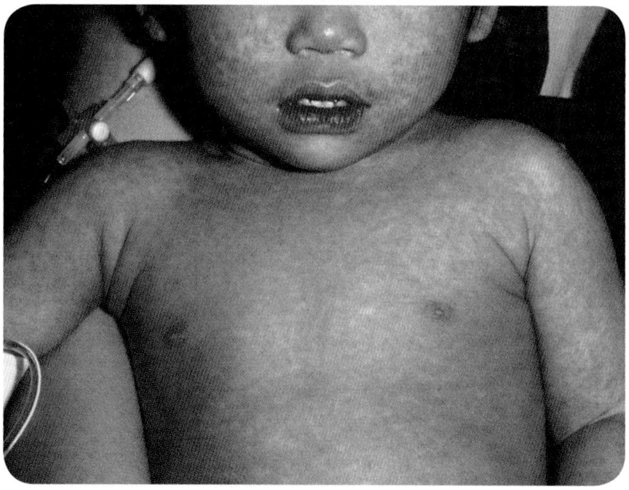

Figure 4-60 Measles in a child with multiple macules and papules.

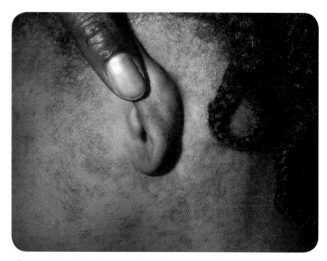
Figure 4-61 Measles eruption often appears behind the ears when it starts on the face.

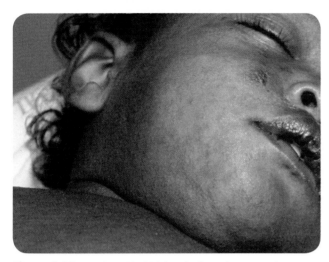

Figure 4-62 Measles with slightly raised papules on the face.

Cytomegalovirus Infection

The dermatologic manifestation most commonly associated with CMV infection is a generalized petechial exanthem (Fig. 4-63). In nonimmunocompromised patients, a morbilliform exanthem may occur in association with antibiotic therapy, similar to that occurring with EBV mononucleosis. Scarlatiniform, follicular, and urticarial eruptions have been seen. A CMV vasculitis, with disseminated palpable purpuric papules, has also been reported. Verrucous growths may have associated ulceration.

Cervical lymphadenopathy is often present.

Asymmetric Periflexural Exanthem of Childhood

Discrete 1-mm erythematous papules with occasional purpuric areas that coalesce into plaques. The lesions begin unilaterally, on the trunk or near large flexural areas (most often

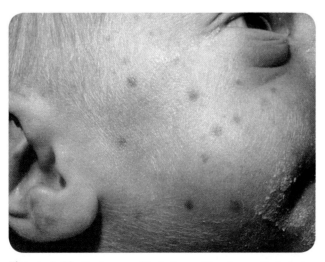

Figure 4-63 Blueberry muffin lesions with cytomegalic inclusion disease.

the axilla followed by inguinal), and spread centrifugally. New lesions appear on the adjacent trunk and extremity, with normal skin in between. A second stage involving the contralateral side occurs in most cases (65% to 70%) over 2 to 4 weeks, but the exanthem remains more prominent on one side. Lesions disappear with moderate desquamation within another 2 to 4 weeks.

Diagnostic Pearls

Rubeola (Measles)

Look for oral lesions called Koplik spots, which are minute red papules with a central bluish-white speck. The spots are usually opposite the second molars. Bluish-gray or white spots can also be seen on the tonsils.

Most populations have been immunized, but the disease should be suspected in migrant workers, those who are recent immigrants from countries with endemic disease, etc.

Cytomegalovirus Infection

In HIV-infected individuals, chronic perianal and lower-extremity ulcers, nodules, and purpura have been reported. The perianal lesions may be difficult to distinguish from other ulcerative processes and, therefore, require biopsy and culture.

Asymmetric Periflexural Exanthem of Childhood

The asymmetry of the eruption extending from a flexural area in combination with the young age suggests the diagnosis. Patients may have had an antecedent febrile viral illness. When patients or their parents show the eruption, it is through a "Statue of Liberty" (one arm extended upward) or "touchdown" (both arms extended upward) motion/position.

?? Differential Diagnosis and Pitfalls

Rubeola (Measles) and Cytomegalovirus Infection

- Morbilliform drug eruption
- Other infectious exanthems, including rubella, parvovirus B19, human herpesvirus-6, and dengue fever; mycoplasma, hepatitis B
- Rocky Mountain spotted fever
- Kawasaki disease
- Syphilis
- Leukocytoclastic vasculitis
- Graft versus host disease
- Before the eruption, it is easy to confuse rubeola with common URIs

- Bacterial sepsis
- Disseminated herpes simplex virus infection
- Primary HIV infection with mononucleosislike symptoms
- Primary toxoplasmosis
- Erythema multiforme
- Drug eruption
- Syphilis

Asymmetric Periflexural Exanthem of Childhood

- Seborrheic dermatitis can present with a flexural distribution.
- Gianotti-Crosti syndrome is a more diffuse papular exanthem that is not limited to one side and occurs more prominently over the knees and elbows as well as extensor surfaces.
- Other eruptive disorders of childhood, either infectious or systemic, may mimic APEC. APEC may be confused with more chronic dermatitis, especially atopic dermatitis, because of the associated pruritus and distribution of lesions during the final stage of eruption. The asymmetry, pruritus, and erythema suggest contact dermatitis in some children.

✓ Best Tests

Rubeola (Measles)

- The diagnosis can be made on clinical grounds, with the characteristic symptoms and cutaneous and oral findings as above.
- Given the rarity of measles in the United States, however, laboratory confirmation should be sought. The CDC has developed a highly specific and sensitive IgM enzyme immunoassay, which is considered the reference test in North America.
- If pneumonia or encephalitis is suspected, consider a chest X-ray or lumbar puncture, respectively.

Cytomegalovirus Infection

- CMV cultures of urine, saliva, semen, vaginal secretions, and tissue biopsies.
- Serological tests include the detection of CMV IgM, rising titers of complement fixation, and indirect fluorescent antibody (IFA) or anticomplement IFA.
- Antigen testing and both quantitative and qualitative PCR tests are now available.
- In the mononucleosis syndrome, atypical lymphocytes and a negative heterophil (monospot) are seen, sometimes with hemolytic anemia and elevated LFTs.

- Microscopically, the hallmark of CMV infection is a large (cytomegalic) cell with large, basophilic intranuclear "owl's eye" and intracytoplasmic inclusion bodies. A skin biopsy may aid in diagnosis.
- In cases of retinitis, funduscopic exam may show necrotic patches with white granular component of retina.
- Imaging and procedural studies that may be needed include chest X-ray, bronchoscopy, endoscopy, and CT scan or MRI.

Asymmetric Periflexural Exanthem of Childhood

This is a clinical diagnosis.

▲▲▲ Management Pearls

Rubeola (Measles)

- The measles vaccine contains live, attenuated virus and is given in concert with vaccinations for mumps and rubella (MMR). It is recommended that children in industrialized nations receive one dose at 12 to 15 months of age and another at 4 to 6 years of age. Claims that implicate the MMR vaccine as the cause of autism remain unproven. Increases in the number of unvaccinated individuals because of such claims are deleterious to herd immunity. Vaccination is contraindicated during pregnancy, however.
- Disease may be mitigated or prevented in nonimmune patients who have experienced an exposure by the administration of vaccine (up to 72 hours after the exposure) or measles immune globulin (may be given up to 6 days postexposure).

Precautions: Standard, contact, droplet, airborne. (Isolate the patient in a negative pressure room, wear respiratory protection [N95 mask], and limit patient transport.) Airborne transmission via aerosolized droplet nuclei has been documented in closed areas (e.g., an office examination room) for up to 2 hours after a person with measles occupied the area.

Note: Susceptible persons should not enter the room of patients known or suspected to have measles if other immune caregivers are available. If susceptible persons must enter the room of a patient known or suspected to have measles, they should wear respiratory protection (N95 respirator). Persons immune to measles need not wear respiratory protection.

Cytomegalovirus Infection

- Persistent perianal lesions may be herpetic, cytomegalic, or even related to amebiasis. Careful histology and cultures are necessary in immunosuppressed patients with such lesions.

- Depending on the clinical scenario, the following consultations may be needed: infectious diseases, neurology, critical care, gastroenterology, and/or ophthalmology.
- Patients with HIV/AIDS and CD4+ counts <50/mm³ should be on HAART with the goal of raising their CD4+ T-cell counts.

Precautions: Standard and contact (Isolate the patient, wear gloves and a gown, limit patient transport, and avoid sharing patient care equipment.)

Asymmetric Periflexural Exanthem of Childhood

APEC is a self-limited illness.

Therapy

Rubeola (Measles)
Treatment is supportive, as there is no specific therapy.

Consider vitamin A supplementation, especially in those who appear clinically deficient or otherwise malnourished. Vitamin A is recommended for hospitalized patients 6 months to 2 years of age or any patient over 6 months who has risk factors for severe involvement (immunodeficiency, impaired intestinal absorption, malnutrition, vitamin A deficiency). Supplementation has been associated with decreased morbidity and mortality in cases of measles in developing countries.

The use of ribavirin is considered experimental.

Passive immunization with human immunoglobulin (0.25 mg/kg) should be considered and can be effective up to 5 days postexposure.

Rest, antipyretics, and antitussives are appropriate adjunctive measures. Pay close attention to fluid balance, and keep the patient well hydrated. Patients who develop complications (pneumonia, encephalitis, severe diarrhea) may require hospitalization.

Identify and treat any complicating infections, such as bacterial pneumonia.

Cytomegalovirus Infection
Patients with healthy immune systems generally require only supportive therapy, as symptoms are self-limited. Immunocompromised patients and those with otherwise severe disease manifestations require active treatment and/or prophylaxis. These patients will most often require hospitalization and intensive supportive care.

Many of the drugs used to treat CMV infection have serious side effects. Consider consulting with a medical professional familiar with their usage prior to instituting therapy.

Prophylaxis in immunocompromised patients:

- High dose acyclovir (800 mg p.o. five times daily) can be used as prophylaxis but is ineffective against the active viral disease. Acyclovir is also not as effective as ganciclovir for prophylaxis.
- Ganciclovir 1 g p.o. three times daily. Oral valganciclovir (a prodrug) has not yet been studied as primary prophylaxis.
- Cidofovir 5 mg/kg IV once weekly for 2 weeks and then once every other week. Given with aggressive hydration and probenecid (2 g p.o. 3 hours before infusion and 1 g p.o. at hours 2 and 8 after infusion), as the drug is nephrotoxic.

Treatment of active disease in immunocompromised hosts:
Intravenous ganciclovir is the drug of choice. Induction therapy consists of 5 mg/kg IV administered over 1 hour every 12 hours for 14 to 21 days. Maintenance therapy consists of either 1 g p.o. three times daily or 5 mg/kg IV daily on 5 to 7 days of the week. Valganciclovir (900 mg p.o. daily) has better oral bioavailability and is largely replacing oral ganciclovir.

Foscarnet is an alternative, used most often in resistant cases. It may work synergistically with ganciclovir. Induction consists of 60 mg/kg IV every 8 hours for 14 to 21 days. Maintenance therapy is 90 to 120 mg/kg IV daily as a single infusion. **Caution:** Foscarnet is also nephrotoxic. Monitor renal function and be sure to keep the patient well hydrated.

CMV-specific immune globulin has been reported to be an effective means of prophylaxis in transplant recipients (especially kidney, lung, liver, pancreas, and heart). It is often given in combination with ganciclovir. Immune globulin has also been given as an adjunctive therapy in cases of CMV pneumonia.

Additionally, evidence exists in the Chinese literature for the possible use of hochu-ekki-to, a traditional Chinese herbal medication, in the treatment of CMV.

Asymmetric Periflexural Exanthem of Childhood
Oral antihistamines, antipruritic agents (e.g., pramoxine), and topical steroids may help with pruritus.

Suggested Readings

Cannon MJ. Congenital cytomegalovirus (CMV) epidemiology and awareness. *J Clin Virol.* 2009;46(Suppl 4):S6–S10. Epub 2009 Oct 2.

Coustou D, Léauté-Labrèze C, Bioulac-Sage P, et al. Asymmetric periflexural exanthem of childhood: A clinical, pathologic, and epidemiologic prospective study. *Arch Dermatol.* 1999;135(7):799–803.

Foti G, Hyeraci M, Kunkar A, et al. Cytomegalovirus infection in the adult. *Minerva Med.* 2002;93(2):109–117.

Hawker JI, Olowokure B, Wood AL, et al. Widening inequalities in MMR vaccine uptake rates among ethnic groups in an urban area of the UK during a period of vaccine controversy (1994–2000). *Vaccine.* 2007;25(43):7516–7519.

Hossain MS, Takimoto H, Hamano S. Protective effects of hochu-ekki-to, a Chinese traditional herbal medicine against murine cytomegalovirus infection. *Immunopharmacology.* 1999;41(3):169–181.

Hutchins SS, Jiles R, Bernier R. Elimination of measles and of disparities in measles childhood vaccine coverage among racial and ethnic minority populations in the United States. *J Infect Dis.* 2004;189(Suppl 1): S146–S152.

McCuaig CC, Russo P, Powell J, et al. Unilateral laterothoracic exanthem. A clinicopathologic study of forty-eight patients. *J Am Acad Dermatol.* 1996;34(6):979–984.

Pasquinelli L. Enterovirus infections. *Pediatr Rev.* 2006;27(2):e14–e15.

Sawyer MH. Enterovirus infections: Diagnosis and treatment. *Curr Opin Pediatr.* 2001;13(1):65–69.

Stalkup JR, Chilukuri S. Enterovirus infections: A review of clinical presentation, diagnosis, and treatment. *Dermatol Clin.* 2002;20(2):217–223.

Taïeb A, Mégraud F, Legrain V, et al. Asymmetric periflexural exanthem of childhood. *J Am Acad Dermatol.* 1993;29(3):391–393.

Yang Y, Sujan S, Sun F, et al. Acute metabolic crisis induced by vaccination in seven chinese patients. *Pediatr Neurol.* 2006;35(2):114–118.

Erythema Infectiosum (Fifth Disease)

Laurie Good

Diagnosis Synopsis

Erythema infectiosum, or fifth disease, is a common illness in young children caused by infection with human parvovirus B19. Infection can result in a mild exanthem, no exanthem, or the typical "slapped cheeks" rash. Children may have a prodromal headache with associated low-grade fever and rhinorrhea beginning 2 days before the onset of the rash. Children recover spontaneously without therapy.

The classic presentation—erythema of the cheeks—occurs most commonly in children. This facial erythema, however, may not be appreciable on more darkly pigmented skin. In fact, in dark-skinned patients without anemia, it may go unnoticed entirely. One study found that asymptomatic infections are more common in black individuals than in whites (68% vs. 20%, respectively). Arthropathy is a fairly common complicating sequela of erythema infectiosum and, when it occurs, usually persists for several months. A meta-analysis conducted in Chinese literature found a significant association between infection with parvovirus B19 and childhood idiopathic thrombocytopenia in China.

Although seropositivity is found among the majority of women of childbearing age, a substantial percentage of women worldwide are still vulnerable to primary infection with human parvovirus B19. Epidemiologic studies in women in Libya, Kuwait, Iran, and Brazil showed anti-B19 IgG seroprevalence in 51%, 53%, 66%, and 71% of women, respectively, demonstrating immunity to primary infection with human parvovirus B19 when in the absence of IgM (only present in 2% to 5%).

When a primary infection occurs in early pregnancy, the consequences on the developing fetus can be devastating. Hydrops fetalis, chronic anemia, and intrauterine death are all possible outcomes, and immunocompromised women are at particularly high risk of having such fetal complications.

Although rare, human parvovirus B19 has gained recognition for its role in persistent anemia in HIV-positive patients and solid organ transplant hosts. Most cases respond to intravenous immunoglobulin (IVIG).

Look For

Erythema of the cheeks is a classic finding (Fig. 4-64); however, this may be subtle or not appreciable in patients with darker pigmentation.

Classically, the rash in children with erythema infectiosum goes through three phases. After several days of a nonspecific flulike illness, an exanthem abruptly begins with the appearance of asymptomatic macular diffuse erythema involving the bilateral cheeks (slapped cheek appearance).

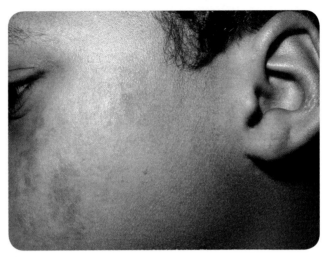

Figure 4-64 The face is a common location for erythema infectiosum and may have multiple papules instead of the classical slapped-face appearance.

One to four days later, a lacy reticulated eruption consisting of discrete erythematous macules and papules appears on the proximal extremities. The trunk later becomes involved. The third stage is marked by a recurrence of a milder form of the eruption after exposure to heat, friction, or sunlight or in response to crying or exercise. Roughly 7% of children with erythema infectiosum develop mild arthralgias that resolve within several weeks.

Diagnostic Pearls

Bright redness of the cheeks, most intense beneath the eyes, is the classic initial sign with sparing of eyelids, chin, and perioral area. This may not be noticeable on more deeply pigmented skin.

Differential Diagnosis and Pitfalls

- Scarlet fever—typically begins on the neck and trunk and then later involves the extremities. Patients also display signs and symptoms of streptococcal pharyngitis.
- Rubella—starts on the face and progresses caudad, covering the entire body in 1 day and resolving by the third day. Red macules or petechiae may be seen on the soft palate and uvula (Forchheimer sign).
- Roseola infantum—3 days of high fever followed by the appearance of a morbilliform erythema upon defervescence consisting of rose-colored macules on the neck, trunk, and buttocks. Mucous membranes are spared.

- Erysipelas of the face—an acute beta-hemolytic Group A streptococcal infection of the skin involving the superficial dermal lymphatics. Skin lesions have a distinctive raised, sharply demarcated advancing edge.
- Rubeola (measles)—is marked by the appearance of morbilliform lesions on the scalp and behind the ears that spread to involve the trunk and extremities over 2 to 3 days. Koplik spots are pathognomonic and appear during the prodromal phase.
- A careful history should help distinguish from a potential drug eruption.

✓ Best Tests

This is usually a clinical diagnosis, and testing in otherwise healthy patients with erythema infectiosum is not indicated; however, in pregnant women, patients with hemolytic disease, or those experiencing arthropathy, serologic testing (RIA or ELISA) in the presence of human parvovirus B19-induced acute exanthems will reveal elevated specific IgM and IgG antibodies. IgM will be positive within days of onset and remain positive for several weeks, while IgG antibodies will be positive 3 weeks after infection and remain positive for life. DNA PCR should be used to test for infection in immunosuppressed and immunocompromised patients.

▲▲ Management Pearls

- Reassure the parents that the eruption can persist and be exacerbated by warmth and sunlight over a period of weeks to months. Patients are infectious from 7 days before the onset of the rash and are not infectious once the exanthem appears.
- Pregnant women up to 21 weeks pregnant, immunocompromised patients, and patients with hemoglobinopathies are at elevated risk for complications. Those with elevated risk who have shared a room for >15 minutes or had face-to-face contact with a laboratory-confirmed case should be evaluated by their physician, and laboratory evaluation (serologies or viral titers) should be considered to rule out infection.

Suggested Readings

Chorba T, Coccia P, Holman RC, et al. The role of parvovirus B19 in aplastic crisis and erythema infectiosum (fifth disease). *J Infect Dis.* 1986;154(3):383–393.

Elnifro E, Nisha AK, Almabsoot M, et al. Seroprevalence of parvovirus B19 among pregnant women in Tripoli, Libya. *J Infect Dev Ctries.* 2009;3(3):218–220.

Maksheed M, Pacsa AS, Essa SS, et al. The prevalence of antibody to human parvovirus B19 in pregnant women in Kuwait. *Acta Trop.* 1999;73(3):225–229.

Ziyaeyan M, Rasouli M, Alborzi A. The seroprevalence of parvovirus B19 infection among to-be-married girls, pregnant women, and their neonates in Shiraz, Iran. *Jpn J Infect Dis.* 2005;58(2):95–97.

Gianotti-Crosti Syndrome

Laurie Good

Diagnosis Synopsis

Gianotti-Crosti syndrome (papular acrodermatitis of childhood, papulovesicular acrolated syndrome) is a self-limiting dermatosis likely triggered by viral infection.

The eruption of Gianotti-Crosti syndrome typically lasts 3 to 4 weeks and is usually seen in preschool children but can be seen in children aged 6 months to 14 years. The lesions can last up to 8 weeks before resolving spontaneously.

Agents thought to be responsible for the typical eruption include hepatitis B virus, hepatitis A and C viruses, cytomegalovirus (CMV), Epstein-Barr virus (EBV), enteroviruses, rotavirus, respiratory syncytial virus, parvovirus B19, vaccinia virus, rubella virus, HIV-1, and parainfluenza virus. The syndrome has also been observed following immunizations against poliovirus, diphtheria, pertussis, Japanese encephalitis, influenza, and hepatitis B virus and measles (together). In regions with low hepatitis B prevalence, the most common trigger is believed to be EBV, while in areas of higher hepatitis B prevalence (Sub-Saharan Africa, Southeast Asia, China, Indonesia, etc.), hepatitis B virus is still the most common cause of Gianotti-Crosti syndrome. The clinical features of the syndrome are identical, independent of the triggering agent.

With widespread immunization, most cases of Gianotti-Crosti syndrome seen in the United States, Canada, Europe, and India are not associated with hepatitis B virus infection. EBV is by far the most common cause in the United States.

Look For

Symmetrically distributed, monomorphous, pink-brown, flat-topped papules or papulovesicles 1 to 10 mm in diameter on the face, extensor limbs, and buttocks (Figs. 4-65 and 4-66). Lesions initially appear on the buttocks and spread distally. The torso is typically spared or minimally affected, and scale is absent. Lesions may be pruritic. Mucous membranes are not involved.

Additional manifestations of the disease include low-grade fever, enlarged inguinal and axillary lymph nodes, and an enlarged spleen. When hepatitis B virus is implicated as a trigger, acute viral hepatitis occurs at the same time or 1 to 2 weeks after the onset of the skin eruption. Hepatomegaly may be prominent in these cases.

Diagnostic Pearls

Monomorphic erythematous to brown papules involve the face, buttocks, and extensor extremities. There is relative sparing of the torso and popliteal fossae.

Differential Diagnosis and Pitfalls

- Erythema multiforme presents with targetoid lesions, often best seen on the palms and soles. The patient may have coexisting herpes orolabialis.

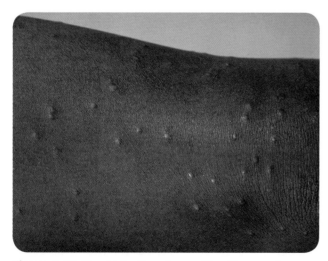

Figure 4-65 Gianotti-Crosti syndrome with uniform papules on an extremity.

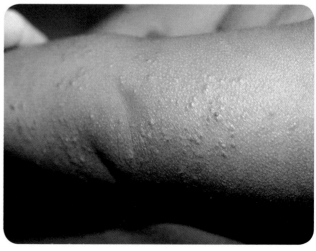

Figure 4-66 Gianotti-Crosti syndrome with uniform slightly red papules on an extremity.

- Henoch-Schönlein purpura presents with palpable purpura over the bilateral lower extremities.
- Lichen planus typically presents with pruritic, flat-topped, polygonal, violaceous papules on the volar wrists and ankles. Mucosal and nail findings frequently aid in the clinical diagnosis.
- Inflamed lesions of molluscum contagiosum may mimic those seen in Gianotti-Crosti syndrome but tend to be concentrated within the groin and axillae as well as antecubital and popliteal fossae. The presence of noninflamed molluscum lesions is a helpful clue.
- A detailed history is helpful in distinguishing this entity from a drug eruption.
- Id reaction (autoeczematization) secondary to a primary severe inflammatory dermatosis elsewhere (allergic contact dermatitis, dermatophytosis, bacterial infection)
- Scabies can present very similarly, but a negative skin scrape and lack of affected contacts can rule it out.

 Best Tests

Liver function tests and hepatitis serologies may be performed if the patient has not been immunized against hepatitis B virus previously.

 Management Pearls

The eruption of Gianotti-Crosti syndrome spontaneously resolves, usually over a period of 3 to 4 weeks. Associated lymphadenopathy may persist for 2 to 3 months. Investigate for triggers such as viral hepatitis, CMV, and EBV only if indicated.

Therapy

The treatment for Gianotti-Crosti syndrome is supportive. No treatment appears to shorten the course of the disease.

Suggested Readings

Baleviciené G, Maciuleviciené R, Schwartz RA. Papular acrodermatitis of childhood: The Gianotti-Crosti syndrome. *Cutis.* 2001;67(4):291–294.

Brandt O, Abeck D, Gianotti R, et al. Gianotti-Crosti syndrome. *J Am Acad Dermatol.* 2006;54(1):136–145. Epub 2005 Dec 2.

Fastenberg M, Morrell DS. Acral papules: Gianotti-Crosti syndrome. *Pediatr Ann.* 2007;36(12):800–804.

Karakaş M, Durdu M, Tuncer I, et al. Gianotti-Crosti syndrome in a child following hepatitis B virus vaccination. *J Dermatol.* 2007;34(2): 117–120.

Lowe L, Hebert AA, Duvic M. Gianotti-Crosti syndrome associated with Epstein-Barr virus infection. *J Am Acad Dermatol.* 1989;20(2 Pt 2): 336–338.

Cellulitis

Mat Davey

▪▪ Diagnosis Synopsis

Cellulitis

Cellulitis is a common bacterial infection of the dermis and subcutaneous tissue characterized by erythema, pain, warmth, and swelling. For discussion on a related condition, omphalitis, see VisualDx online. (If you are a first-time online user, go to www.essentialdermatology.com/pigmented; if you already have your password set up, go directly to www.visualdx.com/visualdx.) It occurs at any age, in both sexes, and in any ethnicity, but it is most commonly found in men aged 45 to 65. Causes of cellulitis are strongly correlated with age and immune status and include the following:

- Immunocompetent adults: *Staphylococcus aureus* (methicillin sensitive or methicillin resistant) and *Streptococcus pyogenes*, less commonly non-group A beta-hemolytic streptococci, and *Pasteurella multocida* (usually acquired from animal bites).
- Immunocompromised individuals, including those with diabetes, venous insufficiency, or decubitus ulcers: mixture of Gram-positive cocci and Gram-negative aerobes including *Streptococcus pneumoniae*, *Campylobacter jejuni*, *Bacteroides fragilis*, *Yersinia enterocolitica*, and *Cryptococcus*. *Haemophilus influenzae* may cause plaques of cellulitis on the face, although in most western countries, this disease has been markedly decreased by the HiB vaccine.

The most common routes of bacterial seeding in immunocompetent and immunocompromised individuals are direct bacterial inoculation and hematogenous seeding, respectively. Risk factors include minor skin trauma, body piercing, tinea pedis infection, injection drug use, animal bites, and surgical procedures. Additional predisposing factors include alcoholism, diabetes, peripheral vascular disease, nephrotic syndrome, and immunocompromised states.

As opposed to impetigo, in cellulitis and erysipelas, systemic symptoms of fevers, chills, and malaise often precede or coincide with the appearance of the skin lesions. Complications are not common but can include glomerulonephritis, lymphadenitis, and subacute bacterial endocarditis. If left untreated, both cellulitis and erysipelas can be complicated by bacteremia and death.

Of note, a rising prevalence of community-acquired methicillin-resistant *S. aureus* (CA-MRSA) has increasingly been identified as a pathogen of skin and soft tissue infections in otherwise healthy individuals lacking the traditional risk factors for such infections (IV drug use, incarceration, participation in contact sports, etc.). Antibiotic coverage must take into account the risk of MRSA. It is helpful to be aware of patterns of antimicrobial resistance within your local community.

Pediatric Patient Considerations

H. influenzae may cause plaques of cellulitis on the face in young children, but the incidence of this infection in western countries has been markedly decreased by the HiB vaccine (**Fig. 4-67**).

Perianal Streptococcal Cellulitis

Perianal streptococcal cellulitis, or perianal streptococcal dermatitis, is a fairly common, often unrecognized variant of cutaneous streptococcal infection. It may present as chronic diaper dermatitis or, alternatively, as an acute symptomatic cellulitis. Affected children usually range in age from 6 months to 10 years, although cases have been reported in both adolescents and adults. Presenting symptoms include painful defecation, fecal hoarding behavior, and incontinence. Blood-streaked stool and anal fissures may also be noted. Balanitis may occur in male patients. Vulvovaginal involvement has been reported in female patients but is less commonly reported than balanitis in male patients.

◉ Look For

Cellulitis

In cellulitis, look for poorly defined borders, erythema, swelling, tenderness, and warmth (**Fig. 4-68**). In the extremities, unilateral edema of the affected limb is not uncommon. Lymphangitis and inflammation of regional lymph nodes often occur. In severe cases, vesicles, bullae, ecchymoses, and petechiae may be present (**Fig. 4-69**).

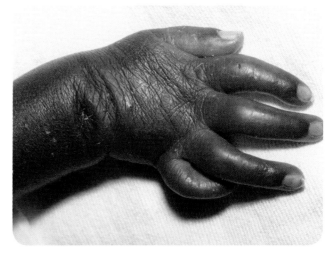

Figure 4-67 *Haemophilus influenzae* cellulitis of the hand. *H. influenzae* skin infections are rare, since *H. influenzae* vaccination is almost universal in some countries. The face was a common location in the past.

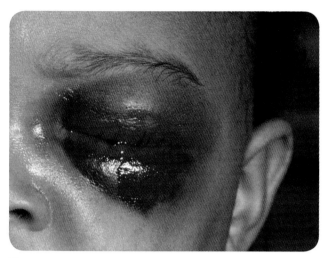

Figure 4-68 Cellulitis with redness and edema of the soft tissues of the eye and the orbit.

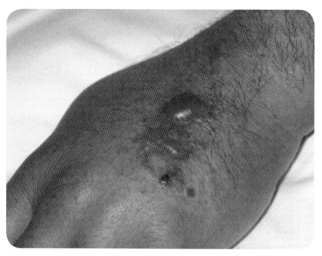

Figure 4-69 Cellulitis, in addition to edema, erythema, and warmth, frequently has purpura or, as in this instance, hemorrhagic vesicles and bullae.

Perianal Streptococcal Cellulitis

In perianal streptococcal cellulitis, look for perianal erythema and moist superficial erosions with well-defined margins. Genitalia may be involved. Fissures and scaling plaques may be present.

 Diagnostic Pearls

Cellulitis

- Presence of bullae and crepitus in the soft tissue infections along with severe localized pain are signs of necrotizing fasciitis, requiring immediate surgical intervention.
- A tender, edematous extremity with minimal overlying erythema strongly suggests a process affecting deeper tissues (Fig. 4-70). Rule out necrotizing infection if there is significant pain, and rule out deep venous thrombosis.
- If redness and involvement of the legs are bilateral in a patient suspected to have cellulitis, consider an alternative diagnosis. Cellulitis virtually never occurs bilaterally at the same time. Stasis dermatitis and contact dermatitis are frequent causes of bilateral severe leg or foot redness.

Perianal Streptococcal Cellulitis

Streptococcal infections may be especially serious in those with sickle cell disease. Guttate psoriasis can appear as a sign of occult streptococcal infection. Poststreptococcal acute nephritis and rheumatism can occur as a result of streptococcal infection.

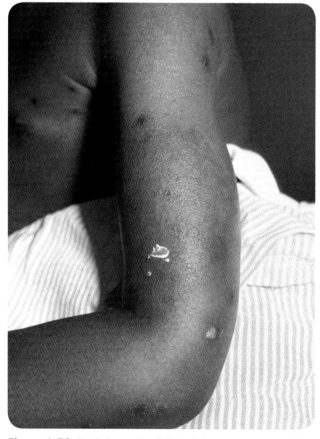

Figure 4-70 Staphylococcal cellulitis of the upper arm area with a sharp border of erythema.

?? Differential Diagnosis and Pitfalls

Impetigo/Cellulitis/Erysipelas

- Stasis dermatitis
- Erythema nodosum (panniculitis)
- Erysipeloid
- Lipodermatosclerosis
- Thrombophlebitis
- Contact dermatitis
- Necrotizing fasciitis
- Deep vein thrombosis
- Herpes zoster
- Erythema chronicum migrans (Lyme disease)
- Vasculitis—polyarteritis nodosa
- Inflammatory carcinoma of the breast
- Eosinophilic cellulitis (Well syndrome)
- Urticaria
- Sweet syndrome

Perianal Streptococcal Cellulitis

- Candidiasis
- Psoriasis
- Seborrheic dermatitis
- Contact dermatitis
- Pinworms
- Sexual abuse

✓ Best Tests

- Diagnosis is most often made clinically. Mark the leading edge of erythema in patients with cellulitis or erysipelas with pen or marker, and check every 4 to 6 hours. If progressive after 24 hours of therapy, consider more aggressive therapy or other etiologies. Surgical consultation is recommended if necrotizing fasciitis is a possibility. MRI can be performed to evaluate deeper tissue involvement.
- Wound cultures for bacterial identification and antibiotic susceptibility should be obtained. Sensitivities should be performed on any *S. aureus* isolates to determine antibiotic resistance. Consider oropharyngeal, nasal, and conjunctival cultures if there is facial involvement. If diagnosis is in doubt, biopsy can be performed and sent for Gram stain and tissue culture.
- A CBC may show normal or elevated white blood cells. Blood cultures are of very little utility in patients lacking signs of systemic toxicity (tachycardia, hypotension).

▲▲ Management Pearls

Cellulitis

- In patients with recurring cellulitis, treatment aims should include the aggressive management of any underlying predisposing condition such as tinea pedis, stasis dermatitis, or other chronic skin disease. Reports of the efficacy of prophylactic antibiotics in such cases are mixed.
- Given the prevalence of MRSA, maintain a high index of suspicion for this diagnosis and make the initial choice of empiric antibiotic therapy accordingly. It is helpful to be aware of patterns of antimicrobial resistance within your community. In patients with recurrent MRSA infections, eradication of MRSA nasal carriage may be accomplished by application of mupirocin 2% cream (twice daily for 5 days) to the nares. The combination of rifampin (600 mg daily for 10 days) plus TMP-SMX (1 double-strength tab twice daily for 10 days) has also been shown to eradicate colonization.

Perianal Streptococcal Cellulitis

- In patients with suspected perianal streptococcal infections, a rapid streptococcal test may yield positive results. Culture perirectal as well as pharyngeal sites for group A streptococci.
- In pediatric patients with known group A streptococcal infection, posttreatment culture should be sent to confirm complete treatment. Additionally, a urinalysis should be obtained around 1 month after treatment is complete to evaluate for poststreptococcal glomerulonephritis.

Therapy

Most of these infections are caused by *S. aureus* or *S. pyogenes*, so the same antibiotic regimen may be used for impetigo, cellulitis, and erysipelas:

- Dicloxacillin 250 to 500 mg p.o. every 6 hours
- Amoxicillin plus clavulanic acid 250 to 500 mg p.o. every 6 hours
- Cephalexin 250 to 500 mg p.o. every 6 hours
- Azithromycin 500 mg p.o. one time, then 250 mg p.o. daily (used for patients with penicillin allergy)

Most patients with mild cellulitis can be treated and followed on an outpatient basis with a 7- to 14-day course of oral antibiotics.

Patients exhibiting signs or symptoms of systemic involvement or with rapidly progressing infections or patients with significant comorbidities (i.e., immunosuppression) should be hospitalized for observation, and initiation of an antibiotic covering MRSA should be pursued as follows:

- Vancomycin 30 mg/kg/d IV divided twice daily or linezolid 600 mg IV or p.o. every 12 hours

Pediatric Patient Considerations

Cellulitis
The majority of cases can be treated on an outpatient basis. Antibiotics should include *S. aureus* and *S. pyogenes* coverage such as those used for impetigo but for 10 to 14 days. Other therapies are discussed online.

For infections in which an organism cannot be identified:

- Cefazolin 50 to 100 mg/kg/d, not to exceed 6 g/d, p.o. divided three times daily for 10 days

For *H. influenzae*:

- Cefotaxime 100 to 200 mg/kg/d p.o. divided three times daily for 7 days
- Ceftriaxone 50 to 100 mg/kg/d IM/IV daily for 7 to 14 days
- Chloramphenicol 75 to 100 mg/kg/d p.o. divided four times daily for 7 to 14 days

Patients with facial/orbital cellulitis along with those exhibiting signs or symptoms of systemic involvement or with rapidly progressing infections or significant comorbidities (i.e., immunosuppressed) should be hospitalized for observation and parenteral antibiotic administration. Suggested regimens include the following:

- Nafcillin or oxacillin 100 to 150 mg/kg/d IV divided into four doses or cefazolin 50 mg/kg/d IV divided into three doses

Critically ill patients with MRSA or suspected MRSA should receive vancomycin or linezolid:

- Vancomycin 40 mg/kg/d IV divided into four doses or linezolid 10 mg/kg IV or p.o. every 12 hours

Perianal Streptococcal Infection
While topical antibiotics may be used as monotherapy for less severe cases, oral antibiotics are recommended as first-line treatment for most patients. Suggest a 10- to 14-day course of antibiotics.

Suggested Readings

Bernard P. Management of common bacterial infections in the skin. *Curr Opin Infect Dis.* 2008;21(2):122–128.

Craft NC, Lee PK, Zipoli, MT, et al. Superficial cutaneous infections and pyodermas. In: Fitzpatrick TB, Wolff K, eds. *Fitzpatrick's Dermatology in General Medicine.* 7th Ed. New York, NY: McGraw-Hill; 2008: 1694–1703.

Elston DM. Community-acquired methicillin-resistant *Staphylococcus aureus. J Am Acad Dermatol.* 2007;56(1):1–16; quiz 17–20.

James WD, Berger TG, Elston DM, eds. *Andrews' Diseases of the Skin: Clinical Dermatology.* 10th Ed. Philadelphia, PA: Saunders Elsevier; 2006:251–264.

Stevens DL, Bisno AL, Chambers HF, et al. Infectious Diseases Society of America. Practice guidelines for the diagnosis and management of skin and soft-tissue infections. *Clin Infect Dis.* 2005;41(10):1373–1406.

Dermatomyositis

Mat Davey

Diagnosis Synopsis

Dermatomyositis (DM) is a multisystem autoimmune disease characterized by a symmetric, proximal, extensor inflammatory myopathy, a characteristic violaceous cutaneous eruption, and pathogenic circulating autoantibodies. Amyopathic DM typically has characteristic cutaneous changes, but subclinical or absent myopathy.

Clinical features of DM can be categorized into cutaneous and systemic manifestations. Cutaneous features are quite characteristic and may precede muscle disease by several weeks to years. Extreme pruritus is common, and sunlight may exacerbate the cutaneous eruption.

Systemic manifestations of DM include fatigue, malaise, and myalgias. In patients with myositis, proximal extensor muscle group inflammation (triceps and quadriceps) leads to muscle pain and weakness. Dysphagia may be seen in patients with scleroderma overlap. Some level of pulmonary involvement will be present in 15% to 30% of patients. The presence of autoantibodies to aminoacyl-tRNA synthetase (anti-Jo-1, anti-PL-7, anti-PL-12, anti-OJ, anti-EJ, and anti-KS) correlates well with the development of pulmonary disease, with manifestations ranging from mild diffuse interstitial fibrosis to severe acute respiratory distress syndrome. Cardiac involvement is usually asymptomatic, although arrhythmias can be seen.

Acute cases of DM may be fatal, with death due to mechanical respiratory failure, aspiration pneumonia, intestinal perforation, and heart failure. Pulmonary hypertension with cor pulmonale has been observed. A chronic fluctuating course is most common, but rapid progression is most common in young patients and malignancy-associated cases.

DM is more likely than polymyositis to be associated with an underlying neoplasm. In women, there may be a particular association with ovarian cancer. Other associations include thymoma, hemolytic anemia, Hashimoto thyroiditis, multiple myeloma, and linear morphea.

DM demonstrates a bimodal incidence, with the adult form most commonly seen in individuals aged 45 to 60 and the juvenile form found in children aged 10 to 15 years. A 2:1 female-to-male incidence ratio exists in adults, and dark-skinned individuals outnumber whites 4:1. Black women of childbearing age are the most frequently affected population. Among Asian populations, men are more likely affected than women.

Pediatric Patient Considerations

Childhood-type DM, also known as juvenile-onset DM, is typically first detected in children aged between 2 and 15 years. Clinical findings are similar to those in adult-onset DM, with the addition of calcinosis cutis, vasculitic lesions (manifested by infarctive or purpuric lesions), and GI ulceration being more common. In juvenile-onset DM, no significant ethnic predilection is present.

Look For

- Heliotrope rash, a violaceous, edematous, periorbital erythema that may be slightly scaly, is considered pathognomonic for DM (Figs. 4-71 and 4-72).
- Poikilodermatous changes with violaceous erythema, hyperpigmentation and hypopigmentation, telangiectasia, and variable atrophy are often present over the posterior neck and shoulders (shawl sign). This can be exacerbated by ultraviolet light (Fig. 4-73).
- Photosensitivity can occur even in those with type IV and type V skin. The upper back is a common location.

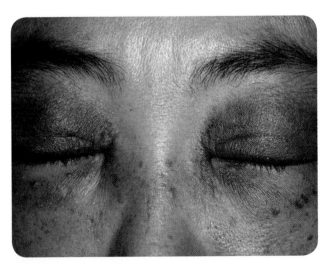

Figure 4-71 Heliotrope eyelid edema in DM.

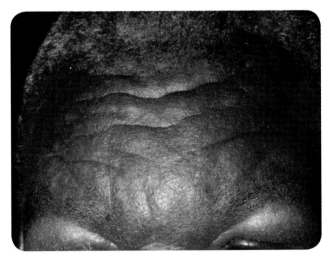

Figure 4-72 DM with forehead and eyelid edema.

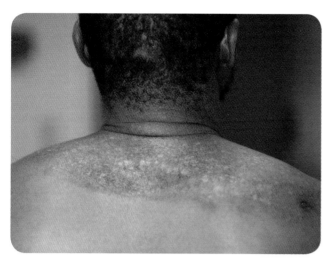

Figure 4-73 DM with diffuse shawl-like hyperpigmentation with some hypopigmentation.

- Gottron papules appear as red to purple, scaly, flat-topped papules on the dorsal knuckles. They may be telangiectatic and may eventually atrophy.
- Erythema and telangiectases at the proximal nail folds are seen with some capillary loops exaggerated. Thickening, roughness, hyperkeratosis, and irregularity of the cuticle with little or no redness are frequent. Fingers may appear more sausage-like than with systemic lupus erythematosus (SLE).
- "Mechanic's hands" refers to the hyperkeratosis, scaling, fissuring, and hyperpigmentation on the ulnar aspect of the thumb and radial side of the fingers.
- Other cutaneous manifestations include vesicles, bullae, lichenoid papules, and calcinosis cutis.
- Lesions are frequently symmetrical (Fig. 4-74).
- Facial lesions involve the nasolabial fold, which is usually spared in lupus erythematosus (Fig. 4-75).
- Scalp involvement may be present in the majority of patients but is frequently misdiagnosed as psoriasis or seborrheic dermatitis. Scalp lesions generally appear as diffuse, atrophic, erythematous, scaly plaques, often with some degree of alopecia.
- In patients with darker skin types, the above violaceous and poikilodermatous changes are less noticeable than in those with lighter skin types.

Pediatric Patient Considerations

Calcinosis cutis is more common in children. Look for cutaneous ulcers and/or infarctive or purpuric lesions.

Diagnostic Pearls

- Gottron papules are specific for DM and are seen in approximately 80% of patients.

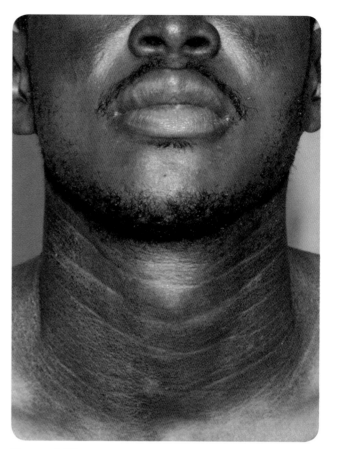

Figure 4-74 DM with symmetrical inflammatory plaques on the face, neck, and upper chest.

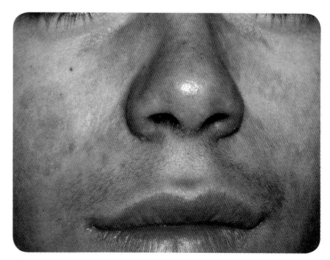

Figure 4-75 Red plaques on the face in DM, not sparing the naso-labial fold.

- The photosensitivity can be pruritic and profound, leading to bullous lesions.
- Nailfold lesions may be present early in the course, and the nails should be carefully examined with good light and magnification.

- Poor prognostic factors include cardiac or pulmonary involvement, dysphagia, severe muscle weakness, older age, delay of therapy, and malignancies.
- The most underdiagnosed form of the disease is the eruption without muscle lesions (amyopathic DM).

Differential Diagnosis and Pitfalls

- Lupus erythematosus
- CREST syndrome
- Polymorphous light eruption
- Contact dermatitis
- Seborrheic dermatitis
- Scleroderma
- Graft versus host disease
- Mixed connective tissue disease
- Generalized morphea
- Polymyositis
- Acute lesions of erythropoietic protoporphyria
- Atopic dermatitis
- Psoriasis
- Lichen planus

For patients with myositis, one must rule out scleroderma, polymyositis, mixed connective tissue disease, and lupus erythematosus.

✓ Best Tests

Skin

- Skin biopsy—mucin deposition in the dermis, lymphocytic infiltrate, epidermal atrophy, vacuolar changes of the basal keratinocytes. Note: Skin biopsy does not distinguish DM from SLE.

Muscle

- Electromyogram—Look for altered electrical conduction.
- MRI (is replacing triceps muscle biopsy: see below)—Look for increased T2-weighted signal density of triceps of quadriceps.
- Serum muscle enzymes (aldolase, CPK, SGOT, AST, and LDH)—Look for elevated levels during exacerbations.
- Triceps muscle biopsy (gold standard)—Look for type II muscle fiber atrophy, lymphocytes in perifascicular and perivascular distribution, necrosis, and sarcolemmal nuclei that are centrally placed.

Pulmonary

- High-resolution CT—Look for interstitial pulmonary fibrosis.
- Pulmonary function tests.

Cardiac

- ECG for conduction and rhythm aberrancies.

Autoantibodies

- Antinuclear antibodies are present in up to 80% of patients.
- Jo-1 antibody (present in 20% of patients) and other autoantibodies to aminoacyl-tRNA synthetase correlate with the development of pulmonary disease.
- Anti-Mi-2 antibody (present in 15% of patients) is associated with acute onset of classic DM and a good prognosis.

Additional studies, for example, dysphagia and barium swallow, should be performed based on symptoms.

Management Pearls

- Once a diagnosis of DM is confirmed, all adults older than 50 years should be screened for underlying malignancy. Initial cancer screening and vigilant serial monitoring for 2 to 3 years postdiagnosis are strongly recommended, as up to 30% of patients have an occult malignancy. The underlying malignancy, when present, can usually be presumptively diagnosed from careful history and physical and routine screening tests appropriate for the age. Cancer screening studies can include colonoscopy, mammography, stool occult blood test, and CBC. Chest, abdomen, and pelvis CT scanning—even in the absence of symptoms—should be considered. Ovarian cancer is more frequently observed, but the other malignancies are similar to those found in the general population.
- Photosensitivity is frequently present and should be managed with 45 SPF or opaque sunscreens when necessary. It is important to impress upon darkly pigmented patients the important role that sun protection and sun-avoidance techniques play in their therapy.
- Exercise should be avoided during acute episodes of myositis.
- Have the patient contact the National Dermatomyositis and Polymyositis Support Group.
- The care of patients with DM is multidisciplinary, including a rheumatologist and/or a neurologist. Patients may benefit from the expertise of a physical or occupational therapist.

Caution: Hydroxyurea, penicillamine, nonsteroidal anti-inflammatory drugs, tryptophan, and practolol have been reported to cause DM-like skin lesions.

Pediatric Patient Considerations

Internal malignancy is uncommon in juvenile-onset DM. Cancer screening is not warranted.

Therapy

Treatment strategy should be primarily dictated by the degree of muscle disease and additional internal organ involvement.

Treatment of Skin Disease

Note that cutaneous disease in DM is notoriously difficult to treat. Sun avoidance and appropriate protection remain key interventions. Sunscreens that contain both UVB and UVA blockers (Parsol 1789 or titanium dioxide) should be used. For lesions on the trunk and extremities, high-potency (classes 1 and 2) topical steroids applied twice daily may control inflammation and itch. These agents should not be used on the face, genitals, or intertriginous areas; low- to moderate-potency (classes 5 to 7) topical steroids should be implemented instead. In some patients, hydroxychloroquine 200 to 400 mg p.o. daily has improved skin lesions.

Treatment of Muscle Disease

Prednisone 1 to 2 mg/kg p.o. daily remains the mainstay of therapy in patients with systemic disease. Treatment should continue until symptoms reside and be followed by a very slow prednisone taper. Methotrexate and azathioprine have been used in patients as steroid-sparing agents. In addition, mycophenolate mofetil, infliximab, intravenous immunoglobulin, and, recently, rituximab have been effective in some patients.

Pediatric Patient Considerations

In the severe systemic juvenile-onset DM, pulse intravenous methylprednisolone (30 mg/kg/d) or high-dose oral prednisone (1 to 2 mg/kg/d) is the mainstay of therapy. In addition, topical treatments and sun-protective methods listed above may improve skin lesions.

Suggested Readings

Abreu Velez AM, Howard MS. Diagnosis and treatment of cutaneous paraneoplastic syndromes. *Dermatol Ther.* 2010;23(6):662–675.

Callen JP, Wortmann RL. Dermatomyositis. *Clin Dermatol.* 2006;24(5): 363–373.

Feldman BM, Rider LG, Reed AM, et al. Juvenile dermatomyositis and other idiopathic inflammatory myopathies of childhood. *Lancet.* 2008;371(9631):2201–2212.

James WD, Berger TG, Elston DM, eds. *Andrews' Diseases of the Skin: Clinical Dermatology.* 10th Ed. Philadelphia, PA: Saunders Elsevier; 2006: 166–171.

Peloro TM, Miller OF, Hahn TF, et al. Juvenile dermatomyositis: A retrospective review of a 30-year experience. *J Am Acad Dermatol.* 2001;45(1):28–34.

Sontheimer RD, Costner MI. Dermatomyositis. In: Fitzpatrick TB, Wolff K, eds. *Fitzpatrick's Dermatology in General Medicine.* 7th Ed. New York, NY: McGraw-Hill; 2008:1536–1553.

Erythema Annulare Centrifugum and Lyme Disease

Naurin Ahmad

Large moving distinctive rashes may be associated with internal diseases, especially arthritis. Two of these eruptions, erythema annulare centrifugum (EAC) and Lyme disease, are discussed in detail. For discussions on juvenile rheumatoid arthritis and erythema marginatum, see VisualDx online. (If you are a first-time online user, go to www.essentialdermatology.com/pigmented; if you already have your password set up, go directly to www.visualdx.com/visualdx.)

EAC usually does not have a rash, but its striking morphologies may lead to confusion with Lyme disease.

▪▪ Diagnosis Synopsis

Erythema Annulare Centrifugum

EAC is characterized by circular or polycyclic lesions that may be superficial or deep. Individual lesions enlarge over days to months and subsequently resolve, but new lesions may continue to develop for weeks to years. They may be anywhere on the body, and usually several are present at once. Superficial lesions may be pruritic. Deep lesions are not itchy. There is no consistent cause.

Lyme Disease

Lyme disease is an immune-mediated inflammatory disease resulting from infection with the spirochete *Borrelia burgdorferi sensu lato*.

In the United States, Lyme disease is primarily seen in New England, the Midwest states, and the West Coast, and it is endemic to most of Europe. *Ixodes* ticks transmit Lyme disease, and mice and deer are the major reservoirs. Transmission occurs most commonly in the spring and summer months.

In a CDC surveillance study in the United States, between 1992 and 2006, 94.1% of patients reported to have Lyme disease were white and 1.7% were African American. This may be attributable to differences in exposure and not susceptibility.

Lyme disease is subdivided clinically into three phases:

1. *Early localized disease*—Early localized disease presents a few days to a month after a tick bite. The characteristic lesion of Lyme disease, erythema migrans, develops at the site of the tick bite in approximately 60% to 90% of those diagnosed. If left untreated, the disease disseminates to lymph nodes and hematogenously. In Europe, early lesions sometimes present as Borrelia lymphocytomas.
2. *Early disseminated disease*—Multiple smaller skin lesions can represent hematogenous spread or, in rare cases, multiple independent primary tick bites. Burning and itching can occur at the site of the tick bite and erythema migrans lesions. Initial infection is typically associated with flulike symptoms, headache, arthralgias, and neck pain. Early neurologic symptoms can include facial nerve paralysis (Bell palsy). Atrioventricular block can develop and persist from several days to a few weeks. Lyme disease–associated arthritis usually develops from a few months to 2 years after initial infection.
3. *Chronic*—Acrodermatitis chronicum atrophicans is a manifestation of chronic Lyme disease in Europe. Untreated cases can also lead to chronic arthritis, encephalopathy, and neuropathy.

◉ Look For

Erythema Annulare Centrifugum

Annular polycyclic plaques that may begin as urticarial lesions and increase in size to 10 cm (Fig. 4-76). As the red outer edge increases in diameter, there is central clearing or duskiness. The outer edge is scaly in superficial lesions; it is more indurated and without scale in deep lesions.

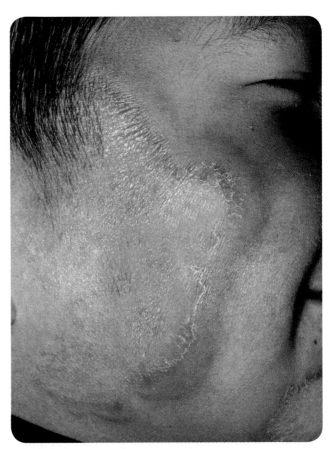

Figure 4-76 Large urticarial lesion with irregular border and wide rim, with fine scale on the inner edge of the lesion, is often present with EAC.

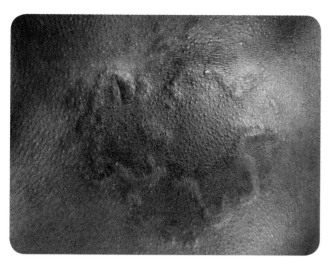

Figure 4-77 EAC with a serpiginous, very urticarial border and dark central pigmentation.

In darker-pigmented skin, lesions may appear more violaceous and may clear with mild postinflammatory hyperpigmentation (Fig. 4-77).

Lyme Disease

In early localized disease, there is a red macule or edematous plaque that initially develops at the site of the tick bite. The lesion expands centrifugally, eventually forming a characteristic large targetoid, or "bull's-eye," lesion. Lymphocytomas can present as bluish-red nodules or plaques on the ear lobe, nipples, or scrotum.

In the early disseminated form, multiple erythematous blanching patches and minimally elevated targetoid plaques can be present in a scattered distribution.

In chronic disease, acrodermatitis chronica atrophicans typically presents with chronic blue-red plaques on the acral extremities, with associated edema and "doughy" texture of the involved skin. Later, involved skin becomes atrophic and shiny. Occasionally, these areas are indurated and can be associated with peripheral neuropathy and local lymphadenopathy.

 ## Diagnostic Pearls

Specifically question the patient about movement of lesions.

Lyme Disease

The characteristic lesion is an expanding targetoid erythematous patch. Transmission of Lyme borreliosis takes 24 to 48 hours of tick attachment and feeding. Therefore, a brief tick exposure (<24 hours) should not be sufficient to contract Lyme disease.

?? Differential Diagnosis and Pitfalls

These diseases also have to be distinguished from the following:

- Tinea corporis—scale present
- Pityriasis rosea—usually scaly
- Cutaneous lupus—thick scale and atrophy present
- Erythema multiforme
- Cutaneous larva migrans
- Urticaria
- Granuloma annulare
- Secondary syphilis—multiple lesions, palm and sole involvement
- Sarcoidosis
- Gyrate erythemas (erythema gyratum repens, erythema migrans, familial annular erythema)
- Southern tick-associated rash illness clinically presents with erythema migrans but is transmitted by the tick *Amblyomma americanum*, possibly caused by *Borrelia lonestari*.
- Erysipelas/cellulitis has a more rapid onset with homogenous erythema as it expands from the site of initial infection.

✓ Best Tests

- Biopsy is essential but may not be specific other than for EAC.
- The diagnosis of Lyme disease is based on a high clinical index of suspicion in an endemic area, with detection of *Borrelia* spirochete from tissues (either lesional or blood). Current serologic tests can be unreliable, especially when the pretest likelihood is low.
- The FDA currently recommends a 2-step testing regimen for suspected cases, which is as follows:
  1. ELISA for either total or IgM or IgG antibodies. If there is a positive or equivocal result, complete step 2.
  2. Perform a western blot (immunoblot) as a second-line test.
- Tests can be falsely negative if taken too early in infection (window period of seroconversion) and should be repeated between 2 and 4 weeks after the initial tick bite if clinical suspicion remains high.
- Biopsy is not specific but can aid in diagnosis.

▲▲ Management Pearls

Erythema Annulare Centrifugum

If KOH scraping and culture are repeatedly negative, EAC may be the diagnosis.

Lyme Disease

Lyme disease is usually a systemic disease after the initial bite, and patients need careful follow-up.

Therapy

(See VisualDX online for more details.)

Erythema Annulare Centrifugum

- Identification and treatment of underlying disease if there is one
- Topical steroids (often mid and high potency) may be necessary.
- Antihistamines for pruritus may be warranted.
- The empirical use of topical antidermatophyte, anti-candidal, and/or antibacterial agents has been suggested by some.

Lyme Disease

Infectious Diseases Society of America Guidelines

Prophylaxis

Within 72 hours of tick bite, doxycycline, 200 mg in a single dose

Prophylaxis is indicated only when *all* of the following conditions are met:

- The attached tick is identified as an *Ixodes scapularis* tick that has been attached for approximately 36 hours (determined by the degree of engorgement of the tick with blood or certainty of the time of exposure).
- Postexposure prophylaxis is started within 72 hours of tick removal.
- The local rate of infection with *B. burgdorferi* is at least 20%.
- Doxycycline is not contraindicated.

Observation is recommended if these criteria are not met.

Treatment

Early Localized Disease

Preferred oral regimens for adults and children aged older than 8 years:

- Doxycycline 100 mg p.o. every 12 hours for 14 to 21 days

Preferred oral regimen for pregnant women and children aged younger than 8 years:

- Amoxicillin 500 mg p.o. every 8 hours for 14 to 21 days

Alternative Regimens

- Cefuroxime axetil 500 mg p.o. every 12 hours for 14 to 21 days
- Azithromycin 500 mg p.o. daily for 7 to 10 days
- Clarithromycin 500 mg p.o. twice daily for 14 to 21 days
- Erythromycin 500 mg p.o. four times daily for 14 to 21 days

Mild Early Disseminated Disease or Chronic Disease

Preferred oral regimen for adults and children aged older than 8 years:

- Doxycycline 100 mg p.o. every 12 hours for 14 to 28 days

Preferred oral regimen for pregnant women and children aged younger than 8 years:

- Amoxicillin 500 mg p.o. every 8 hours for 14 to 28 days

Alternative Regimen

- Cefuroxime axetil 500 mg p.o. every 12 hours for 14 to 28 days

Severe Early Disseminated Disease or Chronic Disease

Preferred parenteral regimen:

- Ceftriaxone 2 g IV daily for 14 to 38 days (duration dependent upon severity of infection)

Alternative Parenteral Regimens

- Cefotaxime 2 g IV every 8 hours for 14 to 28 days (duration dependent upon severity of infection)
- Penicillin G 18 to 24 million U IV daily, in divided doses every 4 hours for 14 to 28 days (duration dependent upon severity of infection)

Suggested Readings

Chagani HS, Aziz K. Clinical profile of acute rheumatic fever in Pakistan. *Cardiol Young.* 2003;13(1):28–35.

da Silva CH. Rheumatic fever: a multicenter study in the state of Sao Paulo, Brazil. *Revista do Hospital das Clinicas.* 1999;54(3):85–90.

Jowi, JO, Gathua, SN. Lyme disease: report of two cases. *East Afr Med J.* 2005;82(5):267–269.

Kim KJ, Chang SE, Choi JH, et al. Clinicopathologic analysis of 66 cases of erythema annulare centrifugum. *J Dermatol.* 2002;29(2):61–67.

Mhalu FS, Matre R. Serologic evidence of Lyme borreliosis in Africa: results from studies in Dar es Salaam, Tanzania. *East Afr Med J.* 1996;73(9): 583–585.

Minni J, Sarro R. A novel therapeutic approach to erythema annulare centrifugum. *J Am Acad Dermatol.* 2006;54(3 Suppl 2):S134–S135.

Tyring SK. Reactive erythemas: erythema annulare centrifugum and erythema gyratum repens. *Clin Dermatol.* 1993;11(1):135–139.

Sarih M, Jouda F, Gern L, et al. First isolation of Borrelia sensu lato from Ixodes ricinus in Morocco. *Vector Borne Zoonotic Dis.* 2003;3(3): 133–139.

Strijdom SC, Berk M. Lyme disease in South Africa. *S Afr Med J.* 1996;86(6 Suppl):741–744.

Wormser GP, Dattwyler RJ, Shapiro ED, et al. The clinical assessment, treatment, and prevention of Lyme disease, human granulocytic anaplasmosis, and babesiosis: clinical practice guidelines by the Infectious Diseases Society of America. *Clin Infect Dis.* 2006;43(9):1089–1134.

Drug Eruption (Morbilliform and Urticarial)

Suzanne Berkman

■■ Diagnosis Synopsis

Exanthematous, or morbilliform, eruptions are the most common of all drug-induced eruptions. Almost any oral agent can cause an exanthematous reaction, but they are most commonly seen with the use of antibiotics (penicillins and sulfas), allopurinol, phenytoin, barbiturates, carbamazepine, gold, and D-penicillamine. Onset is usually within 7 to 14 days of initiating a medication but can even occur 2 to 4 weeks after discontinuing the medication.

The eruption consists of erythematous macules and papules that often arise on the trunk and spread symmetrically to involve the proximal extremities. In severe eruptions, lesions coalesce and may lead to generalized erythroderma (Fig. 4-78). Palms, soles, and mucous membranes may be involved. Pruritus is common, and fever may occur in severe reactions. In dark-skinned patients, postinflammatory hyperpigmentation or hypopigmentation may take weeks to months to resolve. Lesions may have a lichen planus–like morphology (Fig. 4-79). Some drug eruptions can be pustular in nature (acute generalized exanthematous pustulosis [AGEP]) (Fig. 4-80).

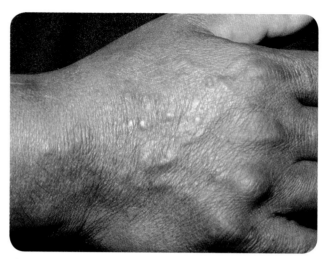

Figure 4-79 Lichen planus drug eruption induced by quinine.

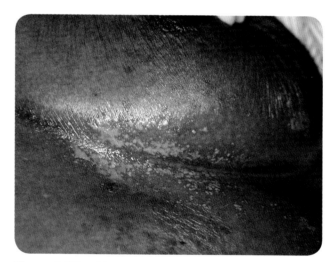

Figure 4-80 Multiple small opaque pustules are characteristic of AGEP.

(◉) Look For

Red macules and papules initially occurring on the trunk with extension to the proximal extremities (Fig. 4-81). Areas of pressure may be more severely affected. Superficial desquamation occurs as the eruption resolves.

●● Diagnostic Pearls

Exanthematous papules blanch with pressure and thus can be differentiated from palpable purpuric lesions, which are indicative of vasculitis. While initial exanthematous papules are not scaly, scale will become apparent upon resolution.

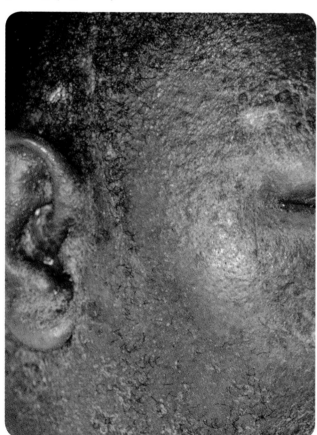

Figure 4-78 Exfoliative erythroderma secondary to dilantin.

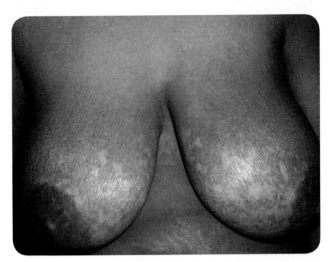

Figure 4-81 Exanthematous drug eruption secondary to allopurinol.

?? Differential Diagnosis and Pitfalls

- Measles
- Papular urticaria
- Early erythema multiforme
- Urticarial bullous pemphigoid
- Juvenile rheumatoid arthritis
- Contact dermatitis

✓ Best Tests

For the most part, this is a clinical diagnosis. Biopsy of the lesions will show the type of drug eruption and will be helpful in diagnosis and to determine life-threatening dermatosis.

▲▲ Management Pearls

Identification and discontinuation of the offending agent(s) are critical. After the medication has been stopped, it may take an additional 7 to 14 days before the eruption completely resolves.

Therapy

Discontinue the offending agent(s). Antihistamines for itching (hydroxyzine 50 mg every 4 to 6 hours or cetirizine 10 to 20 mg twice daily). Avoid systemic corticosteroids if possible. Topical steroids will give relief of pruritus and decrease the inevitable postinflammatory hyperpigmentation in pigmented skin.

Suggested Readings

Bigby M. Rates of cutaneous reactions to drugs. *Arch Dermatol.* 2001;137:765–770.

Edwards IR, Aronson JK. Adverse drug reactions: Definitions, diagnosis and management. *Lancet.* 2000;356:1255–1259.

Shear NH. Diagnosing cutaneous adverse reactions to drugs. *Arch Dermatol.* 1990;126:94–97.

Pityriasis Rosea

Stephanie Diamantis

Diagnosis Synopsis

Pityriasis rosea (PR) is a common cutaneous eruption that arises spontaneously most often in otherwise healthy adolescents or young adults. Although PR can occur year-round, there is usually a higher incidence in the spring and fall. Women are affected more often than men. Most sources note no predilection in any ethnicity; however, some studies report that PR occurs twice as commonly in black individuals compared with whites. Black people tend to show more widespread and atypical forms with hyperpigmentation upon resolution. Black children have also been found to more frequently develop papular lesions (33%) and have scalp (8%) and facial (30%) involvement. While the exact cause is unclear, current investigational efforts have largely focused on the role of human herpesvirus 6 and 7 in this condition. The following observations support a viral etiology: presence of a flulike prodrome in some patients, absence of recurrence (suggesting an immune response with specificity and cell memory to a pathogen), seasonal variation, and case clustering (suggesting possible "outbreaks").

Initially, a solitary pink or flesh-colored patch or scaly plaque appears (the herald patch) followed by a more generalized eruption several days later. The eruption consists of multiple erythematous, scaly papules and plaques that favor the trunk and upper extremities. Lesions follow the lines of cleavage in a characteristic "Christmas tree" distribution. Classically, the face, palms, and soles are spared. Lesions are asymptomatic or pruritic and self-limited in nature. Up to a quarter of patients can experience mild to severe pruritus. Fever, malaise, headache, and nausea may be present in a minority of cases.

PR occurring during pregnancy may be associated with premature birth or fetal demise, especially if erupting during the first 15 weeks of pregnancy.

Look For

Typical lesions are salmon-colored, oval or circular patches and plaques with an associated fine, central scaling (Figs. 4-82–4-84). The condition usually begins with one larger truncal plaque, known as the herald patch. Then, 1 to 3 weeks later, new plaques appear oriented with the long axis of oval lesions along skin fold lines (Christmas tree pattern) (Fig. 4-85), which is better seen on the back. Pruritus is variably present.

There are many variants, including vesicular, pustular, purpuric, and those mimicking urticaria or erythema multiforme. Facial lesions are rare. An inverse form has been described where the lesions occur on the face, neck, groin, axillae, and lower abdomen.

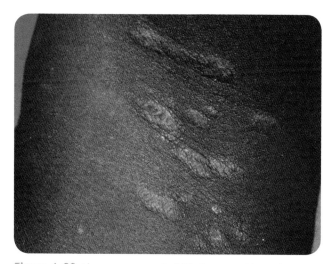

Figure 4-83 Linear arrangement of PR plaques on the neck.

Figure 4-82 Multiple discrete and confluent scaly plaques of PR.

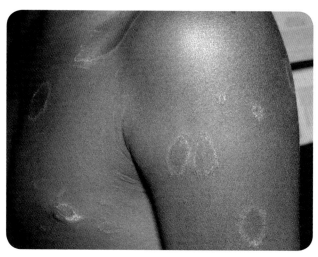

Figure 4-84 Very large annular plaques of PR.

111

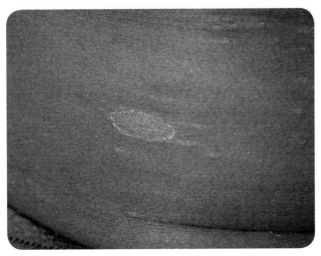

Figure 4-85 Large plaque of PR oriented parallel to skin folds with fine central scale and some smaller papules.

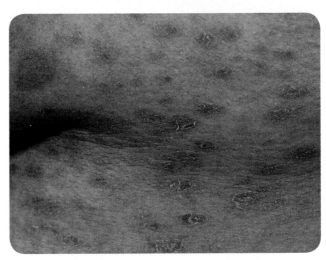

Figure 4-86 PR in pigmented skin often has a purple hue.

The typical "salmon-pink" color is not easily apparent in darkly pigmented skin, and lesions often appear more papular or vesicular in these patients and often have a distinct purple hue (Fig. 4-86). Follicular prominence is evident. PR is more likely to be present in an inverse distribution in black patients. Postinflammatory hypopigmentation or hyperpigmentation is more common in darkly pigmented individuals.

●● Diagnostic Pearls

Patients will usually give a history of an asymptomatic macule that appeared before the rest of the lesions (the herald patch). Lymphadenopathy is a rare finding.

?? Differential Diagnosis and Pitfalls

- Secondary syphilis—Systemic symptoms are more pronounced, including lymphadenopathy, fevers, history of primary chancre, condyloma lata; if remotely suspicious, check syphilis serologies.
- Drug eruption
- Tinea corporis—hyphae present on KOH
- Tinea versicolor
- Nummular eczema—very pruritic
- Guttate psoriasis—smaller size, thicker scale
- Parapsoriasis
- Erythema multiforme
- Urticaria
- Lichen planus
- Pityriasis lichenoides chronica

✓ Best Tests

- Diagnosis is usually made on clinical grounds. Skin biopsy is rarely indicated because histology is nonspecific and the clinical picture is characteristic.
- Syphilis serology with clinical suspicion (systemic symptoms, lymphadenopathy, history of primary chancre, condyloma lata, HIV)
- KOH examination of skin scrapings should be performed when considering tinea infection.

▲▲ Management Pearls

The acute onset and widespread involvement often causes significant concern for the patient or parents. Education and assurance of the benign nature may assist in management.

Therapy

Complete and spontaneous resolution is the rule; management is primarily symptomatic if needed.

Antipruritics (such as lotions containing camphor, menthol, or pramoxine), oatmeal baths, and antihistamines can provide symptomatic relief.

Antihistamines
- Diphenhydramine hydrochloride (25, 50 mg tablets or capsules): 25 to 50 mg nightly or every 6 hours as needed

- Hydroxyzine (10, 25 mg tablets): 12.5 to 25 mg every 6 hours as needed
- Cetirizine hydrochloride (5, 10 mg tablets): 5 to 10 mg/d

Topical corticosteroids may also help improve itch and appearance by decreasing inflammation.

Mid-potency Topical Corticosteroids (Classes 3 and 4)

- Triamcinolone cream, ointment—Apply twice daily (15, 30, 60, 120, 240 g).
- Mometasone cream, ointment—Apply twice daily (15, 45 g).
- Fluocinolone ointment, cream—Apply twice daily (15, 30, 60 g).

Acyclovir may be helpful in patients presenting early and in those with extensive disease/flulike symptoms. Dosing is as follows: acyclovir 800 mg five times a day by mouth for 1 week.

Phototherapy should be used with caution, as it may worsen postinflammatory hyperpigmentation.

Suggested Readings

Amer A, Fischer H, Li X. The natural history of pityriasis rosea in black American children: how correct is the "classic" description? *Arch Pediatr Adolesc Med.* 2007;161(5):503–506.

Blauvelt A. Pityriasis rosea. In: Wolff K, Goldsmith LA, Katz SI, Gilchrest BA, Paller AS, Leffell DJ, eds. *Fitzpatrick's Dermatology in General Medicine.* 7th Ed. New York, NY: McGraw Hill; 2008:362–366.

Broccolo F, Drago F, Careddu AM, et al. Additional evidence that pityriasis rosea is associated with reactivation of human herpesvirus-6 and -7. *J Invest Dermatol.* 2005;124(6):1234–1240.

Drago F, Broccolo F, Zaccaria E, et al. Pregnancy outcome in patients with pityriasis rosea. *J Am Acad Dermatol.* 2008;58(5 Suppl 1):S78–S83.

Drago F, Vecchio F, Rebora A. Use of high-dose acyclovir in pityriasis rosea. *J Am Acad Dermatol.* 2006;54(1):82–85.

Halder RM, Roberts CI, Nootheti PK. Cutaneous diseases in the black races. *Dermatol Clin.* 2003;21:679–687.

Pruritic Urticarial Papules and Plaques of Pregnancy

Chris G. Adigun

■■ Diagnosis Synopsis

Pruritic urticarial papules and plaques of pregnancy (PUPPP), or polymorphous eruption of pregnancy, is the most common dermatosis of pregnancy. It is a benign, intensely pruritic eruption that occurs almost exclusively in primigravidas during the third trimester and resolves around the time of delivery, or shortly thereafter. The lesions typically originate in striae gravidarum (striae distensae), which tend to develop late in pregnancy. Pruritus can be severe, leading to sleep disturbance. It is important to note that this is a benign dermatosis. Additionally, there is no association with adverse fetal or maternal outcomes. Recurrence with subsequent pregnancies is uncommon.

The etiology is unknown, but research has established associations with striae distensae, maternal weight gain, and multiple gestations. Some postulated etiologies include hormonal aberrations, immunologic mechanisms, and skin distension. Immunologic possibilities include the conversion of nonantigenic "self" molecules to antigenic molecules, inducing an inflammatory cascade. Numerous factors, including pregnancies with multiple gestation and excessive maternal-fetal weight gain, have been found to be associated with PUPPP. Significant factors that have shown no association include fetal weight and sex.

The incidence of PUPPP in singleton pregnancies is 1 in 200 (0.5%). Recent studies have confirmed the proposed thought that PUPPP occurred more frequently in multiple gestations and have analyzed the incidence in these populations, with frequencies of 2.9% of twin and 14% of triplet pregnancies. A recent study in a mixed ethnic population found PUPPP to predominantly affect white pregnant women as compared to Asian or African/Afro-Caribbean women.

PUPPP is benign and is not associated with any medical consequences for either the mother or fetus. It does usually require intervention for symptom relief, as pruritus can be severe. In some cases, laboratory workup, histopathology, and immunologic studies should be performed to exclude more serious dermatoses of pregnancy, such as impetigo herpetiformis (pustular psoriasis of pregnancy), pemphigoid gestationis, or intrahepatic cholestasis of pregnancy.

Although PUPPP is a benign condition with no association with adverse fetal outcomes, it is considered to be a risk factor for the development of an epidural abscess, and necessary precautions during delivery should, thus, be addressed.

◉ Look For

The eruption characteristically occurs initially on the abdomen and/or proximal thighs, particularly within or adjacent to striae distensae (91%). It then extends over the legs, back,

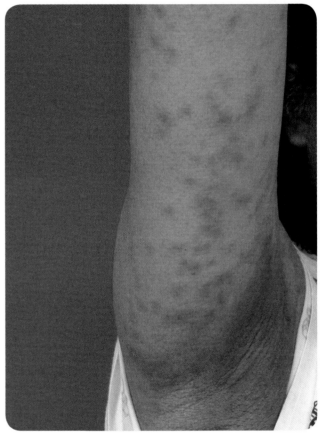

Figure 4-87 Hyperpigmented papules of PUPPP on the upper arms.

buttocks, arms, and breasts. The typical skin findings are erythematous, urticarial papules and plaques (Fig. 4-87). A few vesicles may be noted, as may the rare targetoid lesion or annular wheal. The immediate periumbilical area, face, palms, and soles are spared.

●● Diagnostic Pearls

Initially, lesions are very itchy and are usually very small (1 to 2 mm). PUPPP characteristically spares the periumbilical area, and often—but not always—spares the face, palms, and soles. It is not uncommon for small vesicles to occur, but formation of bullae should be a warning sign, as the finding of frank bullae should suggest the rarer and more prognostically serious disorder pemphigoid gestationis.

?? Differential Diagnosis and Pitfalls

- Impetigo herpetiformis—distinct pustules and/or vesicles
- Prurigo gestationis

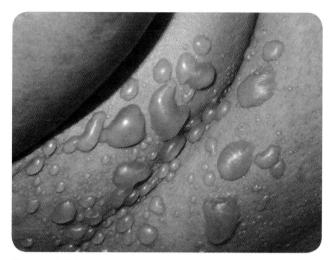

Figure 4-88 Herpes gestationis is rarer than PUPPP and will frequently have significant vesicles or bullae, which are not usually present in PUPPP.

- Pemphigoid (herpes) gestationis—an autoimmune blistering disease that occurs in pregnancy wherein the lesions have definite vesicles and bullae (Fig. 4-88)
- Urticaria
- Intrahepatic cholestasis of pregnancy
- Erythema multiforme
- Drug eruption
- Viral eruption
- Pityriasis rosea
- Insect bites
- Contact dermatitis
- Seabather eruption
- Scabies

✓ Best Tests

- PUPPP is an ill-defined entity because of its variable clinical presentation and lack of specific laboratory abnormalities. Diagnosis can, therefore, be difficult. Most importantly, more prognostically serious dermatoses of pregnancy must be ruled out.
- Although not frequently indicated, if there is a concern for other pregnancy-associated dermatoses, consider skin biopsy for direct immunofluorescence. Histopathological analysis is not specific but helps eliminate pemphigoid gestationis and impetigo herpetiformis. Additionally, serum may also be submitted for indirect immunofluorescence to rule out pemphigoid gestationis. A highly sensitive and specific serologic test is the NC16a enzyme-linked immunosorbent assay. This test is very helpful in differentiating pemphigoid gestationis from PUPPP and may additionally confirm the diagnosis of pemphigoid gestationis.

- Investigation has shown no HLA antigen association in women with PUPPP.

▲▲ Management Pearls

- Patients should be provided with continual reassurance that the itching will eventually clear after delivery and that there is no evidence that the eruption is associated with any fetal distress or poor fetal outcome. There is some recent evidence that demonstrates that some cases of PUPPP can abate entirely during pregnancy with appropriate topical steroid therapy.
- Symptoms typically abate shortly after delivery in most mild cases, although delivery does not usually provide relief of intractable symptoms. Most women have resolution by 6 weeks postpartum.
- Patients should be warned of residual postinflammatory hyperpigmentation that will persist after appropriate intervention and resolution of symptoms. In deeply pigmented patients, this may be more pronounced and may persist for longer periods of time. Furthermore, patients with darker complexions may have the added complication of hypopigmentation in areas in which topical steroids were applied.

Therapy

- Treatment of PUPPP focuses on the mitigation of the intense pruritus. Antihistamines, skin emollients, and topical steroids have been the primary agents used. However, research has shown that therapy is not consistently successful. Other treatment options include cool soaks and cooling emollients, which may provide some symptomatic relief in mild cases.
- For systemic intervention of pruritus, consider the use of a first-generation antihistamine such as diphenhydramine 25 to 50 mg every 6 hours or a long-acting antihistamine once daily such as cetirizine, levocetirizine, loratadine, or fexofenadine (under obstetrical guidance).
- Rarely, severe cases of PUPPP warrant systemic corticosteroids. Consult with an obstetrician first if considering this treatment.

Suggested Readings

Ahmadi S, Powell FC. Pruritic urticarial papules and plaques of pregnancy: Current status. *Australas J Dermatol.* 2005;46(2):53–58; quiz 59.

Brzoza Z, Kasperska-Zajac A, Oleś E, et al. Pruritic urticarial papules and plaques of pregnancy. *J Midwifery Womens Health.* 2007;52(1):44–48.

Buccolo LS, Viera AJ. Pruritic urticarial papules and plaques of pregnancy presenting in the postpartum period: A case report. *J Reprod Med.* 2005;50(1):61–63.

Cummings KC III, Dolak JA. Case report: Epidural abscess in a parturient with pruritic urticarial papules and plaques of pregnancy (PUPPP). *Can J Anaesth*. 2006;53(10):1010–1014.

Elling SV, McKenna P, Powell FC. Pruritic urticarial papules and plaques of pregnancy in twin and triplet pregnancies. *J Eur Acad Dermatol Venereol*. 2000;14(5):378–381.

Halder RM, Bridgeman-Shah S. Skin cancer in African Americans. *Cancer*. 1995;75(2 Suppl):667–673.

Halder RM, Nootheti PK. Ethnic skin disorders overview. *J Am Acad Dermatol*. 2003;48(6 Suppl):S143–S148.

High WA, Hoang MP, Miller MD. Pruritic urticarial papules and plaques of pregnancy with unusual and extensive palmoplantar involvement. *Obstet Gynecol*. 2005;105(5 Pt 2):1261–1264.

Matz H, Orion E, Wolf R. Pruritic urticarial papules and plaques of pregnancy: Polymorphic eruption of pregnancy (PUPPP). *Clin Dermatol*. 2006;24(2):105–108.

Ohel I, Levy A, Silberstein T, et al. Pregnancy outcome of patients with pruritic urticarial papules and plaques of pregnancy. *J Matern Fetal Neonatal Med*. 2006;19(5):305–308.

Powell AM, Sakuma-Oyama Y, Oyama N, et al. Usefulness of BP180 NC16a enzyme-linked immunosorbent assay in the serodiagnosis of pemphigoid gestationis and in differentiating between pemphigoid gestationis and pruritic urticarial papules and plaques of pregnancy. *Arch Dermatol*. 2005;141(6):705–710.

Rudolph CM, Al-Fares S, Vaughan-Jones SA, et al. Polymorphic eruption of pregnancy: Clinicopathology and potential trigger factors in 181 patients. *Br J Dermatol*. 2006;154(1):54–60.

Tunzi M, Gray GR. Common skin conditions during pregnancy. *Am Fam Physician*. 2007;75(2):211–218.

Urticaria, Angioedema, and Dermographism

Alicia Ogram • Adam Tinkelpaugh

■■■ Diagnosis Synopsis

Urticaria

Urticaria (hives) refers to raised erythematous wheals lasting 48 hours and caused by the release of histamine and other vasoactive substances from mast cells. Pruritus, prickling, and stinging sensations or pain may occur with urticaria. Urticaria is defined as acute (<6 weeks) or chronic (>6 weeks). Chronic urticaria is more common in women and middle-aged individuals, whereas acute urticaria is more commonly seen in children. Disease resolves within 12 months in approximately 50% of adults with idiopathic urticaria. In 90% of cases, a cause is never found if it is not one listed below.

Risk factors for urticaria are as follows:

- Systemic illnesses such as infections, collagen vascular diseases, neoplasia, endocrine disorders, and blood dyscrasias
- Environmental stimuli such as insect stings and inhalants (pollen, spores, animal dander, perfumes, detergents)
- Pregnancy
- Foods such as strawberries, nuts, eggs, uncooked shiitake mushrooms, and shellfish
- Physical stimuli such as heat, cold, exertion, sunlight, water, vibration, or pressure
- Drugs such as aspirin, nonsteroidal anti-inflammatory drugs (NSAIDs), morphine and codeine, penicillins, cephalosporins, sulfa, streptomycin, tetracycline, griseofulvin, blood products, radiographic contrast media, angiotensin-converting enzyme inhibitors, and sulfonylureas

Angioedema

Angioedema is potentially life-threatening and demands immediate medical attention.

Angioedema is an allergy-mediated tissue edema characterized by transient dermal swelling. It is a variant of urticaria, with the edema occurring at a deeper level, usually within the dermis and subcutis. Angioedema can be caused by certain medications (e.g., antibiotics, cardiac drugs, immunotherapeutics, chemotherapeutics, ACE inhibitors, calcium channel blockers, and histamine releasers) and foods (e.g., milk, eggs, shellfish, wheat, and nuts), or it may be idiopathic. Serum sickness results from therapeutic, usually nonhuman, proteins (including monoclonal antibodies) or sera; serum sickness-like eruption results from drugs, commonly penicillin and its related drugs, cefaclor, bupropion, and minocycline.

Drug-induced angioedema can be associated with urticaria but can occur alone, with deeper tissue swellings being the only manifestation. Can be life-threatening. The subcutaneous tissues, airway, and gastrointestinal tract are all possible sites of involvement.

Angiotensin-converting enzyme (ACE) inhibitors may be a cause of drug-induced angioedema, especially among African Americans. The reported incidence of ACE-induced angioedema among African Americans is 0.1% to 0.2%, five times more common than in whites.

Hereditary angioedema usually lasts longer (3 to 4 days), is not responsive to standard antihistamine therapy, and usually will not have typical urticarial lesions and often has severe intestinal syndromes. Precipitating factors include minor trauma such as dental manipulations or hormonal factors.

Familial forms begin in adolescence; they have autosomal dominant inheritance and are related to disorders of complement regulation.

Dermographism

Dermographism is an exaggerated wheal and flare reaction to pressure. Inadvertent stroking or rubbing of the skin results in linear wheals. Wheals are transient and persist for 15 to 30 minutes. It is usually asymptomatic, but some forms are associated with pruritus. The exact cause of dermographism is unknown. An increased incidence has been reported during pregnancy and in individuals with Behçet disease, thyroid disorders, infections, and atopic dermatitis. It affects approximately 2% to 5% of the population and is more common in young adults.

Pediatric Patient Considerations

Urticaria

While uncommon in infants younger than 6 months, food (e.g., cow's milk, eggs) and viral infection are the most common cause of urticaria for this population. In infants older than 6 months, infections and drugs (especially the penicillins) are the most common cause of acute urticaria.

Papular Urticaria

Papular urticaria is a chronic or recurrent pruritic eruption believed to be an allergic (hypersensitivity) reaction to insect bites. Very common in urban children, especially in the spring and summer in temperate climates and year round where the weather is warm, and in those of lower socioeconomic status and those with poor hygiene. Common under wet conditions, such as flooding after a hurricane. History of exposure to fleas, mosquitoes, chiggers, mites, bedbugs, or other small insects.

Papular urticaria can occur anywhere on the body but tends to occur on the exposed extensor surfaces of the extremities. The lesions are firm, pink, raised 2- to 8-mm papules, often with a visible central punctum (Fig. 4-89).

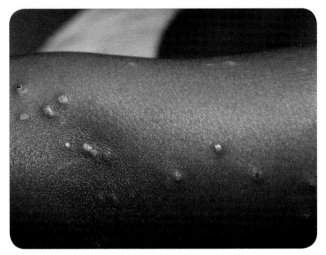

Figure 4-89 Papular persistent lesions of papular urticaria, unlike typical forms of urticaria, are usually attributed to insect bites.

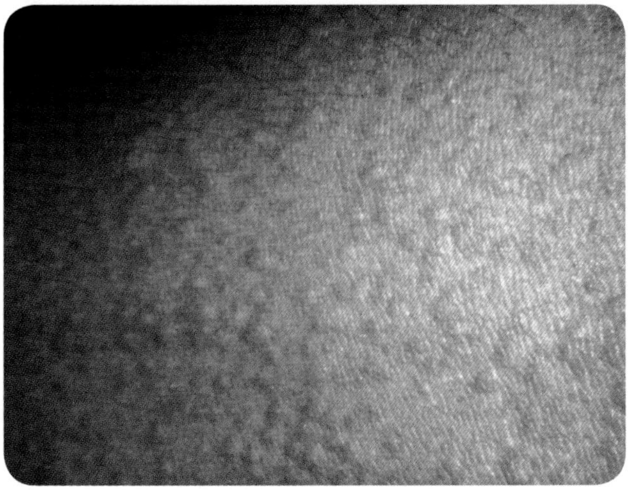

Figure 4-90 Multiple flesh-colored papules lasting less than an hour are typical of cholinergic urticaria.

The lesions are usually grouped in linear clusters and are present on exposed areas with sparing of the genital, perianal, and axillary regions. They may become excoriated or secondarily infected. They can last weeks to months and often recur at the same time each year. Often, only one person in the household is affected and caretakers are disbelieving of the proposed cause.

After resolution of the papule, pigmented (postinflammatory) macules may persist. Permanent hyperpigmentation and/or hypopigmentation may occur, particularly in darkly pigmented individuals.

Cholinergic Urticaria

Cholinergic urticaria is a type of urticaria associated with sweating, exercise, and overheating. Small, transient lesions occur rapidly and typically last less than a few hours. Some patients have reported headache, dizziness, wheezing, and gastrointestinal distress with this condition. It mainly occurs in adolescents and adults. Angioedema is uncommon but can be an associated feature. It can be initiated by injection of a cholinergic agent, for example, acetyl-B-methyl-choline (mecholyl).

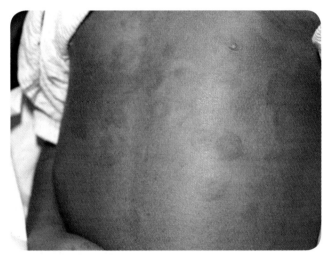

Figure 4-91 Aspirin-induced hives, some of which are annular with central clearing.

- The color of characteristically pink urticarial lesions may be obscured in darker skin. Lesions may appear merely as pruritic nonscaly papules or plaques. The abrupt onset, constantly changing character of the lesions, and intense pruritus help establish the diagnosis.
- Urticaria may occur anywhere on the body but is more common on the trunk.
- Angioedema is seen in approximately 50% of urticaria cases. Familial angioedema usually does not have individual small hives.

⦿ Look For

Urticaria

- Urticaria presents as well-circumscribed, edematous papules, patches, or plaques, often with a pale center; each lesion lasts <24 to 48 hours (Figs. 4-90 and 4-91).
- Lesions vary in size from 2 to 30 cm, are usually sharply marginated, and may be annular, serpiginous, or irregularly shaped. Edema of the mucous membranes may be present.

Papular Urticaria

Crops of papules, especially on the lower extremities and exposed extensor surfaces, may be seen in infants. Target lesions may be seen, particularly in darker-skinned patients.

Cholinergic Urticaria

Small (2 to 4 mm) edematous papules or wheals surrounded by pink or erythematous patches. The lesions most commonly extend from the neck to the thighs but can occur on any body region. Each lesion lasts less than an hour.

Angioedema

Diffuse erythematous swelling of the eyelids, lips, tongue, and sometimes the genitalia (Figs. 4-92 and 4-93). Patients may complain of malaise, fever, arthralgias, respiratory symptoms, fatigue, abdominal pain, and diarrhea and sometimes can have hypotension and shock.

Dermographism

Linear wheals or geometric shapes suggestive of external provocation such as stroking or rubbing of the skin (Figs. 4-94 and 4-95). The extent of the white inner portion and the extent of the wheal are more than the normal triple response of Lewis with peripheral blanching. These color changes may be more difficult to see in darker skin.

Diagnostic Pearls

Urticaria

- Provocative tests (e.g., ice cube test or strenuous exercise) may help establish a diagnosis of physical urticaria.
- Physically induced urticarias are common.
- Delayed urticaria from pressure may occur hours after exposure.
- The pruritus of urticaria rarely leads to excoriations.

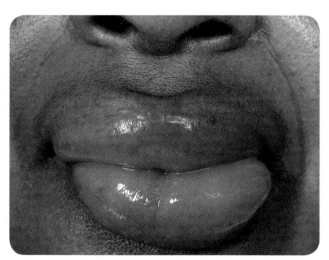

Figure 4-92 Diffusely swollen lips are typical of angioneurotic edema.

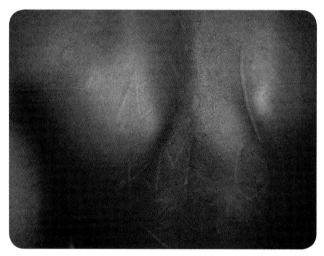

Figure 4-94 Prominent linear dermographism.

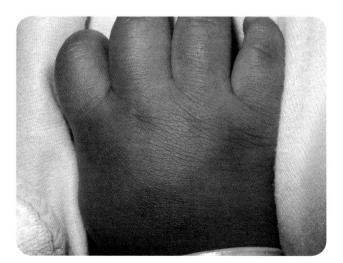

Figure 4-93 Diffuse swelling of the hand and fingers in a serum sickness-like eruption due to penicillin.

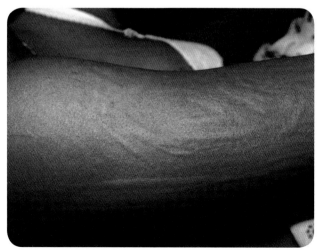

Figure 4-95 Pale lesions of dermographism in dark skin.

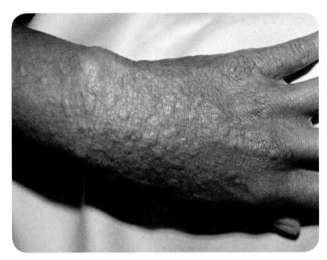

Figure 4-96 Recurrent contact urticaria from rubber gloves, with some lichenification.

- The duration of individual wheals can be helpful in eliciting a cause:
  - Ordinary urticaria (viral, food, or drug): 2 to 24 hours
  - Contact urticaria (latex allergy): <2 hours (Fig. 4-96)
  - Physical urticaria (heat, cold, water, ultraviolet light): <1 hour
  - Urticarial vasculitis: several days
  - Angioedema: several days

Papular Urticaria

History of similar lesions in the past. Intensely pruritic, found in groups of three to five. Fresh insect bites will cause old lesions to "light up."

Cholinergic Urticaria

Typical lesions will have a pink patch with a small central edematous papule.

Angioedema

Angioedema tends to last fewer than 24 hours in any given location, but new lesions can evolve quickly at other locations.

Dermographism

Dermographism may occur concomitantly with other physical urticarias such as cold- or pressure-induced urticaria. Most patients with active urticaria also manifest dermographism.

?? Differential Diagnosis and Pitfalls

Urticarias including the physical urticarias and dermographism can mimic each other, and several conditions should be considered.

- Urticarial vasculitis—Lesions persist over 24 hours and may have associated purpura.
- Dermographism—induced by firmly stroking the skin and persists for 0.5 to 2 hours
- Contact dermatitis—typically an unusual geometric shape and is often urticarial early and often develops blisters
- Drug reactions—may be urticarial
- Herpes zoster—may initially be urticarial, but condition is painful and evolves into blisters and crusts
- Insect bites (papular urticaria)—may last longer than 24 hours
- Serum sickness—may present as urticarial but is accompanied by arthralgias, fever, and malaise
- Angioedema—not pruritic and commonly affects the face
- Anaphylaxis—associated with angioedema and multiple systemic symptoms that usually begin within minutes of exposure
- Lupus erythematosus—often with epidermal changes
- Bullous pemphigoid—may have urticarial plaques without blisters
- Papulovesicular polymorphous light eruption
- Pityriasis lichenoides et varioliformis acuta
- Miliaria crystalline—presents as tiny vesicles rather than urticarial papules
- Exercise-induced anaphylaxis—It usually occurs after ingestion of food prior to exercise. It is characterized by pruritus, whealing, and angioedema that may progress to respiratory obstruction or cardiovascular collapse.
- Strongyloides (cutaneous larva migrans)—Lesions may resemble rapidly moving urticarial wheals.

Angioedema—common mimickers to be considered

- Pressure-induced urticaria—usually localized, and history often reveals local pressure before the lesion appeared
- Serum sickness
- Facial cellulitis—lasts for several days; painful, often associated with fever, followed by peeling
- Crohn disease of mouth and lips—causes granulomatous swelling of lips complicated by lymphoedema. Patients often show cobblestone thickening of buccal mucous membrane.
- Tumid discoid lupus—red edematous plaques on light-exposed areas of the face; persistent; may cause scarring
- Ascher syndrome—recurrent episodes of eyelid edema leading to blepharochalasis

- Melkersson-Rosenthal syndrome—granulomatous swelling of lips that is persistent; can be associated with lingua plicata and/or Bell palsy
- Superior vena cava syndrome—edema of the eyelids, lips; associated with venous engorgement

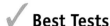 ## Best Tests

Urticaria and Angioedema

- Urticaria typically is a clinical diagnosis.
- In chronic urticaria, perform a CBC with differential, ESR, and thyroid function tests. Persistent lesions require biopsy for urticarial vasculitis. If positive, further lab tests include urinalysis, renal and liver function tests, C3, C4, CH50 levels, hepatitis B and C serologies, ANA, cryoglobulins, immunoglobulin levels, and serum protein electrophoresis/urine protein electrophoresis. Skin testing or radioallergosorbent assays may be useful if hypersensitivity to a particular allergen is suspected. For patients with acquired cold urticaria, check cryoglobulins, a CBC with differential, and hepatitis serologies.
- Urinalysis for proteinuria is useful to rule out serum sickness and urinary tract infection as a source of the urticaria.
- A biopsy may be suggestive in cases of papular urticaria.
- Exercise induction of lesions (e.g., walking stairs) can be diagnostic of cholinergic urticaria.
- If strongly suspecting hereditary angioedema on clinical grounds, C4 is a good screening test. If low, check quantitative and functional levels of C1 inhibitor.
- Dermographism is reproduced by application of firm, slow pressure with the dull end of a pen cap or a ballpoint pen tip (retracted).

▲▲▲ Management Pearls and Therapy

Urticarial Eruptions

- Avoid triggers and physical circumstances (aspirin, heat, pressure, cold, and alcohol). Cooler temperatures may be beneficial.
- In cases of anaphylaxis, immediate intervention is needed to secure the airway and prevent circulatory collapse. For severe reactions (anaphylaxis, severe angioedema, serum sickness-like reaction)—methylprednisolone 1 to 2 mg/kg/d p.o. for 3 days. Consultation with allergist.
- Make the patient an active participant in searching for disease-inducing agents.
- Children with uncomplicated urticaria who respond to antihistamines should be observed by the caregiver for 30 minutes to 2 hours for development of anaphylaxis.
- The detailed workup of chronic urticaria is enhanced by the involvement of a dermatologist or allergist.

Papular Urticaria

Avoid insect bites by covering the skin and using repellant.

Cholinergic Urticaria

Rapid cooling to prevent sweating

Angioedema

- Patients with severe angioedema should be advised to wear a medical alert bracelet and have an EpiPen available.
- ACE inhibitor treatment for hypertension is commonly resumed shortly after an event of angioedema. It is important to warn African American patients of potentially fatal reactions with ACE inhibitors.

Dermographism

Antihistamines can control itch. If treatment is desired by the patient, be sure to warn them about the sedating effects of certain antihistamines.

Nonsedating H1 antagonists are first-line therapy:

- Cetirizine hydrochloride—10 mg p.o. nightly or twice daily
- Loratadine—10 mg p.o. once or twice daily
- Fexofenadine—120 to 180 mg p.o. once daily

Leukotriene inhibitors may be used with antihistamines:

- Montelukast—10 mg p.o. once daily
- Zafirlukast—20 mg p.o. twice daily
- Zileuton—600 mg p.o. four times a day

Tumor necrosis factor-α inhibitors may be effective in recalcitrant urticaria and delayed pressure urticaria.

- Etanercept—25 to 50 mg p.o. twice weekly

In severe cases, systemic corticosteroids (prednisone 0.5 to 1 mg/kg p.o. daily) can be used for 3 to 5 days while introducing antihistamine therapy.

Papular Urticaria

Mild topical corticosteroids and oral antihistamines for the itching. Treat secondary impetigo or cellulitis with appropriate antibiotics.

Cholinergic Urticaria

Hydroxyzine—10 mg/5 mL (240-mL bottle)

Severe cholinergic urticaria may also be treated with scopolamine butylbromide with concomitant antihistamine therapy.

Angioedema

H1 antihistamines may reduce swelling:

- Diphenhydramine hydrochloride—5 mg/kg/d p.o. divided three to four times daily
- Hydroxyzine HCl—2 to 4 mg/kg/d divided three to four times daily
- Cetirizine hydrochloride—2.5 to 10 mg per day p.o.
  - Children aged 6 years and older—5 or 10 mg once daily
  - Children aged 2 to 5 years—2.5 mg once daily
- Loratadine—5 to 10 mg per day p.o.

For resistant cases, H2 blockers can be paired with the H1 blocker:

- Cimetidine—10 to 40 mg/kg/d p.o. divided four times daily
- Ranitidine—2 to 4 mg/dose p.o. divided twice daily
- Doxepin—5 to 10 mg p.o. daily, off-label use in pediatrics

For severely refractory cases, systemic steroids may be warranted:

- Prednisone 1 to 2 mg/kg/d p.o. divided twice daily

Hereditary angioedema has been treated with danazol, fresh frozen plasma, and recently specially treated C1 esterase inhibitor and an inhibitor of kallikrein. Long-term treatment of this disorders requires accurate diagnose and often a consultation with an allergist.

Dermographism

H1 antihistamines may reduce symptoms:

- Diphenhydramine hydrochloride—5 mg/kg/d, nightly to four times daily
- Hydroxyzine:
  - Children aged 6 and older—12.5 to 25 mg, every 6 hours as needed
  - Children up to age 6—12.5 mg every 6 hours as needed

Narrowband ultraviolet B phototherapy may be an effective second-line treatment for patients with recalcitrant dermographism and poor response to fexofenadine.

Suggested Readings

Altraide DD, George IO, Frank-Briggs AI. Prevalence of skin diseases in Nigerian children—(the University of Port Harcourt Teaching Hospital) experience. *Niger J Med*. 2008;17(4):417–419.

Breathnach SM, Allen R, Milford-Ward A, et al. Symptomatic dermographism: natural history, clinical features, laboratory investigations and response to therapy. *Clin Exp Dermatol*. 1983;9:463–467.

Cicardi M, Levy RJ, McNeil DL, et al. Ecallantide for the treatment of acute attacks in hereditary angioedema. *N Engl J Med*. 2010;363:523–531.

Eliason M, Liddle M, Hull C, Powell D. A case series of 3 patients with chronic urticaria who responded well to anti-TNF-alpha biologic agents. *J Am Acad Dermatol*. 2008:58(2, Suppl 2):AB10. Poster Abstracts, American Academy of Dermatology 66th Annual Meeting.

Gibbs CR, Lip GYH, Beevers DG. Angioedema due to ACE inhibitors: increased risk in patients of African origin. *Br J Clin Pharmacol*. 1999;48(6):861–865.

Grattan CEH. Autoimmune urticaria. *Immunol Allergy Clin North Am*. 2004;24:163–181.

Hernandez RG, Cohen BA. Insect bite-induced hypersensitivity and the SCRATCH principles: a new approach to popular urticaria. *Pediatrics*. 2006;118(1):e189–e196. Epub 2006 Jun 2.

Horan RF, Sheffer AL. Exercise-induced anaphylaxis. *Immunol Allergy Clin North Am*. 1992;12:559–569.

Kaplan AP, Greaves MW. Angioedema. *J Am Acad Dermatol*. 2005;53(3):373–388. Retrieved November 27, 2009.

Kelso JM. Pollen-food allergy syndrome. *Clin Exp Allergy*. 2000;30:905–907.

Kontou-Fili K, Borici Mazi R, Kapp A, et al. Physical urticaria: classification and diagnostic guidelines. An EAACI position paper. *Allergy*. 1997;52:504–513.

Magerl M, Philipp S, Manasterski M, et al. Successful treatment of delayed pressure urticaria with anti-TNF-alpha. *J Allergy Clin Immunol*. 2007;119(3):752–754.

Mahoney EJ, Devaiah AK. Angioedema and angiotensin-converting enzyme inhibitors: are demographics a risk? *Otolaryngol Head Neck Surg*. 2008;139(1):105–108. Retrieved November 27, 2009.

Nettis E, Pannofino A, D'Aprile C, et al. Clinical and etiological aspects in urticaria and angioedema. *Br J Dermatol*. 2003;148:501–506.

Noe R, Cohen AL, Lederman E, et al. Skin disorders among construction workers following Hurricane Katrina and Hurricane Rita: an outbreak investigation in New Orleans, Louisiana. *Arch Dermatol*. 2007;143(11):1393–1398.

Ujiie H, Shimizu T, Natsuga K, et al. Severe cholinergic urticaria successfully treated with scopolamine butylbromide in addition to antihistamines. *Clin Exp Dermatol*. 2006;31(4):588–589. Retrieved November 27, 2009.

Volcheck GW, Li JTC. Exercise-induced urticaria and anaphylaxis. *Mayo Clin Proc*. 1997;72:140–147.

Wakelin S. Contact urticaria. *Clin Exp Dermatol*. 2001;26:132–136.

Zuraw BL, Busse PJ, White M, et al. Nanofiltered C1 inhibitor concentrate for treatment of hereditary angioedema. *N Engl J Med*. 2010;363:513–522.

Zembowicz A, Mastalerz L, Setkowicz L, et al. Safety of cyclo-oxygenase 2 inhibitors and increased leukotriene synthesis in chronic idiopathic urticaria with sensitivity to nonsteroidal anti-inflammatory drugs. *Arch Dermatol*. 2003;139:1577–1582.

Drug-Induced Photosensitive Reaction

Suzanne Berkman

Diagnosis Synopsis

Drug-Induced Photoallergic Reaction

Drug-induced photoallergic reactions are manifest by red, scaling, pruritic papules and plaques in photodistributed areas (forehead, malar areas, sides of the neck, and dorsal hands).

Oral agents reported to cause photoallergic reactions include the following: griseofulvin, quinine, quinolone, sulfonamides, quinidine, piroxicam, and pyridoxine hydrochloride. Constituents of sunscreens (benzophenone 3, cinnamates, Parsol 1789, anthranilate, and homosalate) and fragrances (musk ambrette, 6-methylcoumarin, bergamot oil, and sandalwood oil) are also common causes of photoallergic reactions. Careful histories are essential to determine inciting agents.

Drug-Induced Phototoxic Reaction

Drug-induced photosensitivity/phototoxicity results in an eruption similar to sunburn. Drugs that cause such a reaction typically have absorption spectra within the ultraviolet (UV) range. The effects are dependent on both the dose of the drug and the amount of UV light to which the person is exposed. Reactions typically occur 6 to 24 hours after the light exposure. The reaction will cause stinging and burning of the affected areas and can vary in color from red to bluish-red. Blistering may occur with severe reactions.

Drugs known to cause such reactions include nonsteroidal anti-inflammatory drugs (especially benoxaprofen and piroxicam), sulfonamides, trimethoprim, quinidine, thiazide diuretics, some tetracyclines, especially doxycycline, and fluoroquinolones.

Look For

Drug-Induced Photoallergic Reaction

Eczematous red papules in photodistributed areas on the face, neck, arms, and hands (Fig. 4-97). Lesions usually resolve with erythema; they are less likely to result in postinflammatory hyperpigmentation than phototoxic reactions.

Drug-Induced Phototoxic Reaction

A bright red confluent rash in sun-exposed areas, sometimes accompanied by edema, weeping, and blistering and, later, desquamation. It is usually prominent at the forehead, superior cheeks and lips, the "V-area" of the chest, extensor arms, and dorsum of the hands. Vesicles may be present

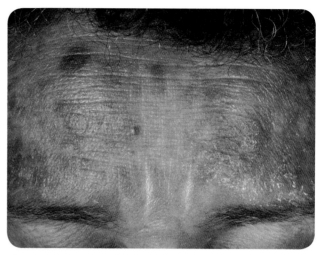

Figure 4-97 Quinine- and light-induced lichenoid lesions on the forehead.

as in severe sunburn. Onycholysis is also seen as a result of phototoxicity.

Diagnostic Pearls

Drug-Induced Photoallergic Reaction

Photoallergic reactions often spare the eyelids, whereas atopic dermatitis and contact dermatitis often involve the eyelids.

Drug-Induced Phototoxic Reaction

Skin under the nose, chin, and other areas protected from direct exposure to the sun may be spared. Drug-induced photosensitivity is often related to acute, intense sun exposure.

?? Differential Diagnosis and Pitfalls

Drug-Induced Photoallergic Reaction

- Atopic dermatitis
- Contact dermatitis
- Subacute cutaneous lupus
- Dermatomyositis
- Pemphigus foliaceus
- Pellagra

Drug-Induced Phototoxic Reaction

- Sunburn
- Systemic lupus erythematosus

- Dermatomyositis
- Porphyria cutanea tarda
- Airborne contact dermatitis

 ## ✓ Best Tests

Drug-Induced Photoallergic Reaction

Skin biopsy will show eczematous changes.

Drug-Induced Phototoxic Reaction

Usually a clinical diagnosis. Biopsy may confirm the diagnosis.

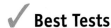 ## ▲▲ Management Pearls

Drug-Induced Photoallergic Reaction

Discontinue the offending agent.

Drug-Induced Phototoxic Reaction

Eliminate the medication and protect the patient from UV light sources with clothing and sunscreens. The eruption generally resolves over 7 to 10 days but in some instances may persist for months.

Therapy

Drug-Induced Photoallergic Reaction
Sunscreens with both UVB and UVA protection are essential. Topical corticosteroids twice daily or topical tacrolimus ointment 0.1% twice daily may be used.

Drug-Induced Phototoxic Reaction
Treatment involves decreasing the dose of or eliminating the use of the drug and limiting exposure to UV sources. Combined UVB/UVA sunscreens are essential.

Suggested Readings

Ferguson J. Photosensitivity due to drugs. *Photodermatol Photoimmunol Photomed.* 2002;18:262–269.

Foti C, Bonamonte D, Cassano N, et al. Photoallergic contact dermatitis. *G Ital Dermatol Venereol.* 2009;144:515–525.

Gould JW, Mercurio MG, Elmets CA. Cutaneous photosensitivity diseases induced by exogenous agents. *J Am Acad Dermatol.* 1995;33:551–573.

Acanthosis Nigricans

Katie L. Osley

■■ Diagnosis Synopsis

Acanthosis nigricans is a localized velvety hyperpigmentation and thickening of the skin that can be related to heredity, endocrine disorders, obesity, certain medications, and malignancy. Acanthosis nigricans can thus be subdivided into these subtypes: hereditary benign, obesity-related, syndromic, acanthosis nigricans maligna, acral acanthosis nigricans, medication-induced, and mixed.

Inherited acanthosis nigricans is rare and is unilateral, unlike the more common forms. This type is thought to be autosomal dominant with variable penetrance and will usually either stabilize or start to regress around puberty. When it is associated with obesity, acanthosis nigricans is typically mild and will regress with weight loss.

A large number of syndromes have been reported to be associated with acanthosis nigricans and are listed in Table 4-1. Most of the syndromes involve an element of either insulin resistance or mutations in fibroblast growth factor receptors. Both metabolic syndrome and polycystic ovarian syndrome have been associated with acanthosis nigricans. This can be attributed to the increased insulin resistance and compensatory hyperinsulinemia seen in those diseases.

Some of the medications that have been identified as causing acanthosis nigricans are insulin, nicotinic acid, oral contraceptives, corticosteroids, and protease inhibitors. The association is based on their tendency to induce hyperinsulinemia. A recent case report further supports insulin's role in acanthosis nigricans by demonstrating that exogenous insulin leads to formation of acanthosis nigricans. It has been shown that excess insulin binding to insulin-like growth factor-1 receptors on keratinocytes and fibroblasts is implicated in the pathogenesis of the hyperproliferative state in acanthosis nigricans.

Acanthosis nigricans can also be a useful marker for serious internal malignancies. It has been suggested that increased serum levels of transforming growth factor-α produced by tumor cells lead to hyperproliferation of keratinocytes-bearing epidermal growth factor receptors.

African Americans are 25 times more likely to have acanthosis nigricans compared to those of European descent. Furthermore, the condition is most common in Native Americans, followed by African Americans, Hispanics, and then non-Hispanic whites. The racial predisposition is evidenced by a study of an unselected population of children that showed acanthosis nigricans in 80 of 601 African Americans, 19 of 343 Hispanics, and 2 of 440 non-Hispanic whites. Studies have also shown that the prevalence of non–insulin-dependent diabetes in African Americans with acanthosis nigricans is higher than for those without acanthosis nigricans.

TABLE 4-1 Syndromes Associated with Acanthosis Nigricans
Acromegaly
Alström syndrome
Ataxia-telangiectasia
Bartter syndrome
Beare-Stevenson syndrome
Benign encephalopathy
Bloom syndrome
Capozucca syndrome
Chondrodystrophy with dwarfism
Costello syndrome
Crouzon syndrome
Dermatomyositis
Familial hypertrophy of the pineal body
Giantism
Hashimoto thyroiditis
Hepatic cirrhosis
Hirschowitz syndrome
Laurence-Moon-Bardet-Biedl syndrome
Lawrence-Seip syndrome
Lupoid hepatitis
Lupus erythematosus
Phenylketonuria
Pituitary hypogonadism
Pituitary basophilism
Prader-Willi syndrome
Pyramidal tract degeneration
Rabson syndrome
Reversible gestational insulin resistance
Rud syndrome
Scleroderma
Streak gonads
Type A syndrome of insulin resistance (HAIR-AN syndrome)
Can include PCOS and hirsutism and/or acral hypertrophy, clitoral hypertrophy, and muscle cramps
Rabson-Mendenhall syndrome, pseudoacromegaly syndrome, and leprechaunism
Can share clinical features of type A syndrome
Type B syndrome of insulin resistance
Diabetes mellitus, ovarian hyperandrogenism, lipoatrophic diabetes
Werner syndrome
Wilson disease

Source: Modified from Table 154-2 in Wolff K, et al. *Fitzpatrick's Dermatology in General Medicine.* 7th Ed. New York, NY: McGraw-Hill Medical; 2008.

Pediatric Patient Considerations

Acanthosis nigricans is usually a benign finding in children (except for a few rare cases) and is most commonly found in conjunction with type II diabetes and obesity. A recent placebo-controlled, randomized trial showed that acanthosis nigricans identifies an at-risk group of children who should be screened for glucose intolerance and who may benefit from early medical intervention. Some lesions are of the congenital subtype and can arise anytime between infancy and adulthood.

Nail changes include striation, brittle nails, longitudinal grooves, thickening, patchy leukonychia, or a completely white appearance. Rarely, pruritus or hair loss due to scalp, eyebrow, limb, or axilla involvement can occur.

Pediatric Patient Considerations

Examination of the neck in children is critical because 99% of children with acanthosis nigricans have involvement in this area. The axillae are also a very common area in children and are involved 73% of the time.

◉ Look For

Look for circumscribed, hyperpigmented brown plaques that can be velvety and verrucous or fine and papillomatous. The symmetric eruption arises most commonly in the axillae and on the posterior and lateral neck (Fig. 4-98). Other areas of involvement include the axillae, inguinal region, antecubital and popliteal surfaces, the umbilical area, and the oral mucosa, although any location on the skin can be affected (Figs. 4-99–4-101). Oral mucosa and lip lesions have thickening and papillation and usually lack hyperpigmentation.

The typical patient will be obese and dark skinned, with a tendency toward developing type II diabetes.

Acanthosis nigricans may also coexist with other cutaneous signs of internal malignancy, such as the sign of Leser-Trélat (acute appearance of multiple seborrheic keratoses), tylosis (hyperkeratosis of the palms and soles), or tripe palms (rugated and thickened appearance of palms).

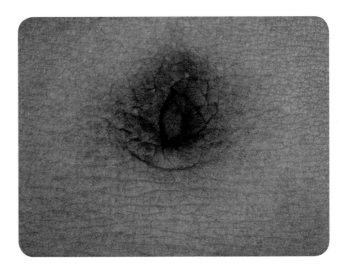

Figure 4-99 Periumbilical acanthosis nigricans.

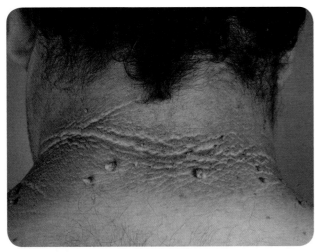

Figure 4-98 Typical location for acanthosis nigricans, with thickened and darkened skin folds.

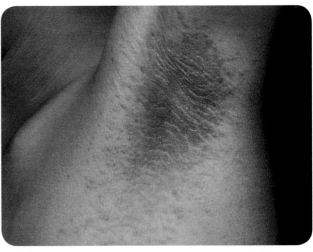

Figure 4-100 Acanthosis nigricans with prominent parallel darkened rows of thickened skin in the axilla.

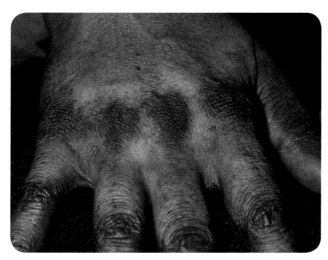

Figure 4-101 A common location for acanthosis nigricans is over metacarpophalangeal and proximal interphalangeal joints.

Diagnostic Pearls

- Acanthosis nigricans classically starts out with a dirty look to the skin, which eventually becomes thickened and papillomatous. The neck is the best location to detect early involvement. It is often associated with overlying acrochordon (skin tag) formation over time.
- Acanthosis nigricans maligna can be distinguished from the benign subtypes by its diffuse skin involvement and rapid onset and prominent oral involvement.
- In patients with deeper skin pigmentation, skin changes will often be a darker black color rather than the gray to brown colors seen in lighter-skinned individuals.

?? Differential Diagnosis and Pitfalls

- Becker nevus—most commonly located on the trunk rather than intertriginous areas
- Linear epidermal nevus—Lesions follow lines of Blaschko and can be either unilateral or bilateral.
- Fox-Fordyce disease—Extreme pruritus and perifollicular papules with central punctum help differentiate this.
- Pellagra—Look for GI upset and dementia. Rule out with successful therapeutic trial of niacin or serum niacin levels.
- Erythema ab igne—Reticulated pattern and history of prolonged exposure to a heat source will be evident.
- Addison disease—Measure serum sodium, potassium, ACTH, and cortisol to help rule out this diagnosis. Hyperpigmentation can occur in axillae but mostly occurs on the sun-exposed face, neck, and hands in addition to areas of chronic pressure like knees and elbows.
- Hemochromatosis—mimics many common conditions, including diabetes, so abnormal serum ferritin and transferrin can help establish diagnosis

- Tinea versicolor—KOH preparation may show classic "spaghetti and meatball" picture of *Malassezia furfur*.
- Cowden disease—As opposed to oral acanthosis nigricans, papillomatous involvement of oral mucosa in Cowden disease will be whitish in color, and papules coalesce to form a cobblestone appearance. Multiple GI hamartomas, macrocephaly, and thyroid or breast cancer will also be clues to this diagnosis.
- Confluent and reticulated papillomatosis, atopic dermatitis, and erythrasma all present a specific challenge when determining the diagnosis of acanthosis nigricans in individuals with deeper skin pigmentation. The following diagnoses are more likely to be confused with acanthosis nigricans in dark-skinned individuals:
  - Confluent and reticulated papillomatosis (Gougerot-Carteaud syndrome)—KOH examination of skin scrapings to identify *Malassezia* species associated with this rash. Wood lamp would also show yellow fluorescence.
  - Atopic dermatitis—Early forms of acanthosis nigricans may lack thickening and resemble this diagnosis. Pruritus and response to topical corticosteroids would be helpful clues here.
  - Erythrasma—Wood lamp will create classic coral red fluorescence, or KOH preparation may show evidence of bacilli in chains.

Pediatric Patient Considerations

- Goltz-Gorlin syndrome—When brown lesions appear on the oral mucosa in a child, other clinical features such as lobster claw deformity and several ocular, craniofacial, and musculoskeletal abnormalities would help distinguish this disease from oral acanthosis nigricans.
- Peutz-Jeghers syndrome—presents at birth with mucocutaneous lentigines. Distinguishing features are that lentigines fade with age and are more discrete than acanthosis nigricans. Both diagnoses often have a positive family history due to autosomal dominant inheritance and have an increased risk of intestinal tumors.
- X-linked ichthyosis—dirty-appearing brown scales with involvement of the flexural surfaces, trunk, neck, and extremities

✓ Best Tests

A crucial first step is identifying the underlying cause of the acanthosis nigricans. It is recommended that the clinician calculate body mass index, measure blood pressure, and obtain fasting glucose, fasting insulin, fasting lipid profile, hemoglobin A1C, and liver enzymes. Polycystic ovarian syndrome can be screened for by asking about menstrual irregularities, acne, hirsutism, and virilization. Cushing syndrome may be evidenced by central obesity and purple striae, which would warrant a 24-hour cortisol test. Due to the prevalence of Hashimoto thyroiditis, a screening of TSH may also be helpful.

The diagnosis of acanthosis nigricans is usually based on clinical presentation; however, a biopsy can be confirmatory if the presentation is atypical or an alternate diagnosis is suspected. Histopathology demonstrates papillomatosis and hyperkeratosis with increased melanocytes at the epidermal basal layer, but the hyperpigmentation is usually attributed to the hyperkeratosis. Note: histopathologic evaluation does not differentiate between benign and malignant subtypes. CT scan imaging of the abdomen and endoscopy should be ordered if acanthosis nigricans maligna is suspected.

Pediatric Patient Considerations

A workup for insulin resistance and metabolic syndrome will suffice unless florid signs of acanthosis nigricans maligna are present.

▲▲▲ Management Pearls

Diet and exercise should be advised in the management of patients with obesity and insulin resistance, but only one case report has shown improvement of the rash with this intervention alone. A nutritionist consult may be advisable. An endocrine consult is also wise if the rash has this type of etiology. Removal of an offending medication has consistently led to clearing of these skin findings.

When acanthosis nigricans is extensive or when it coexists with other skin manifestations of malignancy such as Leser-Trélat sign (explosion of multiple seborrheic keratoses), mucocutaneous papillomatosis, or tripe palms (hyperkeratosis with marked papillary markings), a thorough workup for malignant tumors and consultation with oncology should be set in motion. Adenocarcinomas of the abdomen are the most common associated malignancy (70% to 90%), with gastric cancer making up 55% to 61%. Endoscopy with biopsy should therefore always take place when acanthosis nigricans maligna is diagnosed. The skin changes associated with the malignancy will often regress once the tumor is removed. However, treatment of the skin lesions should also be attempted in order to prevent discomfort and pruritus. Return of acanthosis nigricans in an oncology patient may provide a clue to reappearance of the tumor.

Therapy

Therapy generally involves treating the underlying condition. Benign acanthosis nigricans is treated for cosmetic purposes only.

- Metformin—1,700 to 2,250 mg daily in two or three divided doses for obesity-related and insulin resistance-related acanthosis nigricans (patient and physician should be aware of the side effects)
- Retinoic acid 0.1% cream twice daily for 2 weeks; once per week for maintenance. Considered to be first-line treatment due to ease of use and good safety profile. It can be combined with ammonium lactate 12% creams (Lac-Hydrin).
- Calcipotriene 0.005% twice daily
- Salicylic acid 6% in propylene glycol twice daily
- Oral retinoids—isotretinoin 3 mg/kg/d or acitretin 0.8 mg/kg/d divided twice daily (must consider the side effect profile and risk for toxicity with this medication)
- Oral cyproheptadine
- Dietary fish oil 10 to 20 mg per day
- PUVA (psoralen + UVA treatment)
- Long-pulsed alexandrite laser treatments (fluence 16 to 23 J/cm², spot size 10 to 12.5 mm)

Suggested Readings

Brickman WJ, Huang J, Silverman BL, et al. Acanthosis nigricans identifies youth at high risk for metabolic abnormalities. *J Pediatr.* 2010;156(1):87–92. Epub.

DeWitt CA, Buescher LS, Stone SP. Cutaneous manifestations of internal malignant disease: cutaneous paraneoplastic syndromes. In: Wolff K, Goldsmith LA, Katz SI, et al., eds. *Fitzpatrick's Dermatology in General Medicine.* 7th Ed. New York, NY: McGraw-Hill Medical; 2008.

Higgins SP, Freemark M, Prose NS. Acanthosis nigricans: a practical approach to evaluation and management. *Dermatol Online J.* 2008;14(9):2.

Koyama S. Transforming growth factor-alpha (TGF alpha)-producing gastric carcinoma with acanthosis nigricans: an endocrine effect of TGF alpha in the pathogenesis of cutaneous paraneoplastic syndrome and epithelial hyperplasia of the esophagus. *J Gastroenterol.* 1997;32(1):71–77.

Krawczyk M, Mykała-Cieśla J, Kołodziej-Jaskuła A. Acanthosis nigricans as a paraneoplastic syndrome. Case reports and review of literature. *Pol Arch Med Wewn.* 2009;119(3):180–183.

Mailler-Savage EA, Adams BB. Exogenous insulin-derived Acanthosis nigricans. *Arch Dermatol.* 2008;144(1):126–127.

Paron NG, Lambert PW. Cutaneous manifestations of diabetes mellitus. *Prim Care.* 2000;27:371–383.

Romo A, Benavides S. Treatment options in insulin resistance obesity–related acanthosis nigricans. *Ann Pharmacother.* 2008;42(7):1090–1094. Epub 2008 May 20.

Schwartz RA. Acanthosis nigricans. *J Am Acad Dermatol.* 1994;31(1):1–19; quiz 20–22.

Stuart CA, Gilkison CR, Smith MM, et al. Acanthosis nigricans as a risk factor for non-insulin dependent diabetes mellitus. *Clin Pediatr.* 1998;37:73–79.

Stuart CA, Pate CJ, Peters EJ. Prevalence of acanthosis nigricans in an unselected population. *Am J Med.* 1989;87(3):269–272.

■■ Diagnosis Synopsis

Peutz-Jeghers Syndrome

Peutz-Jeghers syndrome (perioral lentiginosis) is a genetically inherited condition with oral, labial, and perioral hypermelanotic macules and gastrointestinal (GI) polyposis. The condition is inherited in an autosomal dominant fashion, with 50% to 75% of patients carrying a mutation in the STK11/LKB1, a tumor suppressor gene. Forty percent of cases are the result of sporadic mutation. There are no differences between the sexes, and the condition may occur in any ethnic group. Novel mutations have been identified in certain ethnic groups.

Hypermelanotic macules can be found in the oral cavity, on the vermilion, and in the perioral distribution at birth or early in childhood. The lower lip is the favored site of involvement. Similar lesions can appear on the dorsal hands and feet, fingers, toes, and genital mucosa over time.

GI polyps typically form in the second decade, commonly involving the small intestine, particularly the jejunum. Polyp formation, however, can occur at any site along the GI tract. Patients may present with abdominal pain, nausea/vomiting, diarrhea, GI bleeding, intussusception, and/or obstruction. The polyps are benign hamartomas with a low rate (2% to 13%) of malignant transformation, and when this occurs, it is most commonly in the colorectal region, followed by the small bowel; patients also have a generalized increased risk of other cancers (breast, pancreas, and ovarian, among others).

Linear and Whorled Nevoid Hypermelanosis

Linear and whorled nevoid hypermelanosis is a rare pigmentary disorder characterized by streaks and swirls of macular hyperpigmentation following the lines of Blaschko. The onset of hyperpigmentation typically occurs within the first few weeks of life and continues to progress for a year or two before stopping. There is no preceding inflammatory stage. The patterns of pigmentation are segmental, linear, swirled, or a combination of distributions, all following the lines of Blaschko and all with sharp midline cutoffs. Lesions spare the mucous membranes, palms, and soles. Occurrence is sporadic without sex predilection.

Progressive cribriform and zosteriform hyperpigmentation is considered to be a localized, unilateral variant of this disorder that can present later in life.

Associated abnormalities have been reported in a minority of cases, involving primarily the central nervous system and musculoskeletal system. Histologically, involved areas of skin show epidermal melanosis in the basal layer without dermal pigment incontinence.

Etiology may be related to mosaicism. Supporting this hypothesis, underlying chromosomal mosaicism has been demonstrated in some cases. One case report describes a Japanese patient with dysgenetic male pseudohermaphroditism due to sex chromosomal mosaicism who incidentally was found to have linear and whorled nevoid hypermelanosis on the trunk. Another report describes a Japanese mother and daughter with linear and whorled nevoid hypermelanosis on the trunk and extremities; however, chromosomal analysis revealed no evidence of mixoploidy or chimerism.

The emerging opinion is that linear and whorled nevoid hypermelanosis should not be separated as its own single entity but rather grouped with other pigmentary disorders that follow the lines of Blaschko and are thought to be due to genetic mosaicism. The term "pigmentary mosaicism" would thus group together pigmentary abnormalities such as linear and whorled nevoid hypermelanosis, hypomelanosis of Ito, and others.

Pediatric Patient Considerations

Linear and whorled nevoid hypermelanosis typically presents within the first few weeks of life.

◉ Look For

Peutz-Jeghers Syndrome

Flat, oval, pigmented (dark brown, gray-blue, or black) macules <5 mm (and often <1 mm) in diameter usually on the lips, nose, periorbital area, elbows, dorsal aspects of fingers and toes, palms and soles, and buccal mucosa (Figs. 4-102 and 4-103). The skin lesions may fade at puberty or in adulthood, but buccal lesions often persist.

Linear and Whorled Nevoid Hypermelanosis

Linear and whorled nevoid hypermelanosis classically presents with streaks and swirls of macular hyperpigmentation, without preceding inflammation, following the lines of Blaschko (Figs. 4-104 and 4-105). Of note, the lines of Blaschko form a V shape on the back, an S shape on the abdomen, an inverted U shape from the chest to the upper arms, and perpendicular lines on the extremities, all with a characteristic sharp midline cutoff.

●● Diagnostic Pearls

Peutz-Jeghers Syndrome

Premature puberty may occur.

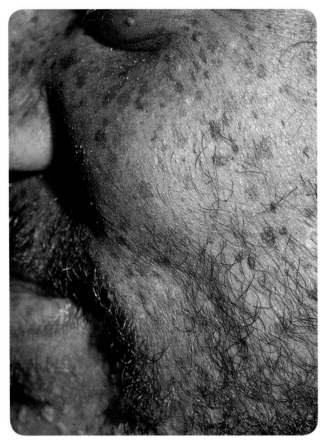

Figure 4-102 Peutz-Jeghers syndrome with facial lentigo and also multiple lesions of dermatosis papulosa nigra.

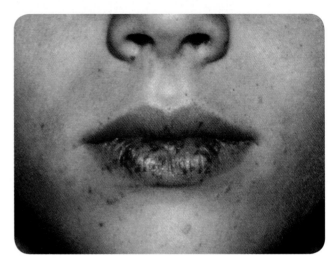

Figure 4-103 Multiple hyperpigmented brown macules on lips and face in Peutz-Jeghers syndrome.

Linear and Whorled Nevoid Hypermelanosis

Macular hyperpigmentation in a linear or whorled pattern following the lines of Blaschko.

Pediatric Patient Considerations

The hyperpigmentation classically presents in the first few weeks of life and continues to progress for a year or two before stabilizing.

?? Differential Diagnosis and Pitfalls

Peutz-Jeghers Syndrome

- LEOPARD syndrome—lentigines, hypertrophic cardiomyopathy, deafness
- Carney complex—lentigines and cardiac myxomas
- Laugier-Hunziker syndrome—mucosal pigmentation and pigmented nail streaks
- Cronkhite-Canada—melanotic macules on fingers, GI polyposis, alopecia, and nail dystrophy

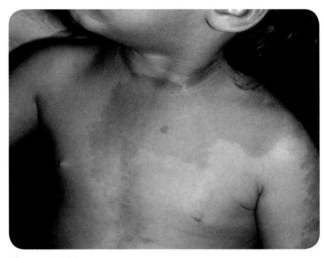

Figure 4-104 Sharply bordered hypopigmented lesions on the face and trunk in nevoid hypermelanosis.

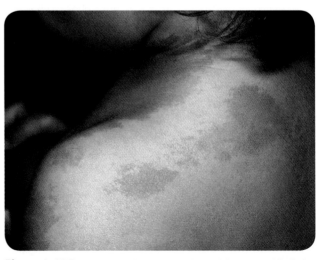

Figure 4-105 Large hypopigmented lesions with some residual pigmentation in nevoid hypermelanosis.

- Bannayan-Ruvalcaba-Riley syndrome—penile lentigines, GI polyposis, lipomas, hemangiomas
- Centrofacial lentiginosis
- Familial benign lentiginosis
- Labial melanotic macules

Linear and Whorled Nevoid Hypermelanosis

- Hypomelanosis of Ito—This is characterized by linear hypopigmentation.
- Incontinentia pigmenti—Characteristic inflammatory vesicular and verrucous stages precede the whorled hyperpigmentation. The hyperpigmented stage is followed by a hypopigmented stage later in life. Also, this is usually lethal in men.
- Inflammatory linear epidermal nevi
- Goltz syndrome—On histopathologic examination, dermal hypoplasia is present.
- Proteus syndrome—Epidermal nevi become elevated and verrucous with time.

 ## Best Tests

Peutz-Jeghers Syndrome

When the diagnosis is suspected, the entire GI tract should be investigated. Skin biopsy is not diagnostic. Intestinal biopsy is diagnostic with smooth muscle arborization.

Linear and Whorled Nevoid Hypermelanosis

Clinical examination coupled with a thorough history is usually the best diagnostic method.

Additionally, dermatoscopic examination reveals a linear or circular arrangement of streaklike pigmentation arranged in parallel fashion, correlating with the clinical appearance. Also, blue-gray dots are absent, correlating histopathologically with the absence of pigment incontinence.

If clinical exam is not conclusive, diagnosis may be confirmed with a biopsy. On histopathological evaluation, hyperpigmentation of the basal layer with prominent melanocytes is seen; however, melanocytes are normal in size and number, indicating that there is no proliferation of melanocytes.

 ## Management Pearls

Peutz-Jeghers Syndrome

Referral to a gastroenterologist is necessary to facilitate monitoring of the GI polyps by upper endoscopy, routine colonoscopy, and capsule endoscopy. Referral to a gynecologist is also useful with monitoring for breast and ovarian cancers. Family members should be examined for skin and intestinal lesions. A genetics referral may be appropriate.

Linear and Whorled Nevoid Hypermelanosis

Patients with linear and whorled nevoid hypermelanosis should have a thorough history taken, and a physical examination should be performed to look for any possible associated extracutaneous abnormalities. If any such abnormalities are present or suspected, further testing may need to be performed by the appropriate specialist.

Pediatric Patient Considerations

It is important to note that associated abnormalities, if present, typically manifest early in childhood.

Therapy

Peutz-Jeghers Syndrome

Individual polypectomy for symptomatic GI polyps. The lentigines do not require treatment but can be lightened with chemical peels or laser. Darkly pigmented patients are at increased risk for posttreatment pigment alteration following these types of cosmetic treatments. However, in one report, the Q-switched alexandrite laser led to successful elimination of oral labial lentigines in several Chinese subjects after only one treatment, with no recurrence or scarring at 2-year follow-up. The lentigines on the lips may disappear with time, but those on the buccal mucosa persist.

Linear and Whorled Nevoid Hypermelanosis

To date, no effective treatments for linear and whorled nevoid hypermelanosis exist. In some cases, hydroquinone cream was applied to lesions in an attempt to lighten the areas; however, results were disappointing as the hyperpigmented areas did not respond to the treatment. Future developments in laser therapy and camouflage cosmetics may prove to be helpful for some patients.

Suggested Readings

Akiyama M, Aranami A, Sasaki Y, et al. Familial linear and whorled nevoid hypermelanosis. *J Am Acad Dermatol.* 1994;30:831–833.

Alrobaee AA, Alsaif F. Linear and whorled nevoid hypermelanosis associated with developmental delay and generalized convulsions. *Int J Dermatol.* 2004;43:145–147.

Brar BK, Mahajan BB, Puri N. Linear and whorled nevoid hypermelanosis. *Indian J Dermatol Venereol Leprol.* 2008;74:512–513.

Ertam I, Turk BG, Urkmez A, et al. Linear and whorled nevoid hypermelanosis: Dermatoscopic features. *J Am Acad Dermatol.* 2009;60:328–331.

Hong SP, Ahn SY, Lee WS. Linear and whorled nevoid hypermelanosis: unique clinical presentations and their possible association with chromosomal abnormality. *Arch Dermatol.* 2008;144:415–416.

Lapeere H, Boone B, De Schepper S, et al. Hypomelanoses and hypermelanoses. In: Wolff K, Goldsmith LA, Katz SI, Gilchrest BA, Paller AS, Leffell DJ, eds. *Fitzpatrick's Dermatology in General Medicine.* 7th Ed. New York, NY: McGraw-Hill; 2008:631–634.

Lernia VD. Linear and whorled hypermelanosis. *Pediatr Dermatol.* 2007;24:205–210.

Pinheiro A, Mathew MC, Thomas M, et al. The clinical profile of children in India with pigmentary anomalies along the lines of Blaschko and central nervous system manifestations. *Pediatr Dermatol.* 2007;24:11–17.

Vélez A, Gaitan MH, Marquez JR, et al. Two novel LKB1 mutations in Colombian Peutz-Jeghers syndrome patients. *Clin Genet.* 2009;75(3): 304–306.

Xi Z, Hui Q, Zhong L. Q-switched alexandrite laser treatment of oral labial lentigines in Chinese subjects with Peutz-Jeghers syndrome. *Dermatol Surg.* 2009;35(7):1084–1088.

Genetic Disorders of Pigmentation

Donna Culton

■■ Diagnosis Synopsis

Cutaneous pigmentation is a complex, multistep process involving melanocyte precursor migration during embryogenesis, synthesis of melanin by melanocytes, packaging of melanin into melanosomes, and subsequent transfer of melanosomes to keratinocytes. Disturbances in any of the multiple steps can lead to hypopigmentation variants. There are several inherited disorders that include partial or a complete lack of pigmentation as part of their clinical findings.

The most classic of these genetic disorders is oculocutaneous albinism (OCA), an autosomal recessive disorder due to a mutation in tyrosinase, an enzyme important in the biosynthesis of melanin. This disease presents with diffuse absence or dilution of pigment in the skin, hair, and retina and can be seen in all races and ethnicities. Reduced visual acuity and nystagmus are often associated findings. Prevalence is estimated at 1 in 20,000 people worldwide and 1 in 16,000 in the United States. In the United States, there is a slightly higher prevalence in African Americans compared to whites.

The OCA group is divided into OCA types 1 through 4. OCA1A (tyrosinase-negative OCA) is due to a mutation in the *TYR* gene, which encodes tyrosinase. These patients have a complete lack of melanin in all tissues and present with white hair, pink skin, and red eyes. OCA1B (yellow-mutant OCA) is due to a point mutation in the *TYR* gene, such that tyrosinase activity is greatly reduced but not completely absent. These patients are indistinguishable from OCA1A patients at birth but slowly accumulate small amounts of pigment in the first few years of life and eventually develop yellow hair with increased pigment in their skin and eyes as well. OCA2 results from mutations in the P gene, which encodes melanosomal membrane protein, which is thought to regulate tyrosinase. The clinical phenotype of these patients is variable. OCA3 is due to a mutation in the *TRP-1* gene and has been described in South African black people with minimal hypopigmentation. Finally, OCA4 results from mutation in the *MATP* gene, which encodes a protein important in melanosome trafficking. OCA4 is very common in Japanese patients and is very rare in whites. The clinical phenotype is variable.

Piebaldism and Waardenburg syndrome (WS) are rare autosomal dominant disorders due to defective melanocyte development and migration during embryogenesis. These diseases present with fixed depigmented patches of the skin (leukoderma) and hair (poliosis or white forelock), which are present at birth. Piebaldism is due to mutations within the *c-kit* or *SLUG* genes, and clinical features include depigmented patches on the midline ventral surface (midforehead, chest, and abdomen) and symmetric involvement of extremities. WS can be caused by mutations within a number of genes including *PAX3* (WS types 1 and 3), *MITF* (WS type 2),

and *Sox10* (WS type 4). Clinically, these patients present with features similar to those seen in piebaldism but also have associated pigmentary abnormalities in the iris (heterochromic irides), widely set eyes (dystopia canthorum), congenital deafness, and Hirschsprung disease (WS type 4). As with many genetic conditions, novel mutations have been identified within certain ethnic groups, and founder effect may be present in certain countries.

Disorders due to melanosome formation and transfer of melanosomes to keratinocytes include Hermansky-Pudlak syndrome (HPS), Chediak-Higashi syndrome (CHS), and Griscelli syndrome. HPS is a rare autosomal recessive disorder caused by mutations in the *HPS* genes, which encode proteins important in lysosome-related organelles like melanosomes. HPS has been identified in almost all ethnic groups, but disease is most common in patients of Puerto Rican, Northern European, Japanese, and Israeli descent. Cutaneous manifestations include reduction in pigment of the skin, hair, and eyes. Extrapigmentary findings include easy bruising with prolonged bleeding due to platelet granule dysfunction and granulomatous colitis and pulmonary fibrosis due to ceroid storage disease. Easy bruising is often difficult to detect in patients with more heavily pigmented skin.

CHS and Griscelli syndrome are also due to defects in melanosome formation and trafficking. These diseases belong to a group of disorders with pigmentary alteration associated with silvery hair, all of which are inherited in an autosomal recessive fashion. CHS is a multisystem immunodeficiency disorder characterized by recurrent infections, mild bleeding diathesis, OCA, and multiple neurologic problems (nystagmus, photophobia, peripheral neuropathy, seizures, problems in the spine and cerebellum). Mutation in the *LYST* gene, which is important in melanosome trafficking, results in giant organelles including melanosomes, lymphocyte granules, and platelet granules. These dysfunctional organelles help to explain the clinical findings that are often present by early childhood. Death in childhood may occur due to infections or an accelerated lymphomalike hemophagocytic phase that occurs in 90% of patients. Griscelli syndrome is caused by mutations in *MYO5A*, *RAB27A*, or *Slac-2a*, all of which are involved in organelle transport. Pigment abnormalities are typically more limited to the silvery hair. Other clinical findings are determined by the particular mutation and include neurologic disorder (*MYO5A*) and hemophagocytic syndrome (*RAB27A*). Elejalde syndrome is allelic to the *MYO5A* form of Griscelli syndrome and is associated with severe neurologic dysfunction.

Hypomelanosis of Ito, more commonly referred to simply as pigmentary mosaicism, is focal whorled depigmented patches present at birth or early in infancy. There are occasional associations with mental retardation, seizures, or developmental delay.

⊙ Look For

Albinism (Figs. 4-106 and 4-107)—Look for lack of or decreased pigment in eyes (gray-blue iris), hair (white to yellow in color), and skin (pink or slightly pigmented/tan). Children with type IA have nystagmus and photophobia and are usually legally blind.

Piebaldism (Fig. 4-108)—White forelock (depigmentation of central frontal scalp and hair) occurs in 80% to 90% of patients. Hypopigmentation of the central face and ventral midline trunk are also seen with occasional symmetrical distribution on the proximal arms and distal legs. Normally pigmented spots may be seen within larger areas of depigmentation.

WS—Look for poliosis (white forelock), leukoderma (white patches of skin), synophrys (confluent eyebrows), heterochromia iridis (pigmentary alteration in the iris), and dystopia canthorum (widely spaced eyes). These cutaneous findings are often in association with sensorineural deafness and megacolon (Hirschsprung, WS type 4).

HPS—Look for lightly colored skin, hair, and eyes in association with prolonged bleeding time, pulmonary fibrosis, and granulomatous colitis.

CHS (Fig. 4-109)—Look for recurrent infections, OCA, and neurologic impairments. A silvery sheen to the hair may be apparent.

Hypomelanosis of Ito (Figs. 4-110 and 4-111)—Look for asymmetric "whorled" hypopigmented macules and patches following lines of Blaschko. There may be a sharp midline cutoff. Occasionally, limb hemihypertrophy and genital abnormalities may be seen.

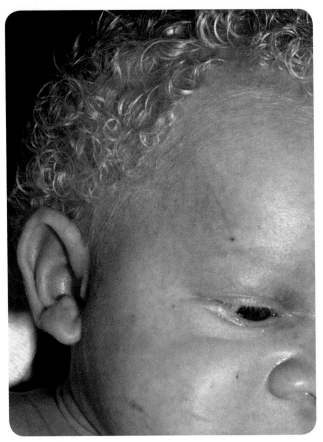

Figure 4-106 Infant with albinism with unaffected family members.

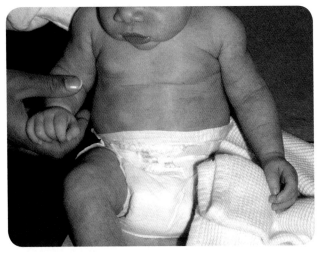

Figure 4-107 Infant with albinism with an unaffected parent's hand.

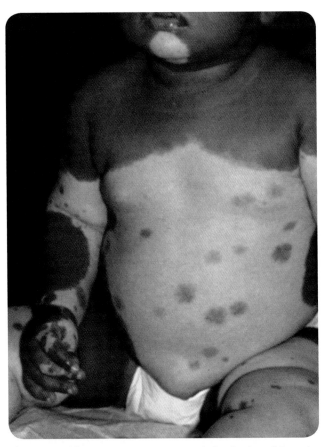

Figure 4-108 Piebaldism with a typical distribution of hypopigmented macules.

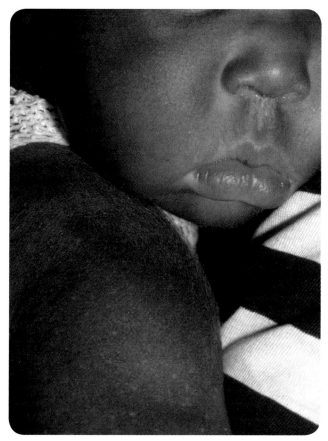

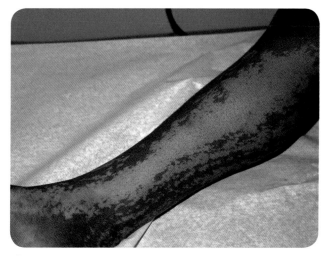

Figure 4-110 Hypomelanosis of Ito in a Blaschko line distribution.

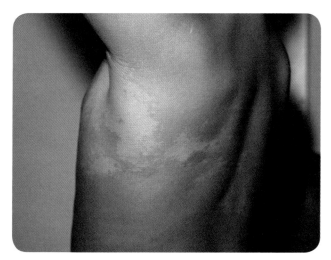

Figure 4-109 One of two siblings with Chediak-Higashi syndrome with moderate pigment dilution.

Diagnostic Pearls

- Use a Wood light (UVA black light) to detect subtle areas of hypopigmentation in light- or fair-skinned infants.
- High clinical suspicion is necessary in any patients presenting with pigmentary alteration, particularly if findings have been present since birth. A thorough review of systems is necessary to correctly diagnose these complex genetic syndromes.

Differential Diagnosis and Pitfalls

- Oculocutaneous albinism
- Nonsyndromic poliosis
- Piebaldism
- Waardenburg syndrome
- Hermansky-Pudlak syndrome
- Chediak-Higashi syndrome
- Griscelli syndrome
- Vitiligo—acquired depigmented patches
- Nevus depigmentosus
- Ash-leaf spots of tuberous sclerosis

Figure 4-111 Hypomelanosis in the dermatome-like distribution.

- Alezzandrini syndrome—unilateral facial hypopigmentation associated with retinal detachment and blindness and hypoacusis in some patients
- Vogt-Koyanagi-Harada syndrome—ocular pain, loss of vision, and hair loss with vitiligo
- Phenylketonuria
- Cross-McKusick-Breen syndrome—severe mental retardation with spastic tetraplegia

Best Tests

- Many of these diagnoses are made by clinical means and confirmed by genetic testing.
- Albinism—Diagnosis is clinical, but PCR and hair bulb tyrosinase assay can be used to differentiate forms of albinism.

- WS—clinical diagnosis, usually with family history; mutations in the *PAX3* gene on chromosome 2q35 (types I and III) and *MITF* gene on chromosome 3p13 (type II)
- CHS—Exam of a peripheral blood smear reveals giant granules in neutrophils, eosinophils, and granulocytes. Laboratory findings include slightly low neutrophil numbers, impaired neutrophil function, and hypergammaglobulinemia. Hair shaft pigment analysis shows evenly distributed pigment granules.
- Griscelli syndrome—irregular large pigmentary clumping

▲▲▲ Management Pearls

- For all disorders with decreased pigmentation, sun avoidance, sun protection, and eye protection are necessary. The use of sunscreen with both UVA and UVB blockers and sun-protective clothing should be emphasized. Patients with darkly pigmented skin are often unaware of their increased risk of actinic damage and nonmelanoma skin cancers. Aggressive counseling is necessary.
- In addition, for any genetic syndrome, genetic counseling should be offered.
- The psychosocial impact of albinism or pigmentary alteration in patients with darkly pigmented skin should not be overlooked. Appropriate referral for counseling should be considered.
- Referral to specialists for management of associated extracutaneous manifestations should be made:
  - OCA—Regular ophthalmologic evaluation is necessary.
  - Waardenburg—Patients should have regular ophthalmologic and auditory evaluations with early intervention for hearing abnormalities.
- HPS—Referral to hematology for management of bleeding diathesis is warranted. Referral to pulmonology and gastroenterology to evaluate for pulmonary fibrosis and granulomatous colitis is necessary.
- CHS—Prophylactic antibiotics are used to prevent infections, with aggressive therapy of bacterial infections as they occur. Bone marrow transplantation can be life-saving. Hematologic and neurologic consultation should be considered.

Therapy

There is no particular treatment for the lack of pigment, as this is a genetic disorder. Patient education is important, including counseling regarding sun protection and sun avoidance. Depending on the extent of the condition, some surgical techniques are available, with varying success: dermabrasion, skin grafting, and minigrafting.

Suggested Readings

deSaxe M, Kromberg JG, Jenkins T. Waardenburg syndrome in South Africa. Part II. Is there founder effect for type I? *S Afr Med J.* 1984;66(8):291–293.

Dessinioti C, Stratigos AJ, Rigopoulos D, et al. A review of genetic disorders of hypopigmentation: Lessons learned from the biology of melanocytes. *Exp Dermatol.* 2009;18(9):741–749.

Okulicz JF, Shah RS, Schwartz RA, et al. Oculocutaneous albinism. *J Eur Acad Dermatol Venereol.* 2003;17(3):251–256.

Thomas I, Kihiczak GG, Fox MD, et al. Piebaldism: An update. *Int J Dermatol.* 2004;43(10):716–719.

Yin XY, Ren YQ, Yang S, et al. A nove KIT missense mutation in one Chinese family with piebaldism. *Arch Dermatol Res.* 2009;301(5):387–389.

Pityriasis Alba

Cynthia Marie Carver DeKlotz

◼ Diagnosis Synopsis

Pityriasis alba is a benign skin disorder that is characterized by hypopigmented macules or patches. Lesions may be asymptomatic or mildly pruritic and range in size from 0.5 to 5 cm. Classically, there is no preceding inflammatory stage, and, on exam, fine scale may be present. Often, the lesions are poorly demarcated; however, at times, the hypopigmentation may be well defined.

Pityriasis alba often has a chronic course, tends to relapse, and usually worsens in the summer with increased sun exposure. It predominately occurs in children between the ages of 3 and 16 years and is found equally in both sexes. In the majority of patients, spontaneous resolution typically occurs before adulthood. Lesions most commonly occur on the face and upper arms. Pityriasis alba is often found in association with atopic dermatitis or in patients with an atopic diathesis. Pityriasis alba tends to be more noticeable in patients with darkly pigmented skin.

The etiology of pityriasis alba is not well established; however, many possible causes or triggers have been implicated. These include microorganisms such as *Pityrosporum*, *Streptococcus*, *Aspergillus*, and *Staphylococcus*, as well as other factors such as temperature, air humidity, and sunlight exposure. Evidence also suggests that pityriasis alba is a mild eczematous dermatitis.

Pediatric Patient Considerations

Pityriasis alba is most often found in the pediatric and adolescent patient population.

◉ Look For

Pityriasis alba classically presents on the face and upper arms as hypopigmented macules or patches with fine overlying scale (Figs. 4-112–4-116).

●● Diagnostic Pearls

Try to elicit a history of an atopic diathesis and look for other signs of atopic dermatitis, as these are strongly associated with pityriasis alba.

?? Differential Diagnosis and Pitfalls

The differential diagnosis of pityriasis alba is numerous and includes other hypopigmented lesions:

- Nevus depigmentosus—This is distinguished histopathologically by its reduction in both the amount of melanin and the number of melanocytes.
- Tinea versicolor—Potassium hydroxide (KOH) smears are positive in tinea and negative in pityriasis alba.
- Vitiligo—depigmented lesions where Wood lamp examination reveals bright white accentuation of the lesion
- Postinflammatory hypopigmentation—This is preceded by an inflammatory stage.
- Corticosteroid-induced hypopigmentation
- Guttate psoriasis
- Idiopathic guttate hypomelanosis
- Ash-leaf spot of tuberous sclerosis

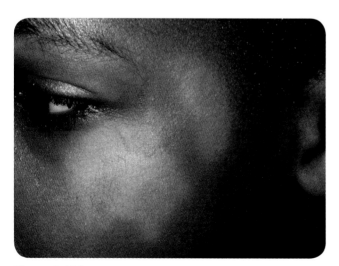

Figure 4-112 Flat, smooth, hypopigmented macules and patches in a typical location for pityriasis alba.

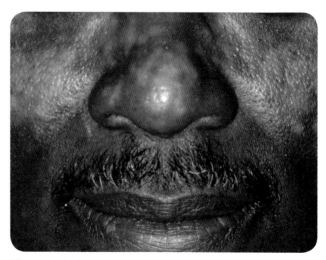

Figure 4-113 Irregular, mottled, hypopigmented lesions of pityriasis alba.

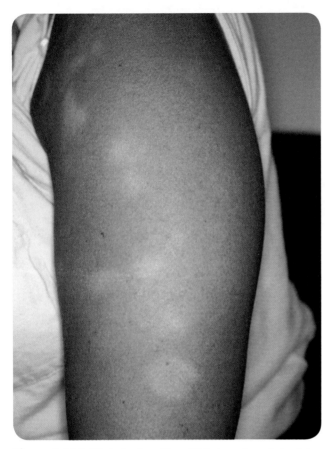

Figure 4-114 Pityriasis alba with multiple hypopigmented patches on an extremity.

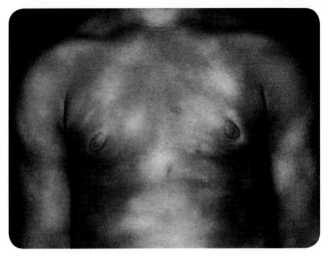

Figure 4-115 Multiple nonscaling flat hypopigmented macules of pityriasis alba.

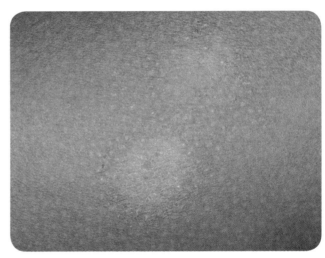

Figure 4-116 Hypopigmented lesion of pityriasis alba surrounded by flat-topped papules suggestive of atopic dermatitis.

- Mycosis fungoides
- Sarcoidosis—Hypopigmented plaques of sarcoidosis would have substance.

✓ Best Tests

- Clinical examination is usually the best diagnostic method.
- Additionally, in-office procedures can aid in the diagnosis. Scrapings tested with KOH will be negative, helping to eliminate tinea in the differential. Additionally, Wood lamp examinations can demonstrate anywhere from slight, off-white, minimal accentuation to no accentuation of the pityriasis alba lesions.
- If clinical exam and in-office tests are atypical, diagnosis may be confirmed with a biopsy. On pathological evaluation, follicular plugging, follicular spongiosis, and atrophic sebaceous glands are often seen. Additionally, spongiosis, hyperkeratosis, and acanthosis may be found in the epidermis, and perivascular lymphocytic infiltrates may be seen in the dermis. Notably, lesional skin of pityriasis alba will have markedly reduced pigment in the epidermis. However, there have been reports of both increased numbers and decreased numbers of melanocytes in lesional skin, and often there can be no significant difference in the melanocyte count between lesional and nonlesional skin. Additionally, degenerative changes in melanocytes can be seen ultrastructurally, and a reduced number of melanosomes can be found within keratinocytes. Overall, histopathologically, pityriasis alba is characterized by reduced melanin pigment and a variable number of melanocytes.

▲▲ Management Pearls

In general, since pityriasis alba is a benign, self-limited process, the most important intervention is reassurance that the hypopigmentation will eventually resolve. However, since pityriasis alba can be both symptomatic and cosmetically displeasing, treatment is often sought and given. This can be particularly true in patients with pigmented skin, as the contrasting hypopigmentation can cause great emotional stress.

Therapy

Despite limited studies, low- or moderate-potency topical corticosteroids are often considered first-line agents in the treatment of pityriasis alba. However, care must be taken to avoid a worsening in the appearance of the lesions secondary to corticosteroid-induced hypopigmentation or atrophy.

Studies in patients with Fitzpatrick type III to IV skin demonstrated that twice-daily tacrolimus ointment 0.1% appears to be an effective and safe treatment for pityriasis alba, improving pruritus, scaling, and hypopigmentation. Standard moisturizers with SPF 20 sunscreen also resulted in mild improvements in that study.

Another study in patients with predominately type IV to V skin demonstrated the effectiveness of twice-daily pimecrolimus cream 1% application in the treatment of pityriasis alba. In this study, patients additionally used a daily facial emollient containing SPF 15 sunscreen.

It can be deduced that good basic skin care with mild cleansers, sun protection, and emollients might be viewed as a treatment of pityriasis alba, improving symptoms but often not producing resolution.

Cosmetic cover-up can additionally be used to help camouflage the lesions.

Suggested Readings

Fujita WH, McCormick CL, Parneix-Spake A. An exploratory study to evaluate the efficacy of pimecrolimus cream 1% for the treatment of pityriasis alba. *Int J Dermatol.* 2007;46:700–705.

In SI, Yi SW, Kang HY, et al. Clinical and histopathological characteristics of pityriasis alba. *Clin Exp Dermatol.* 2008;34:591–597.

Lio PA. Little white spots: An approach to hypopigmented macules. *Arch Dis Child Educ Pract Ed.* 2008;93:98–102.

Plensdorf S, Martinez J. Common pigmentation disorders. *Am Fam Phys.* 2009;79:109–116.

Rigopoulos D, Gregoriou S, Charissi C, et al. Tacrolimus ointment 0.1% in pityriasis alba: An open-label, randomized, placebo-controlled study. *Br J Dermatol.* 2006;155:152–155.

Confluent and Reticulated Papillomatosis

Lynn McKinley-Grant

■■ Diagnosis Synopsis

Confluent and reticulated papillomatosis is a rare cutaneous disorder of as-yet undetermined etiology with clinical features resembling acanthosis nigricans. The disorder typically affects young adults and is more common in women and those with darker skin types. While responsive to treatment, the disease is usually chronic and marked by exacerbations and remissions. The chief complaint is often hyperpigmentation.

Confluent and reticulated papillomatosis is characterized by hyperpigmented, hyperkeratotic, thin papules, usually on the trunk, that coalesce into reticulated plaques. The lesions are usually asymptomatic but may be pruritic.

◉ Look For

Hyperpigmentation is a feature in pigmented skin. Side lighting is helpful to see the papular nature. Lesions begin as hyperkeratotic or very thin, slightly verrucous 1- to 2-mm papules that enlarge and coalesce to form reticulated papules (Fig. 4-117). Skin markings are often accentuated, and there may be slight overlying scale. Early lesions may be red, but they typically become gray-brown over time.

Lesions usually begin on the chest or abdomen and spread centrifugally. The face, neck, and proximal extremities may also be involved.

●● Diagnostic Pearls

- Scraping the lesions may produce a fine scale that is negative.
- The mucous membranes are spared.

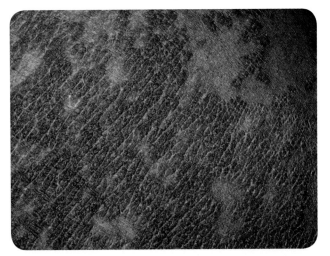

Figure 4-117 The confluent and reticulated papillomatosis of Gougerot and Carteaud is acquired and may mimic forms of ichthyosis.

?? Differential Diagnosis and Pitfalls

- Acanthosis nigricans
- Macular amyloidosis
- Darier disease
- Pityriasis rubra pilaris
- Seborrheic keratoses
- Tinea versicolor
- Dermatopathia pigmentosa reticularis
- Epidermal nevus syndrome
- Erythema dyschromicum perstans
- Dowling-Degos disease (reticulated pigmented anomaly of the flexures)
- Dyskeratosis congenita
- Erythema ab igne
- Prurigo pigmentosa
- Incontinentia pigmenti

✓ Best Tests

- Perform a KOH preparation and fungal culture of skin scraping to rule out a fungal infection. On occasion, concomitant *Pityrosporum* infections may be detected.
- Skin biopsy may be helpful and is consistent with the diagnosis.

▲▲ Management Pearls

- Treatment is for cosmetic reasons.
- Overweight patients with confluent and reticulated papillomatosis have experienced the regression of lesions with weight loss.

Therapy

The most consistently helpful results in the treatment of confluent and reticulated papillomatosis have been achieved with oral minocycline (50 to 100 mg p.o. twice daily).

Other antibiotic regimens have had purported success:

- Azithromycin—250 to 500 mg p.o. three times weekly
- Clarithromycin—500 mg p.o. daily
- Erythromycin—1,000 mg p.o. daily
- Tetracycline—500 mg p.o. twice daily
- Cefdinir—300 mg p.o. twice daily

Retinoids are sometimes useful:

- Topical—tretinoin cream (0.025%, 0.05%, 0.1%), apply nightly; tazarotene, apply nightly
- Systemic—isotretinoin 0.5 to 1 mg/kg p.o. divided twice daily; acitretin 25 to 50 mg p.o. daily

Other topical treatments that have shown mixed results include the following:

- Selenium sulfide—Apply to affected area once daily for 10 minutes and then rinse.
- Ketoconazole—Apply to affected areas twice daily.
- Calcipotriene 0.005% cream—Apply to affected areas twice daily.

Suggested Readings

Atasoy M, Ozdemir S, Aktaş A, et al. Treatment of confluent and reticulated papillomatosis with azithromycin. *J Dermatol.* 2004;31(8): 682–686.

Jang HS, Oh CK, Cha JH, et al. Six cases of confluent and reticulated papillomatosis alleviated by various antibiotics. *J Am Acad Dermatol.* 2001;44(4):652–655.

Montemarano AD, Hengge M, Sau P, et al. Confluent and reticulated papillomatosis: Response to minocycline. *J Am Acad Dermatol.* 1996; 34(2 Pt 1):253–256.

Scheinfeld N. Confluent and reticulated papillomatosis: A review of the literature. *Am J Clin Dermatol.* 2006;7(5):305–313.

Urticaria Pigmentosa and Mastocytoma

Chris G. Adigun

▪▪ Diagnosis Synopsis

Cutaneous mastocytosis (CM) is typically divided into four clinical variants: urticaria pigmentosa (UP), solitary mastocytoma, diffuse CM, and telangiectasia macularis eruptiva perstans (TMEP). Of the CM disorders, UP is the most common in both adults and children. In UP, mast cells accumulate in the skin, causing characteristic yellow-tan to reddish-brown macules or slightly raised papules scattered over the body (Figs. 4-118–4-120). These lesions tend to predominate in sun-protected areas and generally spare the palms, soles, face, and scalp. They characteristically urticate or form wheals with any mechanical stimuli, such as rubbing or scratching (Darier sign). This syndrome presents within the first weeks to months of life and can be expected to spontaneously involute by early childhood or puberty. In adults, UP is typically associated with systemic mastocytosis, most often with indolent systemic mastocytosis (ISM). However, it is very unusual for children to develop systemic disease, and 50% of cases resolve by young adulthood.

Mastocytoma is the second most common form of CM (Fig. 4-121). Mastocytomas will typically occur before age one, with the majority of them presenting within the first 3 months of life. They are usually solitary, although isolated cases of multiple mastocytomas have been reported. Mastocytomas have the highest concentration of skin mast cells compared with the other forms of CM and as many as 150 times more mast cells than normal skin. This increase in mast cells is frequently associated with local symptoms such as a positive Darier sign, pruritus, and even blistering, especially after rubbing the lesion. These symptoms tend to abate over time, and the lesions will completely resolve, generally by adolescence.

Diffuse CM is diagnosed in infancy but may persist into adulthood. Skin is typically thickened, with a reddish-brown discoloration. Discrete lesions are not seen, and formation of blisters is common with mechanical stimuli. TMEP is the least common variant of the CM syndromes and occurs almost exclusively in adults. Patients will present with red-brown telangiectatic macules with irregular borders. Darier sign and pruritus occur less consistently, and the tendency to form blisters is uncommon.

Despite these syndromes being isolated to the skin, patients may experience systemic symptoms secondary to mast cell degranulation and release of mediators into the bloodstream. These symptoms include cutaneous flushing, pruritus, hypotension, GI upset including acid reflux and diarrhea, asthma exacerbations, and shortness of breath.

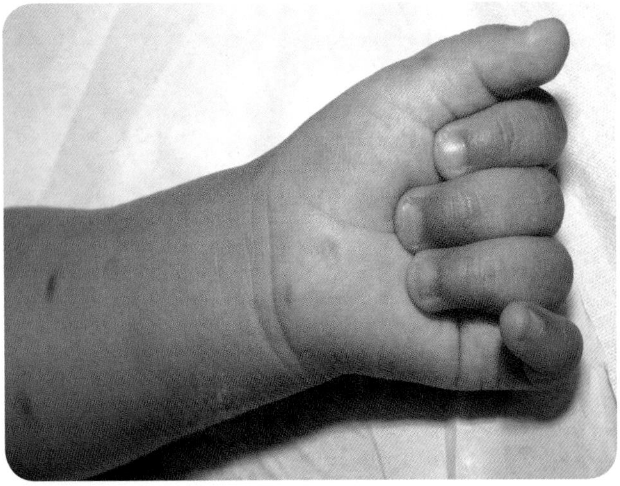

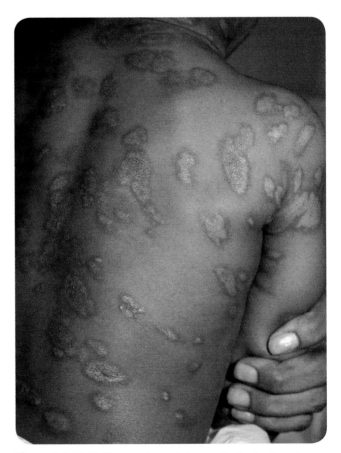

Figure 4-118 Multiple macules, including one on the palm, in urticaria pigmentosum.

Figure 4-119 Multiple papules and plaques of urticaria pigmentosum.

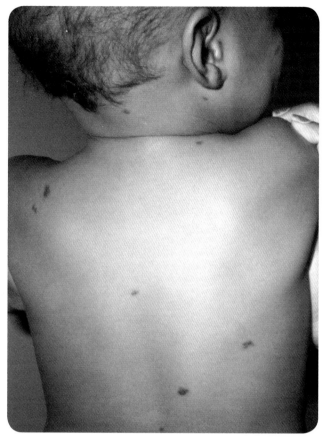

Figure 4-120 Several brownish papules of urticaria pigmentosum; distinguished from nevi by rubbing (Darier sign).

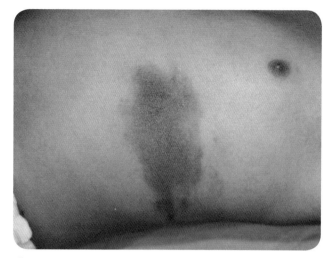

Figure 4-121 Localized mastocytoma.

Pediatric Patient Considerations

Fifty percent of pediatric patients with CM will have complete resolution by adolescence. Of the remaining 50%, most will have significantly reduced symptoms by adulthood. However, 10% to 15% will have symptoms that persist into adulthood.

The other forms of cutaneous and systemic mastocytosis (including diffuse CM, TMEP, systemic mastocytosis, and mast cell leukemia) are very rare in the pediatric population.

⊙ Look For

In UP, larger plaques often have increased skin markings. Firmly stroke a red-brown patch to attempt to elicit a Darier sign. Observe for a wheal or vesicle forming. Severe forms of the condition can present with blisters and sometimes nodules with blisters.

In mastocytoma, look for a brown, yellow, or red lesion that becomes swollen and red with rubbing. It may blister. Observe for a Darier sign by rubbing the skin of a lesion with a blunt object for 10 seconds. If it becomes red or swollen or

blisters in the next 5 minutes, the test is positive. However, to confirm the diagnosis of mastocytoma, the same procedure in adjacent normal-looking skin should be negative.

●● Diagnostic Pearls

- Darier sign typically presents in only 50% of cases. This may be difficult to see in darkly pigmented skin.
- Dermatographism is not a diagnostic test for mastocytosis.

?? Differential Diagnosis and Pitfalls

If localized or multiple macules:

- Café au lait spots
- Neurofibromatosis
- Albright syndrome
- Multiple cutaneous lentiginosis
- Congenital nevus
- Spitz nevus
- Juvenile xanthogranuloma
- Postinflammatory hyperpigmentation
- Secondary syphilis
- Chronic urticaria
- Insect bite reaction
- Leukemia
- Lymphoma
- Neuroblastoma

If bullous lesions:

- Bullous impetigo
- Chronic bullous disease of childhood
- Linear IgA dermatosis
- Drug eruption
- Incontinentia pigmenti
- Bullous pemphigoid

143

In patients with darker skin, diagnosis may be more difficult, as the macules may be intensely pigmented, and Darier sign—if present—may be difficult to detect, as erythema could be undetectable. Furthermore, in deeply pigmented skin, the individual lesions may be very difficult to detect unless surface change is present. There have been reports of cases of UP in pigmented skin where the eruption presented as a dark pink maculopapular exanthem, which contrasts greatly with the typical "tan to yellow-orange macule" that is prototypical with white skin. Additionally, identifying telangiectases in dark skin can be challenging. This is a critical finding in TMEP, which does not also have surface alteration to aid in the diagnosis.

Best Tests

- Skin biopsy
- *Note*: Biopsy in pediatric patients is not required if clinical features are consistent and Darier sign is positive. However, one may consider measuring serum tryptase or urinary histamine levels, as these will be elevated with systemic disease.
- In an adult or adolescent with persistent systemic symptoms, a CBC and serum tryptase measurement are required. If serum tryptase is >20 ng/mL, bone marrow biopsy is needed.

Management Pearls

Treatment is aimed at controlling or decreasing symptoms associated with the skin lesions. Because the majority of the skin lesions and their associated symptoms resolve by adulthood, parents need to be reassured and educated.

Central to therapy is the avoidance of mast cell degranulators/histamine triggers:

- Physical stimuli (e.g., friction, pressure, scratching lesions)
- Medications (e.g., aspirin, cholinergic drugs, opiates, codeine, polymyxin B, radiocontrast with iodine, and some anesthetics)
- Venomous stings (e.g., bees, wasps, jellyfish)

There is no indication to treat asymptomatic lesions, especially in the pediatric population.

Therapy

First-line therapy is with antihistamines. Consider H1 blockers, such as hydroxyzine, dexchlorpheniramine, or doxepin, at recommended doses, to improve itching and flushing symptoms. Second-generation antihistamines can be helpful due to their likelihood to be less sedating. These include cetirizine, loratadine, and mizolastine. For GI side effects, H2 blockers, such as ranitidine or cimetidine, can be very effective.

Topical steroids can be used on individual lesions for symptomatic relief. Choose a midpotency steroid, such as triamcinolone acetonide, and be sure to counsel about side effects of these medications, especially skin atrophy and surrounding hypopigmentation. These medications should only be used locally on the individual lesions.

Prednisone, aspirin, and UV light therapy have been employed in the adult population for those who do not respond to antihistamine therapy.

Keep in mind that for patients with darker skin, postinflammatory hyperpigmentation or hypopigmentation is likely to result at the site of skin lesions. Patients should be counseled to not overuse topical steroids on these lesions, as pigmentary changes due to overuse of the topical steroid may result.

Pediatric Patient Considerations

Oral antihistamines can be used in the pediatric patient for symptom management. Mid- to high-potency topical steroids under occlusion may reduce the severity of the skin lesions.

Cromolyn sodium is most helpful in treating gastrointestinal symptoms, but recent reports have shown that only very high dosages are able to elicit moderate inhibitory effects on mast cells of the GI tract.

For symptoms, consider H1 antagonists.

Hydroxyzine:

- 2 mg/kg/d divided three to four times daily (0.5 mg/kg/dose)

Diphenhydramine:

- 5 mg/kg/24 hours divided in four doses, or
- 2 to 6 years old: 6.25 mg four times daily
- 6 to 12 years old: 12.5 mg four times daily
- Older than 12 years: 25 to 50 mg/dose every 4 to 6 hours

Cetirizine:

- 6 to 12 months old: 2.5 mg daily
- 12 to 24 months old: 2.5 mg once to twice daily
- 2 to 6 years old: 2.5 to 5 mg/d
- 6 to 12 years: 5 to 10 mg/d
- Older than 12 years: 10 mg/d

Also consider H2 blockers such as cimetidine and ranitidine, especially with GI symptoms and symptoms of hyperacidity or peptic ulcer disease. More severe reactions should be managed in conjunction with a dermatologist and allergist and may include topical steroids for blisters. For those with anaphylaxis or anaphylaxislike reactions, an EpiPen is critical.

Suggested Readings

Brockow K. Urticaria pigmentosa. *Immunol Allergy Clin North Am.* 2004;24(2):287–316, vii.

Carter MC, Metcalfe DD. Biology of mast cells and the mastocytosis syndromes. In: Wolff K, Goldsmith LA, Katz SI, et al., eds. *Fitpatrick's Dermatology in General Medicine.* 7th Ed. New York, NY: McGraw Hill, 2008:1434–1443.

Escribano L, Akin C, Castells M, et al. Mastocytosis: current concepts in diagnosis and treatment. *Ann Hematol.* 2002;81(12):677–690.

Izikson L, English JC 3rd, Zirwas MJ. The flushing patient: differential diagnosis, workup, and treatment. *J Am Acad Dermatol.* 2006;55(2):193–208.

Patnaik MM, Rindos M, Kouides PA, et al. Systemic mastocytosis: a concise clinical and laboratory review. *Arch Pathol Lab Med.* 2007;131(5):784–791.

Shaffer HC, Parsons DJ, Peden DB, et al. Recurrent syncope and anaphylaxis as presentation of systemic mastocytosis in a pediatric patient: case report and literature review. *J Am Acad Dermatol.* 2006;54(5 Suppl):S210–S213.

Congenital Nevus Including Giant Congenital Nevus

Stephanie Diamantis

■■ Diagnosis Synopsis

Congenital melanocytic nevi (CMN) are proliferations of melanocytes in the epidermis and/or dermis that are present at birth or shortly thereafter (congenital nevus tardive). No data exist regarding ethnic predilection. CMN are typically grouped according to their size in adulthood: small (<1.5 cm in diameter), medium (1.5 to 19.9 cm), or large/giant (>20 cm). Some authors also define "large" nevi as those that cover more than 1% of the surface of the head or neck or those that cannot be excised in a single operation.

Only large (or giant) CMN have increased potential for malignancy. Multiple satellite lesions surrounding large CMN are a marker for increased risk of neurocutaneous melanocytosis (the presence of benign or malignant melanocytic proliferations in the central nervous system, most commonly involving the leptomeninges). Large nevi over the head or axial skeleton, especially those with many satellite lesions, require assessment for neurocutaneous involvement (developmental delays, seizures, hydrocephalus, increased intracranial pressure).

◉ Look For

Symmetrical, round or ovoid, slightly raised, tan to dark brown plaque ranging in size from smaller than 1 cm to larger than 20 cm that is present at birth (Fig. 4-122). Margins may be irregular or smooth. Lesions can be warty or cobblestoned on the surface. Multiple smaller pigmented lesions, termed satellite lesions, may be associated with larger nevi (Fig. 4-123). The most common locations are the buttocks, thighs, and trunk, but lesions may also occur on the face and extremities and, least often, on the palms, soles, and scalp.

Changes in thickness, color, and hair growth within the nevus occur throughout childhood with acceleration during adolescence. CMN grow proportionally with the child.

●● Diagnostic Pearls

The pigmented lesions are mildly palpable but develop more density with age. Multiple satellite lesions or nevi overlying the posterior midline raise the concern for potential neurocutaneous melanosis.

?? Differential Diagnosis and Pitfalls

- Café au lait macules—flat lesions
- Mongolian spots—flat, blue-gray in color
- Blue nevus
- Nevus sebaceus
- Nevus spilus
- Nevus of Ota
- Nevus of Ito

✓ Best Tests

- Careful, complete skin examination in a fully disrobed patient that includes the scalp, the mouth, behind the ears, and between the toes. Dermoscopy performed by a clinician experienced with this method may be useful.
- For most nevi, the diagnosis can often be made clinically, but suspicious lesions should be biopsied and examined by a dermatopathologist. Complete excisional biopsy provides the pathologist with the best opportunity to make an accurate diagnosis and may obviate the need for a future additional procedure.

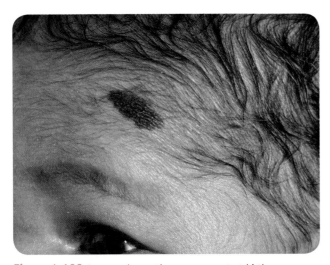

Figure 4-122 Large melanocytic nevus present at birth.

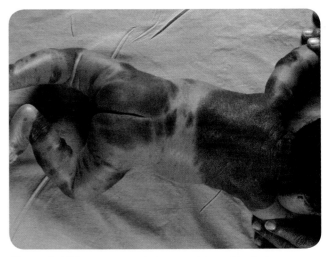

Figure 4-123 Giant congenital nevus with satellite lesions.

Management Pearls

- Consultation and management by a dermatologist with further consultation to a plastic surgeon or dermatologic surgeon is often necessary. May consider removal for cosmetic reasons in smaller lesions.
- Exercise vigilance in following for changes that suggest melanoma, especially in giant congenital nevi. May consider early excision of large nevi because of the increased risk of malignancy.
- Giant congenital nevi are best managed with a multidisciplinary approach, and consultations should be obtained from pediatrics, dermatology, and plastic surgery. Psychiatry should be involved for the parents and caregivers, as well as the patients themselves as they get older. If neurocutaneous melanosis is suspected, neurology and neurosurgery should be consulted as well.

Therapy

Multiple different treatments have been proposed and include surgical excision, curettage, dermabrasion, chemical peel, and laser. Surgical excision, sometimes in conjunction with tissue expansion, is the therapy most often recommended. Decisions are best made on a case-by-case basis after discussion involving the entire treatment team. For patients in whom neurocutaneous melanosis is suspected, an MRI of the brain and spinal cord should be obtained.

Removal, often in stages, is recommended for large lesions because of the increased risk of melanoma. Smaller lesions may be followed clinically with a dermatologist.

Suggested Readings

Barnhill RL, Llewellyn K. Benign melanocytic neoplasms. In: Bolognia JL, Jorizzo JL, Rapini RP, eds. *Dermatology*. 1st Ed. Philadelphia, PA: Elsevier; 2003:1757–1787.

Marghoob AA, Dusza S, Oliveria S, et al. Number of satellite nevi as a correlate for neurocutaneous melanocytosis in patients with large congenital melanocytic nevi. *Arch Dermatol*. 2004;140:171–175.

Spitz S. Melanomas of childhood. *Am J Path*. 1948;24:591–609.

Suh KY, Bolognia JL. Signature nevi. *J Am Acad Dermatol*. 2009;60(3):508–514.

Swerdlow AJ, English JS, Qiao Z. The risk of melanoma in patients with congenital nevi: A cohort study. *J Am Acad Dermatol*. 1995;32(4):595–599.

Drug-Induced Pigmentation

Lynn McKinley-Grant

Diagnosis Synopsis

Drug-induced pigmentation or hyperpigmentation may be caused by multiple drugs and through a number of differing mechanisms. Perhaps the most common reaction is postinflammatory hyperpigmentation as typically seen following inflammatory drug eruptions or fixed drug eruptions (considered separately). Other mechanisms include cutaneous deposition of the drug or its metabolites, increased melanin synthesis, "pigment incontinence" from damage to melanocytes in the basal layer of the epidermis, and increased lipofuscin.

Increased melanin most often produces a brownish pigmentation. When drugs deposit in the dermis, however, there may be blue-black or blue-gray patches on the skin. Drugs known to have such an effect are metals (e.g., silver, gold, mercury, and bismuth), antimalarials, phenothiazines, amitriptyline, oral contraceptive pills, carbamazepine, gabapentin, lamotrigine, clozapine, amiodarone, clofazimine, and minocycline.

Immunocompromised Patient Considerations

Nail and skin hyperpigmentation have been observed in HIV/AIDS patients independent of HAART. Thus, pigmentary alteration in this population may be especially difficult to attribute to drugs. Newer agents used to treat HIV-infected patients have been shown to cause skin and nail hyperpigmentation, with nail hyperpigmentation being one of the most common cutaneous side effects of antiretroviral therapy (see below).

A number of chemotherapeutic agents are also associated with hyperpigmentation. Among them are carmustine, bleomycin, cisplatin, busulfan, doxorubicin, fluorouracil, hydroxyurea, mitoxantrone, vinorelbine, thiotepa, methotrexate, ifosfamide, cyclophosphamide, and docetaxel.

Look For

In darkly pigmented skin, typical colors seen in lighter skin might appear purple, dark brown, and black. Blue-gray, brown, yellow, or red-brown macular skin discoloration as seen in lighter skin can be very subtle in dark skin, particularly when there is not any surface change (i.e., no scale). The pigmentation may be accentuated in certain areas (photodistributed, within scars, etc.) or may be widespread. Early and active lesions might have subtle erythema with a purple hue.

With a number of drugs, the pigmentary change also affects the nail unit (cyclophosphamide, doxorubicin, nucleoside antiretroviral drugs) or the conjunctiva (phenothiazines, etc.). The nail matrix or nail bed may be darkened, and linear dark bands of varying width can occur.

Antiretroviral- and diltiazem-induced skin hyperpigmentation occurs with higher frequency in black individuals. In addition, periocular hyperpigmentation has been reported in black patients using a prostaglandin F2-alpha derivative (latanoprost) for treatment of glaucoma and can be anticipated as this agent is used for enhanced eyelash growth.

Immunocompromised Patient Considerations

Hyperpigmentation of the palms and soles can occur with emtricitabine, a nucleoside reverse-transcriptase inhibitor used to treat HIV-infected individuals.

Diagnostic Pearls

Diffuse hyperpigmentation may indicate drug-induced pigmentation or systemic disease.

Some drugs and typical associated pigmentations:

- Yellow—quinacrine
- Blue-black—antimalarials, chloroquine, hydroxychloroquine, hydroquinone
- Blue-gray—gold, silver
- Blue—minocycline, amiodarone
- Red-brown—clofazimine
- Brown streaks (flagellate or linear)—bleomycin (Fig. 4-124)
- Minocycline may cause pigmentation primarily within scars, especially acne scars.

Immunocompromised Patient Considerations

- Emtricitabine—hyperpigmentation of palms and soles
- Zidovudine—nail and oral hyperpigmentation

Note: generally, hyperpigmentation caused by these antiretroviral agents is dose dependent and reversible.

Differential Diagnosis and Pitfalls

- Jaundice causes a yellow cast to the skin.
- Carotenemia causes an orange color in the skin.

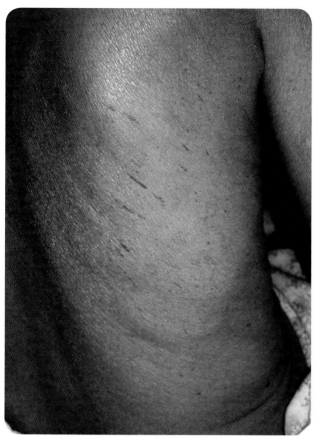

Figure 4-124 Bleomycin-induced pigmentation in a flagellate linear pattern; some typical small seborrheic keratoses are present.

- Generalized hyperpigmentation is also seen in Addison disease, Cushing syndrome, scleroderma, Wilson disease, hemochromatosis, chronic renal failure, porphyria cutanea tarda, vitamin B_{12} deficiency, pellagra, ochronosis, Gaucher disease, and carcinoid.
- Melasma or chloasma
- Erythema ab igne
- Ashy dermatosis (erythema dyschromicum perstans)
- Confluent and reticulated papillomatosis (Gougerot-Carteaud syndrome)
- Longitudinal melanonychia

Immunocompromised Patient Differential Diagnosis

Always have Kaposi sarcoma in the differential diagnosis of hyperpigmentation in HIV-infected individuals (have a low threshold to biopsy).

✓ Best Tests

- This diagnosis can usually be made clinically. Take a careful medication history.

- Antimalarials may fluoresce with a bluish color with a Wood light.
- Skin biopsy can often reveal the type of pigment within the skin and determine whether the pigmentation is dermal or epidermal.
- Other tests may be used to rule out systemic illnesses such as liver or renal function tests, iron studies, ACTH levels, etc.

▲▲ Management Pearls

Discontinuing the responsible drug is the treatment of choice. Patients should be made aware that it may take months to years for the pigment to resolve or that it may never resolve.

Immunocompromised Patient Considerations

In some instances, antiretroviral-induced skin hyperpigmentation will resolve spontaneously without discontinuation of the offending drug. In most cases, however, the offending drug must be discontinued in order for the hyperpigmentation to resolve.

Therapy

- Discontinue the medication if at all possible. Treatment is largely for aesthetic purposes. Consider the use of camouflage cosmetics.
- Some forms of drug-induced pigmentation are worsened by sun exposure. Counsel the patient regarding sun avoidance and the use of barrier clothing and combined UVA/UVB sunscreens.
- Topical corticosteroids, classes 3 and 4 for trunk and classes 6 and 7 for face, may help with some of the hyperpigmentation in the epidermis.

Midpotency Topical Corticosteroids (Classes 3 and 4)
- Triamcinolone cream, ointment—Apply twice daily (15, 30, 60, 120, 240 g).
- Mometasone cream, ointment—Apply twice daily (15, 45 g).
- Fluocinolone cream, ointment—Apply twice daily (15, 30, 60 g).

Low-potency Topical Steroids (Classes 6 and 7)
- Desonide cream, ointment—Apply twice daily (15, 60, 90 g).
- Alclometasone cream, ointment—Apply twice daily (15, 45, 60 g).

Immunocompromised Patient Considerations

Be aware that dermatophyte (tinea) infections can occur in immunosuppressed patients treated with topical corticosteroids.

Suggested Readings

Dereure O. Drug-induced skin pigmentation. Epidemiology, diagnosis and treatment. *Am J Clin Dermatol.* 2001;2(4):253–262.

Granstein RD, Sober AJ. Drug- and heavy metal—induced hyperpigmentation. *J Am Acad Dermatol.* 1981;5(1):1–18.

Hendrix JD, Greer KE. Cutaneous hyperpigmentation caused by systemic drugs. *Int J Dermatol.* 1992;31(7):458–466.

Nikolaou V, Stratigos AJ, Katsambas AD. Established treatments of skin hypermelanoses. *J Cosmet Dermatol.* 2006;5(4):303–308.

Vassallo P, Trohman RG. Prescribing amiodarone: An evidence-based review of clinical indications. *JAMA.* 2007;298(11):1312–1322.

Wiper A, Roberts DH, Schmitt M. Amiodarone-induced skin pigmentation: Q-switched laser therapy, an effective treatment option. *Heart.* 2007;93(1):15.

Erythema Dyschromicum Perstans

Lynn McKinley-Grant

■■ Diagnosis Synopsis

Erythema dyschromicum perstans (ashy dermatosis) is an acquired hypermelanosis of unknown etiology. It was originally described in Latin American individuals of intermediate skin tone but has subsequently been identified in other ethnicities and skin types. Recent studies suggest a cell-mediated immune reaction to antigens located in basal and midepidermal keratinocytes. It is associated with lichen planus as well as with certain exposures, including ammonium nitrate, oral radiographic contrast media, cobalt, and parasitic whipworm infection. Erythema dyschromicum perstans is more common in women. Age of onset is usually in the second or third decade, but all age groups may be affected.

◉ Look For

Erythema dyschromicum perstans presents as asymptomatic or mildly pruritic gray-blue macules of various sizes on the trunk and proximal extremities (Fig. 4-125). There are gray-blue "ashy" macules and patches of various sizes (0.5 to 3.0 cm), concentrated most commonly on the trunk, neck, and proximal extremities. Sometimes, there is a very fine scale. Plaques can have indistinct borders and coalesce to form larger patches with irregular borders.

●● Diagnostic Pearls

Active lesions may have a narrow, difficult-to-discern erythematous border.

?? Differential Diagnosis and Pitfalls

- Lichen planus (including the variant lichen planus pigmentosus)—pruritic
- Lichenoid drug eruptions—usually more erythematous
- Postinflammatory hyperpigmentation
- Fixed drug eruption—multiple
- Macular amyloidosis
- Maculae cerulea (arthropod bites)
- Macular urticaria pigmentosa
- Pinta—late
- Argyria
- Drug-induced pigmentation
- Addison disease
- Melasma

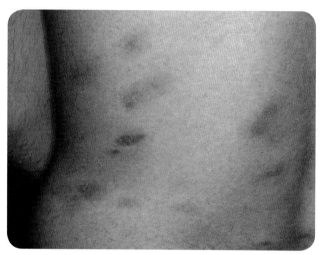

Figure 4-125 Multiple macules with bluish-gray pigmentation are seen in erythema dyschromicum perstans.

- Confluent and reticulated papillomatosis
- Dermal melanosis

✓ Best Tests

- Skin biopsy will demonstrate vacuolar degeneration of the basal layer with pigmentary incontinence and dermal macrophages laden with melanin.
- Serological tests for syphilis should be considered to exclude treponematosis.

▲▲ Management Pearls

- There have been reports of spontaneous resolution.
- Camouflage cosmetics may be used for cosmetic purposes.

Therapy

No treatment is a reasonable option.

In patients desiring treatment, the following have demonstrated variable success:

- Triamcinolone—0.1% cream or ointment twice daily
- Dapsone—100 mg p.o. daily for 3 months; all necessary precautions for dapsone use and initiation of use must be carefully followed

Suggested Readings

Bahadir S, Cobanoglu U, Cimsit G, et al. Erythema dyschromicum perstans: Response to dapsone therapy. *Int J Dermatol.* 2004;43(3):220–222.

Osswald SS, Proffer LH, Sartori CR. Erythema dyschromicum perstans: A case report and review. *Cutis.* 2001;68(1):25–28.

Schwartz RA. Erythema dyschromicum perstans: The continuing enigma of Cinderella or ashy dermatosis. *Int J Dermatol.* 2004;43(3):230–232.

Stratigos AJ, Katsambas AD. Optimal management of recalcitrant disorders of hyperpigmentation in dark-skinned patients. *Am J Clin Dermatol.* 2004;5(3):161–168.

Zaynoun S, Rubeiz N, Kibbi AG. Ashy dermatoses—a critical review of the literature and a proposed simplified clinical classification. *Int J Dermatol.* 2008;47(6):542–544.

Fixed Drug Eruption

Suzanne Berkman

◼◼ Diagnosis Synopsis

A fixed drug eruption is an adverse drug reaction manifested by nonmigratory and recurring fixed plaques. The plaques occur at the same body site each time the individual is reexposed to the specific drug. Lesions are often symptomatic with burning or pruritus. Blisters, which eventually rupture, may occur (bullous fixed drug eruption). Drugs known to cause the condition include pyrazolone derivatives, naproxen, mefenamic acid, sulfonamides, trimethoprim, erythromycin, tetracycline, phenolphthalein, and phenobarbital.

⦿ Look For

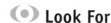

Solitary or multiple sharply demarcated deep red, brown, or black patches recurring in exactly the same location(s) each time the drug is taken (Fig. 4-126). Fixed drug eruptions usually begin as a red patch and frequently leave hyperpigmented patches between acute flares. Flaccid bullae are common (Fig. 4-127). The darker the skin type, the darker the fixed drug lesions. It most frequently occurs on the genitals, with the glans penis being a common location for a plaque, but lesions can occur anywhere (Fig. 4-128). Multiple lesions are not uncommon (Fig. 4-129).

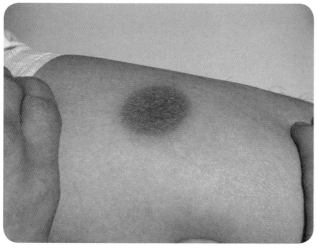

Figure 4-126 Rim of erythema around a central hyperpigmented macule in a fixed drug eruption.

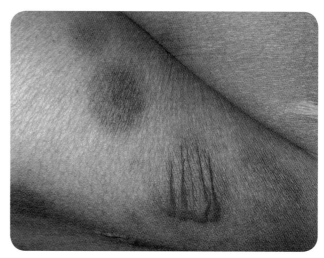

Figure 4-127 Flaccid bullae and hyperpigmented macule in a fixed drug eruption.

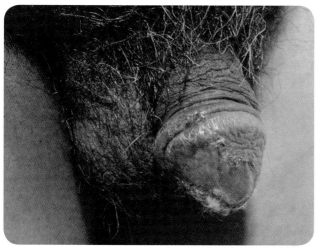

Figure 4-128 Erosion and flaccid bullae on the glans, a characteristic location for a fixed drug eruption.

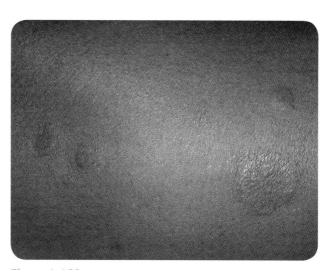

Figure 4-129 Multiple lesions may occur in a fixed drug eruption.

Diagnostic Pearls

Symptoms (e.g., itching and burning) and worsening of the plaques occur within 12 hours of taking the drug.

 ## Differential Diagnosis and Pitfalls

- Insect bite reactions can leave similar hyperpigmented patches.
- Postinflammatory pigmentation
- Contact dermatitis
- Lichen planus
- Erythema multiforme
- Recurrent herpes simplex virus (HSV)
- Cellulitis or erysipelas
- Bullous impetigo
- Cicatricial pemphigoid

 ## Best Tests

Skin biopsy will be suggestive of the diagnosis. Rechallenge to the medication and observing for the characteristic change is possible but is *not* recommended because of the risk of a more severe generalized reaction.

 ## Management Pearls

It is important to consider all prescription medications as well as over-the-counter medications and health food supplements as potential causes. Discontinue the drug and any potential cross-reacting medications.

Therapy

Some experts use topical corticosteroids in pigmented skin to minimize the postinflammatory hyperpigmentation. The best therapy is watchful waiting and avoidance of the drug and its related compounds. The lesions will heal spontaneously; thus, treatment is only needed for any pain or secondary infection. Recovery usually takes 2 to 3 weeks. However, the secondary pigment alteration may be persistent.

Suggested Readings

Kauppinen K, Stubb S. Fixed eruptions: Causative drugs and challenge tests. *Br J Dermatol.* 1985;112:575–578.

Stubb S, Alanko K, Reitamo S. Fixed drug eruptions: 77 cases from 1981 to 1985. *Br J Dermatol.* 1989;120:583.

Lentigo Simplex

Chris G. Adigun

▪ Diagnosis Synopsis

Lentigo simplex is an extremely common hyperpigmented macule located anywhere on the body. They generally occur early in life (may be present at birth) and are not associated with sun exposure. Lentigo simplex lesions result from an increased number of normal melanocytes in the epidermis producing increased amounts of melanin. They differ from common ephelides, because ephelides have normal numbers of melanocytes with increased pigment.

Clinically, these lesions are asymptomatic, well-circumscribed, symmetric, homogeneous light brown to black macules. They are usually 4 to 10 mm in size and are distributed anywhere on the trunk, extremities, genitals, and mucous membranes (Fig. 4-130). Lentigines found on mucous membranes can be deeply pigmented and larger in size, and they can have irregular borders. They occasionally form in cutaneous scars and after therapy with psoralen/ultraviolet light. They differ clinically from solar lentigines in that they appear earlier in life on non–sun-exposed skin. When melanocytes are present—including normal skin—melanoma may arise, but increased risk has not been demonstrated for lentigo simplex.

Lentigo simplex may occur as single or multiple lesions. Occasionally, multiple lentigines are associated with rare genetic disorders. These include the following:

- LEOPARD syndrome—lentigines, EKG changes, ocular hypertelorism, pulmonary stenosis, abnormal genitalia, growth retardation, and deafness
- Carney complex—lentigines (mucous membranes, lips, face, external genitalia), atrial myxoma, mucocutaneous myxoma, and nevi

- Peutz-Jeghers syndrome (PJS)—lentigines (perioral and oral), multiple gastrointestinal polyps, and visceral tumors (pancreas, ovary, testes)
- Xeroderma pigmentosum—lentigines on sun-exposed skin and multiple skin cancers
- Cronkhite-Canada syndrome—lentigines (buccal mucosa, face, palmoplantar), alopecia, nail dystrophy, and intestinal polyps
- Touraine centrofacial lentiginosis—lentigines (central face and lips, spares mucosa, none elsewhere), bone abnormalities, dysraphia, endocrine disorders, neurologic disease
- Inherited patterned lentiginosis in individuals of African descent—lentigines (central face, hands, feet, elbows, knees, buttocks, spares mucous membranes), no other associated systemic abnormalities, and no increased risk of malignancy

Other rare disorders associated with multiple lentigines include generalized lentigines, arterial dissection with lentiginosis, Laugier-Hunziker syndrome, Cantú (hyperkeratosis-hyperpigmentation) syndrome, Cowden disease, and Bannayan-Riley-Ruvalcaba syndrome.

Inherited patterned lentiginosis in individuals of African descent has a similar presentation to centrofacial lentiginosis, Carney complex, and PJS, except these patients have no other associated medical problems, and the lentigines spare mucous membranes and often extend onto other parts of the body beyond the central face. Furthermore, in centrofacial lentiginosis, lentigines regress over time, whereas this does not occur in inherited patterned lentiginosis.

Finally, most patients with centrofacial lentiginosis are of Western European descent, whereas those with inherited patterned lentiginosis are of African descent.

◉ Look For

Look for light brown to almost black, regular, oval or round macules that are usually 4 to 10 mm in size. The edge of the macule can be jagged or smooth.

Pediatric Patient Considerations

Look for brown to almost black, regular, small macules, typically 3 mm or smaller in diameter.

▪▪ Diagnostic Pearls

- Lentigo simplex is more regular than the sun-exposed variant (solar lentigo). The use of a dermatoscope allows

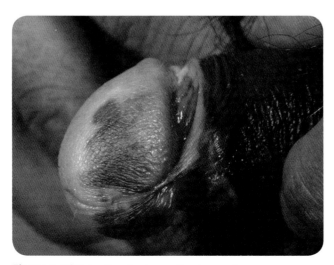

Figure 4-130 Lentigo simplex on the glans and corona.

closer examination of the pigment, which often seems to stream from the center of a lesion.

- Lentigo simplex lesions are typically darker than ephelides and do not darken or increase with sun exposure.

?? Differential Diagnosis and Pitfalls

- African Americans may have centrofacial lentigos that have an autosomal dominant inheritance pattern. These may also be present on the hands, feet, buttocks, and extensor surfaces.
- Solar lentigo typically occurs with increasing age on sun-exposed surfaces and is less regular in appearance.
- A café au lait spot is macular and present from the time of infancy and tends to be larger.
- Labial (lip) and vulvar melanotic macules are deeply pigmented, usually solitary, macules that may be confused with melanoma. Mucosal pigmentation is fairly common in those with darkly pigmented skin.
- An oral mucosal lesion may be difficult to distinguish from an amalgam tattoo and mucosal melanoma.
- Lentigo maligna must be considered in patients with darkly pigmented skin.
- Melanoma must be considered in patients with darkly pigmented skin.
- Ephelides
- Seborrheic keratoses
- Junctional and compound nevi

If multiple:

- Agminated nevi
- Nevus spilus

Pediatric Patient Differential Diagnosis

In children with multiple lentigines, consider LEOPARD syndrome. Also consider PJS, especially with multiple facial and perioral lentigines. GI hamartomatous polyps and a positive family history also tend to be present. Lip and oral mucous membrane lentigines are the hallmark of this syndrome. All ethnicities have been described to have PJS; thus, those with darkly pigmented skin and multiple lentigines must have this in their differential.

✓ Best Tests

- Dermatoscopic examination may help differentiate lentigo simplex from a malignancy. Concerning features include asymmetric pigmented follicular openings and dark (brown or black) rhomboidal structures. If there is doubt, perform a skin biopsy.

- If a skin biopsy is performed, Mart-1, Mel-5, and DOPA immunohistochemistry may be helpful to illustrate increased number of melanocytes confined to the basal layer and lacking nest formation on histopathological analysis.

Pediatric Patient Considerations

Clinical exam is generally sufficient.

▲▲▲ Management Pearls

- Suspicious single lesions should be biopsied or surgically removed because they may be difficult to distinguish from melanoma.
- Multiple facial lentigines, though often benign, can be cosmetically disfiguring. In patients with darkly pigmented skin, treatment options tend to be more limited.

Pediatric Patient Considerations

The ABCDEs of melanoma should be reviewed with the parents (and the patient if he/she is old enough). The patient may be followed annually in the office or at home by the patient or his/her parents with instructions to return if any suspicious changes are noted.

A—asymmetry
B—border irregularity
C—color variation
D—diameter >6 mm
E—evolution (change in appearance)

Therapy

Any suspicious lesions should be surgically excised and sent for histopathologic examination. It is appropriate to periodically follow up on benign-appearing lesions.

Cryosurgery or a combination of tretinoin and hydroquinone cream applied once or twice daily may improve cosmetic appearance. The risk of hypopigmentation secondary to cryosurgery is very high in patients with darkly pigmented skin.

New laser therapies have become available for treatment of pigmented lesions. Laser therapies can be more challenging in darkly pigmented skin due to the risk of pigmentation alterations and scarring. Laser that emits wavelengths that are absorbed by melanin and can destroy pigmented lesions may produce hypopigmentation or reactive hyperpigmentation in patients with darkly pigmented skin.

Some recent trials of new laser therapies have proved promising for this population. These trials include a Q-switched ruby laser (QSRL) to treat a woman of Afro-Caribbean decent with inherited patterned lentiginosis, a long-pulsed alexandrite 755 nm laser for solar lentigines in Japanese patients with phototype IV skin, a Q-switched alexandrite laser for oral labial lentigines in Chinese subjects with PJS, and a QSRL for lentigines in Chinese patients. All subjects in these trials experienced no hypopigmentation, reactive hyperpigmentation, or recurrence.

Pediatric Patient Considerations

For a simple lentigo, no treatment is required. A biopsy (preferably a punch biopsy) should be performed if there is any concern about melanoma. Laser therapies may be employed but are recommended to be used when children are able to tolerate the procedure.

Suggested Readings

Akslen LA, Puntervoll H, Bachmann IM, et al. Mutation analysis of the EGFR-NRAS-BRAF pathway in melanomas from black Africans and other subgroups of cutaneous melanoma. *Melanoma Res.* 2008;18(1):29–35.

Bauer AJ, Stratakis CA. The lentiginoses: Cutaneous markers of systemic disease and a window to new aspects of tumourigenesis. *J Med Genet.* 2005;42(11):801–810. Epub 2005 Jun 15.

Chrousos GP, Stratakis CA. Carney complex and the familial lentiginosis syndromes: Link to inherited neoplasias and developmental disorders, and genetic loci. *J Intern Med.* 1998;243(6):573–579.

Gach JE, James MP. Laser treatment of lentiginosis in an Afro-Caribbean. *J R Soc Med.* 2001;94(5):240–241.

O'Neill JF, James WD. Inherited patterned lentiginosis in blacks. *Arch Dermatol.* 1989;125(9):1231–1235.

Redbord KP, Hanke CW. Case reports: Clearance of lentigines in Japanese men with the long-pulsed alexandrite laser. *J Drugs Dermatol.* 2007;6(6):653–656.

Schiffner R, Schiffner-Rohe J, Vogt T, et al. Improvement of early recognition of lentigo maligna using dermatoscopy. *J Am Acad Dermatol.* 2000;42 (1 Pt 1):25–32.

Xi Z, Hui Q, Zhong L. Q-switched alexandrite laser treatment of oral labial lentigines in Chinese subjects with Peutz-Jeghers syndrome. *Dermatol Surg.* 2009;35(7):1084–1088. Epub 2009 Apr 28.

Melanoma, Acral Lentiginous Melanoma, Lentigo Maligna, and Lentigo Maligna Melanoma

Jennifer Hensley • Suraj Venna

▪▪ Diagnosis Synopsis

Melanoma

Melanoma is a life-threatening skin cancer seen with increasing frequency worldwide. Having a high index of suspicion for melanoma in patients with darker skin types is an important preventative measure. Careful examination of the skin, including non-sun-exposed areas such as the palms, soles, nail bed, scalp, and oral and genital mucosa, enhances the detection of early melanoma. This chapter emphasizes the clinical characteristics of melanoma in more deeply pigmented skin and presents an overview of biopsy and therapeutic guidelines; the surgical treatment, and even biopsy, of melanomas should be done whenever feasible by physicians with direct experience in the care and management of these lesions.

Predisposing factors for melanoma include a family history or prior personal history of melanoma, a history of severe sunburns, or multiple atypical nevi. Other rarer predisposing factors include giant congenital melanocytic nevi, dysplastic nevus syndromes, and xeroderma pigmentosum. Early diagnosis and treatment can lead to complete cure and survival, but in dark-skinned individuals, the diagnosis is made later and the prognosis is thus much worse than for whites. Ethnic minorities are 1.96 to 3.01 times as likely to die from melanoma compared to whites of the same age and sex. In one study, median survival time was found to be 45 months for people of African descent compared to 135 months for whites.

Melanoma is the third most common skin cancer among African American, Asian American, and Latino American ethnic groups. There has been an increasing annual rate of melanoma in Hispanics in the United States over the past 15 years at 2.9%, which is comparable to the rate in white non-Hispanics (3.0%). The most common site of primary melanomas in Native Americans is the trunk, while the lower extremity is most common in African American, Latino American, and Asian/Pacific Islanders. People of African descent have a much higher incidence of acral melanoma, acral lentiginous melanoma (ALM), and subungual melanoma as compared to whites. While Hispanics also have a higher incidence of ALM as compared to whites, the most common histologic subtype in this population is superficial spreading melanoma. In the Asian/Pacific Islander population, ALM is the most common histologic subtype, and the most common sites of melanoma are the extremities. There is also a greater percentage of mucosal melanomas that occur in this population.

While UV light is known to be a major factor in the development of melanoma in whites, the etiology of most melanoma subtypes in ethnic minorities is unknown. Although chronic UV exposure is often sustained by ethnic minorities due to job exposure in the agriculture and construction labor force, they still have a lower risk compared to white individuals with intermittent recreational UV exposure.

Pediatric Patient Considerations

Patients aged 20 years and younger represent 1% of all patients diagnosed with melanoma.

Acral Lentiginous Melanoma

ALM accounts for <5% of all melanoma clinical subtypes. It occurs in all races including individuals of African descent, Hispanics, and Asians and is the most common type of melanoma in darker-complected individuals. Interestingly, the *incidence rate* of ALM is similar in whites and those of African descent, although ALM accounts for a much higher proportion of melanoma subtypes in individuals of African descent (vs. conventional forms of cutaneous melanoma). ALM, compared to other subtypes of melanoma, accounts for about 36% in individuals of African descent, 18% in Asian/Pacific Islanders, 9% in Hispanic whites, and 1% in non-Hispanic whites. There has been an increasing incidence of invasive ALM among Hispanics over the past 15 years. The incidence of ALM in men and women is similar, and the overall incidence of ALM has remained stable over time in the United States.

In dark-skinned individuals the diagnosis is often delayed, and therefore the prognosis is much worse than in whites. Both physicians and patients are often unaware of the fact that darker-complected people are susceptible to a life-threatening form of skin cancer. People of color with ALM are more likely to present with Stage III/IV disease compared to whites. As with conventional types of melanoma, recognizing the disease at an early stage can lead to cure.

ALM presents as a pigmented lesion on the distal extremities, including the palms, soles, and subungual areas. The most common location for ALM is on a lower extremity. It occurs frequently on the hallux and thumb. Because ALM occurs in non–sun-exposed areas, it has been suggested that sun exposure is less of a risk factor than in the other subtypes of melanoma, indicating other possible etiologies such as environmental or immunologic. This has led to the theory that trauma may be a risk factor leading to the development of ALM, as some studies have shown an association with injuries to the foot.

In addition to presenting as an irregular or changing lesion, ALM may also present with inflammation, itching, erosions, or ulcerations. It is often thought to be a fungal infection of the nail and is treated as such until at some point, a biopsy is taken, revealing ALM.

Advances in the molecular analysis of acral melanoma have revealed mutations in a tyrosine kinase, C-KIT, at a rate of approximately 25% to 30%. Inhibitors of this activated oncogene are currently being investigated.

Lentigo Maligna

Lentigo maligna (Hutchinson melanotic freckle) is a noninvasive form of melanoma (melanoma *in situ*) found most commonly on sun-exposed areas of the head and neck in older patients. This precursor lesion has been likened to a "stain" on the skin and occurs most commonly in fair-skinned individuals with a history of significant UV radiation exposure. Lentigo maligna and lentigo maligna melanoma have also been associated with basal cell carcinoma, porphyria cutanea tarda, Werner syndrome, oculocutaneous albinism, and xeroderma pigmentosa.

Lentigo maligna is difficult to distinguish from its invasive counterpart discussed below. The natural history of lentigo maligna is gradual horizontal growth with enlargement at the periphery of the lesion accompanied by a darkening of the lesion and the development of irregular edges. After several years, a vertical growth phase may occur; at that point, the condition becomes lentigo maligna melanoma.

Lentigo Maligna Melanoma

Lentigo maligna melanoma develops when a lentigo maligna (melanoma *in situ*) enters a vertical growth phase and is no longer *in situ* within the epidermis. It is a tumor that extends slightly above the surface of the skin and may be prone to bleeding. This condition generally occurs 5 to 20 years after the lentigo maligna first develops. It is most common on sun-damaged skin (usually facial) and is most frequently found on individuals aged 60 or older. Lentigo maligna melanoma is associated with nonmelanoma skin cancers, fair skin, porphyria cutanea tarda, Werner syndrome, oculocutaneous albinism, and xeroderma pigmentosa.

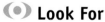 Look For

Melanoma

Morphology will vary somewhat by subtype, but most melanomas share several common features as outlined in the ABCDEs of melanoma (see "Diagnostic Pearls" below). ABC: Asymmetry, Border irregularity, and Color depth and multi-colored features are the classic signs (Fig. 4-131). In dark-skinned patients, subtle color variation can be difficult to see. Distal (hands and feet) melanomas are much more common in dark-skinned patients than white patients. Ulceration and bleeding are universally late signs.

Superficial spreading melanoma—an asymmetric macule with brown variegated pigmentation and notched or ragged borders. May occasionally be somewhat elevated. Usually seen on the trunk in men and the lower extremities in women.

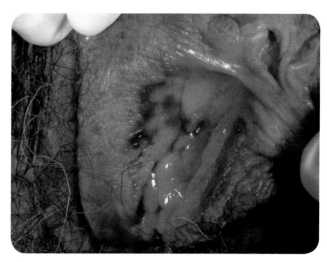

Figure 4-131 Vulval melanoma with irregular dark pigmentation.

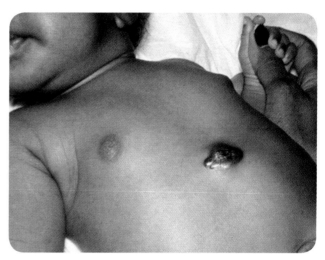

Figure 4-132 A five-week-old patient with melanoma on the abdomen.

Nodular melanoma—a dark brown to bluish-black nodule that grows rapidly (Fig. 4-132). This type of melanoma is most likely to ulcerate or bleed with minor trauma. Found commonly on the trunk, head, and neck.

Pediatric Patient Considerations

Change in size is not often reliable as children are growing, but any lesion that grows out of proportion with the patient raises concern. Lesions that ulcerate, bleed, or change color are also worrisome.

Acral Lentiginous Melanoma

An asymmetric brown to black macule with variegated pigmentation and irregular borders (Figs. 4-133 and 4-134), found on the palms or soles or involving the nail apparatus.

Palms and soles—On the soles, palms, distal digits, or beneath nail beds, look for a black or multicolored (brown,

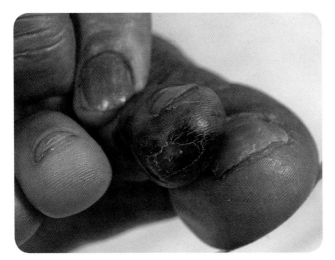

Figure 4-133 Acral lentiginous melanoma with very dark pigmentation on the volar surface of the second toe.

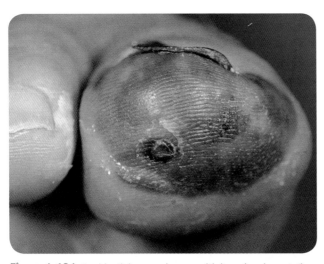

Figure 4-134 Acral lentiginous melanoma with irregular pigmentation.

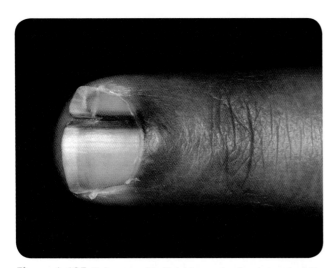

Figure 4-135 Melanoma with Hutchinson sign involvement of the posterior nail fold with black pigmentation.

black, blue, and depigmented pale areas) mole or irregularly shaped patch. ALM most frequently presents on the skin of the lower limb. In people of color, most cases involve the foot, with the hallux being the most common site.

Nail apparatus—On the nail plate, look for periungual hyperpigmentation known as Hutchinson sign, a black discoloration of the proximal nail fold at the end of a pigmented streak (Fig. 4-135). Melanoma arising from the nail matrix can present as a dark streak, multicolored, and wide (at least 3 mm) or widening. A clinical clue to this variant of melanoma is extension of the dark pigment onto the skin of the proximal nail fold and beyond.

A mnemonic for suspicious *nail* pigmentation, analogous to the ABCDEs of conventional melanoma, has been suggested:

- **A**
  - **A**ge—ages 20 to 90 years, peaking in the fifth to seventh decades
  - Race—**A**frican **A**merican, Native **A**merican, **A**sian

- **B**
  - **B**and—nail band
  - Pigment—**b**rown-**b**lack
  - **B**readth—greater than or equal to 3 mm
  - **B**order—irregular or blurred

- **C**
  - **C**hange—rapid increase in size of the nail band or failure of nail dystrophy to improve despite treatment

- **D**
  - **D**igit involved—common digits involved: thumb, hallux, index finger, single digit or multiple digits; sometimes localized to the **d**ominant hand

- **E**
  - **E**xtension—**e**xtension of pigment to involve the proximal or lateral nail fold (Hutchinson sign)

- **F**
  - **F**amily—**f**amily and/or personal history of melanoma or dysplastic nevus syndrome

Lentigo Maligna

Irregularly bordered, hyperpigmented (tan-brown) flat patch, usually on the face of an elderly person. There may be variations in pigmentation throughout. There is a particular predilection for the nose and the cheeks, but the arms, legs, and trunk may be affected. Cutaneous lentigo maligna may spread to mucosal surfaces, in which case hyperpigmented areas may be observed on the conjunctiva and oral mucosa.

Lentigo Maligna Melanoma

An irregularly bordered and pigmented brown to black patch or plaque with color variations, typically on the head and neck region (often on the nose and cheek)—or other sun-exposed area—of an elderly patient. There may be palpable dermal induration or nodularity within the lesion.

Diagnostic Pearls

Melanoma

Primary care physicians may play an important role in preventing mortality from melanoma. By identifying risk factors for melanoma (see introduction) and by applying ABCDE criteria (see below) to lesions brought to clinical attention by patients or via a careful screening during physical exam, the generalist will make the proper decision on the need to refer to a dermatologist.

Decision to biopsy should begin with a history and physical examination. *The surgical treatment, and even the biopsy, of melanomas should be done whenever feasible by physicians with direct experience in the care and management of these lesions. Even the first biopsy if positive for melanoma has information necessary for planning further diagnostic procedures and therapies. Incorrect management of melanomas is a significant cause of malpractice judgments.*

Individual pigmented lesions are evaluated in the physical exam by applying "the ugly duckling rule" and the **ABCDEs** of melanoma:

- **A**—Asymmetry: One half of the lesion does not mirror the other half.
- **B**—Border: The borders are irregular, shaggy, or indistinct.
- **C**—Color: The color is variegated; the pigment is not uniform, and there may be varying shades and/or hues.
- **D**—Diameter: Classically, any pigmented lesion >6 mm in diameter is concerning. Melanomas, however, are often detected at smaller sizes.
- **E**—Evolving: Notable change in a lesion over time raises suspicion for malignancy. Ulceration and bleeding are late signs and should certainly prompt biopsy.

In a patient with multiple pigmented lesions, look for and strongly consider biopsy of "the ugly duckling" lesion, that is, one that strikes the examiner as unlike the others.

Any NEW dark black lesion—no matter the size—should be considered a possible melanoma. However, being exophytic or raised does not make a pigmented papule more suspicious to be a melanoma. The presence of a depigmented "halo" is not a worrisome feature if the nevus in the center has no features of melanoma.

Dark-skinned patients may have pigmented lesions on the palms and soles; lack of uniformity within a lesion is a clue that must be carefully followed.

When suspicion for a melanoma is very high, the best biopsy technique is scalpel excision with 1- to 3-mm radial margins and a deep margin in the fatty subcutis. A deep shave biopsy with 1- to 2-mm margins (also called saucerization) is favored when suspicion for melanoma is lower but enough to warrant biopsy. Likewise, a punch excision is also acceptable in less suspicious lesions that are small enough to be completely removed in this manner. Incisional biopsies and other sampling approaches are less desirable, as they may miss the worst pathology.

Amelanotic melanomas can be very atypical in appearance and will not have the usual color changes seen in other melanomas. Any suspected melanoma will need a biopsy to establish diagnosis.

Acral Lentiginous Melanoma

Have a low threshold for biopsy in any new pigmented acral lesion. If a person of color presents with a persistent lesion of the lower extremity that has been increasing in size, has been darkening in color, or has been previously treated unsuccessfully as a fungal infection, this should increase suspicion for an ALM.

Lentigo Maligna

Use a Wood lamp (UVA lamp) to examine the skin in a darkened room. This will often reveal more extensive disease, showing borders with more clarity than visible light.

Lentigo Maligna Melanoma

- Lesional borders are often very difficult to perceive. A Wood lamp is useful in clarifying the border.
- The discovery of a more deeply pigmented irregular nodule within the lesion is often indicative of dermal invasion.

?? Differential Diagnosis and Pitfalls

Melanoma, Lentigo Maligna, and Lentigo Maligna Melanoma

- Spitz nevi (sometimes called juvenile melanoma)—often a source of confusion for doctor and patients; seen in first and second decades
- Compound nevi
- Seborrheic keratoses
- Pigmented basal cell carcinoma
- Dysplastic nevus
- Congenital nevus
- Blue nevus
- Lentigo simplex
- Solar lentigo
- Pyogenic granuloma—friable, glistening surface
- Angiokeratoma
- Hemangioma—cherry, thrombosed
- Dermatofibroma—firm tan or brown papule with positive dimple sign

- Halo nevus—tan or brown papule with surrounding depigmented patch
- Metastatic carcinoma
- Paget disease
- Tinea nigra
- Nevus
- Melasma
- Pigmented actinic keratosis
- Pigmented Bowen disease

Acral Lentiginous Melanoma

- Pigmented basal cell carcinoma—brown or black waxy nodule
- Dysplastic nevus—variegated macule or papule
- Blue nevus—well-defined blue nodule or papule
- Lentigo—well-defined oval-shaped brown to black macule
- Pyogenic granuloma—solitary small friable papule on the nail bed or soles

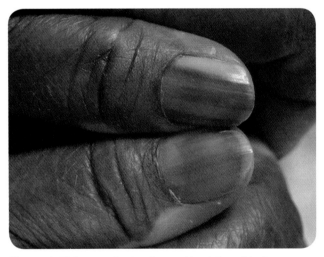

Figure 4-136 Generalized melanonychia of the nail beds.

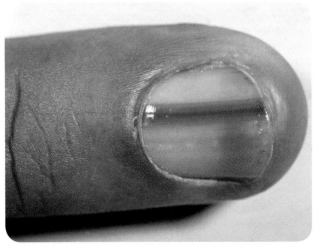

Figure 4-137 Sharply bordered longitudinal melanonychia.

162

- Angiokeratoma—small, warty, blue-black papule on the lower extremity
- Tinea pedis—dark-colored patch on the plantar foot
- Squamous cell carcinoma—ulcerative nodule on the lower extremity
- Subungual hematoma
- Talon noir (black heel)
- Longitudinal melanonychia (a pigmented line along the length of a nail plate) may be a benign finding or a sign of a nail matrix melanoma (Figs. 4-136 and 4-137). Hutchinson sign, the presence of pigment in the proximal nail fold in a patient with longitudinal melanonychia, should prompt consideration of a nail matrix melanoma.

✓ Best Tests

Melanoma

- Full-thickness skin biopsy, preferably excisional or saucerization (see "Diagnostic Pearls" above). Dermatoscopy allows for rapid examination of the pigment pattern in a large number of lesions and may help differentiate between benign and malignant pigmented lesions. Suspicious lesions should always be submitted for histopathologic examination.
- Because melanoma most often metastasizes to the lungs, liver, and brain, the following studies can be considered as part of a metastatic or staging workup once a diagnosis of melanoma is established and if symptoms are present (in the absence of specific symptoms, these are not recommended as screening tools):
  - Chest radiograph
  - Liver function tests and LDH
  - PET scan
  - MRI
  - CT scan(s)

Acral Lentiginous Melanoma

An excisional biopsy will be required, unless the lesion is too large to remove in its entirety. If this is the case, an incisional or punch biopsy should be obtained in order to obtain the Breslow depth.

Lentigo Maligna

- Dermoscopy may help distinguish benign from malignant pigmented lesions, but a full-thickness skin biopsy is indicated for all suspicious lesions.
- A metastatic workup is not indicated for lentigo maligna.

Lentigo Maligna Melanoma

Full-thickness skin biopsy. Dermoscopy may help differentiate between benign and malignant pigmented lesions, but suspicious lesions should always be submitted for histopathologic examination.

▲▲ Management Pearls

Melanoma

- Patients with suspicious pigmented lesions and those with known melanoma should be referred to and followed regularly by a dermatologist, as individuals with one melanoma have a higher frequency of another melanoma occurring. In patients with a melanoma and multiple atypical nevi, family members should be examined.
- All skin biopsy specimens of pigmented lesions should be interpreted by a dermatopathologist.
- All patients with melanoma *except* those with Stage 0 or Stage 1A disease (i.e., nonulcerated lesions ≤1.0 mm and do not extend into or below the papillary dermis) should be offered a referral to an experienced surgical oncologist to consider sentinel lymph node biopsy and possible formal lymph node dissection. Medical oncology should be involved as well. The evaluation of a sentinel lymph node for microscopic disease yields powerful prognostic information.
- Patients may ultimately require a plastic surgery consultation for reconstruction.

Acral Lentiginous Melanoma

Dermatoscopic examination allows rapid examination of the pigment pattern in a large number of lesions. It can be used to differentiate melanocytic lesions from nonmelanocytic lesions involving the acrosyringia. There are several benign dermoscopic patterns of acral nevi: parallel furrow, fibrillar, and lattice. A worrisome dermoscopic pattern is the parallel ridge, which involves pigment along the acrosyringia and may represent acral melanoma.

Lentigo Maligna

- Lesional borders are often very difficult to perceive. A Wood lamp is useful in clarifying the border, but ample margins should be used. If there is suspicion of melanoma, the lesion should be excised fully at the time of the biopsy. If a dermatologist is available, defer to his or her expertise and make sure the specimen is interpreted by a dermatopathologist.
- Patients with lentigo maligna should have periodic (every 4 to 6 months) full-body skin examinations by a dermatologist.

Lentigo Maligna Melanoma

Same as for "Melanoma," above.

Therapy

Melanoma

Definitive Lesion Treatment—These should be performed by those with experience in treating melanoma:

Surgical excision is the treatment of choice. The margins required depend on the depth of invasion of the tumor. Guidelines vary, but the following are suggested:

- *In situ*—margins at least 0.5 cm (larger in the lentigo maligna form of melanoma *in situ*)
- <1 mm—margins 1 cm
- 1 to 2 mm—margins 1 to 2 cm
- 2 to 4 mm—margins 2 cm
- >4 mm—margin at least 2 cm

Mohs micrographic surgery or staged excisions have been used for lentigo maligna melanoma with low local recurrence rates. This technique should be performed only by experienced surgeons.

Patients with nodal metastases will require a full lymph node dissection and adjuvant chemotherapy such as interferon alpha 2b. Chemotherapy for patients with metastatic disease may also consist of temozolomide, IL-2, dacarbazine, or granulocyte macrophage colony-stimulating factor (GM-CSF). The treatment of advanced melanoma is difficult and often does not succeed. Patients with advanced disease stage should be referred to a center with expertise in the multidisciplinary care of melanoma and have access to participation in clinical trials. Immunotherapy, including the use of melanoma-specific therapeutic vaccines, is one exciting area of investigation but has yet to demonstrate improvements in survival.

Close clinical surveillance of patients after a diagnosis of melanoma is imperative, as patients are at risk for local or systemic recurrence as well as for second primary melanomas. Published guidelines vary; one approach is to see patients four times a year in the first 2 years after a new diagnosis and then one to two times a year thereafter. First-degree family members of melanoma patients should also be screened and counseled as to their increased risk.

Acral Lentiginous Melanoma

Treatment of choice for ALM is surgical excision using the following guidelines for excision of suspicious lesions after biopsy: 0.5 cm margin for *in situ* melanoma, 1 cm margins for lesions ≤1 mm in thickness, 1 to 2 cm margins for lesions 1 to 2 mm in thickness, and at least 2 to 3 cm margins for lesions >2 mm in thickness. Amputation may also be required for acral lesions. Patients with lesions thicker than 1 mm in depth

(Continued)

or those with thin melanomas (<1 mm in depth) but having high-risk histologic features (ulceration or high mitotic rate) may be considered for sentinel lymph node biopsy. If positive sentinel lymph nodes are discovered, a full lymph node dissection will be necessary and possibly adjuvant therapy with interferon alpha as well as a metastatic workup.

Lentigo Maligna

Complete surgical excision is the treatment of choice, with margins of 0.5 to 1.0 cm when feasible.

In patients who are not candidates for surgery, successful use of the following modalities has been reported:

- Radiotherapy
- Q-switched ruby laser
- Q-switched Nd:YAG laser
- Topical imiquimod 5% applied daily for 3 months
- Intralesional interferon alpha
- Tazarotene 1% gel applied daily for 6 to 8 months

Lentigo Maligna Melanoma

Surgical excision is the treatment of choice. The margins required depend on the depth of invasion of the tumor:

- *In situ*—margins at least 0.5 cm
- <1 mm—margins 1 cm
- 1 to 2 mm—margins 1 to 2 cm
- 2 to 4 mm—margins 2 cm
- >4 mm—margin at least 2 cm

Mohs micrographic surgery and staged excisions have also been used for lentigo maligna melanoma with low local recurrence rates.

In patients who are not surgical candidates, a number of nonsurgical therapies have been employed. All of the nonsurgical options carry a significant rate of recurrence:

- Cryosurgery
- Radiation therapy
- Laser surgery
- Electrodesiccation
- Topical therapies such as imiquimod

Patients with nodal metastases will require a full lymph node dissection and adjuvant chemotherapy such as interferon alpha 2b. Chemotherapy for patients with metastatic disease may also consist of temozolomide, IL-2, dacarbazine, or GM-CSF.

Many vaccines against melanoma have been developed and are currently under development. As of yet, none has demonstrated an ability to impact survival.

Avoidance of sun and use of sun-protective clothing and sunscreens are strongly recommended.

Suggested Readings

Albreski D, Sloan SB. Melanoma of the feet: Misdiagnosed and misunderstood. *Clin Dermatol.* 2009;27(6):556–563.

Beadling C, Jacobson-Dunlop E, Hodi S, et al. KIT gene mutations and copy number in melanoma subtypes. *Clin Cancer Res.* 2008;14(21): 6821–6828.

Bellows CF, Belafsky P, Fortgang IS, et al. Melanoma in African-Americans: Trends in biological behavior and clinical characteristics over two decades. *J Surg Oncol.* 2001;78(1):10–16.

Bradford PT, Goldstein AM, McMaster ML, et al. Acral lentiginous melanoma: Incidence and survival patterns in the United States, 1986–2005. *Arch Dermatol.* 2009;145(4):427–434.

Byrd-Miles K, Toombs EL, Peck GL. Skin cancer in individuals of African, Asian, Latin-American, and American-Indian descent: Differences in incidence, clinical presentation, and survival compared to Caucasians. *J Drugs Dermatol.* 2007;6(1):10–16.

Bristow IR, Acland K. Acral lentiginous melanoma of the foot and ankle: A case series and review of the literature. *J Foot Ankle Res.* 2008;1(1):11.

Byrd KM, Wilson DC, Hoyler SS, et al. Advanced presentation of melanoma in African Americans. *J Am Acad Dermatol.* 2004;50(1):21–24.

Hu S, Parker DF, Thomas AG, et al. Advanced presentation of melanoma in African Americans: The Miami-Dade County experience. *J Am Acad Dermatol.* 2004;51(6):1031–1032.

Kundu R, Kamaria M, Ortiz S, et al. Effectiveness of a knowledge-based intervention for melanoma among those with ethnic skin. *J Am Acad Dermatol.* 2010;62(5):777–784.

Levit EK, Kagen MH, Scher RK, et al. The ABC rule for clinical detection of subungual melanoma. *J Am Acad Dermatol.* 2000;42(2 Pt 1):269–274.

Rahman Z, Taylor SC. Malignant melanoma in African Americans. *Cutis.* 2001;67(5):403–406.

Rouhani P, Hu S, Kirsner RS. Melanoma in Hispanic and black Americans. *Cancer Control.* 2008;15(3):248–253.

Shoo BA, Kashani-Sabet M. Melanoma arising in African-, Asian-, Latino-, and Native-American populations. *Semin Cutan Med Surg.* 2009;28(2):96–102.

Oral Melanotic Macule

Stephanie Diamantis

Diagnosis Synopsis

A melanotic macule is a benign hyperpigmentation of the mucous membranes occurring in approximately 3% of the general population. There is an increase in focal melanin deposition without an increase in the number of melanocytes. Melanotic macules are most commonly found on the vermilion border of the lip, lower more often than upper. Lesions can also be found on the gingiva or palate or in the vulva, and they may be multiple. Although benign, biopsy may be needed to rule out a diagnosis of melanoma. Oral melanotic macules are common in darkly pigmented patients and are seen more frequently in women. Though these macules may appear at any age, the average age at the time of presentation is 40 years. In darkly pigmented patients, onset typically occurs in adolescence. Some experts prefer to refer to lesions on the lip as "labial melanotic macules" and to lesions in the vulva as "vulvar melanosis," although histopathology is identical to that at any other mucosal site.

Look For

A solitary, flat, brown or grayish-brown discoloration of the lip, vulva, or intraoral mucosal surface (Fig. 4-138). The macule appears slowly and has a uniform color and border. Melanotic macules are typically 2 to 15 mm in diameter and are most commonly located on the vermilion border in the central third of the lower lip.

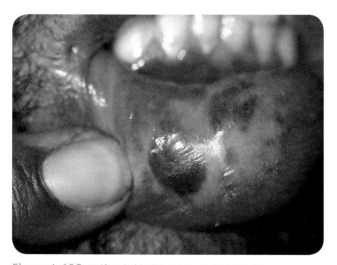

Figure 4-138 Uniformly black lentigo on the buccal mucosa.

Diagnostic Pearls

With a dermatoscope, one sees a very dark linear pattern of pigmented streaks of a uniform width and pigmentation. Within the oral cavity, melanoma is most prevalent on the palate.

Differential Diagnosis and Pitfalls

- Blue nevus
- Melanoma
- Venous lake—purple in color, blanches with diascopy
- Peutz-Jeghers syndrome
- Carney complex
- LEOPARD syndrome
- Drug-induced pigmentation—for example, antimalarials, tetracyclines, some chemotherapeutic agents
- Smoker's melanosis
- Amalgam tattoo
- Heavy metal poisoning
- Addison disease
- Kaposi sarcoma
- Hematoma
- Melanoacanthoma
- Albright syndrome
- Laugier-Hunziker syndrome
- Acanthosis nigricans
- Ephelides (freckles)
- Lentigo simplex

Best Tests

Skin biopsy of a melanotic macule should be performed if melanoma is suspected. Diascopy (pressing on the lesion with a glass slide) can differentiate between a vascular lesion such as a venous lake (which will blanch under the pressure of the slide) and a pigmented melanotic macule.

Management Pearls

- Measure the lesion or use photography to track changes. Lesions that change significantly in size or character over time should be biopsied.
- Lesions occurring in patterns of multiple lentigines (LEOPARD) syndrome or Peutz-Jeghers syndrome should prompt further workup to rule out systemic disease.

Therapy

Clinical observation is generally appropriate for melanotic macules. Treatment is considered cosmetic and may include excision or laser.

Suggested Readings

Barnhill RL, Llewellyn K. Benign melanocytic neoplasms. In: Bolognia JL, Jorizzo JL, Rapini RP, eds. *Dermatology*. 1st Ed. Philadelphia, PA: Elsevier; 2003:1757–1787.

Halder RM, Nandedkar MA, Neal KW. Pigmentary disorders in ethnic skin. *Dermatol Clin*. 2003;21:617–628.

Melasma

Stephanie Diamantis

◼◼ Diagnosis Synopsis

Melasma is an acquired disorder of hyperpigmentation affecting sun-exposed areas, especially the face. The condition is much more common in women (10:1) and is marked by brown patches, which can worsen in pregnancy (termed "chloasma") or with the use of birth control pills. It is rare before puberty, and it occurs most commonly in the reproductive years. It also appears to be more common in darkly pigmented individuals, especially Hispanics but also Asians, African Americans, Africans (especially Ethiopians), and Pacific Islanders. In fact, studies show that up to half of all Mexican women develop melasma in pregnancy. A variant has been described on the forearms of Native American women taking progesterone replacement. Family history is known to confer additional risk.

Melasma is a benign condition mainly of cosmetic concern; treatment consists of sun avoidance and improving the skin's appearance through topical depigmenting agents, physical modalities, or chemical exfoliation.

Melasma is generally thought of as a disorder of epidermal hyperpigmentation, but dermal variants also exist, which tend to be refractory to topical treatments.

◉ Look For

Hyperpigmented patches of the face, typically involving the lateral cheeks, forehead, chin, upper lip, and neck (Figs. 4-139–4-141). The patches are usually symmetric and may have a "moth-eaten" appearance to their borders (Fig. 4-142). A mandibular variant has also been described.

●● Diagnostic Pearls

- Pigment is usually epidermal and, therefore, markedly accentuated with a Wood lamp.
- Areas involved are usually restricted to sun-exposed skin; however, the upper lip can be involved in melasma secondary to oral contraceptive use.

?? Differential Diagnosis and Pitfalls

- Postinflammatory pigmentation from acne or other inflammatory disease
- Lentigo
- Erythema dyschromicum perstans (ashy dermatosis)
- Drug-induced hyperpigmentation from medications such as tetracyclines, phenothiazines, and amiodarone
- Addison disease
- Poikiloderma of Civatte
- Hydroquinone-induced ochronosis, especially in dark-skinned Africans

✓ Best Tests

Melasma is primarily a clinical diagnosis.

▲▲ Management Pearls

- Sun avoidance and protection are of primary importance in melasma management. The use of a broad-spectrum UVA/UVB sunscreen with SPF 30 or higher and long-acting

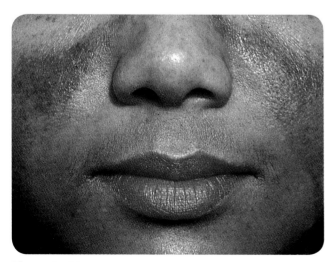

Figure 4-139 Sharply bordered hyperpigmented macule of melasma on cheeks and upper lip.

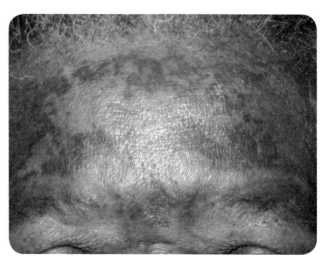

Figure 4-140 Forehead with mottled hyperpigmentation of melasma.

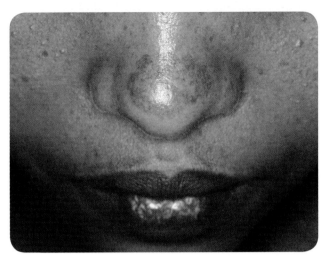

Figure 4-141 Macular hyperpigmentation of melasma on the nose and along the border of the upper lip.

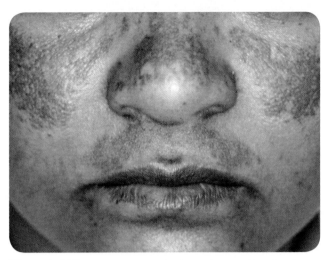

Figure 4-142 Symmetrical macular hyperpigmentation of melasma.

broadband UVA protection is essential. Sunscreen should be used year-round because the skin is very sensitive to small amounts of ultraviolet light, and even penetration through window glass is relevant. To optimize sun protection, protective clothing is also indicated. Sun exposure can also result in relapse of successfully treated melasma.

- If the patient is on oral contraceptive pills (OCPs) and needs to remain on the OCPs, improvement may be difficult. Even if OCPs are discontinued, OCP-induced melasma is challenging to treat and is easily stimulated by small amounts of sunlight.
- Reassure pregnant patients with melasma (chloasma) that the pigmentation will usually fade postpartum.

Therapy

Melasma should be treated in the early stages because increasing severity makes treatment more difficult. In addition to limiting sun exposure, current first-line treatments for melasma include hydroquinone alone or in combination with corticosteroids, tretinoin, retinol, or glycolic acid. A combination formula of hydroquinone 4%, fluocinolone acetonide 0.01%, and tretinoin 0.05% in a cream formulation (Tri-Luma) has been used with good results. There is a recent scale for quantitating melasma.

Bleaching agents (e.g., hydroquinone) should be used carefully and not long term. Hydroquinone is available over the counter in a 2% concentration and by prescription in a 4% concentration. A paradoxical effect of long-term or higher concentrations of hydroquinone (usually in concentrations above that in commercial preparations) is the occurrence of a bluish ochronosislike pigmentation. Other side effects include irritant or allergic contact dermatitis.

Azelaic acid is available in a 20% cream and 15% gel and is used off label for treatment of hyperpigmentation. Noticeable improvement can take up to 4 months. Azelaic acid is safe to use in pregnancy (category B). More common side effects include itching and burning at sites of application.

Kojic acid is increasingly being used in Japanese skin care products. Other topical agents include licorice extract, arbutin, and N-acetylglucosamine.

Adjuvant procedures include superficial chemical peels (glycolic acid, trichloroacetic acid) and microdermabrasion. Laser and other light sources (e.g., intense pulsed light) may offer some additional improvement, but these procedures should be done carefully in darkly pigmented skin because of the higher risk of postinflammatory hyperpigmentation.

Suggested Readings

Grimes PE. Management of hyperpigmentation in darker racial ethnic groups. *Semin Cutan Med Surg.* 2009;28:77–85.

Halder RM, Nandedkar MA, Neal KW. Pigmentary disorders in ethnic skin. *Dermatol Clin.* 2003;21:617–628.

Halder RM, Nootheti PK. Ethnic skin disorders overview. *J Am Acad Dermatol.* 2003;48:143–148.

Pandya AG, Hynan LS, Bhore R, et al. Reliability assessment and validation of the Melasma Area and Severity Index (MASI) and a new modified MASI scoring method. *J Am Acad Dermatol.* 2011;64(1):78–83, 83.e1-2.

Sanchez MR. Cutaneous diseases in Latinos. *Dermatol Clin.* 2003;21:689–697.

Taylor SC. Epidemiology of skin diseases in ethnic populations. *Dermatol Clin.* 2003;21:601–607.

Yang DJ, Quan LT, Hsu S. Topical antibacterial agents. In: Wolverton SE. *Comprehensive Dermatologic Drug Therapy.* 2nd Ed. Philadelphia, PA: Elsevier; 2007:538–539.

Flat Pigmented Lesions

Stephanie Diamantis

Diagnosis Synopsis

Dermal melanocytosis is a term used to describe an increased amount of melanocytes with or without accompanying melanophages in the dermis. This description encompasses many benign skin disorders including the blue-gray (Mongolian) spot, nevus of Ota, and nevus of Ito. Dermal melanocytosis tends to be more common in darkly pigmented individuals. The Tyndall phenomenon is responsible for the blue-gray color observed clinically.

Blue-Gray (Mongolian) Spot

Mongolian spot, also known as congenital dermal melanocytosis, is a benign congenital blue-gray hyperpigmented patch commonly found on the lumbosacral or gluteal area in up to 96% of African American infants, 46% of Hispanic infants, and in a large percentage of Asian American infants (Fig. 4-143). Mongolian spots can occur in other ethnicities and other locations (aberrant Mongolian spot), albeit less commonly. Pigmentary changes become most intense at 1 year of age, peak diameter is attained by 2 years of age, and lesions generally fade completely by adulthood. Rarely, Mongolian spots may persist into adulthood.

Nevus of Ota

Nevus of Ota is a dermal melanocyte hamartoma located on the face in the skin supplied by the first and second division of the trigeminal nerve (Figs. 4.144 and 4-145). Location

(periorbital, malar) differentiates this lesion from the nevus of Ito and Mongolian spot. Nevus of Ota is unilateral in 95% of cases. Dermal melanocytosis may also involve the ocular

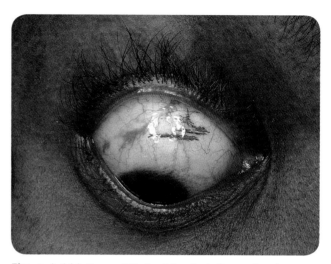

Figure 4-144 Nevus of Ota involving the bulbar conjunctivae.

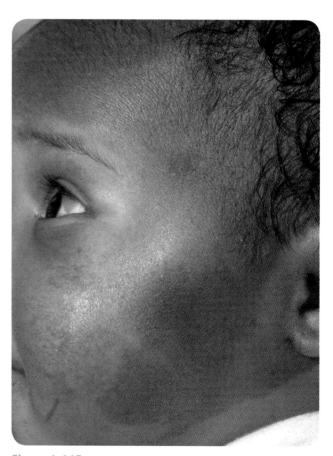

Figure 4-145 Large flat blue macule on forehead and cheek, characteristic of nevus of Ota.

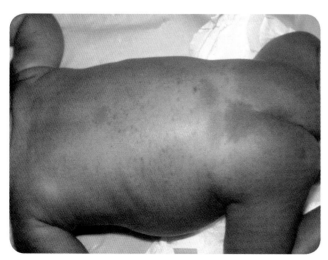

Figure 4-143 A six-month-old male patient with large and small blue macules in a characteristic location.

and oral mucosal surfaces. The incidence is higher in Asians, in black individuals, and in women. The highest incidence is among Japanese women. The lesion typically manifests at birth or infancy, but onset during adolescence has occurred. Acquired bilateral nevus of Ota–like macules (ABNOM), also known as Hori nevus, is found in Asian women in particular. Patients are at risk of developing ipsilateral glaucoma. Rare cases of melanoma arising within nevus of Ota have been described.

Nevus of Ito

Nevus of Ito is a unilateral dermal melanocyte hamartoma that is clinically differentiated from a nevus of Ota and a Mongolian spot by its speckled or mottled appearance and its location. It is analogous to nevus of Ota and may in fact coexist in the same patient. A nevus of Ito presents as a blue to gray patch located over the supraclavicular, deltoid, or scapular area and is often present at birth or develops shortly thereafter (Figs. 4-146 and 4-147). There may be associated sensory changes in the involved skin. Lesions are present for the lifetime of the patient. Melanoma can rarely appear within a nevus of Ito.

Look For

Blue-Gray (Mongolian) Spot

Evenly pigmented blue to gray macules ranging in size from 1 cm to >10 cm. They are typically round to oval but may be polymorphous. Infants may have one or multiple macules of varying shades of gray and blue. Borders are typically irregular to indistinct. A lumbosacral location is most common.

Nevus of Ota

Confluent blue or brown macules resulting in an ill-defined, mottled patch involving the forehead, temple, periorbital region, nose, and superior cheek, typically in a trigeminal distribution. In women, the intensity of pigmentation can vary and increase during menstruation. The pigmentation may involve the sclera as well. Lesions may enlarge and darken over time.

Nevus of Ito

Blue to gray confluent or mottled patch in a supraclavicular, deltoid, or scapular location.

Diagnostic Pearls

Blue-Gray (Mongolian) Spot

Blue-gray patches on the lumbosacral location at birth are highly suggestive of this diagnosis.

Nevus of Ota

Look for ipsilateral, patchy, blue discoloration of the sclera and conjunctiva in conjunction with a blue to brown pigmented lesion distributed within the first and second divisions of the trigeminal nerve.

Nevus of Ito

Patients are almost always of Asian, and in particular Japanese, descent. However, lesions have been reported in those

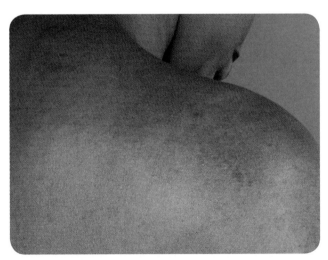

Figure 4-146 Nevus of Ito involving the upper shoulder.

Figure 4-147 Large flat blue macule on shoulder characteristic of nevus of Ota.

of African and East Indian descent. The location in the region of the shoulder/upper arm is diagnostic.

?? Differential Diagnosis and Pitfalls

Blue-Gray (Mongolian) Spot

Similar differential diagnosis as nevus of Ota and Ito, but also consider the following:
- Congenital melanocytic nevus
- Deep infantile hemangioma—Overlying telangiectases often represent superficial component; may swell or deepen in coloration when dependent or crying; rapidly elevates over days to weeks

Nevus of Ota

Similar differential diagnosis as nevus of Ito, but also consider the following:
- Melasma
- If change occurs, consider the onset of melanoma or a malignant blue nevus, which rarely occurs within the nevus of Ota.

Nevus of Ito

- Blue nevus—similar blue to gray pigmentation, but smaller and well demarcated
- Nevus of Ota—trigeminal distribution of the face
- Tattoo—diagnosed by history
- Mongolian spot—typically overlies buttocks or lumbosacral area
- Melanoma—usually presents later in life, more focal distribution
- Lentigo
- Café au lait macule
- Ochronosis
- Phytophotodermatitis—acute onset, diagnosed by history
- Drug-induced hyperpigmentation
- Ecchymoses—history of trauma
- Vascular malformation
- Nevus spilus—darker speckled pigmentation within
- Becker nevus—similar distribution but often has coarse hair within

Best Tests

Diagnosis of nevus of Ito, nevus of Ota, and Mongolian spot can usually be made clinically. Skin biopsy will show an increased number of dendritic melanocytes in the dermis.

▲▲ Management Pearls

Blue-Gray (Mongolian) Spot

Document the presence of blue-gray spots to prevent false accusations of child abuse by unknowing persons. Blue-gray spots have no increased risk for the development of melanoma or other skin cancers.

Nevus of Ota

- Consider an ophthalmology referral because of the association of nevus of Ota with elevated intraocular pressure and glaucoma.
- Skin biopsy is indicated if there is suspicion for malignant transformation.

Nevus of Ito

Cosmetic makeup can be used.

Therapy

- Mongolian spots usually resolve spontaneously, so treatment is not recommended prior to adulthood.
- Nevus of Ito and nevus of Ota lesions can be covered with opaque makeup with good cosmetic results. Q-switched lasers (ruby, alexandrite, or neodymium:yttrium-aluminum-garnet [Nd:YAG] laser) can also be effective in fading lesions over several treatments.

Suggested Readings

Barnhill RL, Llewellyn K. Benign melanocytic neoplasms. In: Bolognia JL, Jorizzo JL, Rapini RP, eds. *Dermatology*. 1st Ed. Philadelphia, PA: Elsevier; 2003:1757–1787.

Cordova A. The Mongolian Spot: A study of ethnic differences and a literature review. *Clin Pediatrics*. 1981;20(11):714–718.

Halder RM, Nandedkar MA, Neal KW. Pigmentary disorders in ethnic skin. *Dermatol Clin*. 2003;21:617–628.

Harrison-Balestra C, Gugic D, Vincek V. Clinically distinct form of acquired dermal melanocytosis with review of published work. *J Dermatol*. 2007;34:178–182.

Lee CS, Lim HW. Cutaneous diseases in Asians. *Dermatol Clin*. 2003;21: 669–677.

Park JM, Tsao H, Tsao S. Acquired bilateral nevus of Ota-like macules (Hori nevus): Etiologic and therapeutic considerations. *J Am Acad Dermatol*. 2009;61:88–93.

Spitz Nevus

Stephanie Diamantis

Diagnosis Synopsis

Spitz nevi (spindle and epithelioid cell nevi, benign juvenile melanoma) are benign melanocytic nevi of childhood and adolescence. The majority of lesions are solitary, but, rarely, they can be multiple and localized in one area (agminated). No ethnic predilection has been documented. An atypical variant has been described that exhibits larger size and asymmetry clinically and deeper infiltration into the dermis, frequent mitoses, and lack of maturation histologically.

The importance of these lesions lies in their frequent histopathologic confusion with melanoma. Lesions can develop slowly or appear quite rapidly. Without excision, lesions may remain stable for years, evolve into compound nevi, flatten over time, or involute spontaneously.

Look For

Red, red-brown, or blue-red dome-shaped papules, 3 to 6 mm in size, typically located on the face or extremities, but any location is possible. Head and neck lesions predominate in children (Fig. 4-148).

Diagnostic Pearls

Lesions are usually more red than brown and can be clinically mistaken for a pyogenic granuloma.

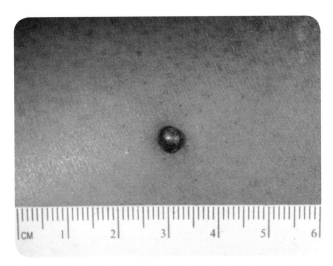

Figure 4-148 A 13-year-old Hispanic girl with a 5-mm pedunculated nodule that has slowly been expanding in size.

Differential Diagnosis and Pitfalls

- Melanoma
- Atypical melanocytic nevus
- Juvenile xanthogranuloma
- Blue nevus
- Combined nevus (blue nevus and compound nevus together)
- Dermatofibroma
- Pyogenic granuloma
- Multiple Spitz nevi should be distinguished from urticaria pigmentosa, familial atypical multiple mole and melanoma syndrome.

Best Tests

- Careful, complete skin examination in a fully disrobed patient that includes the scalp, the mouth, behind the ears, and between the toes. Dermoscopy performed by a clinician experienced with this method may be useful.
- For most nevi, the diagnosis can often be made clinically, but suspicious lesions should be biopsied and examined by a dermatopathologist. Complete excisional biopsy provides the pathologist with the best opportunity to make an accurate diagnosis and may obviate the need for a future additional procedure.

Management Pearls

Complete excision is recommended, as histopathologic diagnosis can be difficult and childhood melanoma can be missed.

Therapy

Complete excision is recommended. Adequate margins should be obtained (~1 cm) when excising the atypical variant, and the patient should be followed on a regular basis to monitor for recurrence.

Suggested Readings

Spitz S. Melanomas of childhood. *Am J Path.* 1948;24:591–609.

Spatz A, Calonje E, Handfield-Jones S, et al. Spitz tumors in children: A grading system for risk stratification. *Arch Dermatol.* 1999;135(3):282–285.

Suh KY, Bolognia JL. Signature nevi. *J Am Acad Dermatol.* 2009;60(3):508–514.

Becker Nevus

Stephanie Diamantis

 ## Diagnosis Synopsis

A Becker nevus (Becker melanosis) is typically a large, hyperpigmented patch with increased hair growth on the upper trunk in men. This lesion is not uncommon and is found in all ethnicities. Lesions are usually present before puberty but often have increased coarse hair growth and a slightly raised texture during adolescence due to androgen stimulation. Rarely, there is associated hypoplasia of the underlying tissues (e.g., breast hypoplasia, pectoralis hypoplasia, or limb hypoplasia). Most Becker nevi have no associated abnormalities. Becker melanosis is a benign lesion, and treatment is only required in rare cases for cosmetic or psychosocial reasons.

 ## Look For

Becker nevi present as large, hyperpigmented, solitary patches with associated hypertrichosis, typically distributed on the shoulder, upper chest, or back in men (Fig. 4-149). Borders are well defined but can be irregular. The coarse, dark hair found within is more noticeable several years after the hyperpigmented patch appears (during puberty). In women, Becker nevi can present as multiple lesions. Becker nevi may have a distinct papular quality due to associated underlying smooth muscle hamartoma.

Diagnostic Pearls

Large hyperpigmented, hypertrichotic patch on the upper trunk in men. Lesions on the ipsilateral arm and chest that

appear to be separate may actually be the same dermatome. The borders of the lesion are not as distinct as a café au lait macule.

 ## Differential Diagnosis and Pitfalls

- Congenital nevi—darker and with distorted hair pattern
- Epidermal nevi—more epidermal change, dermatomal distribution
- Giant café au lait macule—clinically resembles a Becker nevus in preadolescent patients but can usually be distinguished later by the development of hypertrichosis and epidermal/dermal changes in a Becker nevus

 ## Best Tests

- Careful, complete skin examination in a fully disrobed patient that includes the scalp, the mouth, behind the ears, and between the toes. Dermoscopy performed by a clinician experienced with this method may be useful.
- For most nevi, the diagnosis can often be made clinically, but suspicious lesions should be biopsied and examined by a dermatopathologist. Complete excisional biopsy provides the pathologist with the best opportunity to make an accurate diagnosis and may obviate the need for a future additional procedure.

 ## Management Pearls

Observation is sufficient, as the risk for malignant degeneration is extremely low. For cosmetic reasons, associated hypertrichosis can be treated with laser.

Therapy

Reassure the patient that the lesion is benign and no treatment is necessary. For cosmetic or psychosocial reasons, laser treatments may improve hyperpigmentation and/or hypertrichosis. Electrolysis and depilatories are also effective in hair removal.

Suggested Readings

Barnhill RL, Llewellyn K. Benign melanocytic neoplasms. In: Bolognia JL, Jorizzo JL, Rapini RP, eds. *Dermatology.* 1st Ed. Philadelphia, PA: Elsevier; 2003:1757–1787.

Suh KY, Bolognia JL. Signature nevi. *J Am Acad Dermatol.* 2009;60(3): 508–514.

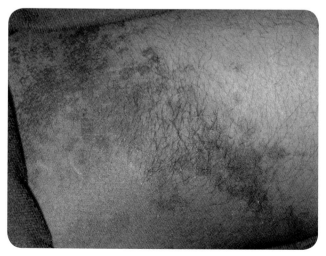

Figure 4-149 Becker nevus with hyperpigmentation and hypertrichosis.

Nevi (Moles)

Stephanie Diamantis

◼◼ Diagnosis Synopsis

Benign and Common Nevi

Common acquired melanocytic nevi ("moles") are aggregations of melanocytes (pigment-producing cells) in one of three locations: the junction of the epidermis and dermis (junctional nevus), completely within the dermis (intradermal nevus), or a combination of the above (compound nevus). Unlike junctional nevi, which are flat, compound nevi are elevated relative to the surrounding skin (papular). Nevi typically arise during childhood, adolescence, or very early adulthood and peak in number by the third decade. Their formation may be stimulated by sunlight. Compound nevi are more common in individuals with fair skin; however, other forms of nevi (those on palms, soles, conjunctiva, and in the nail bed) are more common in individuals of African descent and Asians.

Atypical Nevi

Atypical nevi (dysplastic nevi or Clark nevi) are aggregates of melanocytes that display clinical and/or histologic features that distinguish them from common melanocytic nevi. They may be familial with autosomal inheritance. Clinical features of atypical nevi include asymmetry, large size, irregular or ill-defined borders, and varied coloration. Histologically, they show abnormal architecture and cellular atypia. An atypical nevus may be a marker for risk of developing a future melanoma. Atypical nevi usually arise *de novo* or in an existing nevus. They are more common in fair-skinned individuals. The incidence of atypical nevi in individuals with skin types IV to VI is not known.

The risk of developing melanoma increases with a positive family history and an increasing number of lesions. Persons with a first- or second-degree relative with melanoma and a large number of nevi including atypical nevi define the dysplastic nevus syndrome (familial atypical multiple mole-melanoma syndrome) and are at increased risk of developing melanoma.

Clinicians chiefly excise atypical nevi for one of three reasons: to exclude the possibility of melanoma, to relieve symptoms of physical irritation, or for a cosmetic reason.

◉ Look For

Benign and Common Nevi

Compound nevi are usually well-circumscribed, uniformly pigmented papules that can be warty or smooth at the surface (Figs. 4-150–4-152). These lesions vary in color from skin-colored to dark brown and may or may not have associated hair (Fig. 4-153). They may occur anywhere on the body. Nevi may regress with a hypopigmented halo ("halo nevi") (Fig. 4-154); halo nevi rarely are a precursor of vitiligo.

Atypical Nevi

Atypical nevi can vary in size and/or color. They are often larger than common nevi. They may have variations in color within the lesion ranging from pink to reddish-brown to

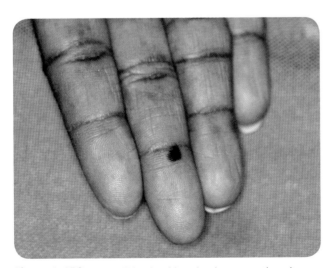

Figure 4-150 Flat, well-bordered junctional nevus on the volar surface of the middle finger.

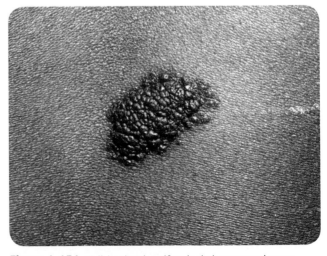

Figure 4-151 Well-bordered, uniformly dark compound nevus.

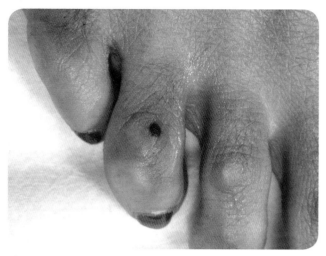

Figure 4-152 Junctional nevus that is uniformly dark and has a regular border.

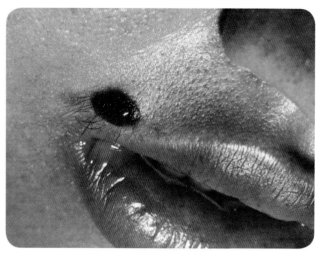

Figure 4-153 Dermal nevus that is uniformly dark and has several hairs growing from it.

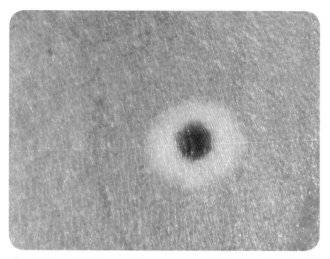

Figure 4-154 Nevi sometimes regress with inflammation and with an associated halo of depigmentation (halo nevus).

dark brown. Borders are often irregular and/or ill defined. They may also have either a darker brown center or periphery. In the atypical nevus syndrome, hundreds of nevi of varying size and color are seen.

Dysplastic nevi may occur anywhere, but they occur more often on sun-exposed areas. Clinical variations include the following: "fried-egg" compound atypical nevus, targetoid, lentigo-like, seborrheic keratosis–like, erythematous, and melanoma-like variants.

In atypical nevus syndrome, hundreds of nevi of varying size and color are seen. The syndrome is rarely reported in Hispanics and African Americans.

 ## Diagnostic Pearls

Benign and Common Nevi

The occurrence of a new pigmented lesion in an adult is unusual after the age of 50. Maintain a low threshold of suspicion for new pigmented lesions in adults, and biopsy early to rule out atypical nevus or melanoma. New nevi in children are common. Melanomas may regress by losing all or a part of their pigmentation.

Atypical Nevi

Apply the ABCDEs of suspicious pigmented lesions:

A—Asymmetry: One-half of the lesion does not mirror the other half.
B—Border: The borders are irregular or indistinct.
C—Color: The color is variegated; the pigment is not uniform, and there may be varying shades and/or hues.
D—Diameter: Classically, any pigmented lesion >6 mm in diameter is a cause for concern.
E—Evolving: Notable change in a lesion over time raises suspicion for malignancy. Ulceration and bleeding should certainly prompt biopsy.

- In a patient with multiple pigmented lesions, look for "the ugly duckling" sign (i.e., one lesion that strikes the examiner as being unlike the others).
- Any new dark black lesion—no matter the size—should be considered a possible melanoma, especially in the older patient population. Maintain a very low threshold of

suspicion for new pigmented lesions in adults, and biopsy early to rule out melanoma.

- Ask about family history of melanoma or personal history of multiple dysplastic nevi, as this can indicate increased risk for future melanomas.
- There is a high incidence of clinically appearing atypical nevi on the scalp and forehead in children and adolescents. Most pediatric dermatologists feel that these lesions have worse clinical appearance than their biologic behavior. Careful clinical examination and monitoring is prudent.

?? Differential Diagnosis and Pitfalls

Benign and Common Nevi

- Melanoma
- Blue nevus
- Combined nevus (blue nevus and compound nevus together)
- Pigmented basal cell carcinoma
- Dermatofibroma
- Atypical nevus
- Junctional nevus
- Acrochordon
- Wart
- Neurofibroma

Atypical Nevi

- Seborrheic keratosis—"stuck-on-" or waxy-appearing, tan to dark-brown papule.
- Pigmented basal cell carcinoma
- Melanocytic nevus
- Lentigo simplex
- Solar lentigo
- Lentigo maligna
- Ephelides (freckles)
- Supernumerary nipple

✓ Best Tests

Careful, complete skin examination in a fully disrobed patient that includes the scalp, the mouth, behind the ears, and between the toes. Dermoscopy performed by a clinician experienced with this method may be useful.

For most nevi, the diagnosis can often be made clinically, but suspicious lesions should be biopsied and examined by a dermatopathologist. Complete excisional biopsy provides the

pathologist with the best opportunity to make an accurate diagnosis and may obviate the need for a future additional procedure.

Management Pearls

Benign and Common Nevi

- Removal is indicated when the nevus becomes symptomatic or when marked asymmetry, border irregularity, or changes in shape or color are noted.
- Refer individuals with suspicious pigmented lesions to a dermatologist, and educate patients regarding the ABCDEs of melanoma.

Atypical Nevi

Atypical nevi frequently run in families, so family history is important. Use of a dermatoscope in experienced hands enhances the ability to discern normal from atypical pigment patterns. Patients with multiple nevi should be examined by a dermatologist every 3 to 12 months, depending on their past medical and family history as well as the morphology of their lesions. Digital photography of nevi may be useful to track changes.

Therapy

Benign and Common Nevi
No treatment is necessary. If the patient requests removal for cosmetic reasons, shave excision is often adequate.

Complete excision with histopathologic examination is indicated when the nevus becomes symptomatic or changes in shape or color.

Atypical Nevi
Observation is a reasonable approach to a clinically atypical nevus that has remained unchanged for many years. Surgical removal is indicated for a changing or suspicious lesion or in the case of suspicious lesions that are difficult to follow or whose past behavior is unknown.

The treatment of atypical nevus is excision, but because there is still controversy present regarding the adequate margins, these patients should be referred to a dermatologist with experience in treating these lesions.

Frequency of follow-up for persons with an atypical nevus ranges from every 3 months to every year.

Recommend regular use of sunscreen (SPF 30 at a minimum) and sun-protective clothing coupled with other sun-protective measures (e.g., avoidance of midday sun and tanning bed use). Provide education regarding sun protection and regular self-examination of the skin.

Suggested Readings

Barnhill RL, Llewellyn K. Benign melanocytic neoplasms. In: Bolognia JL, Jorizzo JL, Rapini RP, eds. *Dermatology.* 1st Ed. Philadelphia, PA: Elsevier; 2003:1757–1787.

Spitz S. Melanomas of childhood. *Am J Path.* 1948;24:591–609.

Suh KY, Bolognia JL. Signature nevi. *J Am Acad Dermatol.* 2009;60(3): 508–514.

Blue Nevus

Stephanie Diamantis

▪▪ Diagnosis Synopsis

Blue nevi are small blue-gray or blue-black papules caused by an aggregate of melanocytes (pigment-producing cells) in the upper and mid dermis. Dermal melanocytes reflect low-wavelength blue light and absorb higher-wavelength light (Tyndall effect), accounting for the blue color.

Blue nevi are more common in women and in those of Asian ancestry. They usually develop in young adulthood. Two variants have been described: the common blue nevus and the cellular blue nevus. Common blue nevi do not require excision, but a skin biopsy may be obtained to confirm the diagnosis. The clinical differential diagnosis includes melanoma.

Cellular blue nevi are typically larger than common blue nevi (1 to 3 cm in diameter), are solitary, and show a predilection for the buttocks or sacrococcygeal region. Malignant blue nevi are rare and tend to arise in cellular blue nevi (especially those on the scalp).

◉ Look For

Common blue nevi are blue-black or blue-gray papules that favor the hands, feet, face, and scalp (50% are found on the dorsal hands and feet) (Fig. 4-155). They are typically 0.5 to 1.0 cm in diameter. The pigmentation is very uniform. Some lesions are a combination of blue nevi and compound nevi, and these may have a more complex clinical morphology. Cellular blue nevi are similar to common blue nevi in morphology but are usually larger and found on the buttocks/sacrococcygeal area.

●● Diagnostic Pearls

Examine under bright light and look tangentially to see the definite blue hue. Rapid growth, size larger than 2 cm, or clinically atypical appearance (e.g., multinodularity) should prompt an excisional biopsy to assess for malignant transformation. A dermatoscope may facilitate visualization of the dense color but does not demonstrate enough detail to avoid biopsy of suspicious lesions in most instances.

?? Differential Diagnosis and Pitfalls

- Melanoma
- Nevus of Ota and nevus of Ito—lesions typically flat, larger, and found in characteristic locations
- Tattoo
- Dermatofibroma

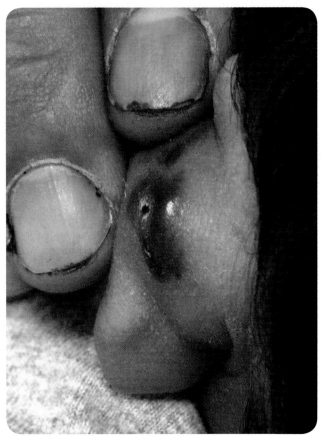

Figure 4-155 Retroauricular blue nevus with uniform, very dark pigmentation.

- Melanocytic nevus
- Venous lake
- Angiokeratoma
- Sclerosing hemangioma
- Pigmented basal cell carcinoma
- Glomus tumor
- Spitz nevus

✓ Best Tests

- Careful, complete skin examination in a fully disrobed patient that includes the scalp, the mouth, behind the ears, and between the toes. Dermoscopy performed by a clinician experienced with this method may be useful.
- For most nevi, the diagnosis can often be made clinically, but suspicious lesions should be biopsied and examined by a dermatopathologist. Complete excisional biopsy provides the pathologist with the best opportunity to make an accurate diagnosis and may obviate the need for a future additional procedure.

Management Pearls

Blue nevi are benign lesions, and no therapy is necessary. Melanoma has rarely been associated with cellular blue nevi, but this fact does not imply that these lesions should be preemptively excised. Biopsy is appropriate in changing lesions to rule out malignant degeneration.

Therapy

No therapy is necessary. If removal is desired, a small elliptical excision is recommended.

Suggested Readings

Barnhill RL, Llewellyn K. Benign melanocytic neoplasms. In: Bolognia JL, Jorizzo JL, Rapini RP, eds. *Dermatology*. 1st Ed. Philadelphia, PA: Elsevier; 2003:1757–1787.

Spitz S. Melanomas of childhood. *Am J Path*. 1948;24:591–609.

Suh KY, Bolognia JL. Signature nevi. *J Am Acad Dermatol*. 2009;60(3): 508–514.

Postinflammatory Hyperpigmentation and Notalgia Paresthetica

Mat Davey • Lynn McKinley-Grant

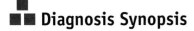 Diagnosis Synopsis

Postinflammatory Hyperpigmentation

Postinflammatory hyperpigmentation describes localized darker skin areas as a consequence of trauma and/or inflammation. The inflammatory process may be incited by an infection, allergy, drug reaction, mechanical or thermal injury (exposure to heating pads or fireplaces), moderate to severe sunburn, phototoxic eruption, or an intrinsic skin disease. Although biologically benign, patches of postinflammatory hyperpigmentation can cause significant cosmetic and psychosocial distress.

Histologically, there is an increased production of melanin without an increase in the number of melanocytes. This increased pigment may be deposited in the epidermis or the dermis. This reaction is much more pronounced in darkly pigmented individuals and patients with lichenoid dermatoses (such as lichen planus). There is no predilection in any age group or ethnicity.

The lesions of postinflammatory hyperpigmentation may be accentuated by sunlight or exposure to certain chemicals or drugs, including tetracycline, antimalarial drugs, hormones, some metals (silver, gold), and chemotherapeutic agents (doxorubicin, bleomycin, 5-fluorouracil, busulfan).

In dark skin, resolution of hyperpigmentation can be prolonged, lasting for months to years. Pigment deposited in the dermis will have a blue-gray color.

Notalgia Paraesthetica

Notalgia paresthetica usually occurs on the skin of the upper back just below or medial to the scapula and is a localized area of extremely pruritic skin. Notalgia paresthetica is felt to be secondary to spinal nerve impingement, causing the persistent itch. Pain, paresthesias, and hyperesthesias may coincide with itch. Hyperpigmented or lichenified skin changes, if present, are attributable to chronic rubbing and scratching.

Notalgia paresthetica can affect people of any age, any race/ethnicity, and either sex. However, it is thought to be most common in middle-aged to older adults. Women develop notalgia paresthetica more frequently than men.

Though the etiology of notalgia paresthetica is not entirely certain, some studies have demonstrated, radiographically, vertebral spine disease correlating to the level of the nerve root affecting the pruritic skin, typically T2-T6.

⊙ Look For

Postinflammatory Hyperpigmentation

Asymptomatic, ill-defined, darkened macules or patches. Lesions will often define an area of previous skin insult or inflammation of any kind. It can occur anywhere on the body (including the mucosa and within the nail unit) (Figs. 4-156–4-160).

Pigment deposited in the epidermis is often light brown, while dermal pigment appears more blue-gray in color.

Notalgia Paraesthetica

Notalgia paresthetica most typically manifests with a unilateral, hyperpigmented patch just below the scapula at the upper back. The patch is noninflammatory, is usually not scaly, and follows the area of skin that the patient has constantly been rubbing.

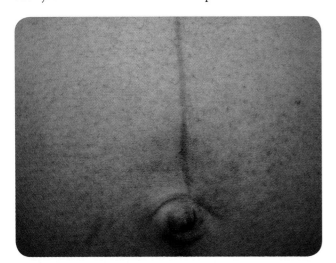

Figure 4-156 Linea nigra is benign; it often begins during pregnancy and is permanent afterward.

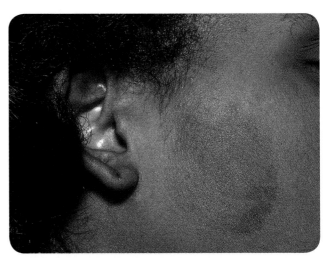

Figure 4-157 Circular macular hyperpigmentation from applying perfumes with oil of bergamot (berlock dermatitis).

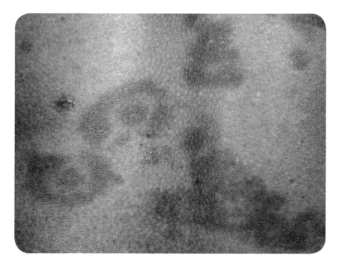

Figure 4-158 Postinflammatory hyperpigmentation secondary to the blistering of pemphigus vulgaris.

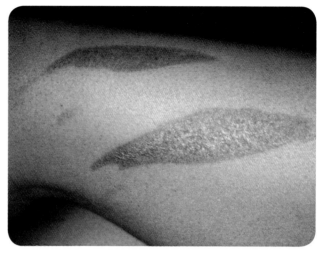

Figure 4-159 Postinflammatory hyperpigmentation from trauma.

 ## Diagnostic Pearls

Postinflammatory Hyperpigmentation

If the pigment is in the dermis, it will not be accentuated with a Wood light, whereas if epidermal pigmentation is increased, this will absorb more of the Wood light and appear darker or more accentuated than the surrounding skin. This difference may have therapeutic implications, as epidermal pigmentation is more successfully treated with topical therapy (see below).

Notalgia Paraesthetica

Notalgia paraesthetica is a clinical diagnosis, with localized macular pigmentation just below the scapula being almost pathognomonic for this condition.

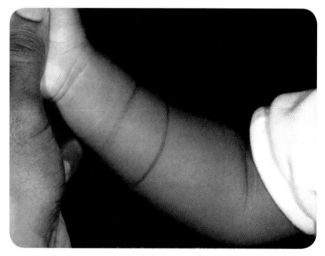

Figure 4-160 Linear postinflammatory hyperpigmentation from trauma.

?? Differential Diagnosis and Pitfalls

Postinflammatory Hyperpigmentation

- Melasma
- Drug-induced pigmentation
- Addison disease
- Acanthosis nigricans
- Tinea versicolor
- Lichen planus
- Lichen amyloidosis
- Peutz-Jeghers syndrome
- Erythema dyschromicum perstans

Pediatric Patient Differential Diagnosis

For single lesions, consider the following:
- Fixed drug eruption
- Blue-gray spot (Mongolian spot)
- Drug-induced pigmentation

Notalgia Paraesthetica

- Postinflammatory hyperpigmentation
- Nummular dermatitis
- Fixed drug eruption
- Macular amyloidosis
- Drug-related hyperpigmentation

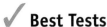

✓ Best Tests

Postinflammatory Hyperpigmentation

- Usually a clinical diagnosis based on history of an antecedent inflammatory skin disease, trauma, or chronic rubbing in the area of pigmentation
- Skin biopsy may be performed in equivocal cases. The biopsy specimen should be stained with Fontana-Masson silver stain to localize the melanin deposition.

Notalgia Paraesthetica

Notalgia paresthetica is a clinical diagnosis. Laboratory studies and skin biopsy are not helpful.

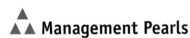

▲▲ Management Pearls

Postinflammatory Hyperpigmentation

- Prevention of the inciting dermatoses will help control the development of the condition. Conservative skin care is often best, with emphasis placed on the importance of allowing the skin to heal itself. Discourage any picking, scratching, or rubbing by the patient.
- The patient should follow sun-protective measures, using clothes and/or sunscreens (with both UVB and UVA blockers) on affected areas to prevent further darkening. Small amounts of UVA (even through window glass) can exacerbate the condition. In darkly pigmented individuals, postinflammatory hyperpigmentation may take many months to fade.
- Camouflage cosmetics may be helpful.

Notalgia Paraesthetica

- Management of notalgia paresthetica can be challenging. A low-cost therapy is treatment with topical capsaicin (topical extract of red pepper). Capsaicin depletes substance P in the cutaneous nerve endings, sometimes resulting in relief of the itch. Patients must be cautioned that the skin will burn and feel worse before it feels better. Patients must also be cautioned to wash their hands carefully after applying capsaicin.
- The understanding that the pathogenesis of the disease frequently involves impingement of the posterior rami of spinal nerves T2-T6 provides the rationale for therapies typically used for peripheral neuropathies (e.g., gabapentin or nerve blocks).

Therapy

Postinflammatory Hyperpigmentation

Sun-protection measures and education as described above

A variety of topical agents are available; these tend to work best on epidermal hyperpigmentation. Oftentimes, a combination of various treatments is needed to achieve a significant result. The following regimens can be tried:

- Hydroquinone 4% applied to lesions twice daily
- Hydroquinone 4% and tretinoin 0.025% applied to lesions twice daily
- Hydroquinone 4%, hydrocortisone 1%, and tretinoin 0.025% applied to lesions twice daily
- Higher concentrations of tretinoin (0.05%, 0.1%) and more potent steroid preparations (betamethasone) may also be used, as tolerated. Use only low-potency topical corticosteroids on the face.

Azelaic acid applied to lesions twice daily may also have a bleaching effect.

Alpha hydroxy acid peels, gentle cryotherapy, and microdermabrasion have all been used with variable results. Caution should be exercised with these modalities because overly aggressive treatment may lead to depigmentation and/or scarring.

Laser therapy for these lesions is in the investigational phase. The Nd:YAG laser may be tried but is not recommended for use in patients of color because treatment can lead to depigmentation.

Notalgia Paraesthetica

- Capsaicin 0.025% cream five times daily for 1 week followed by three times daily for 3 to 6 weeks—may require long-term continuation of therapy
- Transcutaneous electrical nerve stimulation
- Gabapentin 300 to 900 mg daily
- Botulinum toxin A
- Topical anesthetics such as lidocaine, pramoxine, or EMLA cream
- Paravertebral local anesthetic block

Suggested Readings

Bulengo-Ransby SM, Griffiths CE, Kimbrough-Green CK, et al. Topical tretinoin (retinoic acid) therapy for hyperpigmented lesions caused by inflammation of the skin in black patients. *N Engl J Med.* 1993;328(20):1438–1443.

Hexsel D, Arellano I, Rendon M. Ethnic considerations in the treatment of Hispanic and Latin-American patients with hyperpigmentation. *Br J Dermatol.* 2006;156(Suppl 1):7–12.

Inaloz HS, Kirtak N, Erguven HG, et al. Notalgia paresthetica with a significant increase in the number of intradermal nerves. *J Dermatol.* 2002;29(11):739–743.

Lacz NL, Vafaie J, Kihiczak NI, et al. Postinflammatory hyperpigmentation: a common but troubling condition. *Int J Dermatol.* 2004;43(5):362–365.

Loosemore MP, Bordeaux JS, Bernhard JD. Gabapentin treatment for notalgia paresthetica, a common isolated peripheral sensory neuropathy. *J Eur Acad Dermatol Venereol.* 2007;21(10):1440–1441.

Lynde CB, Kraft JN, Lynde CW. Topical treatments for melasma and postinflammatory hyperpigmentation. *Skin Therapy Lett.* 2006;11(9):1–6.

Raison-Peyron N, Meunier L, Acevedo M, et al. Notalgia paresthetica: clinical, physiopathological and therapeutic aspects. A study of 12 cases. *J Eur Acad Dermatol Venereol.* 1999;12(3):215–221.

Savk E, Savk O, Bolukbasi O, et al. Notalgia paresthetica: a study on pathogenesis. *Int J Dermatol.* 2000;39(10):754–759.

Savk E, Savk SO. On brachioradial pruritus and notalgia paresthetica. *J Am Acad Dermatol.* 2004;50(5):800–801.

Savk O, Savk E. Investigation of spinal pathology in notalgia paresthetica. *J Am Acad Dermatol.* 2005;52(6):1085–1087.

Stratigos AJ, Katsambas AD. Optimal management of recalcitrant disorders of hyperpigmentation in dark-skinned patients. *Am J Clin Dermatol.* 2004;5(3):161–168.

Weinfeld PK. Successful treatment of notalgia paresthetica with botulinum toxin type A. *Arch Dermatol.* 2007;143(8):980–982.

Weisshaar E, Fleischer AB, Bernhard JD. Pruritus and dysesthesia. In: Bolognia J, Jorizzo JL, Rapini RP, eds. *Dermatology.* 2nd Ed. St. Louis, MO: Mosby/Elsevier; 2008:100.

Yosipovitch G, Samuel LS. Neuropathic and psychogenic itch. *Dermatol Ther.* 2008;21(1):32–41.

Seborrheic Keratosis and Dermatosis Papulosa Nigra

Naurin Ahmad

■■ Diagnosis Synopsis

Seborrheic keratosis (SK) is a benign epidermal neoplasm with many variants and clinical presentations. African and Caribbean Americans commonly refer to SKs as moles or warts.

Patients may present with a few or hundreds of these raised, "stuck-on"-appearing papules and plaques with well-defined borders. Their etiology is unknown, although there is a familial trait for the development of multiple SKs with an autosomal dominant mode of inheritance. SKs are typically noninflammatory (unless traumatized) and usually arise slowly over time. They may be pruritic, and in these cases, the patient may scratch or rub the lesions, causing redness, bleeding, or secondary infection to develop.

Onset can occur in those as young as 25 years old. SKs tend to increase in incidence and number with increasing age and can exceed 100 in number in some people. SKs are one of the most common skin growths in populations aged 65 and older. SKs can be dark brown, irregular in shape, and raised, thus resembling a malignant melanoma. SKs tend to occur as tan lesions in whites; however, in darker skin, they will present as a darker melanoacanthotic variant.

Six subtypes of SK have been identified:

- Dermatosis papulosa nigra (DPN)
- Stucco keratosis
- Inverted follicular keratosis
- Large cell acanthoma
- Lichenoid keratosis
- Flat SK

In addition, six histologic types of SK have been classified: acanthotic, hyperkeratotic, reticulated, irritated, clonal, and melanoacanthoma.

Relatively rapid onset of numerous SKs can be a cutaneous sign of internal malignancy. Multiple eruptive SKs in association with a visceral cancer are referred to as the sign of Leser-Trélat. The most common associated malignancy is adenocarcinoma of the gastrointestinal tract. Closely monitor for any atypical changes, as several of the subtypes may act as cutaneous markers for internal malignancy.

One of the most common variants of SK is called DPN, which often arises in the neck, including the folds of the neck, and the face, including the cheeks, in patients with skin types III to VI. Lesions are benign epidermal growths similar to SKs. They are typically asymptomatic. DPN is considered to be a form of SK with a specific localization and affecting people of African and Asian descent.

DPN is common in individuals of African and Asian descent. It is less frequently described in the white population, where SKs are more common. A recent study in Senegal of 30 patients with DNP found a genetic predisposition in 93%.

According to one study among African Americans, more fair-complexioned participants (skin type V or less) had the lowest frequency of involvement. In addition to those with African heritage, the condition has also been reported in Filipinos, Vietnamese, Europeans, and Mexicans.

The onset of DPN is typically during adolescence, and women are affected more often than men. There may be a family history of similar lesions. It tends to have an earlier age of onset than that of SK. The number of lesions typically increases with age; up to one-third of African American adults have some of these lesions. Approximately 25% of patients with facial lesions will also have lesions at other body locations.

DPN is a cosmetic concern only. In contrast to SKs, multiple DPNs are not related to any systemic disease or syndrome.

◉ Look For

SKs may present as pink, skin-colored, or yellow-brown to brownish-black, waxy, "stuck-on"-appearing, round or oval papules and plaques (Figs. 4-161 and 4-162). Pigmentation may be variable within a single lesion. Scratching the surface usually shows a scaling, rough appearance. The surface may appear verrucous. Lesions are usually well circumscribed. They may occur on any body site, with the exception of the palms, soles, and mucous membranes.

They can range in size from 1 mm to several centimeters and have a wide range of pigment, from tan to black. They are typically flat, sharply demarcated areas of hyperpigmentation. Dermatoscopy and close exam will reveal horn cysts (small round collections of keratin).

The distribution is widespread and, if present on the trunk, may become aligned with the direction of skin folds and Langer lines.

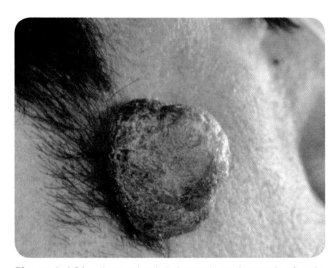

Figure 4-161 A large seborrheic keratosis on the temple of a Hispanic man.

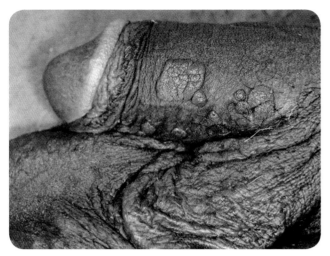

Figure 4-162 Seborrheic keratoses may occur on the shaft of the penis and may be confused with condylomata acuminate.

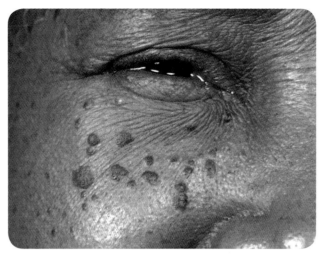

Figure 4-163 Elevated rough papules of dermatosis papulosa nigra with individual lesions resembling typical seborrheic keratoses.

DPNs are often considered a variant and are most often seen as dark brown, 1- to 3-mm, hyperkeratotic papules on the faces of African Americans. The papules are small, round, skin-colored or hyperpigmented, and they are typically located on the cheeks (Figs. 4-163–4-166). The lesions do not appear until adolescence and initially look like freckles. These pigmented papules are often distributed symmetrically across the malar eminences and forehead. Less often, lesions are on the neck, chest, and back.

DPNs become more numerous and larger with age. The papules usually appear during adolescence, gradually increasing in size and number over time and peaking in the sixth decade. As time passes, the lesions spread from just below the eyes to other parts of the face, the neck, and, rarely, the upper chest.

 ## Diagnostic Pearls

The growths have a coarse, waxy scale that can be removed to show a raw, moist base. Individual lesions grow rapidly and reach a static size without further growth. Close examination with a magnifying device such as a magnifying lens or an episcope can show the pluglike structure that is the gross manifestation of the microscopic horn cyst.

 ## Differential Diagnosis and Pitfalls

Differential diagnosis for SKs:
- Melanoma is always in the differential of pigmented solitary lesions and may go undetected, concealed between multiple SKs
- Lentigo maligna
- Warts
- Epidermodysplasia verruciformis
- Epidermal nevus

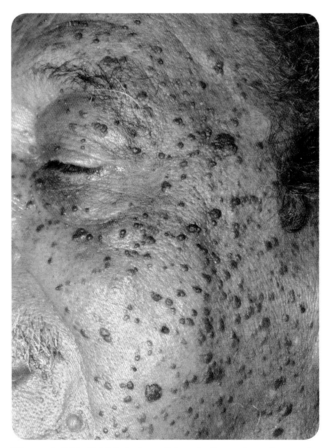

Figure 4-164 Multiple lesions of dermatosis papulosa nigra on the face, which is not a typical location for multiple seborrheic keratoses in an individual with lightly colored skin.

- Pigmented basal cell carcinoma
- Melanocytic nevus
- Bowen disease
- Bowenoid papulosis
- Stucco keratosis

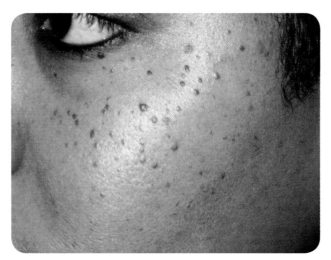

Figure 4-165 Dermatosis papulosa nigra can occur in African Americans with Fitzpatrick type II skin pigmentation.

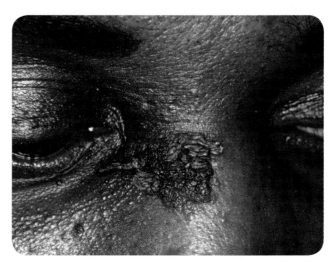

Figure 4-166 Lesions of dermatosis papulosa nigra may have confluent papules in a plaquelike configuration.

- Fibroepithelioma of Pinkus
- Acrokeratosis verruciformis of Hopf
- Cutaneous horn
- Arsenical keratosis
- Acrochordon
- Lentigo
- Nevus sebaceus
- Warts—filiform lesions
- Epidermal nevus
- Melanocytic nevus

The differential diagnosis of DPN primarily includes multiple SKs and acrochordons. Occasionally, melanocytic nevi, lentigines, verrucae, trichoepitheliomas, trichilemmomas, follicular hamartomas, syringomas, and angiofibromas might be considered clinically.

✓ Best Tests

- This diagnosis can usually be made clinically. If there is any concern for malignancy, however, the lesion must be biopsied and sent for histopathology.
- Also, multiple eruptive SKs should prompt a search for underlying internal malignancy, especially if patient history or review of systems is suspicious for cancer.

▲▲ Management Pearls

- Refer to a dermatologist for biopsy or removal of irritated lesions or for cosmetic removal. Patient reassurance regarding the chronic and benign nature of these lesions is key.
- In patients with multiple SKs, a suspicious pigmented lesion may be overlooked. If the diagnosis of SK is in doubt, biopsy of the lesion should be obtained to rule out more serious conditions such as melanoma.

Therapy

Seborrheic Keratosis
All methods of destruction of SKs in pigmented skin will cause hyper- or hypopigmentation. If it is an irritated SK (bleeding or painful), it can be removed by any of the methods below. If it is being removed for cosmetic reasons, the dermatologist and the patient must decide which dyspigmentation or scar will be the most acceptable to the patient.

Electrodesiccation and Curettage
One treatment modality is curettage and electrodesiccation; however, prior to electrotherapy, a topical anesthetic (e.g., lidocaine-prilocaine) should be applied for 1 to 1.5 hours. After electrodesiccation at a very low setting, the lesions should be kept dry for 24 hours. Darkly pigmented patients may still develop postprocedure hyperpigmentation of the skin if this is done too vigorously.

Cryotherapy
Cryotherapy with liquid nitrogen is the first-line therapy for very thick SKs and is also the most common modality, as it is affordable, effective, and quick to perform. However, be aware that melanocytes are very sensitive to temperature, and freezing will cause hypopigmentation, although cryotherapy may leave an area of dyspigmentation (hypo or hyper) and scarring.

Hypopigmentation after cryotherapy is especially seen in type IV and higher skin types if the lesion is frozen more than 25 seconds. If frozen 18 to 25 seconds, hyperpigmentation, which lasts 3 to 6 months, may develop.

Laser Therapy

There are reports that laser therapy may carry a lower risk of pigmentary changes or scarring compared with cryotherapy and electrodesiccation. Laser therapy (pulsed CO_2 and Er:YAG) have demonstrated some efficacy. *Note*: a correct assessment of skin type is necessary, and laser therapy for skin types greater than type III should be approached with caution.

Chemical Destruction

Chemical peels (e.g., trichloroacetic acid, glycolic acid, salicylic acid) have been used for removal of small and superficial SKs.

Excision

Shave excision can be used for larger lesions.

Dermatosis Papulosa Nigra

No treatment is necessary unless the patient requests it for cosmetic reasons. The use of cryotherapy, electrocautery, etc., may pose a risk of dyspigmentation.

For small lesions, snip excision with scissors, curettage, and light electrodesiccation are the most common treatment modalities.

There have been some successful case reports of treating DPNs in African American patients using a single treatment with a long-pulsed 1,064-nm Nd:YAG laser.

Electrodesiccation

Treat with electrodesiccation at a low setting after applying a topical anesthetic (e.g., lidocaine-prilocaine). Allow the desiccated crust to remain, and have the patient apply an ointment daily.

Cryotherapy

Before treating numerous lesions, test a few for postinflammatory hypopigmentation with very cautious use of liquid nitrogen. Freezing more than 25 seconds often causes hypopigmentation, lasting 6 to 12 months, and shorter freezing (15 to 25 seconds) may cause hyperpigmentation, lasting 3 to 6 months.

Suggested Readings

Dunwell P, Rose A. Study of the skin disease spectrum occurring in an Afro-Caribbean population. *Int J Dermatol.* 2003;42(4):287–289.

Grimes P, Arora S, Minus H, et al. Dermatosis papulosa nigra. *Cutis.* 1983;32:385–392.

Hafner C, Vogt T. Seborrheic keratosis. *J Dtsch Dermatol Ges.* 2008;6(8):664–677. (Article in English and German.)

Lupo MP. Dermatosis papulosis nigra: Treatment options. *J Drugs Dermatol.* 2007;6(1):29–30.

Niang SO, Kane A, Diallo M, et al. Dermatosis papulosa nigra in Dakar, Senegal. *Int J Dermatol.* 2007;46(Suppl 1):45–47.

Noiles K, Vender R. Are all seborrheic keratoses benign? Review of the typical lesion and its variants. *J Cutan Med Surg.* 2008;12(5):203–210.

Roberts W. Dermatologic problems of older women. *Dermatol Clin.* 2006;24(2):271–280, viii.

Schaffer JV, Bolognia JL. The clinical spectrum of pigmented lesions. *Clin Plast Surg.* 2000;27(3):391–408, viii.

Schwartz RA. Sign of Leser-Trélat. *J Am Acad Dermatol.* 1996;35(1):88–95.

Schweiger ES, Kwasniak L, Aires DJ. Treatment of dermatosis papulosa nigra with a 1064 nm Nd:YAG laser: Report of two cases. *J Cosmet Laser Ther.* 2008;10(2):12.

Vitiligo

Lynn McKinley-Grant

■■ Diagnosis Synopsis

Vitiligo is an acquired idiopathic type of leukoderma characterized by circumscribed depigmented macules or patches. The lesions are usually chalk-white in color and are surrounded by normal skin, creating well-demarcated margins. Vitiligo is usually asymptomatic, and lesions can range in size from millimeters to centimeters. While any part of the body can be affected, vitiligo often demonstrates distinct patterns including symmetric involvement of the face, upper chest, hands, ankles, axillae, groin, and around orifices (eyes, nose, mouth, urethra, and anus).

Vitiligo occurs in all ages. It occurs in all ethnicities and in both sexes in equal proportions. Despite a common misconception, vitiligo is *not* more common in African Americans; greater perceived prevalence stems from a bigger cosmetic problem in this population. The natural progression of the disease is unpredictable, ranging from insidious to rapid in onset. Years of stable, nonprogressive disease can be observed with the disease subsequently taking an unexpected rapid, exacerbated trajectory.

While the majority of vitiligo patients are otherwise healthy, an association with autoimmune thyroid dysfunction (hyperthyroidism or hypothyroidism) has been demonstrated. In new-onset vitiligo patients with systemic symptoms, thyroid screening with antithyroid peroxidase (TPO) antibody and a serum thyroid-stimulating hormone (TSH) is recommended. Additional endocrinopathy associations include diabetes mellitus, Addison disease, myasthenia gravis, and gonadal failure. It may exist as part of polyglandular autoimmune syndrome, particularly type III (Hashimoto thyroiditis, vitiligo or alopecia areata, and/or another organ-specific autoimmune disease).

Vitiligo is associated with ocular abnormalities including uveitis.

Variants of vitiligo include the following:

- Vitiligo with raised inflammatory borders—Margins of vitiligo lesions have a raised, erythematous border.
- Segmental vitiligo—vitiligo in a dermatomallike distribution
- Blue vitiligo—when vitiligo develops on a postinflammatory hyperpigmented lesion, giving a bluish tint
- Confetti-type vitiligo—multiple small, depigmented macules resembling confetti

While the etiology of vitiligo remains unclear, several theories exist. These can be divided into host attack on normal melanocytes versus intrinsic melanocyte defects. The "host attack" theories are centered on autoimmune destruction of melanocytes via autoantibodies or cytotoxic T lymphocytes. The "intrinsic defects" theories include decreased melanocyte survival due to deficiencies in cellular maintenance proteins, an intrinsic defect in TYRP1 processing in melanocytes, and an intracellular metabolic disorder in affected melanocytes that results in the accumulation of oxidized pteridines and subsequent cell death.

◉ Look For

Sharply demarcated, depigmented macules and/or patches (Figs. 4-167–4-170). There is no associated skin textural change, and erythema surrounding the lesions is rare. Hair may eventually turn white if the affected area is hair bearing. Look for an occasional associated halo nevus, a nevus surrounded by depigmented skin. Trichrome vitiligo, containing a band of intermediate color separating normal skin and the typical depigmented patch, is more common in individuals of African descent.

Vitiligo can be classified into three general schemes: localized, generalized, and universal. Localized forms may be segmental or focal, neither crossing the midline. Areas of predilection include the face, neck, and scalp, as well as areas of repeated trauma (bony prominences, dorsal hands, extensor forearm, fingers) and periorificial areas (around

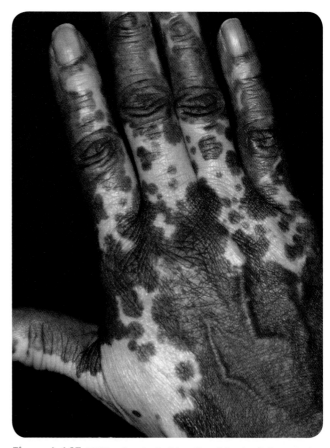

Figure 4-167 Vitiligo in a typical location. Islands of pigmentation within a white area are sometimes signs of repigmentation.

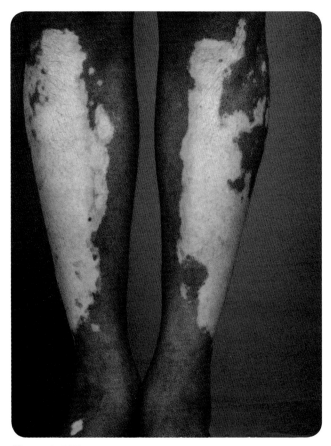

Figure 4-168 The lesions of vitiligo are frequently symmetrical.

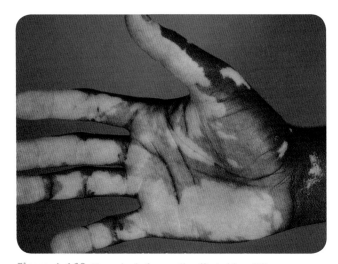

Figure 4-169 The palm is frequently affected by vitiligo.

the lips, genitals, eyes, etc.). Mucous membrane involvement is not uncommon in generalized cases. Generalized forms include vulgaris (widely distributed, scattered macules and patches) and acrofacial (distal extremities and face). In the universal form, nearly 100% of the body surface area is depigmented.

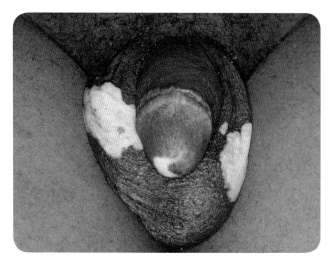

Figure 4-170 Genitals are frequently involved by vitiligo, and patients may be reluctant to discuss lesions in this location unless directly questioned.

Diagnostic Pearls

- Use a Wood lamp to demonstrate depigmentation as opposed to hypopigmentation, which will not be as pronounced under illumination. Under Wood lamp, vitiligo lesions give a yellow-green or blue fluorescence.
- In vitiligo, there is a notable absence of elevation, erythema, purpura, scale, or any textural changes to the skin.
- Some cases of vitiligo begin as halo nevi phenomenon.

?? Differential Diagnosis and Pitfalls

- Idiopathic guttate hypomelanosis—seen commonly in adults as very small polygonal depigmented macules often on the lower extremities. The lesions do not progress and are mainly of cosmetic concern to the patient (Fig. 4-171).
- Tinea versicolor—KOH positive; mild scale noted; often seen in the shoulders, upper trunk
- Pityriasis alba—typically affects the cheeks of atopic individuals; presents with hypopigmented, not depigmented, macules with ill-defined borders
- Discoid lupus erythematosus—presents with atrophy, telangiectasia, and follicular plugging, which are absent in vitiligo
- A history of prior trauma or skin inflammation can usually be elicited in cases of postinflammatory hypopigmentation. These lesions are not depigmented.
- Sarcoidosis—Look for indurated papules and plaques that are hypopigmented, not depigmented; visual changes and shortness of breath on review of systems; biopsy if needed
- Leprosy—Lesions are usually hypopigmented, not depigmented. Some can have an erythematous border. Lesions are anesthetic. The patient must have recently lived in an endemic area.

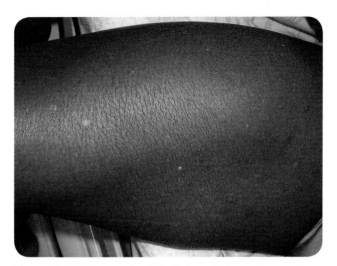

Figure 4-171 Very small white depigmented macules, usually on the extremities, that do not get larger are characteristic of idiopathic guttate hypomelanosis.

- Nevus depigmentosus—common on the trunk; usually present since birth
- Cutaneous T-cell lymphoma (mycosis fungoides)—can have an associated scale. Lesions are usually hypopigmented, not depigmented.
- Scleroderma—Look for sclerotic skin. Check ANA with nucleolar or speckled pattern, anticentromere, anti-Scl-70 antibody; associated with Raynaud phenomenon, arthralgias, mat telangiectases, and CREST.
- Albinism, piebaldism, and other genetic disorders—begin in infancy
- Morphea—Look for sclerotic plaques.
- Lichen sclerosus—Look for sclerotic plaques, often in the genital area; can be severely pruritic.
- Chemical leukoderma—Look for history of chemical use and/or topical corticosteroids.
- Onchocerciasis—Shins are common site of involvement. Suspect if the patient is coming from endemic area (Africa, Central and South America).

✓ Best Tests

Diagnosis can usually be made clinically, particularly when areas elsewhere on the body are affected. Skin biopsy specimens will reveal absence of melanocytes.

Consider the following tests to screen for autoimmune disorders:

- Antinuclear antibodies
- CBC with red blood cell indices
- Thyroid-stimulating hormone level
- Fasting blood glucose

▲▲ Management Pearls

- Take a detailed personal and family history of autoimmune disease, and consider a workup if the review of systems is suggestive.
- Sun avoidance and use of sunscreens are recommended so as not to enhance the contrast between pigmented and nonpigmented areas.
- Spontaneous repigmentation occurs in a few patients but is usually incomplete.
- Check TSH and anti-TPO antibody to screen for thyroid involvement if symptoms are suggestive.

Therapy

The goals of treatment include halting progression of disease and inducing repigmentation. There are many treatment options.

Steroid Therapy
Systemic steroids have been anecdotally reported to be efficacious in rapidly progressive vitiligo. A relatively short course may be useful in the setting of rapidly progressive vitiligo.

Oral Corticosteroids
Prednisone—Dosage and schedule guidelines have not been established. Consider a conservative dose (20 to 40 mg once daily), tapered over 2 weeks.

Topical Corticosteroids
Midpotency Topical Corticosteroids (Class 3–4)

- Triamcinolone cream, ointment—Apply twice daily (15, 30, 60, 120, 240 g).
- Mometasone cream, ointment—Apply twice daily (15, 45 g).
- Fluocinolone cream, ointment—Apply twice daily (15, 30, 60 g).

Low-potency Topical Steroids (Class 6–7)

- Desonide cream, ointment—Apply twice daily (15, 60, 90 g).
- Alclometasone cream, ointment—Apply twice daily (15, 45, 60 g).

Intralesional corticosteroids (triamcinolone acetonide 10 mg/mL) can also be tried for the most recalcitrant lesions. However, its use remains controversial due to risk of skin atrophy and the pain associated with injection.

Phototherapy

- Systemic phototherapy has demonstrated satisfactory repigmentation in a large percentage of patients with early disease.
- The favored regimen is narrow-band UVB phototherapy. An emission spectrum of 310 to 315 nm and a maximum wavelength of 311 nm are used. Use two to three times weekly. This treatment can be used in children, pregnant women, and lactating women.
- Photochemotherapy with 8-methoxypsoralen and UVA (PUVA) may be used, with systemic PUVA reserved for generalized cases. If no response to therapy is seen in 3 to 4 months, PUVA should be discontinued and tried again in 6 or 8 months. Narrow-band UVB may also be tried twice weekly for a maximum of 1 year.

Topical Calcipotriene

Can be used in combination with phototherapy or topical corticosteroids. Apply after phototherapy to affected areas twice daily; apply thin film, avoiding eyes and lips.

Laser Therapy

The 308-nm excimer laser and monochromatic excimer light treatments (twice weekly for 6 months) are newer treatment modalities with some promising results.

Immunomodulators

- Tacrolimus ointment 0.03% or 0.1%—Apply to the affected area twice daily; can continue for 1 week after lesions repigment.
- Pimecrolimus 1% cream—Apply to affected area twice daily.
- Note that immunomodulators are often preferable to topical corticosteroids in the periocular and genital area. Topical tacrolimus has been used in combination with the 308-nm excimer laser as well.

Depigmentation Therapy

For very extensive lesions in deeply pigmented patients, depigmentation of the normal skin with 20% monobenzyl ether of hydroquinone (applied twice daily for 9 to 12 months) is an option. This is not to be undertaken lightly, as it is permanent and easy sunburning is a consequence.

Surgical Therapy

- Superficial autologous skin grafts (split-thickness and suction blister epidermal grafting) have successfully been used, especially in recalcitrant locations (e.g., over joints).
- For patients with facial areas and other visible areas, cosmetic tattooing or Dermablend, a cosmetic cover-up makeup, may be used.

Suggested Readings

Dell'Anna ML, Mastrofrancesco A, Sala R, et al. Antioxidants and narrow band-UVB in the treatment of vitiligo: a double-blind placebo controlled trial. *Clin Exp Dermatol.* 2007;32(6):631–636.

Lee TH, Lerner AB, Halberg RJ. Water soluble vitamins in normal human skin. *J Invest Dermatol.* 1953;20(1):19–26.

Ortonne JP. Vitiligo and other disorders of hypopigmentation. In: Bolognia J, Jorizzo JL, Rapini RP, eds. *Dermatology.* 2nd Ed. St. Louis, MO: Mosby/Elsevier; 2008:913–920.

Silverberg JI, Silverberg AI, Malka E, et al. A pilot study assessing the role of 25 hydroxy vitamin D levels in patients with vitiligo vulgaris. *J Am Acad Dermatol.* 2010;62(6):937–941.

Silverberg NB, Lin P, Travis L, et al. Tacrolimus ointment promotes repigmentation of vitiligo in children: a review of 57 cases. *J Am Acad Dermatol.* 2004;51(5):760–766.

Souza Leite RM, Craveiro Leite AA. Two therapeutic challenges: periocular and genital vitiligo in children successfully treated with pimecrolimus cream. *Int J Dermatol.* 2007;46(9):986–989.

Whitton ME, Ashcroft DM, Barrett CW, et al. Interventions for vitiligo. *Cochrane Database Syst Rev.* 2006;(1):CD003263.

Physical Abuse

Chris G. Adigun

■■ Diagnosis Synopsis

Physical abuse affecting children, domestic partners, and the elderly is a serious public health problem. Cutaneous injury frequently represents the most recognizable form of physical abuse. There are key elements to the clinical exam that aid in correctly distinguishing physical signs of intentional injury or neglect from skin conditions that mimic maltreatment.

Physical and sexual abuse may occur at any age.

The skin is the most commonly injured organ system in the context of physical abuse. Abrasions and bruises are the most common signs of abuse in all ages. Scratches and bites are less common. Burns, hematomas, edema, and marks from physical implements are also less common but should not be missed. The latter are typically recognized by the characteristic patterns of injury left behind after the insult. Blisters and erosions are not uncommon on the genitals and buttocks (Figs. 4-172 and 4-173).

It is often challenging to differentiate findings attributable to physical abuse from those of other benign skin conditions. One hallmark of physical abuse is the presence of numerous bruises in multiple stages of healing. Healing stages are differentiated based on color changes. However, in darkly pigmented skin, healing stages of bruising may be more difficult to discern, as details in color changes are less apparent. This poses a potential problem, as abuse may be missed if cutaneous manifestations are not detected.

In addition, certain benign skin conditions may mimic signs of abuse in darkly pigmented skin, especially those conditions that occur almost exclusively in more deeply pigmented individuals. Certain skin conditions that predominate in ethnic skin, such as blue-gray spots (dermal melanosis), formerly known as Mongolian spots, are commonly misinterpreted as bruises from child abuse. Furthermore, pigmentation abnormalities from inflammatory conditions may also be tricky for the clinician to evaluate.

An astute clinician who detects the signs of sexual abuse, physical abuse, or neglect in a patient has the potential to save lives of children, adults, and the elderly.

◉ Look For

There may be scars, hyperpigmented patches, and bruises in different stages of development. Bruises age in characteristic color: initially red-blue, then purple at 3 to 5 days, then green at about a week, and finally yellow at 8 to 12 days. Detecting the evolution of color change of bruises may be a challenge in more deeply pigmented skin, but on close inspection, it can be achieved. Evidence of previous injury via scratching, whipping, or even bruising may be indicated by hyperpigmented patches in skin of darker pigmentation.

Bruises

Look for ecchymoses in areas that are typically protected, such as the buttocks, back, trunk, genitalia, inner thighs, cheeks, ears, neck, or philtrum, as these areas are much less likely to incur bruises by accident. Bruises that occur over bony prominences are significantly less likely to occur secondary to physical abuse. Characteristics of bruising that increase the likelihood of abuse include the following:

- Multiple bruises in clusters
- Bruises in a defined pattern or at different stages of healing
- Bruises in a child aged younger than 9 months who is not independently mobile
- Bruising away from bony prominences
- Cutaneous and physical injuries other than bruises

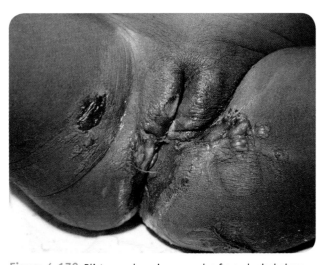

Figure 4-172 Blisters and erosions on vulva from physical abuse.

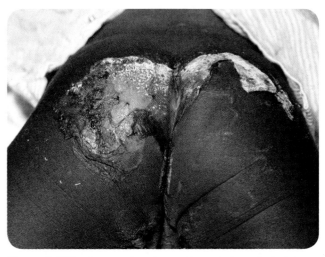

Figure 4-173 Blisters and erosions on buttocks from physical abuse.

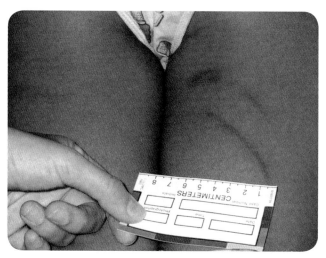

Figure 4-174 Linear bruise from a metal-containing belt.

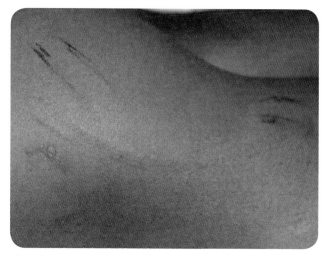

Figure 4-175 Linear purpura from abuse with an extension cord.

Look for geometric patterns, such as from belt buckles, loops from electric cords, the imprint of the hand, ropes, or linear marks from sticks or rods (Figs. 4-174 and 4-175). For example, slapping produces a negative imprint when capillaries break between the fingers, causing petechial bruising as blood is pushed away from the point of impact, leaving an outline of the hand. These are difficult to incur through normal childhood activities and are, therefore, suggestive of abuse. A blow to the ear can result in "cauliflower ear" secondary to a subperichondrial hematoma, which may be associated with retinal hemorrhage and even cerebral edema.

Burns

Cigarette burns classically present as punched-out ulcerations of about 8 to 10 mm with hemorrhagic crust and a nonexpanding dry base with multiple-layer involvement of the skin leading to rolled-appearing edges. Cigarette burns are typically full-thickness, third-degree, painless burns with slow healing and eventual scar formation. Patients may have multiple new and old lesions. In pigmented skin, perfectly round, hyperpigmented macules clustered with newer lesions may be suspicious.

Hot water immersion injuries predominate in children and are typically symmetrical and have sharp lines or drops from splashes, referred to as the "zebra stripe sign." Characteristic sparing of the body areas that come in contact with the cooler bath tub surface is called the "doughnut sign." Any burns in protected areas, such as the buttocks, perineum, head, or back should be investigated further. Diapers provide good protection against full-thickness scald injury, and it is unlikely that severe buttock burns would result from nonintentional immersion in hot water. In both adults and children, symmetrically distributed burn injuries are very suspicious of abuse.

Head and skeletal injuries should raise the question of abuse and are discussed online on VisualDx. (If you are a first-time online user, go to www.essentialdermatology.com/

pigmented; if you already have your password set up, go directly to www.visualdx.com/visualdx.)

Cultural Practices

It is important to note that cultural practices such as cupping and coining lead to ecchymosis formation in distinctive patterns that can mimic physical abuse. Proper evaluation is necessary because the use of cultural practices does not exclude the potential for physical abuse. Cultural practices are discussed in greater detail online on VisualDx.

Neglect

Physical signs include the following:

- Marked subcutaneous wasting
- Severe dermatitis (often diaper dermatitis)
- Scaling and xerosis of the skin due to chronic avitaminosis
- Extensive dental caries
- Poorly treated wounds
- Poor hygiene often with associated pediculosis capitis
- Areas of alopecia that may be associated with traumatic alopecia or severe nutritional deficits
- Multiple untreated injuries
- Inappropriate medications or failure to monitor medications (especially in elderly)
- Presence of preventable infectious diseases (especially in children, as neglected children are often not immunized)

Sexual Abuse

Sexual abuse should be suspected when the physical signs suggest an external etiology of the lesions, especially from blunt trauma. However, signs may be more subtle, and simply the presence of a sexually transmitted infection may be the only symptom. A positive test for *Chlamydia trachomatis*, gonorrhea, *Trichomonas vaginalis*, HIV, syphilis, or herpes simplex virus (HSV), especially in children or the elderly, is highly suspicious for sexual abuse. Sexual abuse in a domestic context is associated with recurrent urinary tract infections, irregular menstrual cycles, and pelvic pain independent of menses in women.

 ## Diagnostic Pearls

- Investigate injuries with minimal or no explanation or unlikely mechanism. A changing history elicited should also be considered suspicious.
- In the context of sexual abuse, if condyloma is detected in a child older than 2 years, perinatal transmission of human papillomavirus (HPV) infection should not be considered the cause, and further investigation is warranted.

?? Differential Diagnosis and Pitfalls

- Dermatologic mimics of bruising and blistering and fractures from genetic diseases must be considered; they are extensive and are detailed online on VisualDx.
- In darkly pigmented skin, previously treated skin disorders or resolved skin disorders may manifest with postinflammatory hyperpigmentation, usually with hyperpigmented macules or patches. These hyperpigmented areas may have bizarre shapes and be located in protected areas, such as the trunk, buttocks, and thighs. This can be disconcerting to the practitioner, who may be concerned that previously treated plaques of psoriasis or atopic dermatitis in private areas are actually manifestations of physical abuse. In this context, a detailed history should aid in the correct diagnosis.

 ## Best Tests

- The evaluation of a victim suffering from possible abuse should begin with a complete history, physical exam, and observation of the caregivers/domestic partner with the victim.
- If child abuse is suspected, a protocol is recommended for a proper evaluation. A complete skeletal survey should be done in all children aged 2 years and younger when abuse is suspected, children aged 12 months and younger who have a fracture, or any child with multiple or severe fractures. Anterior-posterior and lateral views should be obtained on any area of concern. A CT scan of the head should be obtained if head injury is suspected.

 ## Management Pearls

- Given the legal implications of abuse, it is absolutely critical to document correctly and thoroughly. This frequently involves photographing and documenting all injuries, using rulers in photographs where appropriate. Legalities differ greatly in cases involving children and the elderly versus cases of spousal, or domestic, abuse. In these cases, even a suspicion for abuse (including neglect) warrants referral to an expert medical provider in child/elder abuse. This also includes immediate reporting to appropriate authorities to safeguard the child/elder from further injury.

- To report suspected child abuse, the clinician should contact his/her state or local Child Protective Services (CPS) agency. The national number, 1-800-4-A-CHILD, is available to help locate regional departments. If unsure whether to report, consultation with other health care professionals or CPS is recommended to help determine if the incident is reportable. It is important to remember that the duty to report requires only a reasonable suspicion that abuse has occurred and not certainty.

- Reporting of domestic abuse depends on the state in which the abuse occurs. Consulting local legal experts can aid in the decision making in this circumstance. This situation may be especially frustrating, as safeguarding victims of domestic violence is considerably more difficult than safeguarding children and elders. Many hospitals have programs in place to assist this victim population once they make it to a health care facility.

- Depending on the circumstance, admitting the victim to the hospital may be reasonable if the victim is not able to return to a safe location.

Therapy

The victim's injuries should be treated accordingly. In the case of child abuse, it is reasonable to involve a team of experts from different fields that may include ophthalmology, neurology, and pediatric radiology, and consider referral to a specialized pediatric center.

Seek out resources that are likely in place, either in the hospital or community, to aid in the further protection of victims of domestic abuse. Suggest these resources to victims, and get them in contact with these professionals as soon as possible after the medical needs have been addressed.

Suggested Readings

Halder RM, Nootheti PK. Ethnic skin disorders overview. *J Am Acad Dermatol.* 2003;48(6 Suppl):S143–S148.

Halphen JM, Varas GM, Sadowsky JM. Recognizing and reporting elder abuse and neglect. *Geriatrics.* 2009;64(7):13–18.

Kos L, Shwayder T. Cutaneous manifestations of child abuse. *Pediatr Dermatol.* 2006;23(4):311–320.

Mark H, Bitzker K, Klapp BF, et al. Gynaecological symptoms associated with physical and sexual violence. *J Psychosom Obstet Gynaecol.* 2008;29(3):164–172.

Swerdlin A, Berkowitz C, Craft N. Cutaneous signs of child abuse. *J Am Acad Dermatol.* 2007;57(3):371–392.

Wiglesworth A, Austin R, Corona M, et al. Bruising as a marker of physical elder abuse. *J Am Geriatr Soc.* 2009;57(7):1191–1196. Epub 2009 Jun 3.

Stasis Dermatitis, Stasis Ulcer (Venous Ulcer), and Capillaritis

Tess Nasabzadeh

▪▪ Diagnosis Synopsis

Stasis dermatitis, commonly referred to as venous dermatitis, venous eczema, varicose eczema, stasis eczema, or gravitational eczema, is an inflammatory skin condition of the lower legs resulting from venous hypertension. Stasis dermatitis resides along the continuum of cutaneous disease related to lower extremity venous hypertension. This spectrum of disease is clinically graded on a scale from C0 to C6 according to the clinical, etiologic, anatomic, and pathophysiologic (CEAP) framework. It includes telangiectases (C1), varicose veins (C2), edema (C3), hyperpigmentation and stasis dermatitis (C4a), lipodermatosclerosis and atrophie blanche (C4b), and, in the most severe cases, healed or active venous ulcers (also known as stasis ulcers) (C5 and C6).

Lower extremity venous hypertension is caused by valve dysfunction, outflow obstruction, muscle pump failure, or congenital venous disease. In the presence of high venous pressure, leukocytes accumulate in the dermis and produce inflammatory cytokines and metalloproteinases that cause tissue destruction and fibrosis. In addition, high levels of vascular endothelial growth factor (VEGF) lead to capillary proliferation and elongation, while extravasation of red blood cells with hemosiderin accumulation within macrophages and melanin deposition leads to the hyperpigmentation of capillaritis. Stasis dermatitis is often closely linked to irritant contact dermatitis from venous ulcer fluid abutting intact skin and to allergic contact dermatitis from sensitization to topical medications.

The incidence of stasis dermatitis and other manifestations of lower extremity venous hypertension increases with age. Upward of 20% of nursing home patients are affected by stasis dermatitis, and 1% of the general population has a healed or active venous leg ulcer. Risk factors include female sex, obesity, congestive heart failure, pregnancy, pelvic tumor, family history, and an occupation that involves standing. Racial/ethnic differences have been found, with varicose veins being most prevalent in Hispanics and least prevalent in Asians. Rates of edema, hyperpigmentation, lipodermatosclerosis, and venous ulcers are highest among non-Hispanic whites and lowest among African Americans.

Patients may present with symptoms of lower extremity venous hypertension such as achy, throbbing, or tired legs; burning or pruritus; and nocturnal leg cramps. Symptoms improve with exercise and leg elevation.

◉ Look For

Stasis dermatitis is characterized by erythematous, scaly plaques (Figs. 4-176 and 4-177). The plaques are diffusely located on the distal aspect of both legs and are ill defined. They may be warm and tender to touch. There is often exudation of serum causing weepy crusts. Generalized autosen-

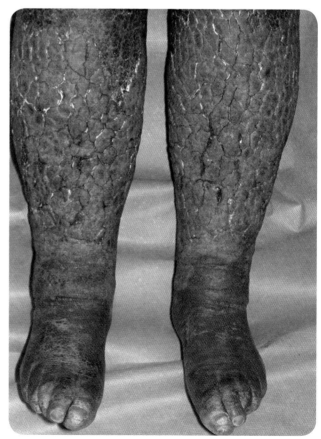

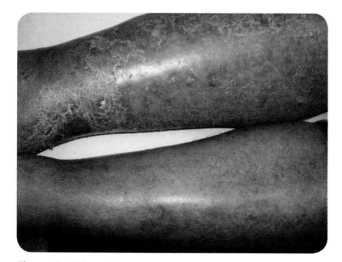

Figure 4-176 Erythema, scaling, and edema in stasis dermatitis.

Figure 4-177 Edema, scale, extensive crust, and retention keratosis in bilateral stasis dermatitis.

sitization dermatitis with a pruritic vesicular eruption on the palms, extremities, or trunk may occur with associated intense local inflammation.

Venous ulcers typically begin above the medial malleoli and may extend to become circumferential (Figs. 4-178– 4-181). They are rarely above the midcalf or on the feet. They have irregular sloping edges and a central region composed of thick yellow fibrinous and bright red granulation tissue. Venous ulcers have significant drainage; drainage that is malodorous and purulent signifies infection.

Dilated blood vessels are commonly seen in patients with lower extremity venous hypertension. Telangiectases are <1 mm in diameter, nonpalpable, and red or purple in color. Telangiectases cluster around the medial ankle and may converge toward a reticular vein. Phlebectasias are <2 mm in diameter, palpable, and red or purple in color. They tend to bleed with minor trauma. Reticular veins are <4 mm in diameter,

nonpalpable, and blue or green in color. Varicose veins are often located on the back of the calf or medial aspect of the leg. They are of variable diameter and color, tortuous, and palpable.

Diagnostic Pearls

- Venous disease must be demonstrated before attributing a patient's signs and symptoms to a manifestation of elevated lower extremity venous pressure.
- It is important to discern the etiology of the lower extremity venous hypertension. Ask about family history; occupation; coexisting arterial or lymphatic disease; hypercoagulability; history of trauma such as leg fracture, malignancy, cardiac or liver disease; and medications that cause peripheral edema such as calcium channel blockers.

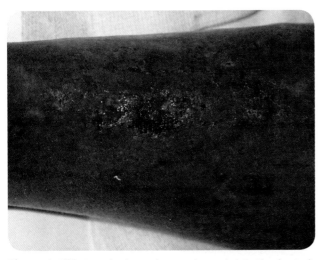

Figure 4-178 Irregular hyperpigmentation and ulceration in stasis dermatitis.

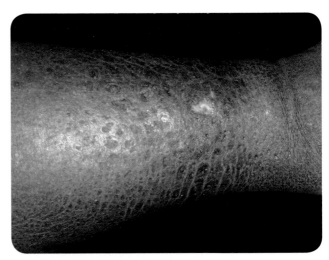

Figure 4-180 Stasis dermatitis with ichthyosis-like scaling and a clean ulceration.

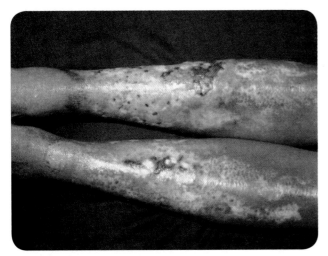

Figure 4-179 Stasis dermatitis with multiple irregular ulcerations.

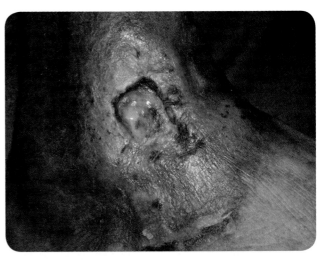

Figure 4-181 Ulceration with yellow crust and surrounding erythema and hyperpigmentation.

?? Differential Diagnosis and Pitfalls

Stasis Dermatitis

- Cellulitis is differentiated from stasis dermatitis by its unilateral location, well-demarcated borders, lymphatic streaking, lack of itchiness and scale, more rapid onset, and presence of fever, lymphadenopathy, or leukocytosis.
- Additional dermatologic findings in a patient with lower extremity venous hypertension are edema, capillaritis, lipodermatosclerosis, and atrophie blanche.
- Edema begins at the ankles and may extend to—but not above—the knee.
- Capillaritis appears as red, yellow, or dusky brown purpuric macules and patches on the distal lower legs.
- Lipodermatosclerosis consists of dermal and subcutaneous induration and fibrosis with atrophy of hair follicles and sweat glands. The skin in patients with lipodermatosclerosis may actually look "hard," and the leg may bear semblance to an "inverted champagne bottle."
- Progressive fibrosis leads to atrophie blanche, marked by areas of white scarring.
- Allergic contact dermatitis often presents in association with stasis dermatitis and venous ulcers; allergy testing with an open patch test, a use test, or a closed patch test on the legs results in itching and erythema.
- Irritant contact dermatitis often presents in association with stasis dermatitis and venous ulcers.
- Tinea corporis or pedis—KOH preparation demonstrates septate hyphae.
- Asteatotic dermatitis
- Lichen simplex chronicus
- Nummular eczema
- Psoriasis
- Necrobiosis lipoidica
- Pretibial myxedema
- Cutaneous T-cell lymphoma

Venous Ulcer

- Pyoderma gangrenosum
- Arterial ulcer—located on the toes or lateral aspect of the lower leg and having a "punched-out" appearance; the patient may complain of claudication and have decreased peripheral pulses and skin that is cool, shiny, and hairless
- Neuropathic ulcer—located on pressure points of the foot and surrounded by a ring of hyperkeratosis
- Ulcers from vasculitis

Edema

- Lymphedema—characterized by edema that begins on the toes and dorsal foot and extends to the entire leg; textural skin changes are hypertrophic, such as verrucous papules (rather than sclerotic and atrophic)

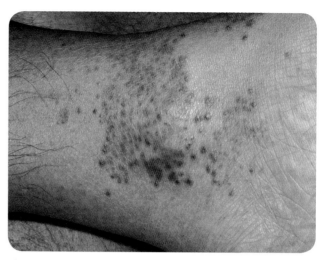

Figure 4-182 Multiple deep red and brownish papules and macules on the ankle, a typical location for a pigmented purpura.

Capillaritis

- Pigmented purpuric dermatoses (Schamberg disease, Majocchi disease, Gougerot-Blum disease, lichen aureus)—often found on the lower legs and may be associated with venous hypertension (Fig. 4-182). These diseases often itch and their pigmentary changes are persistent, but they do not progress to ulceration.
- Vasculitis

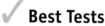

✓ Best Tests

Doppler auscultation is a sensitive screening tool for detecting the presence of retrograde venous blood flow. Noninvasive tests that provide further anatomic and quantitative information include duplex ultrasound and photoplethysmography. Invasive tests that can distinguish between valvular reflux and obstruction and take detailed images of the vessels are contrast venography, MR angiogram, and CT angiogram.

Capillary microscopy in patients with chronic lower extremity venous hypertension demonstrates increased capillary convolution and decreased capillary density. These changes may be difficult to appreciate in darkly pigmented patients.

▲▲ Management Pearls

- The use of compression devices is central to the effective management of the dermatologic manifestations of lower extremity venous hypertension. Compression devices are designed so that the pressure is higher at the ankle and lower at the knee, thereby facilitating venous blood flow.

A number of different types of compression devices are available, such as stockings (Jobst, Juzo, Sigvaris, Truform), inelastic bandages (CircAid, Comprilan), elastic bandages (Setopress, SurePress), and pneumatic pumps. In general, the pressure of the compression device should be prescribed according to the severity of venous disease. With regard to compression stockings, class I (20 to 30 mm Hg at ankle) stockings are sufficient to control edema, while class II (30 to 40 mm Hg at ankle) or class III (>40 mm Hg at ankle) stockings are needed to manage stasis dermatitis and venous ulcers.

- Noncompliance with prescribed use of compression devices is a significant problem and the primary reason for treatment failure. Patient participation in the selection of the compression device may improve compliance.
- Before instituting compression therapy, rule out arterial insufficiency with Doppler studies or an ankle brachial index (ABI). Also, inform patients to remove the compression device and call their physician if they experience numbness, tingling, pain, or dusky toes.
- Additional ways a patient can help fight the effects of lower extremity venous hypertension include walking, weight loss, smoking cessation, eating a well-balanced diet, lower leg exercises, leg elevation when sitting or lying, and avoiding prolonged standing and constrictive clothing.
- Referral to a vascular surgeon may be warranted for patients whose symptoms or cosmetic concerns persist following conservative treatment. However, patients with darkly pigmented skin should be informed that they are at a greater risk of experiencing postinflammatory hyperpigmentation (PIH) following sclerotherapy and surgical incisions.

Therapy

Stasis Dermatitis

Patients should use a daily moisturizer in order to help treat the dryness and scaling of stasis dermatitis. Using a moisturizer that contains an occlusive agent prevents water evaporation from the skin. Occlusives include petrolatum ointment, zinc oxide cream or paste, and dimethicone cream. It is important to avoid products that contain fragrances and preservatives, as these may cause an allergic contact dermatitis. In addition, patients may require intermittent treatment with topical corticosteroids during flares. Prolonged use of topical corticosteroids can result in cutaneous atrophy. Corticosteroid ointments aid in moisturizing the skin, while corticosteroid creams aid in drying out moist lesions. However, creams often contain more preservatives than ointments.

One suggested treatment regimen is as follows:

- Mild dermatitis: midpotency topical corticosteroid for 3 to 4 weeks
- Severe dermatitis: high-potency topical corticosteroid for 3 to 4 weeks
- Weeping dermatitis: high-potency topical corticosteroid and antiseptic and astringent such as potassium permanganate (1 in 10,000)
- Impetiginized dermatitis: high-potency topical corticosteroid, antiseptic and astringent such as potassium permanganate (1 in 10,000), and oral antibiotics with good *Staphylococcus* and *Streptococcus* coverage; examples include cephalexin, amoxicillin, and dicloxacillin

Venous Ulcers

To facilitate wound healing, necrotic tissue needs to be débrided by surgical, mechanical, or enzymatic methods. Persistently nonhealing ulcers may require excision and grafting. Recent evidence suggests that the peripheral vasodilator pentoxifylline at a dose of 1,200 mg p.o. daily may be a useful adjunct to compression in the treatment of venous ulcers due to its capacity to reduce plasma viscosity and inflammation. The ulcer should be dressed according to the amount of drainage the wound produces. For example:

- Venous ulcers with moderate to severe drainage: hydrofiber (Aquacel), alginate (Sorbsan, Tegagen, Kaltostat), or foam (Allevyn, Copa) dressing
- Venous ulcers with minimal drainage: hydrogel dressing (3 M Tegagel Hydrogel Wound Filler, Vigilon Primary Wound Dressing)

Capillaritis

The yellow-brown pigmentation of capillaritis can be difficult to treat. Success has been reported with noncoherent intense pulsed light therapy (IPL). While the use of light or laser therapy generally raises a concern regarding the risk of PIH in darkly pigmented patients, it has been suggested that IPL poses a lower risk of PIH for people of color and thus may be a viable treatment option.

Suggested Readings

Bergan JJ, Schmid-Schönbein GW, Coleridge Smith PD, et al. Mechanisms of disease: Chronic venous disease. *N Engl J Med.* 2006;355(5):488–500.

Calianno C, Holton SJ. Fighting the triple threat of lower extremity ulcers. *Nursing.* 2007;37(3):57–63.

Criqui MH, Denenberg JO, Bergan J, et al. Risk factors for chronic venous disease: The San Diego Population Study. *J Vasc Surg.* 2007;46(2):331–337.

Gosnell AL, Nedorost ST. Stasis dermatitis as a complication of amlodipine therapy. *J Drugs Dermatol.* 2009;8:135–137.

Grey JE, Enoch S, Harding KG. ABC of wound healing: Venous and arterial leg ulcers. *Br Med J.* 2006;332:347–350.

Hess CT. Identifying and managing venous dermatitis. *J Wound Care.* 2005;18(5):242–243.

Middleton H. Exploring the aetiology and management of venous eczema. *Br J Commun Nurs.* 2007;12(9):S16–S23.

Nguyen TH. Evaluation of venous insufficiency. *Semin Cutan Med Surg.* 2005;24:162–174.

Pimentel CL, Rodriguez-Salido MJ. Pigmentation due to stasis dermatitis treated successfully with a noncoherent intense pulsed light source. *Dermatol Surg.* 2008;34(7):950–951.

Raju S, Neglén P. Chronic venous insufficiency and varicose veins. *N Engl J Med.* 2009;360:2319–2327.

Cutis Marmorata

Alicia Ogram • Adam Tinklepaugh

◼◼ Diagnosis Synopsis

Cutis marmorata refers to the netlike violaceous pattern seen in newborns as a result of transient shifts in cutaneous blood flow. It occurs more frequently in premature infants and may persist to the fourth week of life. Trisomy 18, Down syndrome, Cornelia de Lange syndrome, and hypothyroidism have been associated with cutis marmorata that persists beyond early infancy. In Turkey, the incidence is approximately 10.6%.

◉ Look For

A symmetric, blanchable, reticular (netlike), violaceous pattern that preferentially affects the extremities over the trunk. The pattern is more exaggerated with cooling of the skin, and it lessens with warming.

●● Diagnostic Pearls

It may be associated with cold-induced acrocyanosis, which is a bluish discoloration secondary to peripheral vasoconstriction of hands and feet.

?? Differential Diagnosis and Pitfalls

Cutis marmorata telangiectatica congenita—asymmetric, well-localized, and often associated with cutaneous and/or underlying limb atrophy (Fig. 4-183).

✓ Best Tests

This is a clinical diagnosis. Lesions should be blanchable and improve on warming of the infant.

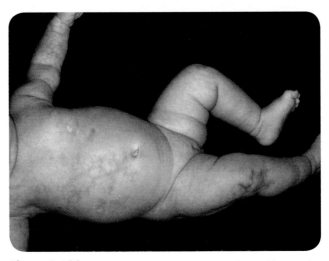

Figure 4-183 Cutis marmorata on abdomen and atrophic vascular lesion consistent with cutis marmorata telangiectatica congenita on leg.

▲▲ Management Pearls

Consider an evaluation for systemic disease (hypothyroidism) in infants with cutis marmorata that does not respond to rewarming or that lasts beyond 6 months of age.

Therapy

Maintain a warm environment for the infant.

Suggested Reading

Ferahbas A, Utas S, Akcakus M, et al. Prevalence of cutaneous findings in hospitalized neonates: A prospective observational study. *Pediatr Dermatol.* 2009;26(2):139–142.

Vascular Malformations

Alicia Ogram • Adam Tinklepaugh

There are a variety of vascular malformations that appear very similar. The more common arteriovenous malformations (AVMs), infantile hemangioma (IH), Kasabach-Merritt syndrome (KMS), and Sturge-Weber syndrome are discussed in detail in this chapter. Discussions of cutis marmorata telangiectatica congenita, diffuse neonatal hemangiomatosis, and Klippel-Trenaunay syndrome are available on VisualDx online. (If you are a first-time online user, go to www.essentialdermatology.com/pigmented; if you already have your password set up, go directly to www.visualdx.com/visualdx.)

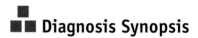 Diagnosis Synopsis

Arteriovenous Malformations

AVMs are vascular anomalies that typically occur in the head/neck area and are often present at birth (40%). They are considered fast-flow anomalies, compared to venous malformations, which are slow flow. AVMs may worsen over time, causing disfigurement through local bone and soft tissue overgrowth, pain, hemorrhage, and possibly death.

Infantile Hemangioma

IHs are the most common tumor of childhood. They occur in up to 10% of infants. In Turkey, they represent approximately 86% of all vascular lesions. Hemangiomas are usually solitary (focal), involving the head and neck region, but they may also be segmental or disseminated. Female sex, light skin, history of chorionic villus sampling, prematurity, placenta previa, and preeclampsia are the risk factors for the development of hemangiomas. Segmental lesions occur more commonly among Hispanic infants, particularly on mucosal surfaces. Associated complications, abnormalities, and PHACES syndrome (posterior fossa malformations, hemangiomas, arterial anomalies, coarctation of the aorta and other cardiac defects, eye abnormalities, sternal defects, and supraumbilical raphe) are more common among Hispanic infants.

Kasabach-Merritt Syndrome

KMS is characterized by an enlarging vascular lesion, profound thrombocytopenia, consumptive coagulopathy, and often a microangiopathic hemolytic anemia. Affected infants typically present with a solitary cutaneous lesion either at birth or within the first year of life, though multiple cutaneous or visceral vascular tumors are also encountered in affected infants.

Sturge-Weber Syndrome

Sturge-Weber syndrome is a neurocutaneous disorder characterized by an extensive unilateral port-wine stain usually involving the cranial nerve V1 area, retinal detachment, and cerebral calcification as the result of leptomeningeal and choroidal angiomatosis. It is a congenital, noninherited condition of unknown cause with a sporadic inheritance pattern. The incidence is estimated at 1 in 50,000. Men and women are equally affected.

◉ Look For

Arteriovenous Malformations

Erythema, localized warmth, atypical segmental distribution, and localized infiltration typically in the cephalic area (Fig. 4-184).

Infantile Hemangioma

IHs are classified as superficial, deep, or mixed and focal, segmental, or indeterminate (Figs. 4-185 and 4-186). Superficial IHs are well-defined bright red lobulated or smooth papules or plaques. Deep IHs present as subcutaneous compressible bluish plaques or nodules with overlying telangiectases or surrounding venous networks. Mixed IHs have features of both superficial and deep components. Focal IHs are discrete papules, nodules, or plaques that appear to arise from a central focus. Segmental IHs are small or large plaques that affect an embryological or developmental

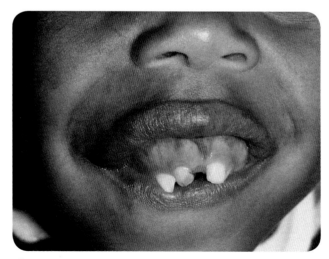

Figure 4-184 Arteriovenous malformation on the right side of the face with associated hypertrophy, including that of the jaw and gingivae.

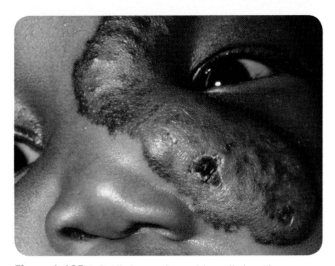

Figure 4-185 Infantile hemangioma with small ulceration.

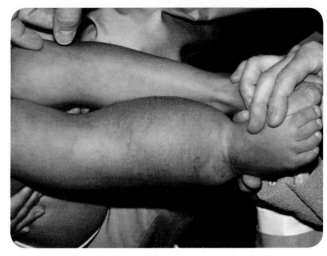

Figure 4-187 Kasabach-Merritt syndrome in a patient receiving prednisone and then Coban wrapping.

segment of the body. Segmental IHs often have many surface telangiectases and irregular, ill-defined borders. Indeterminate IHs are lesions that cannot be distinguished as segmental or focal.

Kasabach-Merritt Syndrome

The clinical phenotype varies depending on the underlying vascular lesion. Cutaneous kaposiform hemangioendothelioma (KHE) lesions are typically single, shiny, purple, indurated, tender, and poorly delineated plaques or nodules with a predilection for the trunk, extremities, and retroperitoneum. Cutaneous tufted angiomas (TAs) are commonly dusky red to violaceous indurated plaques or nodules, ranging from

2 to 5 cm in size, that may be tender. TAs are thought to arise most commonly on the head and neck, though they have also been noted on the abdomen, groin, and lower limbs (Fig. 4-187). TAs may also present as red to violaceous macules or papules.

Sturge-Weber Syndrome

The port-wine stain is commonly a pink to bright red macular area overlying the forehead, eyelids, and temple and is usually present at birth (Fig. 4-188). Though typically unilateral, it may involve both sides of the face. The stain varies from light pink to deep purple, and it darkens and thickens with age.

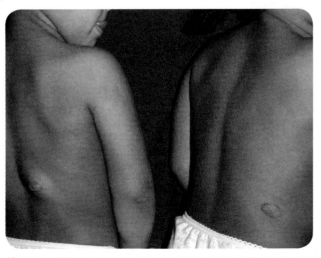

Figure 4-186 Identical twins with hemangiomas in different stages of regression.

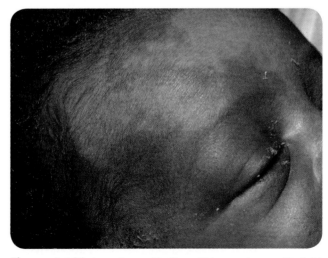

Figure 4-188 A newborn with Sturge-Weber syndrome with facial hemangioma in the distribution of the first branch of the trigeminal nerve.

Diagnostic Pearls

Arteriovenous Malformations

A vascular mass with tense draining veins, a thrill, and bruit are commonly found on auscultation.

Infantile Hemangioma

- Infants with multiple or segmental IHs are more likely to have extracutaneous hemangiomas. The liver is the most commonly affected site; however, any organ may be involved.
- Segmental hemangiomas are more likely associated with structural malformations. PHACES syndrome is characterized by the association of **P**osterior fossa malformation, **H**emangiomas, **A**rterial anomalies, **C**oarctation of the aorta and other cardiac defects, **E**ye abnormalities, **S**ternal defects, and **S**upraumbilical raphe. Sacral lesions can also have underlying spinal dysraphism.

Kasabach-Merritt Syndrome

Tender lesions often distinguish KHE and TA from non-ulcerated hemangiomas of infancy. KMS due to a visceral, particularly retroperitoneal, vascular tumor should be considered in infants presenting with unexplained thrombocytopenia and consumptive coagulopathy.

Sturge-Weber Syndrome

The port-wine stain is usually limited to a branch of the trigeminal nerve.

Differential Diagnosis and Pitfalls

These diseases have similar differential diagnoses.

- Hemangioma
- Physiologic cutis marmorata—less severe vascular pattern that occurs with cold
- Livedo reticularis—prominent vascular pattern related to underlying vasculitis
- Benign neonatal hemangiomatosis—cutaneous lesions with no visceral involvement
- Congenital hemangioma (CH)—fully formed vascular tumors at birth
- Port-wine stain—Early lesions of hemangioma may be confused with port-wine stains.
- TA and KHE—present as extensive brownish vascular plaques with deep fibrotic consistency
- Deep hemangiomas—present similar to venous malformations, which do not go through a phase of rapid proliferation
- KHE

- TA
- Hepatic hemangioma
- Klippel-Trenaunay syndrome
- Consumptive coagulopathy of other etiology
- Parkes Weber syndrome—may present with multiple A-V shunts that can be associated with high-output cardiac failure at birth
- Nevus of Ota

✓ Best Tests

Arteriovenous Malformations

Ultrasonographic (color Doppler) exam or MR with angiography may be necessary to define extent.

Infantile Hemangioma

MRI is the most useful technique to confirm the diagnosis and also to differentiate it from vascular malformations. Doppler studies are less useful than MR imaging. Skin biopsy is indicated only to exclude other vascular or soft tissue tumors.

Kasabach-Merritt Syndrome

CBC with platelets
Peripheral blood smear
Prothrombin time and activated partial thromboplastin time
Fibrinogen and D-dimer
Ultrasound of lesion
MRI of lesion

Sturge-Weber Syndrome

X-rays, MRI, and other neuroimaging modalities may be necessary to establish the location and extent of central nervous system and meningeal involvement. Ophthalmological evaluation and measurement of intraocular pressure are necessary. The diagnosis of a port-wine stain can often be made on clinical grounds.

Management Pearls

Arteriovenous Malformations

Multidisciplinary approach is necessary when multiple organs are involved.

Trauma may worsen condition.

Infantile Hemangioma

- Treat lesions that interfere with feeding, vision, cosmesis, or that obstruct the airways. Evaluate children with large, segmental, or multiple hemangiomas. Look for complications such as high-output failure, hypothyroidism, and visceral hemorrhage.

- Ulceration is common in the intertriginous areas, such as genitalia, perineum, and perianal region, and should be treated immediately.

Kasabach-Merritt Syndrome

- Prompt referral to a pediatric hematologist is recommended. If the underlying vascular tumor is amenable to surgical excision, a pediatric or vascular surgeon should be consulted.
- Management is two-pronged: obtaining/maintaining hemostasis and treating the underlying vascular lesion. Securing hemostasis is paramount and requires frequent monitoring throughout treatment. Platelet transfusions should be performed in actively bleeding patients.

Sturge-Weber Syndrome

A multidisciplinary team is necessary to coordinate the care of individuals with Sturge-Weber syndrome and often includes specialists of neurology, psychiatry/psychology, dermatology, plastic surgery, ophthalmology, and neurosurgery.

Therapy

Arteriovenous Malformations
Percutaneous sclerotherapy is the treatment of choice, particularly for small AVMs. Refer to online discussion for additional details.

Infantile Hemangioma
Most hemangiomas in children do not need treatment. Topical and intralesional steroids can be useful for localized lesions requiring treatment. For more intense therapies, see online discussion.

Kasabach-Merritt Syndrome
First- and second-line therapies can be found online.

Sturge-Weber Syndrome
Pulsed-dye laser (PDL) is the treatment of choice. It is important to begin PDL treatments early, before the local areas of hypertrophy develop. An intense pulsed light source and the potassium titanyl phosphate (KTP) laser have also been used with success.

Suggested Readings

Akyuz C, Yaris N, Kutluk MT, et al. Benign vascular tumors and vascular malformations in childhood: A retrospective analysis of 1127 cases. *Turkish J Pediatr.* 1997;39(4):435–445.

Chen WL, Ye JT, Xu LF, et al. A multidisciplinary approach to treating maxillofacial arteriovenous malformations in children. *Oral Surg Oral Med Oral Pathol Oral Radiol Endod.* 2009;108(1):41–47.

Chiller KG, Passaro D, Frieden IJ. Hemangiomas of infancy: Clinical characteristics, morphologic subtypes, and their relationship to race, ethnicity, and sex. *Arch Dermatol.* 2002;138(12):1567–1576..

Denoyelle F, Leboulanger N, Enjolras O, et al. Role of propranolol in the therapeutic strategy of infantile laryngotracheal hemangioma. *Int J Pediatr Otorhinolaryngol.* 2009;73(8):1168–1172.

Gottschling S, Schneider G, Meyer S, et al. Two infants with life-threatening diffuse neonatal hemangiomatosis treated with cyclophosphamide. *Pediatr Blood Cancer.* 2006;46(2):239–242.

Pandey A, Gangopadhyay AN, Gopal SC, et al. Twenty years' experience of steroids in infantile hemangioma—a developing country's perspective. *J Pediatr Surg.* 2009;44(4):688–694.

Sebai NE, Badri T, Rajhi H, et al. Experience of a multidisciplinary team in the management of superficial venous malformations: 99 cases [French]. *Tunisie Medicale.* 2009;87(4):283–284 [English Abstract. Journal Article].

Vlahovic A, Simic R, Djokic D, et al. Diffuse neonatal hemangiomatosis treatment with cyclophosphamide: A case report. *J Pediatr Hematol Oncol.* 2009;31(11):858–860.

Kaposi Sarcoma

Ivy Lee

◼◼ Diagnosis Synopsis

Kaposi sarcoma (KS) is a malignancy of vascular endothelial cells that occurs in several forms: classic KS, endemic KS, iatrogenically induced KS, and HIV-associated KS. All four types can be linked to coinfection with human herpesvirus type 8 (HHV-8), and the cutaneous lesions are morphologically and histologically indistinguishable among the types. KS may be a reactive process rather than a true neoplasm because it does not produce conventional metastases but spreads in a multifocal way.

Classic (traditional) KS is seen almost exclusively in people of Mediterranean and Ashkenazi Jewish descent, with age of onset typically between 50 and 70 years. Older literature describes classic KS as occurring more often in men, with a male-to-female ratio of approximately 12:1. However, more recent studies suggest that the gender gap may not be so significant. Classic KS most commonly runs an indolent course for 10 to 15 years or more with slow enlargement of tumors and the gradual development of additional lesions. After many years, asymptomatic systemic lesions can develop along the gastrointestinal tract, in lymph nodes, and in other organs. Up to one-third of the patients with classic KS develop a second primary malignancy, most frequently non-Hodgkin lymphoma.

Endemic KS is seen in equatorial black Africans, is unrelated to HIV infection, and is more aggressive in disease course. Areas of highest prevalence include Uganda, the Democratic Republic of Congo, and Zambia. There are two major forms: a benign nodular variant and a fulminant lymphadenopathic variant, typically seen in children. The male-to-female ratio is nearly equal among children but increases with age.

Iatrogenic KS is the result of long-term systemic immunosuppression and is common in transplant recipients, especially renal. It may resolve when immunosuppressive medications are discontinued. This variant is mostly limited to the skin with infrequent visceral involvement.

The AIDS- or HIV-associated epidemic form of KS is the most common neoplasm in HIV-seropositive patients, is an AIDS-defining illness, and traditionally has been associated with CD4 counts <500. Recent studies show that incidence of KS occurs independently of the degree of immunosuppression. This form of KS disproportionately affects men who have sex with men (MSM), African Americans (regardless of sexual orientation), and heterosexual black Africans. Patients with AIDS-associated KS often have multifocal cutaneous disease and concomitant widespread visceral KS, which places these patients at risk for hemorrhage from gastrointestinal lesions, cardiac tamponade, and pulmonary obstruction. The introduction of highly active antiretroviral therapy (HAART) has dramatically decreased the incidence, morbidity, and mortality of AIDS-associated KS.

◉ Look For

Deep red, brown, or purple macules, plaques, and nodules may develop anywhere on the skin. In darker skin types, the violaceous hue may be less conspicuous, and postinflammatory hyperpigmentation is common (Figs. 4-189 and 4-190). Koebnerization (lesions occurring in areas of trauma) occasionally takes place.

In classic KS, the disease is often limited to the lower extremities, especially the ankles and feet. Venous stasis and lymphedema of the involved lower extremity are frequently seen.

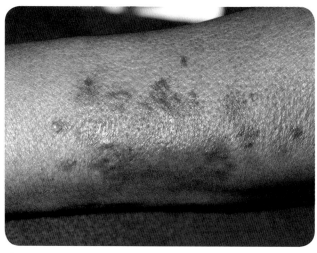

Figure 4-189 Purple plaque and papules in non–AIDS-associated Kaposi sarcoma.

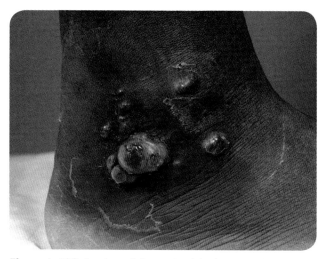

Figure 4-190 Papules and ulcerated nodules in non–AIDS-associated Kaposi sarcoma.

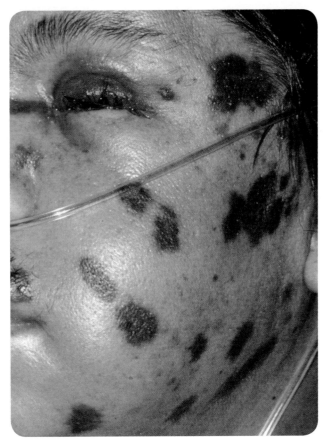

Figure 4-191 Multiple purple facial plaques from AIDS-associated Kaposi sarcoma.

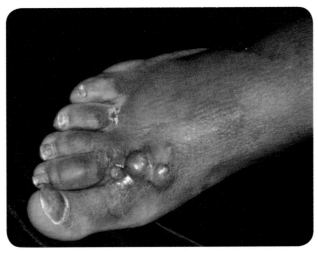

Figure 4-192 Foot nodules and papules of Kaposi sarcoma in a woman with AIDS.

AIDS-associated KS most commonly presents with violaceous nodules or plaques that may occur anywhere on the body with a predilection for the face, posterior neck, earlobes, nose, and oral cavity (hard palate) (Figs. 4-191 and 4-192). Often, lesions will have a linear morphology following skin tension lines. Acral lesions may become hyperkeratotic with psoriasiform scale or verrucous. Twenty percent of patients will have visceral involvement.

 Diagnostic Pearls

Classic Kaposi favors the lower extremities, while AIDS-associated KS lesions have multiple locations.

?? Differential Diagnosis and Pitfalls

- Cat-scratch fever (bacillary angiomatosis)
- Single lesions with rapid onset are consistent with a pyogenic granuloma.
- Dermatofibroma or dermatofibrosarcoma protuberans
- Hemangioma
- Angiokeratoma
- Lichen simplex chronicus
- Hypertrophic lichen planus
- Prurigo nodularis
- Metastatic carcinoma or melanoma
- Pigmented basal cell carcinoma
- Blue rubber bleb nevus syndrome
- Tufted angioma
- Cavernous hemangioma
- Arteriovenous malformation
- Lymphoma
- Angiosarcoma
- Sarcoidosis
- Early KS may resemble a large junctional nevus or port-wine stain.

✓ Best Tests

- Skin biopsy is diagnostic. Consider HIV testing if the patient's HIV status is unknown.
- Additional studies may be warranted to ascertain the extent of disease, including, but not limited to, CT scans, plain films, CBC, and fecal occult blood testing.

▲▲ Management Pearls

- The treatment of advanced KS often necessitates a multidisciplinary approach. Medical or radiation oncologists may be needed to administer systemic chemotherapy or radiation therapy, respectively.
- In elderly patients or those with multiple comorbidities and limited disease, the risks and benefits of pursuing aggressive treatment should be weighed carefully.
- Reduction or cessation of immunosuppressive medications in patients with iatrogenic KS may be all that is

necessary in the way of treatment. Attempt this first before moving on to other forms of therapy.

- In AIDS-associated KS, an infectious disease/HIV specialist should be involved in the treatment of HIV and opportunistic infections. Treatment of AIDS with HAART results in a dramatic reduction in KS lesions and incidence.

Therapy

Solitary Lesions

- Cryosurgery (two freeze-thaw cycles) every 3 weeks. There is increased risk of postinflammatory dyschromia in darker skin types.
- Radiation therapy, such as electron beam, can control these exquisitely radiosensitive tumors. Disease recurrence in adjacent untreated skin may be controlled when extended field radiation is used instead.
- Excisional or laser surgery with risk of local recurrence
- Topical alitretinoin 0.1% applied to the lesion(s) twice daily. Topical imiquimod 5% cream daily may also be tried.
- Intralesional bleomycin (1.5 mg), intralesional interferon-alpha (3 to 5 million units three times per week), or intralesional vinblastine (0.1 mg)

Widespread Skin Disease

- Radiation therapy can be effective in controlling widespread disease. The type of radiation (i.e., photon vs. electron) and fields used must be tailored to suit the distribution of the lesions in the individual patient.
- Chemotherapy is occasionally used. Some commonly employed regimens include weekly IV vinblastine (4 to 6 mg) or vinblastine alternating with vincristine (2 mg IV) on a weekly basis. Combination regimens include doxorubicin, bleomycin, and vincristine.

Suggested Readings

Dawkins FW, Delapenha RA, Frezza EE, et al. HIV-1-associated Kaposi's sarcoma in a predominantly black population at an inner city hospital. *South Med J.* 1998;91(6):546–549.

Hoover DR, Black C, Jacobson LP, et al. Epidemiologic analysis of Kaposi's sarcoma as an early and later AIDS outcome in homosexual men. *Am J Epidemiol.* 1993;138(4):266–278.

Mora RG, Lee B. Cancer of the skin in blacks. A review of nineteen black patients with Kaposi's sarcoma. *JAAD.* 1984;11(4);563–567

Mosam A, Carrara H, Shaik F, et al. Increasing incidence of Kaposi's sarcoma in black South Africans in KwaZulu-Natal, South Africa (1983–2006). *Int J STD AIDS.* 2009;20(8):553–556.

Mosam A, Hurkchand HP, Cassol E, et al. Characteristics of HIV-1 associated Kaposi's sarcoma among women and men in South Africa. *Int J STD AIDS.* 2008;19(6):400–405.

Wahman A, Melnick SL, Rhame FS, et al. The epidemiology of classic, African, immunosuppressed Kaposi's sarcoma. *Epidemiol Rev.* 1991;13:178–199.

Livedo Reticularis and Erythema Ab Igne

Randa Khoury

■■ Diagnosis Synopsis

Livedo reticularis and erythema ab igne are both characterized by reticular, or netlike, discoloration. In livedo reticularis, this discoloration is caused by decreased blood flow to the skin or impaired outflow in the dermal venous plexus and stagnation of the blood within these vessels. The darker discolored areas represent accumulation of deoxygenated blood. These characteristic pigmentary changes may be the result of physiologic livedo reticularis (cutis marmorata), a primary disease (as in idiopathic cases), or associated with collagen vascular diseases. Etiologic categories include vasospasm, vessel wall dysfunction (for example, vasculitis), and vascular flow compromise as in coagulopathies. Livedo reticularis is exacerbated by cold temperatures and is frequently seen in patients with Raynaud disease. In severe cases, the extremities are cold and ulcers may form. Sneddon syndrome is a special case characterized by extensive diffuse livedo reticularis in a typical racemose pattern with cerebrovascular disease (from transient ischemic attacks to frank cerebrovascular accidents); hypertension and antiphospholipid antibodies are often present.

In erythema ab igne, however, the pigmentary change is attributed to long-term exposure to a heat source insufficient to cause burns. This exposure produces cutaneous hyperthermia which, in turn, results in histopathologic changes similar to those seen in solar-damaged skin. Recent studies also suggest that this external heat acts synergistically with ultraviolet radiation to denature DNA in squamous cells *in vitro*, correlating with the increased risk of squamous cell carcinoma arising from erythema ab igne. Although burns do not occur from the heat exposure, the skin develops a coarse pigmentation consisting of mottled patches of pink, purple, and eventually brown from melanin deposition. There may be pruritus or mild burning paresthesias. The resultant pigmentation changes can be permanent. Prolonged use of hot water bottles, heating pads, or electric blankets, or sitting near a wood stove or fireplace can trigger the formation of this disorder. Additionally, there have been case reports of erythema ab igne caused by sitting for long periods of time with a laptop computer on the lap.

Livedo reticularis and erythema ab igne are readily appreciated in skin of color. The prevalence of collagen vascular diseases and connective tissue disorders in the African American population makes livedo reticularis an important diagnostic clue. Cultural practices, such as sitting by a stove or fireplace or use of hot water bottles for arthritis, may contribute to development of erythema ab igne.

Look For

Livedo reticularis—reticular violet to bluish patches on the trunk or extremities (Figs. 4-193–4-195).
Erythema ab igne—reticular or mottled red to brown pigmentation in areas of heat exposure (Fig. 4-196). Telangiectasia and other changes may also be apparent in long-standing cases.

●● Diagnostic Pearls

- To distinguish livedo reticularis from erythema ab igne and other reticular pigmentary changes, it is necessary to take a careful history. Seeing the clinical pattern should lead to specific questions regarding direct heat exposure

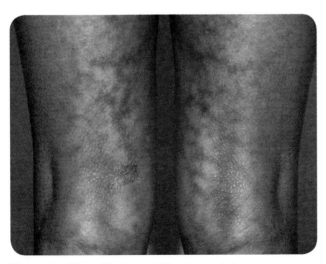

Figure 4-193 Netlike pattern of livedo reticularis.

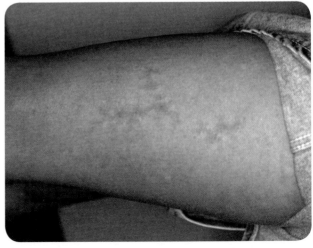

Figure 4-194 Focal network pattern of livedo reticularis.

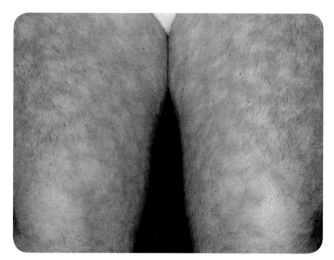

Figure 4-195 Livedo reticularis with a large, open netlike pattern.

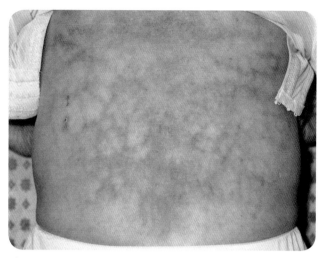

Figure 4-196 Erythema ab igne from chronic external heating.

(e.g., use of a heating pad or hot water bottle, or exposure from radiant heat such as a stove, fireplace, or laptop computer).

- In erythema ab igne, the pattern on the face may be finer and appear more diffuse. With livedo reticularis, elevating the extremity may lessen the color change by increasing venous outflow. The physiologic form of livedo reticularis responds to warming.

?? Differential Diagnosis and Pitfalls

The differential diagnosis for erythema ab igne primarily consists of the following:

- Livedo reticularis
- Livedoid vasculitis
- Acanthosis nigricans
- Reticular erythematous mucinosis

The differential for the cause of livedo reticularis is quite broad, including the following:

- Collagen vascular diseases or vasculitides (polyarteritis nodosa, SLE, rheumatoid arthritis, dermatomyositis)
- Hematologic or hypercoagulable conditions (antiphospholipid antibody syndrome, cryoglobulinemia, polycythemia vera, protein C or S deficiency, heparin-induced thrombocytopenia, thrombotic thrombocytopenic purpura/hemolytic-uremic syndrome, paroxysmal nocturnal hemoglobinuria)
- Livedoid vasculopathy
- Embolic phenomena (cholesterol, fat, septic)
- Deposition diseases (calciphylaxis, oxalosis)
- Medications (amantadine, quinidine, catecholamines, bismuth, arsphenamine, warfarin, interferon, gemcitabine)
- Infections (hepatitis C, mycoplasma, endocarditis, meningococcemia, syphilis, *Rickettsia*, *Mycobacterium leprae* [known as Lucio phenomenon])

- Neoplasms (renal cell carcinoma, pheochromocytoma, some hematologic malignancies)
- Neurologic disorders (multiple sclerosis, Parkinson disease, reflex sympathetic dystrophy, Sneddon syndrome)
- Endocrine/metabolic conditions such as hypercalcemia, hypothyroidism, and carcinoid
- Miscellaneous chronic pancreatitis, heart failure, Degos disease
- Pernio is cold-induced distal blisters or ulcers associated with cold and high humidity.

Reticular erythematous mucinosis is a form of cutaneous mucinosis affecting the upper chest with prominent redness. Erythema ab igne is a form of fixed reticulate dyspigmentation in skin with chronic repeated heat exposure.

✓ Best Tests

Erythema ab igne is best diagnosed from a detailed history. Skin biopsy may be performed if the diagnosis is in doubt, and may also be helpful to rule out vasculitis if evaluated under microscopy and direct immunofluorescence.

Important labs for determining the etiology of livedo reticularis include the following:

- CBC with differential
- Complete metabolic panel
- Coagulation profile
- Serum lipid profile
- Cryoglobulins
- Cold agglutinins
- Hypercoagulable workup including antiphospholipid antibodies, protein C and S, antithrombin III, factor V Leiden mutation, homocystine levels
- Paraproteins
- ANA, rheumatoid factors, anti-neutrophilic cytoplasmic antibodies

Management Pearls

- In livedo reticularis, management is highly dependent on etiology, as treatment of the underlying disease is paramount. In cases of physiologic livedo reticularis, minimize cold exposure and encourage the use of warm clothing. Gently rewarm the affected area or areas.
- With erythema ab igne, eliminate the source of the chronic heat exposure. In patients with mild cases, the hyperpigmentation may remit.

Therapy

The cutaneous manifestation of livedo reticularis is difficult to treat and does not, in and of itself, require any treatment. Identification and treatment of the underlying etiology is most important. Withdraw any medications that may be offending, if possible. Sneddon syndrome patients will require antithrombotic treatment. Those with livedo reticularis resultant from cholesterol emboli should be placed on statin therapy. Pentoxifylline has been proven effective in livedoid vasculopathy. Two patients with ulcer development related to recalcitrant livedo reticularis/livedoid vasculopathy responded to psoralen plus UVA (PUVA).

The hyperpigmentation of erythema ab igne may fade slightly over time, but there is no definitive treatment. The neodymium: yttrium-aluminum-garnet (Nd:YAG), ruby, and alexandrite lasers have been used with some success to improve the appearance of lesions.

Suggested Readings

Chatterjee S. Erythema Ab Igne from prolonged use of a heating pad. *Mayo Clin Proc.* 2005;80(11):1500.

Gibbs MB, English JC, Zirwas MJ. Livedo reticularis: An update. *J Am Acad Dermatol.* 2005;52(6):1009–1019.

Hayes BB, Cook-Norris RH, Miller JL, et al. Amantadine-induced livedo reticularis: A report of two cases. *J Drugs Dermatol.* 2006;5(3):288–289.

Levinbook WS, Mallet J, Grant-Kels JM. Laptop computer-associated erythema ab igne. *Cutis.* 2007;80(4):319–320.

Thiagarajah R, Shrotia S. Erythema ab igne. *J Plast Reconstr Aesthet Surg.* 2998;61(4):446.

Port-Wine Stain

Alicia Ogram • Adam Tinklepaugh

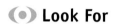 Diagnosis Synopsis

Port-wine stain is a congenital benign capillary malformation typically found on the head and neck, though it may be present anywhere on the body, and may be unilateral (Fig. 4-197). In some individuals, a port-wine stain may become more violaceous and take on a cobblestoned texture with age. Port-wine stains are less common in children of darker skin types. In Turkey, the incidence is approximately 19.2% compared with the United States, where they are found in approximately 3 people in 1,000. Port-wine stains may be isolated or may occur as part of Sturge-Weber and Klippel-Trenaunay syndromes. Port-wine stains are truly malformations of capillaries and will never spontaneously improve.

Look For

At birth, port-wine stain appears as a segmental, flat, irregular vascular patch. Initially, the macules are pink or light red. Rarely, they may be familial (Fig. 4-198). With age, they darken and may thicken and develop a rubbery, cobblestone quality.

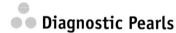 Diagnostic Pearls

Pyogenic granulomas may develop within the lesion. Capillary malformations typically appear in a dermatomal/segmental

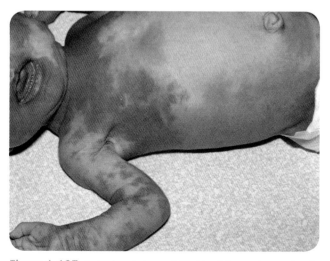
Figure 4-197 Port-wine stain on right side of face and upper trunk, with incidental dermal melanocytosis.

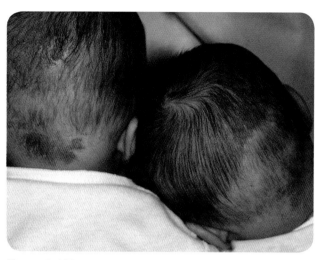
Figure 4-198 Twins with port-wine stains.

distribution on the head and neck. Lesions in the V1 distribution are more likely to be associated with the Sturge-Weber syndrome.

?? Differential Diagnosis and Pitfalls

- Salmon patches—present as small capillary dilatations
- Early infantile hemangiomas
- Sturge-Weber syndrome

✓ Best Tests

- Port-wine stain is a clinical diagnosis. Perform an MRI of the head with gadolinium if Sturge-Weber syndrome is suspected. Consider an MRI or ultrasound in patients with lumbar lesions.
- An ophthalmologic examination with tonometry is indicated for patients with a port-wine stain that involves the periocular area (V1 distribution).

▲▲ Management Pearls

- Camouflage makeup can be used effectively (Dermablend or Covermark).
- Regular ophthalmologic examinations are recommended in patients with V1 port-wine stains.
- Consider a neurologic consultation for patients with suspected Sturge-Weber or those with lumbar lesions.

211

Therapy

Pulsed-dye laser (PDL, 585 to 595 nm) offers the most effective treatment of capillary malformations in light and dark skin. PDL combined with topical imiquimod has shown superior blanching of port-wine stains in recent studies. Darkly pigmented patients (Fitzpatrick skin types V and VI) should not be excluded from PDL therapy due to minimally increased risk of hyperpigmentation and scarring.

PDL has been shown to offer significant improvement in Indian patients and Korean patients (Fitzpatrick skin types III and V) with port-wine stains. Flashlamp-pumped pulsed dye (FLPD) laser therapy is effective in treating vascular malformations of port-wine stain in pigmented skin.

Suggested Readings

Chang CJ, Hsiao YC, Mihm MC Jr, et al. Pilot study examining the combined use of pulsed dye laser and topical Imiquimod versus laser alone for treatment of port wine stain birthmarks. *Lasers Surg Med.* 2008;40(9): 605–610.

Ferahbas A, Utas S, Akcakus M, et al. Prevalence of cutaneous findings in hospitalized neonates: A prospective observational study. *Pediatr Dermatol.* 2009;26(2):139–142.

Garrett AB, Shieh S. Treatment of vascular lesions in pigmented skin with the pulsed dye laser. *J Cutan Med Surg.* 2000;4(1):36–39.

Sharma VK, Khandpur S. Efficacy of pulsed dye laser in facial port-wine stains in Indian patients. *Dermatol Surg.* 2007;33(5):560–566.

Sommer S, Sheehan-Dare RA. Pulsed dye laser treatment of port-wine stains in pigmented skin. *J Am Acad Dermatol.* 2000;42(4):667–671.

Woo S-H, Ahn H-H, Kim S-N, et al. Treatment of vascular skin lesions with the variable-pulse 595 nm pulsed dye laser. *Dermatol Surg.* 2006;32(1):41–48.

Pyogenic Granuloma

Pooja Sodha • Lynn McKinley-Grant

■■ Diagnosis Synopsis

Pyogenic granuloma, also known as lobular capillary hemangioma, is a rare, benign, acquired vascular proliferation of the skin and mucous membranes. Histologically, it is a lobular capillary hemangioma.

The etiology remains unclear. It has been suggested that the lesion is in fact a hyperproliferative vascular response to a myriad of stimuli, including infectious organisms, eczematous dermatitis, penetrating or chronic injury, hormonal fluctuations, and retinoid therapy. Certain angiogenic factors may also play a role in the evolution of this lesion.

The majority of patients appear to have no predisposing factors to the development of pyogenic granulomas, which may be cutaneous, mucosal, subcutaneous, or intravascular, the latter two of which have been reported rarely.

Common cutaneous sites are the trunk, head and neck, and extremities, particularly the hands and fingers. Common mucosal sites are gingiva, cheeks, and lips. Pyogenic granulomas can occur in various races and ethnicities; most reports focus on oral lesions. In a study of the Brazilian population, an incidence of approximately 3% was found, with predominance among white patients, which may be attributable to access to care. In examining oral lesions in 38 Nigerian patients over 11 years at one center, it was found that most lesions were large tumors, suggesting that most patients did not present until incapacitated. This may explain the lower incidence and rarity of the lesion in this population. In a study of cases in India, an incidence of 21% with female predominance was found. Since pyogenic granulomas can present in areas of active inflammation or injury, gingivitis and periodontal health, a socioeconomic indicator, are directly correlated with the lesion.

Reports suggest that the lesion is most common in children and young adults, but most studies focus on these two populations. Moreover, pyogenic granulomas have been cited in nearly every age group, with mean age of presentation in the second and third decades of life. Cutaneous pyogenic granulomas appear to have a slight predilection for men, whereas mucosal pyogenic granulomas are nearly two times more common in women than in men. Some studies suggest that a hormonal influence on mucosal tissue may account for this difference. Nearly 5% of pregnant women develop the lesion on the oral mucosa (granuloma gravidarum) in the second or third trimester. Vulvar pyogenic granulomas have also been reported.

These typically painless lesions are prone to ulceration and bleeding after mild trauma, which, along with cosmetic complaints, often precipitate visits to the clinician.

Pediatric Patient Considerations

As with adults, most pediatric patients do not have any known inciting cause of pyogenic granulomas, which comprise 0.5% of all skin nodules in children. These lesions may arise within other vascular malformations, such as larger hemangiomas or superficial telangiectases. Trauma may also precipitate these lesions.

◉ Look For

Single, small, smooth, rapidly growing, red to deep-purple, sessile or pedunculated papule (Figs. 4-199 and 4-200).

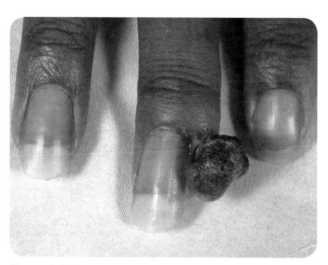

Figure 4-199 Large pyogenic granuloma near the lateral nail fold.

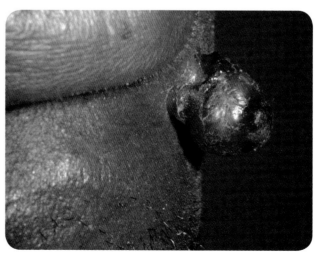

Figure 4-200 Large, friable pyogenic granuloma on the chin.

Painless to palpation. Lesions may appear on head and neck, trunk, upper limb, lower limb, and perineal/vulvar region. Initially soft in consistency, they become firmer over time with deposition of collagen. They are prone to ulceration and hemorrhage, so may present with red crust. They may rarely spontaneously regress. Recurrent pyogenic granulomas with multiple satellite lesions (satellitosis) may occur at sites of chronic irritation or after treatment of the primary lesions.

Diagnostic Pearls

Rapidly (within weeks) evolving single nodular lesion with predilection for the face, mucous membranes, and extremities with tendency to bleed is very suggestive of this diagnosis.

?? Differential Diagnosis and Pitfalls

Pyogenic granulomas (lobular capillary hemangiomas) can best be differentiated by dermatoscopic and histopathologic examination.

Nonvascular

- Basal cell carcinoma
- Squamous cell carcinoma
- Amelanotic melanoma
- Spitz nevus

These lesions are typically nonvascular and will likely present with melanocytes or epithelial cells.

Vascular

- Kaposi sarcoma
- Angiosarcoma
- Hemangioendothelioma
- Bacillary angiomatosis—typically affects immunocompromised patients; Warthin-Starry stain should reveal clumps of organisms.
- Granulation tissue
- Common warts
- Glomus tumor
- Inflamed seborrheic keratosis
- Atypical spindle cell nevus
- Venous lake
- Poroma
- Clear cell acanthoma
- Angiokeratoma—initially red to black, soft, nonpulsating, nonkeratotic papules and plaques, 1 to 5 mm, discrete or in clusters (Figs. 4-201 and 4-202). Lesion grows larger,

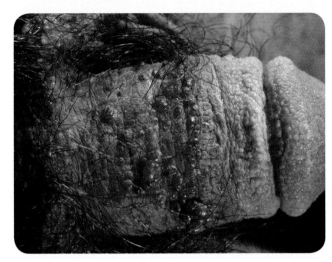

Figure 4-201 Multiple angiokeratomas of different sizes in a characteristic location.

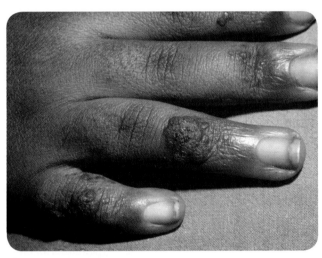

Figure 4-202 Angiokeratoma of Mibelli is usually on the extremities with grouped vascular lesions.

approximately 2 cm, and becomes firm, blue-black, elevated, keratotic, and verrucous. Tender to palpation in later stages. Prone to bleed with trauma.

The five types of angiokeratoma lesions and their most common presentation:

1. Angiokeratoma of Mibelli—verrucous telangiectasic nodules, blue-red or gray. May have central hemorrhagic crust, measuring 2 to 5 mm; typically present on the dorsa of hands and feet
2. Angiokeratoma of Fordyce—verrucous telangiectases measuring 1 to 5 mm; limited typically to the scrotum or vulva; prevalent among men typically in the second and third decades

3. Fabry disease/angiokeratoma corporis diffusum—worldwide prevalence is between 1 in 40,000 and 1 in 117,000, with no known racial or ethnic predilection. It is an X-linked lysosomal storage disease caused by deficiency of alpha-galactosidase A. As the predominant cutaneous manifestation of the disease, angiokeratomas are present in 66% of men and 36% of obligate carrier women. Present at median age of 14 to 16 years. Multiple 1- to 7-mm, slightly elevated, red to purple, hyperkeratotic and coalescing papules in "bathing trunk" distribution, including groin, trunk, and periumbilical regions (less commonly around mouth or breasts). May present with other dermatologic findings associated with this disease including telangiectases (23% men, 9% women), lymphedema (25% men, 17% women), hypohidrosis (53% men, 28% women), or anhidrosis. Thought to present prior to renal or cardiac disease manifestations.
4. Angiokeratoma circumscriptum—present at birth, typically unilateral lesion on lower extremity; may have zosteriform arrangement and evolve to solitary plaque of hyperkeratotic nodules
5. Solitary angiokeratoma—predilection for lower extremity, but can occur on any part of body; larger (2 to 10 mm) and more keratotic than other variants

While these are all vascular lesions, the underlying vessel network has a different morphology. On histology, there will likely be greater mitotic activity and varying cellular infiltrate. Kaposi patients will likely test positive for latent nuclear antigen-1 antibody of human herpesvirus-8 (HHV-8). An angiokeratoma may have an overlying white-yellow tone suggestive of hyperkeratosis.

Pediatric Patient Differential Diagnosis

- Infantile hemangioma
- Common warts
- Insect bite
- Nevus
- Amelanotic melanoma

 ## Best Tests

Dermatoscopic evaluation is an effective noninvasive technique in the initial workup of this lesion, especially since distinction from other benign and malignant lesions is clinically indicated.
Common findings include the following:

- Uniformly reddish area
- White-brown collarette that surrounds the lesion

- White "rail lines" that intersect the lesion
- Ulceration or superficial hemorrhagic crust

Histopathologic examination will show proliferation of capillary-sized blood vessels in lobular arrangement separated by fibrous bands; mitotic activity, though not on the order of malignancy; and hyperkeratosis with acanthosis.

 ## Management Pearls

Since the etiology of the lesion is still not entirely clear, there is no regimen for prevention. If there is concern for complicated lesion or malignancy, refer to dermatologist for further evaluation. Risk of recurrence after treatment exists, but can be managed conservatively. Spontaneous regression has been reported, and is more likely in the early stages of development. Mature lesions are less likely to regress, and some have been reported to last for years if not treated.

Therapy

- Histologic identification of the lesion should be a mandatory step in clinical practice.
- Many consider full-thickness surgical excision with linear closure as standard treatment. Recurrence rate is 3% to 4%. Studies have been pursued to better identify effective therapies that not only minimize the risk of recurrence but also offer the best cosmetic result.
- Shave excision with electrocautery—safe, but prone to recurrence, reported in one study as 43.5%
- Cryotherapy—safe and effective. One study reported complete resolution after no more than three therapeutic sessions. Technique involved 2-mm rim of frozen normal tissue around the lesion.
- Curettage with electrodesiccation—safe and effective. When compared with cryotherapy, offered complete resolution with no more than two therapeutic sessions. Curettage offered better cosmetic results with lower rates of hypopigmentation than cryotherapy, which may be of greater importance in pigmented skin.
- 585-nm pulsed dye laser—well-known therapy for vascular dermatoses. Safe for small (<5 mm), minimally elevated (<5 mm) lesions. Shown to be effective with minimal scarring in fair-skinned individuals, with a failure rate in one study of 9%. In another study of 18 patients, 16 patients demonstrated no posttherapy complications or permanent scarring/pigment change. Study of one patient with skin type V–VI treated with this modality also showed complete resolution of the lesion without any side effects.
- CO_2 laser—effective for larger lesions (>10 mm)

(Continued)

- In one retrospective study of 128 pediatric patients, all parents contacted for telephone follow-up were pleased with the cosmetic results independent of what therapy was used.
- For recurrent lesions, treatment with the primary modality may be tried again. One report showed complete resolution of a recurrent pyogenic granuloma with a 3-week course of topical imiquimod 5% cream under occlusion without local or systemic side effects.

Pediatric Patient Considerations

Because of its ease, efficiency, and cost-effectiveness, one retrospective study of 128 pediatric patients suggested that uncomplicated pyogenic granulomas be initially treated with shave excision and electrocautery, since there were no reported recurrences, although scarring was seen in nearly 50% of cases.

Suggested Readings

Al-Khateeb T, Khansa A. Oral pyogenic granuloma in Jordanians: A retrospective analysis of 108 cases. *J Oral Maxillofacial Surg.* 2003;61: 1285–1288.

Georgiou S, Monastirli A, Pasmatzi E, et al. Pyogenic granuloma: Complete remission under occlusive imiquimod 5% cream. *Clin Exp Dermatol.* 2008;33:454–456.

Ghodsi SZ, Raziei M, Taheri A, et al. Comparison of cryotherapy and curettage for the treatment of pyogenic granuloma: A randomized trial. *Br J Dermatol.* 2006;154:671–675.

Giblin AV, Clover AJP, Athanassopoulos A, et al. Pyogenic granuloma—The quest for optimum treatment: Audit of treatment of 408 cases. *J Plast Reconstruct Aesth Surg.* 2007;60:1030–1035.

Gordón-Núñez MA, Marianne De VC, Benevenuto TG, et al. Oral pyogenic granuloma: A retrospective analysis of 293 cases in a Brazilian population. *J Oral Maxillofacial Surg.* 2010;68(9):2185–2188.

Harris MN, Desai R, Chuang T-Y, et al. Lobular capillary hemangiomas: An epidemiologic report, with emphasis on cutaneous lesions. *J Am Acad Dermatol.* 2000;42:1012–1016.

Larralde MM, Luna PC. Fabry disease. In: Wolff K, Goldsmith LA, Katz SI, et al., eds. *Fitpatrick's Dermatology in General Medicine.* 7th Ed. New York, NY: McGraw-Hill; 2008:1281–1288.

Lawoyin JO, Arotiba JT, Dosumu OO. Oral pyogenic granuloma: A review of 38 cases from Ibadan, Nigeria. *Br J Oral Maxillofacial Surg.* 1997;35: 185–189.

Paliai KA, Cohen BA. Pyogenic granuloma in children. *Pediatr Dermatol.* 2004;21(1):10–13.

Saravana GHL. Oral pyogenic granuloma: A review of 137 cases. *Br J Oral Maxillofacial Surg.* 2009;47:318–319.

Tay Y-K, Weston WL, Morelli JG. Treatment of pyogenic granuloma in children with the flashlamp-pumped pulsed dye laser. *Pediatrics.* 1997;99(3):368–370.

Zaballos P, Llambrich A, Cuellar F, et al. Dermatoscopic findings in pyogenic granuloma. *Br J Dermatol.* 2006;154:1108–1111.

Spider Angioma

Lowell A. Goldsmith

■■ Diagnosis Synopsis

A spider angioma, also known as a spider vein or spider nevus, is the most prevalent of the telangiectases. Clinically, there is a central arteriole from which numerous small, twisted vessels radiate. The ascending central arteriole appears as a spider's body, and the radiating vessels resemble the spider's legs, hence the spider appearance that is visible on the skin.

This common benign, acquired lesion usually appears spontaneously and is present in 40% of normal children up to age 8. Prevalence drops to about 10% to 15% of healthy adults. Many women develop lesions during pregnancy or while taking oral contraceptives, likely due to high estrogen levels in their blood. These lesions usually disappear following parturition or cessation of the contraceptives.

Spider angiomas may be indicative of underlying systemic disease, especially when found in large numbers. Liver dysfunction due to hepatic cirrhosis or hepatic tumors impairs the metabolism of estrogen, which may play a role in increased nevus formation. In addition, elevated levels of serum vascular endothelial growth factor and young age are predictive of spider angioma formation in patients with cirrhosis. Patients with alcoholic cirrhosis are more likely to develop spider angioma than those with viral or idiopathic cirrhosis. In patients with diseases of the liver, regression of the nevus may occur following improvement of the underlying condition, although this is not usually so. They are also associated less frequently with thyrotoxicosis and in patients on estrogen therapy.

Spider angiomas usually appear on the upper half of the body, frequently on sun-exposed areas. It is very uncommon for lesions to occur below the level of the umbilicus. The lesion ranges in size from that of a pinhead to 2 cm.

Pyogenic granuloma developing within a large spider angioma is a possible complication of these benign vascular malformations.

◉ Look For

Spider angiomas appear to be less frequent in patients with darker skin. However, epidemiologic studies are limited.

Spider angiomas occur most commonly on the face, neck, and upper part of the trunk and arms. Also look for lesions on the hands, forearms, and ears. Rarely, they may be visible in the mucous membrane of the nose, mouth, or pharynx.

Spider angiomas are bright red with a small central papule surrounded by small radiating vessels (Fig. 4-203).

Pressure applied to the angioma will lead to its disappearance. Blanching is quickly reversed when pressure is lifted, resulting in a rapid refill from the central arteriole. The refill

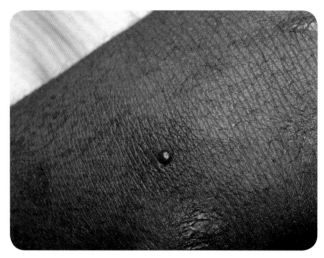

Figure 4-203 Spider angioma with raised central punctum and a red rim without discernible discrete spider "legs."

pattern occurs from the center to the periphery due to the arteriolar origin of the spider nevus.

●● Diagnostic Pearls

- The typical spider appearance of the lesion is unmistakable. Pressure applied to the central arteriole causes blanching of the entire lesion. When pressure is released, these vessels quickly refill with blood. This can be easily seen with diascopy using a glass slide.
- In patients who appear to have many spider angiomas, particularly on mucosal or acral sites, the diagnosis of hereditary hemorrhagic telangiectasia should be considered. Scleroderma (especially CREST syndrome) may also present with multiple matlike telangiectases on the face and acral sites.

?? Differential Diagnosis and Pitfalls

- Hereditary hemorrhagic telangiectasia
- Scleroderma (CREST syndrome)
- Cherry hemangioma
- Angiokeratoma corporis circumscriptum
- Ataxia telangiectasia
- Insect bites
- Essential telangiectasia
- Rosacea
- Pyogenic granuloma
- Capillary malformation—arteriovenous malformation syndrome

Best Tests

- The classic refill pattern remains the diagnostic marker for the identification of spider angiomas. Press down on the lesion and watch for refill radiating from the central vessel outward.
- Liver function tests to assess severity of liver disease, if present

 Management Pearls

Treatment of spider angiomas is usually done for cosmetic purposes, especially when they present on the face.

Therapy

Laser treatment and electrodesiccation are both effective methods, and the lesion is usually completely removed.

Electrodesiccation
The central arteriole can be ablated using fine needle electrodesiccation. This involves sealing of the blood vessels by monopolar high-frequency electric current.

Laser Treatment
Treatment with lasers is very effective but may be more costly than electrodesiccation. Potassium-titanyl-phosphate (KTP), pulsed dye, and argon lasers have all successfully been used in the treatment of spider angiomas. Local anesthesia may be used prior to the procedure. One must be careful not to blanch and obscure the spider vein when infiltrating the anesthesia.

Results are excellent with both types of treatment, and recurrence is infrequent.

Suggested Readings

Bernstein EF. The new-generation, high-energy, 595 nm, long pulse-duration, pulsed-dye laser effectively removes spider veins of the lower extremity. *Lasers Surg Med.* 2007;39(3):218–224.

Bernstein EF, Lee J, Lowery J, et al. Treatment of spider veins with the 595 nm pulsed-dye laser. *J Am Acad Dermatol.* 1998;39(5 Pt 1):746–750.

Goldman MP, Weiss RA, Brody HJ, et al. Treatment of facial telangiectasia with sclerotherapy, laser surgery, and/or electrodesiccation: A review. *J Dermatol Surg Oncol.* 1993;19(10):899–906; quiz 909–910.

Okada N. Solitary giant spider angioma with an overlying pyogenic granuloma. *J Am Acad Dermatol.* 1987;16(5 Pt 1):1053–1054.

Requena L, Sangueza OP. Cutaneous vascular anomalies. Part I. Hamartomas, malformations, and dilation of preexisting vessels. *J Am Acad Dermatol.* 1997;37(4):523–549; quiz 549–552.

Subacute Bacterial Endocarditis

Lowell A. Goldsmith

▪▪ Diagnosis Synopsis

Bacterial endocarditis can be divided into either acute or subacute disease. Acute bacterial endocarditis (ABE) refers to abrupt onset of symptoms occurring for <2 weeks, whereas subacute bacterial endocarditis (SBE) evolves over several weeks or months. Overall, streptococci cause the majority of valvular endocarditis. Staphylococci cause the majority of disease in IV drug abusers, and a combination of staphylococci and streptococci causes a significant number of cases of late prosthetic valve endocarditis.

Clinically, the patient may appear acutely ill or chronically ill and wasted. There are two major cutaneous findings: Osler nodes and Janeway lesions. Osler nodes are painful erythematous nodules located on the fingertips. Janeway lesions are nontender hemorrhagic macules and papules on the palms. Both findings are thought to result from septic embolization from a source of infective endocarditis. Other cutaneous findings include palpable purpura (cutaneous small vessel vasculitis) and splinter hemorrhages. Most patients will have a cardiac murmur at some stage, although in early stages, and especially with right-sided ABE, up to 15% of patients will have no murmur. Splenomegaly is seen in about 30% to 50% of patients.

The number of patients with prior cardiac surgery, immunosuppression, and drug abuse has increased. Mitral valve prolapse is a risk factor for endocarditis only when associated with a precordial systolic murmur. In recent years, an increase in endocarditis in men and elderly patients; acute endocarditis; and endocarditis caused by Gram-negative bacteria, fungi, and miscellaneous microbes has occurred. Endocarditis may be "culture-negative" when caused by *Candida* or *Aspergillus*. Tricuspid valvular disease is associated with IV drug abuse. Veterinarians in California have been shown to be at risk for Q fever endocarditis.

Immunocompromised Patient Considerations

HIV-infected patients with advanced immunosuppression are more likely to develop infective endocarditis and have higher morbidity and mortality.

◉ Look For

Petechiae or palpable purpura on the distal extremities, fingers, and toes can appear as very deep purple to brown or black in darkly pigmented patients (Fig. 4-204). On the palms and soles where there is less melanin, the macules and subtle

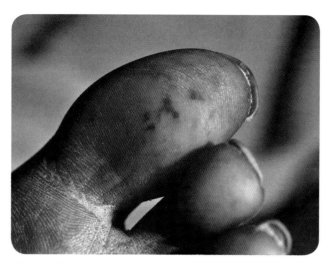

Figure 4-204 Distal purpuric papules in subacute bacterial endocarditis.

papules can appear red to purple. Splinter hemorrhages will be 1 to 3 mm purpuric macules in the nail bed. These are best seen by transilluminating the distal volar finger with a flashlight. Janeway lesions are erythematous, nontender macules on the palms and soles of a few patients with SBE. Osler nodes occur in 10% to 20% of patients and are tender, erythematous nodules often located on the fingertips. Retinal hemorrhages are found in 10% to 25% of patients with SBE and ABE. Roth spots have an ivory or white center surrounded by a red halo.

●● Diagnostic Pearls

Petechiae are often discrete. Look for 2 to 5 mm "splinter petechiae" on distal extremities.

?? Differential Diagnosis and Pitfalls

- Bacterial sepsis
- Candidemia
- Ecthyma gangrenosum
- Leukocytoclastic vasculitis from another cause
- Rocky Mountain spotted fever
- Gonococcemia
- Cholesterol emboli
- Other causes of endocarditis include *Coxiella burnetii* (the cause of Q fever), mycobacteria, and chlamydia.

Immunocompromised Patient Differential Diagnosis

Disseminated fungal infection

219

✓ Best Tests

Blood cultures, obtained as recommended in three venous cultures on the first hospital day, and two more venous cultures on the second day if clinically indicated. On the third day, if indicated, draw two more venous cultures and one arterial culture. Blood cultures are positive in the majority of patients, with multiple blood cultures sometimes needed before the organism is grown. Transesophageal echocardiography is useful in detecting perivalvular abscesses and vegetations. Positive tourniquet test may be present. Anemia, mild leukocytosis, elevated erythrocyte sedimentation rate (almost always), hematuria, RBC casts in urine, biological false-positive syphilis tests, and elevated gamma globulins may occur.

▲▲▲ Management Pearls

Patients may have their course complicated by arrhythmias and myocarditis. Close monitoring is advised. Obtain blood cultures early in therapy to insure efficacy of therapy. Monitor blood levels of drug.

Therapy

Prolonged administration of relatively high intravenous doses of bactericidal antibiotics based on culture results and sensitivities.

Suggested Readings

Bauer A, Jabs WJ, Süfke S, et al. Vasculitic purpura with antineutrophil cytoplasmic antibody-positive acute renal failure in a patient with Streptococcus bovis case and Neisseria subflava bacteremia and subacute endocarditis. *Clin Nephrol.* 2004;62(2):144–148. PubMed Id: 15356972.

Suhge d'Aubermont PC, Honig PJ, Wood MG. Subacute bacterial endocarditis presenting with necrotic skin lesions. *Int J Dermatol.* 1983;22(5):295–299. PubMed Id: 6874187.

Verhagen DW, Vedder AC, Speelman P, et al. Antimicrobial treatment of infective endocarditis caused by viridans streptococci highly susceptible to penicillin: Historic overview and future considerations. *J Antimicrob Chemother.* 2006;57(5):819–824. PubMed Id: 16549513.

Raynaud Phenomenon

Stephanie Diamantis

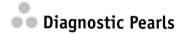 Diagnosis Synopsis

Raynaud phenomenon is a vascular disorder characterized by intermittent arteriolar vasospasm of the digits and occurs in two settings. Primary Raynaud phenomenon, or Raynaud disease, is characterized by the occurrence of vasospasm without ischemic injury or underlying associated disease. This variant is most commonly encountered in otherwise healthy adolescent girls and young women. Individuals suffer from digital pallor, cyanosis, and sharply bordered redness, and the disease is often associated with numbness of the fingers. Vasoconstriction is most often triggered by cold exposure and stress. Patients with primary Raynaud phenomenon have a younger age of onset, normal nail fold capillaries, and negative or low titers of autoantibodies. Primary Raynaud phenomenon usually involves all fingers in a symmetric distribution, and pain is usually absent to minimal. Smoking is contraindicated in these patients, as it may worsen the condition.

Secondary Raynaud phenomenon is characterized by an underlying disease where vasospasm can result in ischemic injury. It is commonly seen in patients with collagen vascular disorders, particularly systemic sclerosis, and in approximately 20% of lupus patients. Additional associations include rheumatoid arthritis, pulmonary hypertension, frostbite, hematologic malignancies, polyvinyl chloride exposure, cryoglobulinemia, reflex sympathetic dystrophy, repeated trauma/vibration, arteriovenous (AV) fistulae, intra-arterial drug administration, thoracic outlet syndrome, thromboangiitis obliterans, and Takayasu arteritis.

Look For

Affected digits commonly demonstrate at least two color changes—white (pallor), blue (cyanosis), and/or red (hyperemia)—and usually, but not always, in that order (Fig. 4-205). Ulcers and necrosis may form due to ischemia in secondary Raynaud phenomenon.

Diagnostic Pearls

Primary Raynaud Phenomenon

Symmetric, absent to minimal pain, normal nail fold capillaries, negative or low titers of autoantibodies, absence of ulcers and necrosis.

Secondary Raynaud Phenomenon

Asymmetric, significant pain with ulcers and necrosis, high titers of autoantibodies, dilated nail fold capillaries. If digital ulcers and necrosis are present secondary to ischemia, aggressively

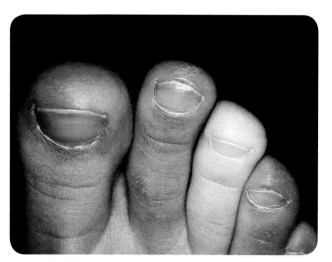

Figure 4-205 A 22-year-old woman with Raynaud phenomenon with toe blanching (white) and hyperemia (red) during cold weather.

pursue an underlying cause. Primary Raynaud phenomenon is not associated with these irreversible findings.

?? Differential Diagnosis and Pitfalls

- Carpal tunnel syndrome
- Reflex sympathetic dystrophy
- Paroxysmal hemoglobinuria
- Deep vein thrombosis (Paget-von Schrötter syndrome)
- Cryoglobulinemia
- Waldenstrom macroglobulinemia, multiple myeloma, and other hematology malignancies
- Various hypercoagulable disorders, including antithrombin deficiency, antiphospholipid antibody syndrome, protein C or S deficiency, etc.
- Effects from drugs such as ergot drugs, vinblastine, methysergide, beta-blockers, caffeine, nicotine, oral contraceptives, and bleomycin
- Toxicity from arsenic, PVC, cocaine, cyanide, or lead
- Livedo reticularis
- Acrocyanosis
- Atherosclerosis
- Thromboangiitis obliterans
- Vasculitis
- Erythromelalgia

✓ Best Tests

- Take a thorough medication history. Nail fold capillaroscopy in the appropriate setting may be beneficial.
- Obtain basic hematologic studies, such as a CBC, chemistry panel, and a coagulation profile.

- If an autoimmune connective tissue disease is suspected, check the following: ANA, anti-dsDNA, anti-Scl-70 (anti-topoisomerase I), anti-centromere, anti-Ro, anti-La, anti-ribonucleoprotein, rheumatoid factor antibodies, erythrocyte sedimentation rate, and cryoglobulins.

▲▲▲ Management Pearls

- Avoidance of exposure to cold temperatures and smoking cessation (if applicable) are essential.
- In cases of secondary Raynaud phenomenon, maximize treatment of the underlying disorder. Eliminate any environmental, occupational, or drug exposures.
- Patients with secondary Raynaud phenomenon may require consultation with a rheumatologist, hematologist, or vascular surgeon.

Therapy

Treatment regimens can be divided based on the severity of digital ischemia and whether the patient has primary or secondary Raynaud phenomenon.

Primary Raynaud Phenomenon
Lifestyle modification is key. Smoking cessation, minimizing exposure to cold environments, avoidance of caffeine, and discontinuing medications that cause vasoconstriction are important in initial management.

Vasodilating drugs may be helpful, such as nifedipine 10 to 30 mg three times daily (gold standard). Other oral treatment options include sildenafil 50 mg twice daily, and for refractory cases losartan 50 mg daily or fluoxetine may be helpful. Topical 2% nitroglycerin in an ointment base has been shown to have some effect.

Secondary Raynaud Phenomenon
Treat the underlying disease. Treatment regimens can be further divided into etiology. Complete discussion of these options is beyond the scope of this text, and referral to the appropriate specialist is recommended.

Suggested Readings

Bakst R, Merola JF, Franks AG, et al. Raynaud's phenomenon: Pathogenesis and management. *J Am Acad Dermatol.* 2008;59(4):633–653.

Boin F, Wigley FM. Understanding, assessing and treating Raynaud's phenomenon. *Curr Opin Rheumatol.* 2005;17(6):752–760.

Bowling JC, Dowd PM. Raynaud's disease. *Lancet.* 2003;361(9374):2078–2080.

Cooke JP, Marshall JM. Mechanisms of Raynaud's disease. *Vasc Med.* 2005;10(4):293–307.

Pope J. Raynaud's phenomenon (primary). *Clin Evid.* 2005;(13):1546–1554.

Raynaud's disease. Cold hands, slowed blood flow. *Mayo Clin Health Lett.* 2007;25(5):7.

Raynaud's Treatment Study Investigators. Comparison of sustained-release nifedipine and temperature biofeedback for treatment of primary Raynaud phenomenon. Results from a randomized clinical trial with 1-year follow-up. *Arch Intern Med.* 2000;160(8):1101–1108.

Thompson AE, Pope JE. Calcium channel blockers for primary Raynaud's phenomenon: A meta-analysis. *Rheumatology (Oxford).* 2005;44(2):145–150.

Vinjar B, Stewart M. Oral vasodilators for primary Raynaud's phenomenon. *Cochrane Database Syst Rev.* 2008;(2):CD006687.

Dermatofibromas

Cynthia Marie Carver DeKlotz

■■ Diagnosis Synopsis

Dermatofibroma, also known as benign fibrous histiocytoma, is a common cutaneous lesion. Clinically, dermatofibromas present as dome-shaped papules or nodules that can vary in color from white-tan to red-purple to reddish-brown. A dermatofibroma is most often a solitary, slowly growing, 1- to 2-cm papule located on the lower extremities. Histologically, dermatofibromas represent a well-circumscribed proliferation of fibrohistiocytic spindle-shaped cells interspersed among thickened dermal collagen bundles. The epidermis may show some acanthosis with basal layer hyperpigmentation. Immunohistochemistry typically reveals positive staining with factor XIIIa.

Dermatofibromas are typically asymptomatic; however, at times, the lesions may be pruritic.

Rarely, multiple eruptive dermatofibromas (MEDFs) may occur in patients. MEDFs are arbitrarily defined as the presence of a minimum of anywhere from 5 to 15 or more dermatofibromas developing in less than a 4-month period. MEDFs have been reported to occur in the setting of HIV disease; in autoimmune disease, most frequently systemic lupus erythematous; and in neoplastic diseases.

Multiple clustered dermatofibroma (MCDF) is an entity where 15 or more dermatofibromas cluster together to form a plaque, most often on the lower half of the body in the first to third decades.

The exact etiology of dermatofibromas remains unclear. However, it has been proposed that dermatofibromas may be the result of an abortive immunoreactive process mediated by dermal dendritic cells. It is possible that a suppressed immune system may not be able to clear some unspecified pathogen, and as a result, dermal dendritic cells may react by increasing fibrohistiocytic proliferation, resulting in the production of a dermatofibroma. This theory is supported by the fact that MEDFs are frequently found in the setting of immunosuppression.

◉ Look For

Patients will give the history of previous trauma, particularly insect bites, shaving, or other minor traumas that they may not remember.

Clinically, dermatofibromas present as dome-shaped papules or nodules that can vary in color from white-tan to red-purple to reddish-brown (Figs. 4-206–4-209).

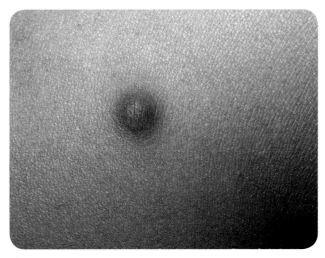

Figure 4-207 Early dermatofibromas may have a rim of surrounding erythema.

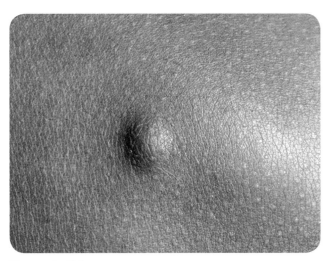

Figure 4-206 Single hyperpigmented papules without pigment extension are frequently dermatofibromas.

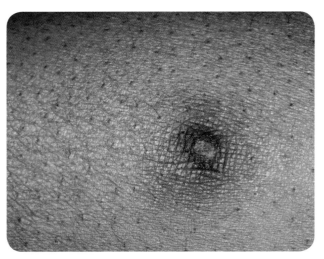

Figure 4-208 Dermatofibroma with some lichenification of surrounding skin shown by accentuated skin markings.

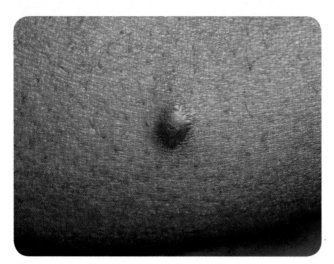

Figure 4-209 Uniform pigmentation without pigment spread leads away from the diagnosis of melanoma.

A dermatofibroma is most often a solitary, slowly growing, 0.5- to 2-cm papule located on the lower extremity.

Clinical variants include MEDF and MCDF as discussed above. Halo eczema has been reported to occur around a dermatofibroma. Additionally, in a case of acute leg edema, halo asteatotic eczema has been reported to occur localized around a dermatofibroma. It is thought that the tethering effect of the dermatofibroma may limit the extensibility of the skin in the surrounding area, resulting in localized fissuring.

Diagnostic Pearls

Lateral compression of the adjacent skin next to the dermatofibroma causes retraction of the lesion, known as a "dimple sign."

Differential Diagnosis and Pitfalls

The differential diagnosis of dermatofibroma is numerous and includes other papular lesions:

- Dermatofibrosarcoma protuberans (DFSP)—DFSP is composed of densely packed spindle cells that often infiltrate the subcutis. Traditionally, DFSP is factor XIIIa negative and CD34 positive, while dermatofibroma is factor XIIIa positive and CD34 negative.
- Pigmented DFSP or Bednar tumors—This comprises 1% to 5% of all DFSP cases.
- Kaposi sarcoma
- Bacillary angiomatosis
- Blue nevus
- Giant cell fibroblastoma
- Keloid
- Hypertrophic scar

Best Tests

Clinical examination is usually the best diagnostic method. However, if clinical exam is atypical, diagnosis may be confirmed with a biopsy. On pathological evaluation, a dermatofibroma shows a well-circumscribed proliferation of fibrohistiocytic spindle-shaped cells interspersed among thickened dermal collagen bundles.

Additionally, dermoscopy may prove useful. In a recent study evaluating suspicious lesions on patients with more deeply pigmented skin, it was incidentally found that dermoscopy aided in the diagnosis of a dermatofibroma. Specifically, on dermoscopy, the dermatofibroma was characterized by a white central patch and a fine peripheral network.

Management Pearls

If a patient presents with MEDF, it is prudent to check HIV status and perform an ANA test to rule out systemic lupus erythematous, as both these diseases are strongly associated with MEDF.

Therapy

If asymptomatic, dermatofibromas do not need to be treated; rather, the patient may simply be reassured and the lesion monitored clinically.

If symptomatic, dermatofibromas may be treated with liquid nitrogen and intralesional corticosteroid injection or topical corticosteroid application. In patients with dark skin, these treatments must be used with caution, as cryotherapy and intralesional triamcinolone injections may result in hypopigmentation.

Suggested Readings

Cox NH. Halo asteatotic eczema localized around a dermatofibroma in acute-onset leg oedema. *Br J Dermatol.* 2008;159:496.

De Giorgi V, Trez E, Salvini C, et al. Dermoscopy in black people. *Br J Dermatol.* 2006;155:695–699.

Gershtenson PC, Krunic AL, Chen HM. Multiple clustered dermatofibroma: Case report and review of the literature. *J Cutan Pathol.* 2010;37(9):e42–e45.

McAllister JC, Recht B, Hoffman TE, et al. CD34+ pigmented fibrous proliferations: The morphologic overlap between pigmented dermatofibromas and bednar tumors. *Am J Dermatopathol.* 2008;30:484–487.

Ogawa R, Akaishi S, Hyakusoku H. Differential and exclusive diagnosis of diseases that resemble keloids and hypertrophic scars. *Ann Plastic Surg.* 2009;62:660–664.

Tan AWH, Tan SH. Dermatofibrosarcoma protuberans: A clinicopathological analysis of 10 cases in Asians. *Aus J Dermatol.* 2004;45:29–33.

Zaccaria E, Rebora A, Rongioletti F. Multiple eruptive dermatofibromas and immunosuppression: Report of two cases and review of the literature. *Int J Dermatol.* 2008;47:723–727.

Solitary Neurofibroma

Kristina L. Demas • Lynn McKinley-Grant

Diagnosis Synopsis

Solitary neurofibromas are the most common of the peripheral nerve tumor type. This well-circumscribed, benign tumor is derived from a mixture of neuromesenchymal tissue including Schwann cells, mast cells, and perineural fibroblasts. In general, these dermal lesions appear primarily during adolescence and adulthood and may increase in size and number with age. Although cutaneous neurofibromas are one of the hallmark signs of von Recklinghausen neurofibromatosis (NF), they are not an indication for NF. Certain melanocytic macules such as café au lait or café-Albright may be considered variants of neurofibromas. Typically, the order of appearance of clinical features in NF is café au lait spots, axillary freckling, Lisch nodules, and neurofibromas.

Look For

Neurofibromas can range in size from 0.2 to 2.0 cm. Various morphologies of neurofibromas exist. Look for large skin-colored papules, pedunculated papules, or dome-shaped nodules on general skin and mucosal regions (Fig. 4-210). Areas most commonly affected include the head, neck and upper body.

Diagnostic Pearls

With direct pressure, the lesion seems to "button hole" or invaginate into the underlying dermis as if it is being pushed

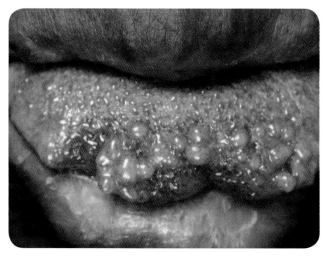

Figure 4-210 Irregular neurofibromas at the tip of the tongue.

deeper into the skin. Subcutaneous neurofibromas are tender and sometimes painful. Lesions may be pruritic. Typically soft centrally, these lesions can be single or multiple. When multiple, they may be indicative of the presence of NF and further workup is highly recommended. However, café au lait macules are not always associated with NF. Malignant transformation of solitary neurofibromas is possible, but highly uncommon.

Differential Diagnosis and Pitfalls

The diagnosis is usually self-evident. Some of the most common masqueraders are the following:

- Neural nevi
- Skin tag
- Lipoma
- Dermatofibroma
- Acrochordon

Best Tests

Skin biopsy. Keep in mind that solitary neurofibromas demonstrate the same histopathology as neurofibromas associated with NF. Molecular testing for NF1 is available.

Management Therapy

Solitary neurofibroma not associated with NF is surgically excised and associated with a low rate of recurrence. Do not perform an extensive NF workup for a solitary neurofibroma if other clinical features such as café au lait spots or axillary freckling are not present.

Therapy

Simple excision of lesion is curative.

Suggested Readings

Boyd KP, Korf BR, Theos A. Neurofibromatosis type 1. *J Am Acad Dermatol.* 2009;61(1):1–14.

Gottfried ON, Viskochil DH, Fults DW, et al. Molecular, genetic, and cellular pathogenesis of neurofibromas and surgical implications. *Neurosurgery.* 2006;58(1):1–16; discussion 1–16.

Theos A, Korf BR. Pathophysiology of neurofibromatosis type 1. *Ann Intern Med.* 2006;144:842–849.

Basal Cell Carcinoma

Mat Davey

Nonmelanoma skin cancers are less common in those with pigmented skin, but the diagnosis of skin cancer should never be excluded on the basis of an individual's pigmentation.

◼◼ Diagnosis Synopsis

Basal cell carcinoma (BCC), a neoplasm of basal keratinocytes, is the most common type of skin cancer. The four major subtypes of BCC are nodular, pigmented, superficial, and infiltrating. The nodular variant is the most common subtype overall; however, pigmented BCC remains the most common variant among individuals of African, Hispanic, and Asian descent. Superficial BCC is the second most common form of BCC, and it tends to occur more often on the sun-exposed areas of the trunk and extremities and in slightly younger patients. Infiltrating or morpheaform BCCs can be extensive and locally destructive and require extensive plastic surgical repair if not treated early.

BCC is primarily a disease of fair-skinned individuals and individuals with a lifetime of sun exposure. In patients with darker skin types, BCC is uncommon secondary to the protective effect of pigmentation. In these patients, secondary risk factors may include exposure to arsenic and therapeutic radiation; immunosuppression; and genetic syndromes such as xeroderma pigmentosum, Bazex syndrome, and basal cell nevus syndrome (BCNS). The incidence of BCC increases in older adults. It is largely a nonmetastasizing form of cancer. Prognosis is excellent with prompt identification and treatment.

Pediatric Patient Considerations

BCNS, also known as Gorlin syndrome and nevoid basal cell carcinoma syndrome (NBCC), is an autosomal dominant condition characterized by the development of multiple BCCs, often at an early age. Mutations associated with tumor suppressor gene Patched-1 are responsible for this syndrome. In addition to the development of multiple BCCs, associated abnormalities of the bones, soft tissue, eyes, CNS, and endocrine organs occur.

Patients with BCNS may develop complications including developmental delay and physical impairments. In addition, tumors may arise (e.g., medulloblastoma of the brain) that carry significant morbidity. No large-scale studies regarding long-term mortality rate among these patients have been completed. The condition occurs in a wide variety of cultural groups and does not have a particular ethnic or racial predilection. Spontaneous mutations occur, and penetrance is variable; therefore, lack of family history does not preclude this diagnosis.

◉ Look For

BCCs are most commonly found on sun-exposed areas—head and neck, upper chest and back, and upper extremities—but can occur on areas usually thought to be sun-protected such as the scalp (Fig. 4-211). A benign skin hamartoma or nevus sebaceus may be a precursor to a BCC.

Nodular BCCs have a pearly or translucent quality, with small telangiectases and a rolled edge or border (Fig. 4-212). As the growth enlarges, crusting usually appears over the central depression, and bleeding with minor trauma is frequent. With time, a nonhealing erosion or ulcer may form (Fig. 4-213).

Pigmented BCCs often mimic melanoma. Look for a brown, blue, or black macule, papule, or nodule with border irregularities and possible color variegation found on sun-exposed areas (Fig. 4-214). Pigmented BCCs will often have telangiectases and/or a certain degree of translucency. A rolled edge with an umbilicated (depressed) center may also be present.

Superficial BCCs typically appear as dry, scaly, flat papules or plaques that enlarge slowly and sometimes develop a

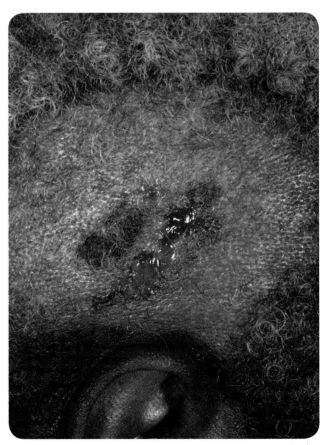

Figure 4-211 Basal cell carcinoma on scalp (hair shaved before surgery).

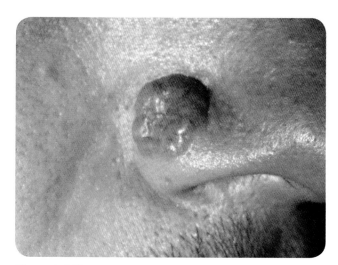

Figure 4-212 Nodular basal cell carcinoma on the side of the nose.

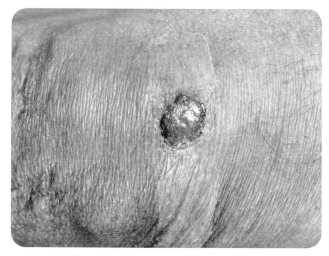

Figure 4-213 Eroded nodular basal cell carcinoma.

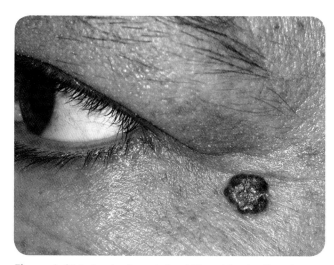

Figure 4-214 Deeply pigmented umbilicated basal cell carcinoma.

raised border (Fig. 4-215). They are typically well defined and pink to red in color, making them difficult to discern in darkly pigmented patients. This variant is encountered on the trunk more often than other subtypes of BCC.

Infiltrating or morpheaform BCCs tend to be subtle. Look for a shiny or scarlike, indurated lesion, sometimes with telangiectases, erosions, or small crusts (Fig. 4-216).

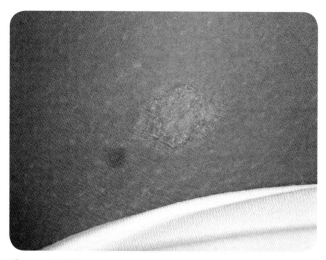

Figure 4-215 Well-bordered superficial basal cell carcinoma.

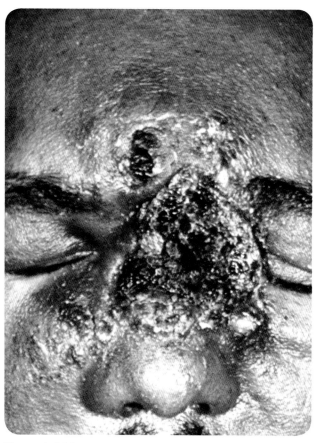

Figure 4-216 Morpheaform basal cell carcinoma in the midface.

227

Some patients present with a hypopigmented or "white" area, which is found to be a firm plaque on palpation.

Pediatric Patient Considerations

In patients with BCNS, the principal lesions (carcinomas) are 1 to 10 cm flesh-colored or pigmented papules and nodules. Carcinomas on the eyelids, axillae, and neck tend to be pedunculated. The lesions are usually symmetric about the body. They begin to appear in young children and continue to appear throughout life. They can become invasive, requiring removal.

There are distinctive small, asymmetric pits on the palms (70%) and soles (50%) that are best seen after the hand or foot has been soaked in warm water (Fig. 4-217). These pits increase in number with age and are permanent. Unilateral or bilateral mandibular jaw cysts can coexist with other bony lesions including bifid ribs, pectus excavatum, short fourth metacarpals, scoliosis, and kyphosis.

These patients have characteristic facies with hypertelorism, frontal bossing, and broad nasal root. Other anomalies include undescended testes, hydrocephalus, strabismus, dystopia canthorum, blindness from coloboma, and glaucoma. Agenesis of the corpus callosum, medulloblastoma, and mental retardation are rare.

Diagnostic Pearls

More than one BCC before the age of 30 may suggest BCNS or exposure to therapeutic ionizing irradiation. Usually, these lesions are larger than they appear clinically. Development of BCC in patients with darkly pigmented skin also warrants consideration of underlying genetic defect or secondary risk factor.

A variant of albinism present in Puerto Ricans and known as Hermansky-Pudlak syndrome results in increased incidence of BCC and is associated with hemorrhagic diathesis secondary to platelet dysfunction.

?? Differential Diagnosis and Pitfalls

- A scar may present similar to infiltrating BCC.
- Merkel cell carcinoma
- Melanoma
- Microcystic adnexal carcinoma
- Other adnexal neoplasms
- Amelanotic melanoma
- Dermatofibrosarcoma protuberans
- Morphea, localized
- Trichoepithelioma
- Seborrheic keratosis
- Bowen disease
- Fibrous papule of the face
- Molluscum contagiosum
- Vascular proliferation—e.g., hemangioma

✓ Best Tests

- Skin biopsy. If infiltrating BCC is suspected, perform a deep or large enough biopsy to allow the dermatopathologist to adequately subtype the tumor.
- A careful past medical and family history should be conducted to evaluate for secondary risk factors (e.g., radiation exposure) or for other affected family members.

Pediatric Patient Considerations

If BCNS is suspected, a full history and physical exam is necessary to evaluate for associated findings (e.g., palmar pits, broad nasal root with frontal bossing). Genetic studies to evaluate for 9q22-31 mutation may be performed. Radiographs of the chest, skull, and jaw are useful. Lamellar calcification of the falx cerebri is usually seen.

▲▲ Management Pearls

- Proper care cannot be delivered if the specific subtype is not known and the treating physician does not understand the natural course of the disease.

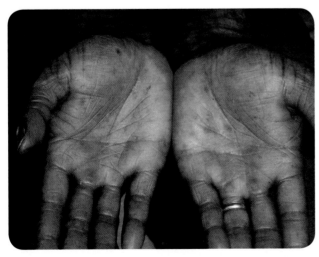

Figure 4-217 Palm pits in a patient with basal cell nevus syndrome.

- Infiltrating BCCs are a subtype of BCC that must be treated appropriately and often require Mohs micrographic surgery. Delayed or inappropriate surgery can lead to further tumor infiltration. Small "strands" of tumor cells can infiltrate widely in the skin and be indistinct from normal skin (tip of the iceberg phenomenon). The diagnosis is made by initial biopsy, and if reports from the pathologist do not mention the subtype of basal cell, then proceed with caution.
- Advise sun avoidance and sun-protection measures such as sunscreen and protective clothing. Patients with BCC should be followed by a dermatologist to assess for recurrence and the appearance of new lesions.

Pediatric Patient Considerations

- Patients with BCNS should be followed closely and taught to be aware of skin changes. They should avoid sun exposure and use sunblock (SPF > 50). Avoid radiation exposure, as radiation leads to tumor growth. At-risk or affected children should be screened clinically; imaging should be used sparingly. Consultation with a dermatologist, dentist, cardiologist, oncologist, and orthopedic surgeon is important. The parents and patient should be offered genetic counseling.
- The prognosis for this condition is good. Rarely do patients develop medulloblastomas or deep epitheliomas.
- Multiple excisions can cause significant scarring.

Therapy

Treatment must be individualized, but simple electrodesiccation and curettage (ED&C), excision, or cryosurgery is often effective for nodular and superficial BCCs. X-ray therapy is an accepted treatment modality for patients who are not good candidates for surgical removal but should be used cautiously and with circumscription since BCCs have been induced in skin after X-ray therapy for internal malignancy.

BCCs that are recurrent, primary BCCs occurring in the nasolabial fold areas, and BCCs with the morpheaform histopathology should be referred for Mohs micrographic surgery so that clear margins can be established intraoperatively by frozen section.

The following therapies may have lower cure rates than surgical removal, but when used correctly in selected patients, they can offer significant advantages:

- Topical imiquimod 5%
- Photodynamic therapy
- Topical 5-fluorouracil has been used with some success, but penetration is an issue. It may not destroy malignant cells in the superficial dermis.
- Cryosurgery
- CO_2 laser

Suggested Readings

Carucci JA, Leffell DJ. Basal cell carcinoma. In: Fitzpatrick TB, Wolff K, eds. *Fitzpatrick's Dermatology in General Medicine.* 7th Ed. New York, NY: McGraw-Hill; 2008:1036–1042.

Garcia C, Holman J, Poletti E. Mohs surgery: commentaries and controversies. *Int J Dermatol.* 2005;44(11):893–905.

Oro AE. Basal cell nevus syndrome. In: Fitzpatrick TB, Wolff K, eds. *Fitzpatrick's Dermatology in General Medicine.* 7th Ed. New York, NY: McGraw-Hill; 2008:1042–1048.

Pruvost-Balland C, Gorry P, Boutet N, et al. Clinical and genetic study in 22 patients with basal cell nevus syndrome. *Ann Dermatol Venereol.* 2006;133(2):117–123.

Rubin AI, Chen EH, Ratner D. Basal-cell carcinoma. *N Engl J Med.* 2005;353(21):2262–2269.

Taylor SF, Cook AE, Leatherbarrow B. Review of patients with basal cell nevus syndrome. *Ophthal Plast Reconstr Surg.* 2006;22(4):259–265.

Pilomatricoma

Saurabh Singh

■■ Diagnosis Synopsis

Pilomatricoma, also known as calcifying epithelioma of Malherbe or pilomatrixoma, is a benign, cutaneous neoplasm derived from cells of the hair matrix. Mutations in the gene that encode for beta-catenin are present in these lesions. Pilomatricomas tend to arise during early childhood as a solitary, asymptomatic, firm, skin-colored to blue nodule or cyst. Although usually sporadic in incidence, familial cases of pilomatricomas have been reported. Additionally, multiple pilomatricomas have been observed in patients with myotonic dystrophy, Rubinstein-Taybi syndrome, Turner syndrome, and Gardner syndrome.

Pediatric Patient Considerations

Pilomatricomas have been reported in infants but tend to arise during early childhood, usually before puberty.

(●) Look For

Usually single, small tumors or cystlike lesions, with either normal overlying skin or a bluish surface color (Fig. 4-218). Lesions typically range between <1 and 3 cm in size. These hard nodular growths are most commonly found on the face, arms, or upper trunk. There is no skin type or ethnic predilection, and cases of pilomatricomas have been reported in many countries worldwide.

●● Diagnostic Pearls

When superficial, pilomatricomas may have a chalky-white appearance. Often, the lesions assume a multifaceted, angulated appearance when the overlying skin is stretched over (tent sign). If deeper within the skin, the lesion may look blue-colored. Upon palpation, pilomatricomas have an irregular "meteorite"-like topography.

?? Differential Diagnosis and Pitfalls

- Epidermal inclusion cysts can frequently be identified by observing an overlying punctum.
- A pilomatricoma is typically firmer and less regular in shape than a dermoid cyst.
- Glomus tumor is painful and tends to involve the nail unit.
- Osteoma cutis presents as a firm dermal nodule and may be clinically indistinguishable from pilomatricoma (Fig. 4-219).
- Calcinosis cutis also presents as a firm dermal nodule and may be clinically indistinguishable from pilomatricoma.

Pediatric Patient Differential Diagnosis and Pitfalls

- Epidermoid cyst
- Dermoid cyst
- Glomus tumor
- Osteoma cutis
- Calcinosis cutis
- Dermatofibroma

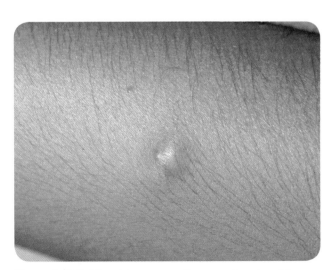

Figure 4-218 Pilomatricoma presenting as an irregular white papule on the arm.

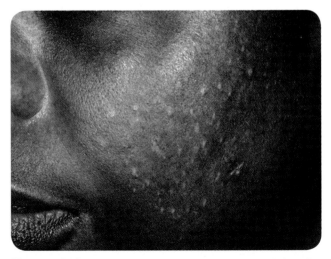

Figure 4-219 Individual lesions of osteoma cutis can mimic a pilomatricoma.

230

Best Tests

Skin biopsy specimen will reveal an encapsulated dermal tumor with characteristic "ghost" or "shadow" cells.

Management Pearls

Incompletely excised lesions may recur. If multiple recurrences are observed, excision with negative margins should be undertaken to rule out the possibility of a pilomatrical carcinoma.

Therapy

Simple excision is the best method of removing this benign neoplasm.

Suggested Readings

Al-Khateeb TH, Hamasha AA. Pilomatricoma of the maxillofacial area in the northern regional Jordanian population: Report of 31 cases. *J Oral Maxillofacial Surg.* 2007;65(2):261–266.

Golpour M. Evaluation of characteristics of patients with pilomatricoma in Mazandaran Province, 1996–2006. *Pak J Biol Sci.* 2009;12(6):548–550.

Holme SA, Varma S, Holt PJ. The first case of exophytic pilomatricoma in an Asian male. *Pediatr Dermatol.* 2001;18(6):498–500.

Jayalakshmi P, Looi LM. Cutaneous adnexal neoplasms in biopsy specimens processed in the Department of Pathology, University of Malaya. *Ann Acad Med (Singapore).* 1996;25(4):522–525.

Lan MY, Lan MC, Ho CY, et al. Pilomatricoma of the head and neck: a retrospective review of 179 cases. *Arch Otolaryngol Head Neck Surg.* 2003;129(12):1327–1330.

Noguchi H, Hayashibara T, Ono T. A statistical study of calcifying epithelioma, focusing on the sites of origin. *J Dermatol.* 1995;22(1):24–27.

Zamanian A, Farshchian M, Farschchian M. Clinical and histopathologic study of pilomatricoma in Iran between 1992 and 2005. *Pediatr Dermatol.* 2008;25(2):268–269.

Keloid and Hypertrophic Scar

Lynn McKinley-Grant

■■ Diagnosis Synopsis

Keloids are dense, fibrous tissue nodules, typically found at areas of previously traumatized skin (burns, lacerations, incision scars), or arising spontaneously on normal skin. Lesions may be single or multiple. Over weeks to months, these large nodules can become painful, tender, and pruritic and grow to become very large (up to 30 cm). They can cause chronic discomfort, be disfiguring, and restrict normal tissue motion. Most patients start developing keloids in their twenties.

Keloids are most frequent in individuals of African descent and those of Mediterranean ancestry, but they can appear in any race or ethnicity. Darker skin types have significantly higher tendency to form keloids, with an incidence as high as 16% in black Africans. There is likely a genetic basis for the tendency to develop keloids.

A distinction should be made between a keloid and a hypertrophic scar. All trauma that involves the dermis will heal with a scar; however, in certain individuals, the scar is much larger and thicker than what is considered normal. These lesions are termed hypertrophic scars. In contrast to keloids, hypertrophic scars are always preceded by trauma and always confined to the margin of the wound (Fig. 4-220). Also, hypertrophic scars appear immediately after trauma and show a tendency to gradually regress, whereas keloids can be delayed in appearance and are thought to very rarely spontaneously resolve.

◉ Look For

Keloids usually appear smooth and shiny. They can be red, hyperpigmented, or skin-colored, have regular or irregularly shaped ridges, and are usually firm to the touch. They

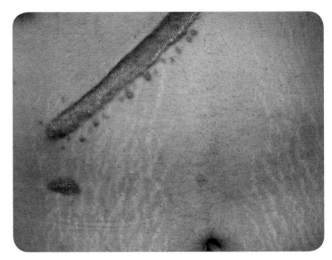

Figure 4-221 Keloid at an incision site with multiple tiny keloids at suture sites.

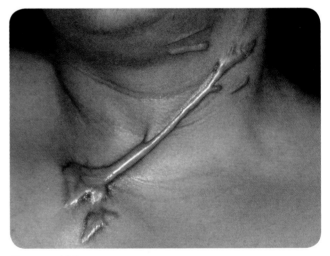

Figure 4-222 Linear keloids from the spilling of a caustic substance.

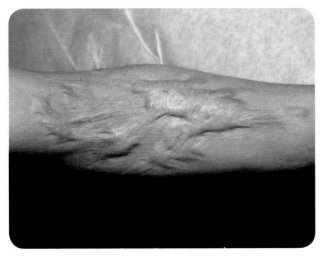

Figure 4-220 Hypertrophic irregular burn scar.

232

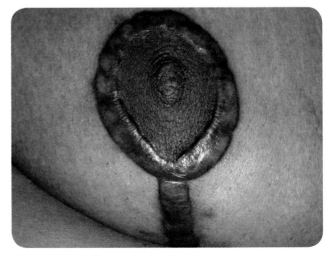

Figure 4-223 Circumareolar keloid.

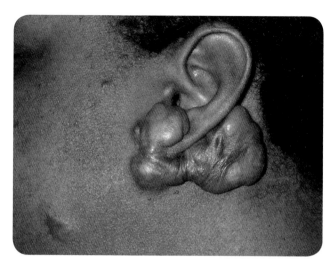

Figure 4-224 A common location for keloids, which may extend beyond the site of an ear lobe piercing.

develop projections that extend beyond the area of original trauma (Figs. 4-221–4-223). The growths can mostly be found on the neck, ears, extremities, and upper trunk, especially the chest (Fig. 4-224). Keloids are rarely found on the central face, eyelids, and genitals.

Diagnostic Pearls

- Keloids very rarely involute and are not confined to the margins of trauma.
- They commonly will occur in acne scars on the chest and back.
- Growth of keloids can be accompanied by pruritus.

?? Differential Diagnosis and Pitfalls

- Hypertrophic scars—See "Diagnosis Synopsis" above.
- Sarcoidosis—can localize in scars and form nodules clinically similar to keloids
- Foreign body reaction—should be associated with a history of trauma to the site
- Dermatofibroma
- Dermatofibrosarcoma protuberans
- Morphea
- Xanthoma disseminatum (sclerotic form)
- Scleroderma
- Leukemia cutis
- Lobomycosis (keloidal blastomycosis)—infection with *Lacazia loboi*

✓ Best Tests

The diagnosis is often made using history and appearance. If there is doubt, a biopsy will confirm the clinical diagnosis.

▲▲ Management Pearls

Surgical excision of keloids is inevitably fraught with the possibility of the keloid recurring in larger size than before the excision. Surgical excision is advised only if there is a post-op plan that includes regular follow-up for adjunctive therapy such as intralesional corticosteroids (5 to 20 mg/mL), pressure bandages, and/or silicone sheeting.

Therapy

Keloids are extremely difficult to treat.

Prevention and patient education are very important. Surgical wounds should parallel skin creases as much as possible, and wounds should be closed with minimal tension. Avoid making incisions overlying joints. Elective cosmetic surgery should be avoided in patients who are known keloid formers. The use of buried sutures and the application of pressure dressings and garments immediately postoperatively may reduce the likelihood of keloid formation.

- There has been some success in treating small earlobe keloids with pressure "clip-on" earrings.
- Some keloids and hypertrophic scars respond to topically applied silicone sheeting.
- Erythematous and inflamed keloids often respond to intralesional triamcinolone (10 to 40 mg/kg), depending on the density of the keloid tissue and the ability to infiltrate the lesion. Use small quantities of high-concentration triamcinolone (>20 mg/mL) to avoid skin atrophy.

Other therapies include the following:

- Intralesional interferon, alpha and gamma
- Cryosurgery plus intralesional steroids (caution: may result in hypopigmentation)
- Surgery plus local radiation therapy
- Laser therapy: argon, CO_2, Nd:YAG, or pulsed dye laser to actively expanding lesions
- Imiquimod or intralesional verapamil postexcision
- Intralesional 5-FU
- Radiation therapy
- Topical tamoxifen

Suggested Readings

Gragnani A, Warde M, Furtado F, et al. Topical tamoxifen therapy in hypertrophic scars or keloids in burns. *Arch Dermatol Res.* 2010;302(1):1–4. Epub 2009 Jul 28.

Shridharani SM, Magarakis M, Manson PN, et al. The emerging role of antineoplastic agents in the treatment of keloids and hypertrophic scars: a review. *Ann Plast Surg.* 2010;64(3):355–361.

Xanthelasma Palpebrarum

Chris G. Adigun

Diagnosis Synopsis

Xanthelasma palpebrarum is a type of plane xanthoma of the eyelids, and it is the most common type of xanthoma. Approximately half of patients with xanthelasma have a lipid disorder, with the remainder being normolipemic. Women are affected more than men. Although xanthomas themselves are often asymptomatic, investigations into and treatment of any underlying cause are warranted to prevent morbidity from lipid disorders and to prevent xanthelasma from progressing.

Note: See "Xanthomas" for information on other types of xanthomas.

Look For

Soft, yellow-to-orange, oblong macules, papules, and plaques, primarily on the superior eyelids near the medial canthus (Fig. 4-225). They frequently occur symmetrically and may be present on all four eyelids. In darkly pigmented skin, they may appear hypopigmented or hyperpigmented, with or without a faint yellowish hue.

Diagnostic Pearls

When xanthelasma palpebrarum is present, be careful to check for other visible signs of hyperlipidemia, such as cutaneous xanthomas over joints and in intertriginous locations, as well as arcus senilis in the cornea.

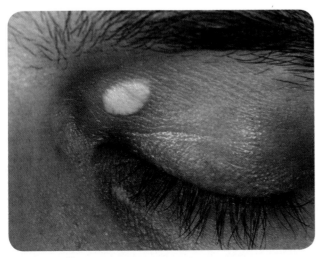

Figure 4-225 Xanthelasma palpebrarum usually is a yellow well-circumscribed plaque presenting medially on the upper lid.

Differential Diagnosis and Pitfalls

- Sebaceous hyperplasia
- Syringoma
- Adnexal cysts
- Epidermoid cysts—typically unilateral and not as yellow or orange in color
- Appendageal tumors—less obviously yellow
- Molluscum contagiosum
- Amyloidosis
- Lipid proteinosis
- Necrobiotic xanthogranuloma

Best Tests

Xanthelasma palpebrarum is usually a clinical diagnosis. However, if necessary, biopsy will confirm it. Xanthelasma is present at least 50% of the time in the absence of any other disease process. However, all new patients presenting with xanthelasma should be evaluated with a complete lipid profile, including fasting serum lipid panel consisting of cholesterol, triglycerides, VLDL, LDL, and HDL.

Management Pearls

- For patients with xanthomas that have an underlying lipid abnormality, reduction of the fat content of the diet is critical. It is recommended to keep total triglyceride levels under 1,500 mg/dL. Medium-chain triglycerides (MCTs) can be substituted for dietary fat. In addition, exercise and dietary modifications should be recommended to all patients with lipid abnormalities.
- For patients seeking mechanical removal of their xanthomas, they should be adequately counseled that recurrence is common after surgical or other mechanical removal. Recurrence is not as common with xanthelasma, however.

Therapy

For hyperlipemic patients, dietary modifications and exercise should be implemented. Many will need systemic lipid-lowering therapy in the form of statins, fibrates, nicotinic acid, or bile-acid binding resins. While these measures are important in the treatment of hyperlipidemia, they typically do not cure the cutaneous xanthomas.

Xanthelasma is unique among the xanthomas in that mechanical intervention is often successful. For the cosmetic treatment of the lesions themselves, the following treatments are options:

- Surgical excision
- Laser ablation—carbon dioxide, argon, Er:YAG, Nd:YAG, or pulsed dye
- Chemical cauterization with topical dichloroacetic or trichloroacetic acid (TCA). Pigmentary changes and scarring (uncommonly) are possible side effects of TCA treatment.
- Light electrodesiccation

Patients should be advised that there is a risk of scarring and recurrence after definitive treatment. For patients with darkly pigmented skin, the chance for either transient or permanent pigmentation abnormalities is very high. Patients with darker skin should, thus, be counseled on these risks prior to intervention.

Suggested Readings

Bergman R. The pathogenesis and clinical significance of xanthelasma palpebrarum. *J Am Acad Dermatol.* 1994;30(2 Pt 1):236–242.

Jialal I, Omar MA, Bredenkamp B, et al. Type III hyperlipoproteinaemia in a black patient. A case report. *S Afr Med J.* 1981;59(8):267–268.

Juvenile Xanthogranuloma
Rodolfo E. Chirinos

■■ Diagnosis Synopsis

Juvenile xanthogranulomas (JXGs) are usually benign, self-limited, regressing, fibrohistiocytic lesions occurring mostly in infancy and early childhood and less commonly in adolescents and adults, who usually present in their third or fourth decade. Lesions are ten times more common in whites and usually appear early in infancy, with up to one-fourth of patients presenting at birth. In childhood, male patients may be affected more often than female patients, whereas adult patients show no sexual predilection.

In both children and adults, JXGs are primarily solitary lesions occurring most often on the head and neck as well as the upper trunk and in very rare cases the palms, soles, digits, anogenital, and intertriginous areas. Oral lesions are exceedingly uncommon but have been reported in both whites and Asians. Like the cutaneous lesions, they typically present as a solitary lesion in infancy and childhood, with a slight male predominance, and occur more frequently in the midline of the palate, lower lip, tongue, and gingiva. Although uncommon, multiple skin lesions may be seen in adults and children, especially on the head and neck of infants <6 months of age.

In infants, lesions characteristically regress within 3 to 6 years, and nearly one-third of children will have complete resolution within 6 months of onset. Lesions may resolve with a trace or leave behind wrinkled, atrophic, or anetodermalike changes to the skin with or without hyperpigmentation. In patients with multiple JXGs, regression may occur at different rates over time. Solitary lesions in adults are typically excised, making spontaneous involution patterns difficult to ascertain, and around one-half may regress in adults with multiple lesions. Spontaneous resolution of oral lesions is rare.

Systemic involvement is rare, particularly in adults, but can occur with or without cutaneous lesions, with the eye being the most common extracutaneous site (0.3% to 0.5%). Children with multiple cutaneous lesions, regardless of size, and those <2 years of age are at highest risk for intraocular lesions.

◉ Look For

JXGs present as discrete, well-demarcated, waxy, nontender, smooth, dome-shaped or flat-topped, round to oval papules or nodules—typically 0.3 to 2 cm in diameter—that are firm and rubbery in consistency with occasional superficial telangiectases and rarely umbilicated (Figs. 4-226–4-229). Early lesions appear skin-colored or pink to red, gradually becoming more yellow over time and eventually reddish-orange to yellow-brown, with larger lesions occasionally having a reddish hue to their base.

The most common location is the head and neck, followed by the upper torso and arms. Most children have a solitary lesion, but some are affected with multiple lesions that may be few in number or range in the hundreds. Various cutaneous variants have been reported including clustered, plaquelike, infiltrative, pedunculated, and lichenoid lesions. Another less common variant is the giant JXG, which is typically a solitary nodule (>2 cm in diameter) present at birth (i.e., congenital giant JXG) and located on the upper back or proximal extremities with a strong female predominance. Lesions may show rapid growth over several weeks to months, resulting in ulceration and crusting and followed by spontaneous regression. None has been associated with systemic JXGs.

Children with ocular involvement almost always have multiple cutaneous JXGs with onset of eye lesions usually

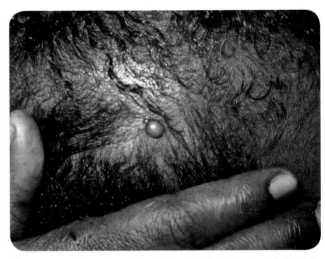

Figure 4-226 Single smooth orange-red papule of juvenile xanthogranuloma in a typical location.

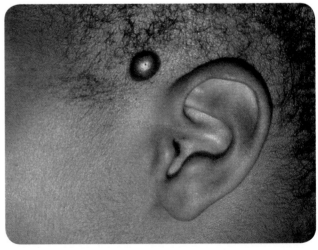

Figure 4-227 Dermal nevus-appearing lesion of juvenile xanthogranuloma.

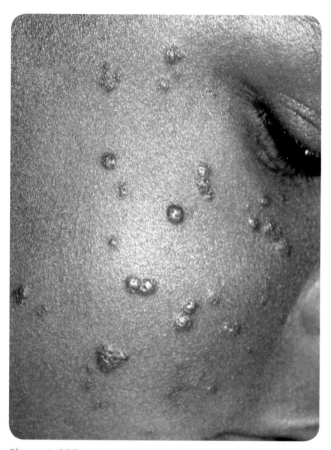

Figure 4-228 Multiple juvenile nevoxanthogranulomata on the face.

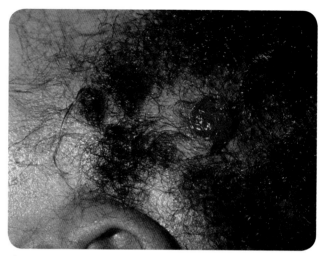

Figure 4-229 Very red, ulcerated lesion of juvenile xanthoma granuloma.

within the first 2 years of life and primarily unilateral. In adults, intraocular JXG is extremely rare and typically presents without skin lesions. Multiple skin lesions—even in the absence of eye symptoms—should prompt an ophthalmic evaluation, as patients are often asymptomatic except adults, who are often symptomatic with hyphema and/or inflammation at clinical presentation. Ocular signs may develop in 10% of patients and most commonly involve the uvea, primarily the iris and ciliary body, followed by the eyelid (which has a tendency to present later). Frequent presenting signs include an asymptomatic mass in the iris with a change in its color (heterochromia iridis), typically a yellowish iridic mass; secondary glaucoma, spontaneous hyphema (hemorrhage into the anterior chamber); iridocyclitis (anterior uveitis); as well as redness of the eye (indicating hyphema or uveitis) and tearing. Other sites of involvement include the conjunctiva, sclera, limbus, cornea, retina, and optic nerve. Involvement of the limbus and sclera has been reported in individuals of African descent and often presents as an elevated, fixed, telangiectatic/vascular skin-colored, pink, yellow-orange, or salmon-colored lesion. Slit-lamp examination is required for proper evaluation, as involvement of the iris may be diffuse and subclinical. Hemorrhages are generally spontaneous because of the extreme friability of the lesions, particularly

those involving the iris, with a risk of hyphema and uncontrolled glaucoma. Parents should be taught to recognize these acute signs, as prompt diagnosis and intervention are required in order to minimize complications. Any patient with a lesion of the iris or hyphema associated with elevated intraocular pressure should be evaluated for JXG, and the absence of skin lesions should not rule out JXG, as lesions can often regress spontaneously. Routine screening does not appear to be indicated in patients with solitary lesions.

Systemic JXG may occur in up to one-fifth of patients, often without evidence of cutaneous disease, and frequently affects two or more organ systems. Adults do not appear to present with systemic disease, and in children, extracutaneous lesions occur more often in male infants. When present, cutaneous JXGs usually precede the development of visceral complications. The most commonly reported site—regardless of skin involvement—is the eye, with the subcutis being the second most common site, followed by similar incidence in the central nervous system (CNS), lung, liver, and spleen. Other sites of involvement include the salivary glands, oropharynx, larynx, pericardium, omentum, retroperitoneum, colon, kidneys, ovaries, testes, penis, and skeletal muscle—most commonly the paraspinal muscles of the back. Significant involvement of other extracutaneous organs will present with clinical findings consistent with mass effects from the infiltrated lesion (e.g., proptosis, uveitis). In those patients with infiltration of vital organs such as the CNS and liver, JXG behaves aggressively and may cause death. Most patients with CNS involvement exhibit a latent period months to years between the recognition of skin manifestations and the onset of neurological findings, which include ataxia, seizures, subdural effusions, increased intracranial pressure, developmental delay, diabetes insipidus, and other neurologic deficits. It is uncertain whether occult disease discovered during routine staging warrants therapy, as most visceral lesions spontaneously regress over time.

Isolated cases have been reported of JXG occurring in children with insulin-dependent diabetes mellitus, urticaria pigmentosa, solitary mastocytoma, Niemann-Pick disease, aquagenic pruritus, and monocytic leukemia. It remains uncertain whether these diseases are truly associated with JXG or simply coincidental in their occurrence.

 Diagnostic Pearls

There should be no pigment in a JXG. The presence of a pigment network or any pigmented globules on magnification (i.e., dermoscopy) favors a Spitz nevus over JXG.

?? Differential Diagnosis and Pitfalls

The primary differential of red-to-yellow papules on a young child are JXG, Spitz nevus, and mastocytoma. Mastocytomas have a similar color to JXGs but develop an urticarial wheal when rubbed or stroked (i.e., positive Darier sign). A Spitz nevus is pigmented and does not regress over time. Information about oral and ocular lesion differentials can be found on VisualDx online. (If you are a first-time online user, go to www.essentialdermatology.com/pigmented; if you already have your password set up, go directly to www.visualdx.com/visualdx.)

Differential Diagnosis of Cutaneous Lesions

- Non-Langerhans cell histiocytoses
- Langerhans cell histiocytoses
- Mastocytoma
- Spitz nevus
- Diffuse normolipemic plane xanthoma
- Plexiform xanthoma
- Hyperlipemic xanthomas
- Dermatofibroma
- Epidermoid cyst
- Amelanotic melanoma
- Fibroma
- Molluscum contagiosum
- Cryptococcosis
- Dermal nevus
- Neurofibroma
- Necrobiotic xanthogranuloma
- Keratoacanthoma
- Schwannoma
- Leiomyoma
- Pyogenic granuloma
- Hemangioma
- Nodular fasciitis (pseudosarcomatous)

- Fibrosarcoma
- Rhabdomyosarcoma
- Malignant fibrous histiocytoma
- Lymphoproliferative conditions
- Alopecia mucinosa (clustered JXG of the scalp)
- Alopecia neoplastica (clustered JXG of the scalp)
- Rhabdomyosarcoma (giant JXG)
- Giant cell fibroblastoma (giant JXG)
- Juvenile nodular fasciitis (giant JXG)
- Dermatofibrosarcoma protuberans (giant JXG)

 Best Tests

Histopathological features are dependent on stage of evolution, as xanthomization, inflammation, and fibrosis are later developments. Early lesions show a monomorphous, non–lipid-containing histiocytic infiltrate in the upper half of the dermis. Mature lesions demonstrate nodular, dense, sheet-like collections of lipid-containing macrophages with foamy cytoplasms (foam cells) and Touton-type giant cells, mainly distributed in the superficial dermis and on the border of the infiltrate. The overlying epidermis tends to be thin, and there may be eosinophils, lymphocytes, and rarely, plasma cells sparsely scattered throughout the lesion. Fibrosis is a variable feature, increasing in older, regressing lesions. Extension into the subcutaneous tissue, fascia, and peripheral muscle may occur in up to one-third of cases and contains fewer Touton-type giant cells and more abundant eosinophils. Immuno-histochemistry is characteristically negative for S100 and CD1a while positive for vimentin, CD68, and factor XIIIa. On electron microscopy, histiocytes show absence of Birbeck granules.

 Management Pearls

- Referral for ophthalmologic examination should be obtained in children, especially those <2 years of age, presenting with multiple JXGs followed by yearly or semiannual ophthalmic screening. Physical and mental development is normal as are serum lipid levels.
- Examine children with JXG for multiple café au lait macules and review their family history for signs of neurofibromatosis. Those with multiple JXGs or a family history of neurofibromatosis should undergo a total body skin exam regularly to check for the presence of café au lait macules. Although uncommon, children with con-current neurofibromatosis type 1 (NF-1) and JXG carry a 20- to 32-fold higher risk of developing juvenile chronic myelogenous leukemia than do patients with NF-1 without JXG. Other hematologic malignancies reported to occur in association with JXGs—prior to, simultaneously, or after their presentation—include acute lymphoblastic

leukemia, monocytic leukemia, histiomonocytic reticulosis, and juvenile myelomonocytic leukemia.

- Adults over 65 years of age who present with multiple JXGs should undergo a complete hematologic workup to screen for hematologic abnormalities. Similarly, lesions may develop before, during, or following presentation of a hematologic disorder; essential thrombocytosis, monoclonal gammopathy, B-cell acute lymphoblastic lymphoma, large B-cell lymphoma, chronic lymphocytic leukemia, and adult T-cell leukemia/lymphoma have been reported.

Therapy

In the majority of patients, cutaneous JXG remains an uncomplicated, self-healing disorder, regardless of appearance. Therefore, conservative management is recommended with excision reserved for symptomatic lesions. Parents should be reassured that lesions tend to resolve spontaneously.

Intraocular JXG is most responsive to treatment when diagnosed early and in the absence of hyphema. Symptomatic ocular lesions may be treated with topical, intralesional, or systemic corticosteroids as well as methotrexate and, for those refractory to local and systemic therapy, low-dose radiation therapy or excision. Iridectomy should be kept as last resort since lesions are relatively vascular and can bleed profusely.

Visceral JXG requires treatment in patients who are either symptomatic or develop organ dysfunction, and clinicians must weigh the risks of uncertain efficacy of anti-JXG therapy against the capacity of lesions to regress even in patients with multisystem involvement. Such visceral lesions may be treated with a combination of systemic corticosteroids and cyclosporine, vinblastine, methotrexate, etoposide, or 6-mercaptopurine. Overall, clinicians should strongly emphasize supportive care and reserve chemotherapy or irradiation for unresectable disease that is life threatening or progressive, utilizing the least toxic modality.

Suggested Readings

Chang MW. Update on juvenile xanthogranuloma: Unusual cutaneous and systemic variants. *Semin Cutan Med Surg.* 1999;18(3):195–205.

Freyer DR, Kennedy R, Bostrom BC, et al. Juvenile xanthogranuloma: forms of systemic disease and their clinical implications. *J Pediatr.* 1996;129:227–237.

Hernandez-Martin A, Baselga E, Drolet BA, et al. Juvenile xanthogranuloma. *J Am Acad Dermatol.* 1997;36:355–367.

Kwan CY, Min LL, Chung LC, et al. Intraoral juvenile xanthogranuloma. A case report and literature review. *Oral Surg Oral Med Oral Pathol Oral Radiol Endod.* 1996;81(4):450–453.

Larson MJ, Bandel C, Eichhorn PJ, et al. Concurrent development of eruptive xanthogranulomas and hematologic malignancy: two case reports. *J Am Acad Dermatol.* 2004;50(6):976–978.

Nayak S, Acharjya B, Devi B, et al. Multiple xanthogranuloma in an adult. *Indian J Dermatol Venereol Leprol.* 2008;74(1):67–68.

Newman B, Hu W, Nigro K, et al. Aggressive histiocytic disorders that can involve the skin. *J Am Acad Dermatol.* 2007;56:302–316.

Parmley VC, George DP, Fannin LA. Juvenile xanthogranuloma of the iris in an adult. *Arch Ophthalmol.* 1998;116(3):377–379.

Shimoyama T, Horie N, Ide F et al. Juvenile xanthogranuloma of the lip: case report and literature review. *J Oral Maxillofac Surg.* 2000;58(6):677–679.

Shoo BA, Shinkai K, McCalmont TH, et al. Xanthogranulomas associated with hematologic malignancy in adulthood. *J Am Acad Dermatol.* 2008;59(3):488–493.

Stover DG, Alapati S, Regueira O, et al. Treatment of juvenile xanthogranuloma. *Pediatr Blood Cancer.* 2008;51(1):130–133.

Vendal Z, Walton D, Chen T. Glaucoma in juvenile xanthogranuloma. *Semin Ophthalmol.* 2006;21(3):191–194.

Yanoff M, Perry HD. Juvenile xanthogranuloma of the corneoscleral limbus. *Arch Ophthalmol.* 1995;113(7):915–917.

Molluscum Contagiosum

Saurabh Singh

■■ Diagnosis Synopsis

Molluscum contagiosum is a communicable disease caused by infection with a DNA poxvirus. It manifests as smooth, firm papules with central umbilication. Molluscum contagiosum may be spread by direct contact (most often in children) or via sexual contact in adults. Higher rates of infection have been linked to young age, crowded living conditions, skin-to-skin contact, sharing of fomites, and living in tropical climates. No association has been demonstrated with sex, seasonality, or hygiene. Molluscum contagiosum infections have also been associated with swimming pools.

Many cases are asymptomatic, but there can be surrounding irritation in association with pruritus. The disease is relatively chronic and may persist for several months and up to 2 years before disappearing. Autoinoculation allows the spread of lesions prior to resolution. In the immunocompetent host, the disease tends to be self-limited. This condition can be found worldwide and has been reported in many different ethnic populations.

Pediatric Patient Considerations

Molluscum contagiosum predominately affects children. It can be spread through intimate contact in sexually active teens.

Immunocompromised Patient Considerations

An increasing number of adults have been afflicted with this virus since the advent of HIV/AIDS. Molluscum lesions often have an atypical appearance in individuals with HIV/AIDS, such as "giant molluscum" or a furunclelike presentation. In addition, molluscum lesions can become widespread in immunocompromised patients.

◉ Look For

Presents with smooth, whitish or skin-colored, 2- to 6-mm pearly papules with a central umbilication (depression),

often clustered together (Figs. 4-230–4-233). (Central umbilication, which can be absent and is not a required morphologic feature, is similar to that of the vesicles of herpes; however, molluscum lesions are solid papules as opposed to the fluid-filled vesicles of herpes infections.) With excoriation, lesions can be spread directly, forming a linear array of mollusca.

In adults, molluscum contagiosum is usually sexually transmitted, and lesions are, therefore, more commonly distributed on the mons pubis, genitalia, perineum, inner thighs, and lower abdomen (Fig. 4-234). This is not true in children.

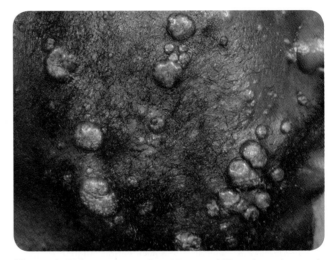

Figure 4-230 Multiple small and large umbilicated papules: a mix of molluscum contagiosum and giant molluscum contagiosum.

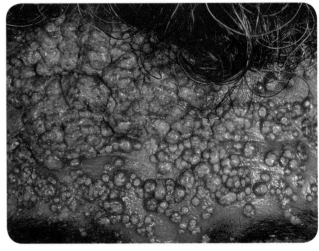

Figure 4-231 Forehead with almost confluent molluscum contagiosum papules.

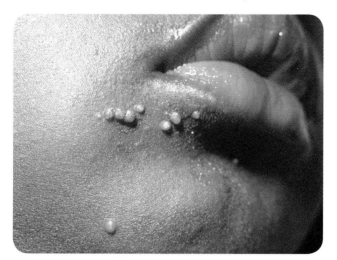

Figure 4-232 Smooth linear papules of molluscum contagiosum, some of which are linear and closely grouped from autoinoculation.

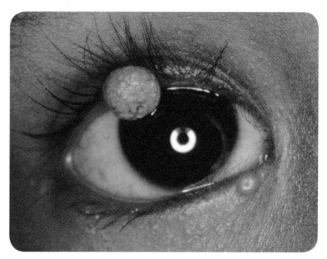

Figure 4-233 Large molluscum on upper lid and a small one on the lower lid; this is not an unusual location for the disease in children.

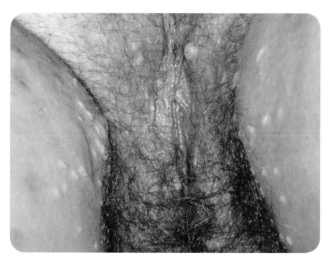

Figure 4-234 Mollusca are very common in the genital regions of both sexes.

Lesions are rarely found in the mouth or on the palms or soles. As lesions resolve, they may become more inflamed and erythematous, causing a characteristic "molluscum dermatitis."

In skin of color, mollusca can appear hyperpigmented.

Immunocompromised Patient Considerations

A variant is giant molluscum (sometimes >3 cm), which can be seen in AIDS patients but can also occur in those with normal immunity.

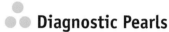

Diagnostic Pearls

- The central umbilication within a firm papule is highly suggestive of molluscum contagiosum. The umbilication may be difficult to see but becomes more obvious when the lesion is gently frozen with liquid nitrogen. Larger lesions will frequently have more than one umbilication.
- Lesions may have a linear distribution due to local inoculation and spread. Lesions can become inflamed (and resemble secondary infection) as the host immune system starts to fight the infection.

Pediatric Patient Considerations

Molluscum is more common in children with atopic dermatitis, but it can trigger an eczematous response in those with or without underlying atopic eczema.

Differential Diagnosis and Pitfalls

- Herpes simplex lesions can resemble molluscum with a central umbilication, but lesions are fluid filled rather than solid as with molluscum contagiosum.
- Warts (verrucae) tend to have a verrucous or jagged surface, whereas molluscum contagiosum lesions are smooth.
- Milia tend to be whiter and more concentrated on the face.
- Nevi

- Pyogenic granuloma is vascular in appearance with frequent overlying ulceration.
- Lichen planus lesions are purple pruritic planar papules that can also spread in a linear pattern.
- Basal cell carcinoma tends to be solitary.
- Keratoacanthomas have a central keratin core and grow rapidly.
- Sebaceous hyperplasia primarily occurs on the face and has a white- to yellow-colored, lobular appearance.

Pediatric Patient Differential Diagnosis

With a pediatric patient, consider the following:

- Folliculitis
- Large cell acanthoma
- Cellulitis (when inflamed)

Immunocompromised Patient Differential Diagnosis

Cutaneous cryptococcal infection in an immunocompromised patient can present with umbilicated papules similar in appearance to molluscum.

✓ Best Tests

- This diagnosis can often be made clinically based on the characteristic clinical appearance.
- Extracting the central core of the molluscum and viewing with light microscopy can confirm molluscum bodies (which appear red using Wright stain). Methylene blue may also be used to stain smears made from lesions.
- Skin biopsy of a lesion can confirm the diagnosis when in doubt.

Immunocompromised Patient Considerations

Skin biopsy should be used in immunocompromised patients to rule out deep fungal infections.

▲▲ Management Pearls

- The condition is self-limited in immunocompetent patients. However, treatment is often desirable and will help to prevent autoinoculation and further spread.

- In cases of sexually transmitted molluscum contagiosum, consider the possibility of other concomitant sexually transmitted diseases.
- Instruct patients to avoid communal bathing, sharing of bath towels, and shaving if lesions are present on the face of men or legs of women.

Pediatric Patient Considerations

- If there are just a few molluscum lesions, treating early to prevent autoinoculation and further spread is recommended if the child is older and/or amenable to treating the few lesions. Conversely, if lesions are widespread or the child cannot tolerate any of the destructive procedures, treatment is not a necessity, as this infection is self-limited and healing occurs without scarring.
- Be sure to caution parents who choose a conservative approach that the lesions frequently spread and increase in number before resolution.

Therapy

- Cryotherapy with liquid nitrogen. Use with caution in darker-skinned patients because of the risk for hypopigmentation.
- Curettage of central core/umbilication followed by gentle hyfrecation
- Imiquimod cream—Apply to affected area three to seven times per week for 4 to 12 weeks.
- Cantharidin solution can be applied to individual lesions with a cotton-tipped applicator and washed off after 4 hours. Be sure to inform patients that the lesions will later blister. Protect unaffected areas with petroleum jelly.
- Tazarotene 0.05% cream or gel—Apply daily to affected area for 4 to 12 weeks.
- Another topical therapy that has been used is 0.5% podophyllotoxin once daily.

Pediatric Patient Considerations

- Freeze with liquid nitrogen or remove lesions with a sharp curette.
- Imiquimod cream or topical tretinoin cream daily, applied at bedtime, for up to 4 weeks (or longer) has been successful, but they are off-label uses.
- Cantharidin (an extract from the blister beetle) is an effective, pain-free method of treating molluscum lesions. As with imiquimod cream and tretinoin cream, cantharidin is off label as well.

Suggested Readings

Braue A, Ross G, Varigos G, et al. Epidemiology and impact of childhood molluscum contagiosum: A case series and critical review of the literature. *Pediatr Dermatol.* 2005;22(4):287–294.

Laxmisha C, Thappa DM, Jaisankar TJ. Clinical profile of molluscum contagiosum in children versus adults. *Dermatol Online J.* 2003;9(5):1.

Mahe A, Bobin P, Coulibaly S, et al. Skin diseases disclosing human immunodeficiency virus infection in Mali. *Annales de Dermatologie et de Venereologie.* 1997;124(2):144–150.

Mahe A, Simon F, Coulibaly S, et al. Predictive value of seborrheic dermatitis and other common dermatoses for HIV infection in Bamako, Mali. *J Am Acad Dermatol.* 1996;34(6):1084–1086.

Reynolds MG, Holman RC, Yorita Christensen KL, et al. The incidence of molluscum contagiosum among American Indians and Alaska Natives. *PLos One.* 2009;4(4):e5255.

Saral Y, Kalkan A, Ozdarendeli A, et al. Detection of molluscum contagiosum virus subtype I as a single dominant virus subtype in molluscum lesions from a Turkish population. *Arch Med Res.* 2006;37(3): 388–391.

Yamashita H, Uemura T, Kawashima M. Molecular epidemiologic analysis of Japanese patients with molluscum contagiosum. *Int J Dermatol.* 1996;35(2):99–105.

Sarcoidosis

Cynthia Marie Carver DeKlotz

■■ Diagnosis Synopsis

Sarcoidosis is a multisystem disorder of unknown etiology characterized histologically by noncaseating granulomas involving almost any organ system. The disease most commonly involves the lungs, lymph nodes, liver, eyes, and skin. Although pulmonary disease is the most frequent manifestation, between 20% and 35% of patients with systemic sarcoidosis have some form of cutaneous involvement, and skin lesions can be the presenting sign. Approximately 30% of patients with the initial diagnosis of cutaneous sarcoidosis will eventually develop systemic sarcoidosis.

Etiology

The etiology of sarcoidosis has not yet been elucidated; however, numerous theories have been considered that include environmental exposures to chemical and metal materials, exposures to water damage or high humidity in the workplace, infectious agents such as *Mycobacterium tuberculosis*, drugs, and autoimmune processes. It is unclear whether socioeconomic status may play a role in these possible exposures. It has been suggested that the development of sarcoidosis probably depends on immune responses to various ubiquitous environmental triggers. Genetic predisposition seems to play a role. Specifically, HLA class II antigens, encoded by HLA-DRB1 and DQB1 alleles, have consistently been associated with sarcoidosis. Genomewide scans have shown linkage signals at chromosomes 3p and 6p in white Germans and strong signals at chromosomes 5p and 5q in African Americans. Subsequent fine-mapping studies of African Americans suggest that sarcoidosis susceptibility genes may exist on chromosomes 3p and 5q11.2, while protective genes may be present on a region of 5p15.2. Whatever the true underlying etiopathogenesis, the immunopathogenesis of sarcoidosis is known to involve the activation of alveolar macrophages in the lung and T-cells, leading to inflammation and, ultimately, granuloma formation.

Epidemiology

Sarcoidosis occurs throughout the world in people of all ages and ethnicities and in both sexes, with a slight female predominance. The incidence peaks between the second and third decades, with a second peak occurring in Scandinavian and Japanese women over the age of 50. Some data suggest that patients with darkly pigmented skin are up to 17 times more commonly affected with sarcoidosis than white patients in different parts of the world.

The ethnic difference in incidence in the American population is impressive. The annual age-adjusted incidence of new cases is highest in African American women (39.1 per 100,000), followed by African American men (29.8 per 100,000) and white women (12.1 per 100,000); it is lowest in white men (9.6 per 100,000). Overall, African Americans have about a threefold to fourfold higher incidence of sarcoidosis compared with white Americans. Sarcoidosis tends to be more severe, extensive, and progressive in African Americans than in whites. Specifically, there is more frequent involvement of the eyes, liver, bone marrow, extrathoracic lymph nodes, and skin in African Americans compared to whites. African Americans also have a lower likelihood of clinical recovery compared to whites, particularly in the presence of extrathoracic involvement.

The European prevalence is estimated at 40 cases per 100,000, with northern European countries reporting higher incidences than southern European countries. The prevalence in India has been estimated to vary from minimal to 150 cases per 100,000. In a recent study of patients in Tunisia, sarcoidosis was found to be much more frequent, extensive, and severe in black West Indian, African, Indian, and Pakistani patients than in native white patients. Sarcoidosis appears to be rare in East Asians, and specifically, cutaneous sarcoidosis is rare in Asia.

Cutaneous lesions of sarcoidosis are broadly categorized as either specific granulomatous lesions or nonspecific lesions. Specific lesions contain noncaseating granulomas and can be macules, papules, plaques, hypopigmented sarcoid, lupus pernio, scar sarcoidosis, alopecia, ulcers, subcutaneous lesions, nail dystrophy, and ichthyosis. In general, these lesions are asymptomatic; pruritus may be present in 10% to 15% of patients. Nonspecific lesions do not contain granulomas.

Specific Cutaneous Lesions

The most frequent specific cutaneous sarcoidosis lesion is the papule. Papules can vary from reddish-brown in color (most often) to violaceous, yellowish, or brown in color (Figs. 4-235

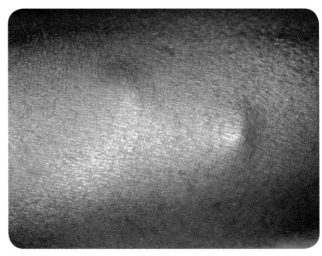

Figure 4-235 Sarcoidosis can present as multiple skin-colored nodules.

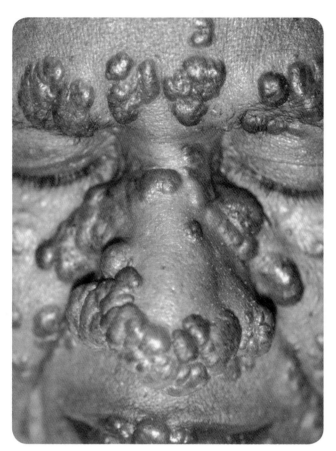

Figure 4-236 Sarcoidosis with multiple-sized nodules on the skin and vermilion border.

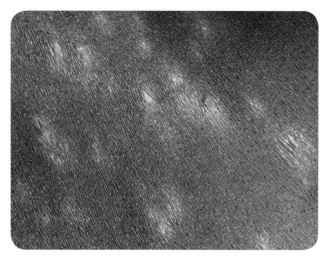

Figure 4-237 Red papules of sarcoidosis often have a rim of hypopigmentation.

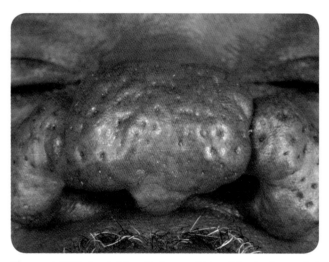

Figure 4-238 Nasal deformity by sarcoidal nodules is often called lupus pernio.

and 4-236). Palpation can reveal some induration. These lesions usually erupt on the face but may also involve any part of the body. Pruritus is rare. Papular sarcoidosis is generally associated with less severe systemic manifestations.

The plaque form is rarer and can involve the extremities, face, and the body. The lesions also vary from a reddish-brown color to skin color and are associated with chronic forms of the disease and can result in scarring upon resolution.

A hypopigmented variant of cutaneous sarcoidosis is found almost exclusively in patients with dark skin types (Fig. 4-237). Clinically, hypopigmented sarcoid presents as well-demarcated round to oval patches or barely elevated plaques that are lighter in color than normal skin. Erythematous or skin-colored papules can sometimes be present in the center of the lesions.

Lupus pernio is one of the few characteristic cutaneous findings of sarcoidosis (Fig. 4-238). Clinically, it consists of chronic, indurated, reddish-brown to violaceous, shiny papules, nodules, and plaques distributed around the central face, especially the alar rim of the nose. The ear lobes can also be involved. Lupus pernio tends to be chronic and can be associated with granulomatous inflammation of the upper respiratory tract. Pernio lesions on the nasal rim have been associated with sarcoidosis of the lungs in up to 75% of cases

and the upper respiratory tract in up to 50% of cases. Lupus pernio is most commonly seen in African Americans. In a recent case series in Asia, no patients had lupus pernio.

Scar sarcoidosis occurs when sarcoidal granulomas infiltrate preexisting scars. This results in an increase in thickness of the area that can be violaceous in color and can clinically resemble hypertrophic scars or keloids.

Scalp sarcoidosis can cause both a reversible alopecia and an irreversible cicatricial alopecia. Often, this initially presents as an erythematous or skin-colored patch or plaque of scarring alopecia. This is most commonly reported to occur in African American patients.

Ulcerative sarcoidosis presents as ulcerative atrophic plaques with violaceous rolled borders, most commonly on the pretibial area. Approximately two-thirds of cases occur in women, and about 60% of cases occur in African Americans.

Most patients with ulcerative sarcoidosis also have systemic involvement of the disease, and their clinical course is often treatment resistant.

Subcutaneous sarcoid eruptions (Darier-Roussy sarcoidosis) can present as skin-colored, deep-seated, firm nodules, most commonly on an upper extremity.

Although uncommon, involvement of the nails may occur and can manifest clinically as nail plate distortion. Bony erosions and cystic changes of the underlying bones of the involved fingers are often present. When nail dystrophy in sarcoidosis is present, it signifies a chronic course of disease. Eighty-six percent of patients with affected digits will also have pulmonary involvement.

Some atypical yet specific cutaneous lesions of sarcoidosis (which contain granulomas histologically) include ichthyosiform changes on the lower legs, erythroderma, and verrucous sarcoidosis.

Nonspecific Cutaneous Lesions

Erythema nodosum, a septal panniculitis, is the most common nonspecific cutaneous lesion of sarcoidosis. These lesions, which have been reported in up to 25% of sarcoid cases, consist of tender, erythematous subcutaneous nodules most commonly on the anterior lower legs. The presence of erythema nodosum in cases of sarcoidosis is a good prognostic sign and often represents the hallmark of acute benign disease, implying a more rapid spontaneous resolution of the disease. Erythema nodosum affects younger patients and is more common in patients of northern European descent. Other nonspecific manifestations such as calcifications, prurigo, and Sweet syndrome are uncommon.

Variants

Specific sarcoidosis syndromes include Heerfordt syndrome and Löfgren syndrome. Heerfordt syndrome is the combination of chronic inflammation of the parotid glands and lacrimal glands, subfebrile temperatures, and cranial nerve palsies. Löfgren syndrome is a type of sarcoidosis that presents with bilateral hilar lymphadenopathy, erythema nodosum, and arthritis. Similar to sarcoid-associated erythema nodosum, the presence of Löfgren syndrome implies a good prognosis.

Pediatric Patient Considerations

Sarcoidosis is extremely rare in children younger than 6 years. In adolescents, the cutaneous manifestations of sarcoidosis are similar to those seen in adults, with the exception of lupus pernio and erythema nodosum which are rare. When sarcoidosis presents in children younger than 6 years, it is characterized by a triad of skin rash, uveitis, and arthritis, without intrathoracic involvement.

⦿ Look For

Although the clinical presentations of cutaneous sarcoidosis are protean, in general, specific lesions—whether macular, papular, plaquelike, or nodular—typically have a reddish-brown to violaceous color and classically have an "apple jelly" appearance on diascopy. Some lesions such as lupus pernio, which occurs most commonly in African Americans, favor the face, whereas others such as alopecia favor the scalp. In patients with darkly pigmented skin, hypopigmented patches or plaques can be a manifestation of sarcoidosis. Nonspecific reactions such as erythema nodosum can suggest the diagnosis. The diagnosis must be confirmed with a biopsy of specific lesions.

Pediatric Patient Considerations

In children younger than 6 years, look for the classic triad of skin rash, uveitis, and arthritis, without intrathoracic involvement.

⦿⦿ Diagnostic Pearls

- Diascopy, in which pressure is applied over cutaneous lesions with a glass slide, classically reveals a yellow-brown color or "apple jelly" appearance in cutaneous sarcoid lesions. This finding, however, is not pathognomonic for sarcoidosis as it can be present in other granulomatous diseases.
- Examine the patient for enlarged lacrimal glands by everting the upper eyelid.

?? Differential Diagnosis and Pitfalls

The differential diagnosis of cutaneous sarcoidosis can be quite extensive and varied. Hence, it seems best to group differentials based on either the categories of potential skin conditions or the primary morphology of the sarcoidosis lesions.

In general, four main categories of skin conditions can clinically mimic sarcoidosis: infectious diseases such as tuberculosis and atypical mycobacterium, immunological and allergic processes such as discoid lupus and atopic dermatitis, granulomatous diseases such as granuloma annulare and foreign body granuloma, and pseudolymphomas and lymphomas.

Alternatively, grouping of differentials based on the primary morphology of the lesions results in the following:

Papules, Plaques, and Nodules

- Granulomatous rosacea
- Benign appendageal tumors, such as trichoepitheliomas

- Psoriasis
- Lichen planus
- Mycobacterial infection
- Leprosy
- Discoid and tumid lupus
- Granuloma annulare
- Erythema induratum of Bazin
- Plaque stage cutaneous T-cell lymphoma (CTCL)
- Atopic dermatitis
- Mycobacterial infection
- Lymphoma
- Foreign body granuloma
- Subcutaneous granuloma annulare

Alopecia

- Discoid lupus erythematosus
- Lichen planopilaris
- Pseudopelade

Lupus Pernio

- Discoid lupus erythematosus
- Nodular rosacea
- Pseudolymphoma

Ulcerative Lesions

- Vasculitis
- Necrobiosis lipoidica
- Vascular insufficiency

Annular Lesions

- Granuloma annulare
- Leprosy

Scar Sarcoidosis

- Keloids
- Hypertrophic scars

Pediatric Patient Differential Diagnosis

Polyarticular juvenile rheumatoid arthritis must be considered in the differential, given the combination of skin, eye, and joint manifestations in children <6 years of age.

 Best Tests

- Any presumptive lesion must be confirmed histologically with demonstration of noncaseating, epithelioid cell granulomas. Tuberculosis generally needs to be excluded, whether via culture, special stains, PCR, or PPD testing.
- Serologic levels of angiotensin-converting enzyme and soluble interleukin-2 levels as well as urinary calcium levels can all serve as useful auxiliary studies in the evaluation of sarcoidosis. However, such tests are often best used for monitoring the activity of disease. Laboratory tests are more often utilized in monitoring systemic disease rather than cutaneous disease.

 Management Pearls

Thirty percent of patients with the initial diagnosis of cutaneous sarcoidosis will eventually develop systemic sarcoidosis. Hence, once a diagnosis of cutaneous sarcoidosis is made, it is extremely important that patients be evaluated for possible systemic involvement, regardless of the patient's symptoms. Initial tests include a chest X-ray and often a pulmonary and ophthalmologist evaluation.

Therapy

To date, there is no cure for sarcoidosis. However, numerous immunosuppressive and immunomodulatory drugs can be used to control the disease. For cutaneous disease, medium- to high-potency topical corticosteroids, such as triamcinolone, fluocinonide, and clobetasol, are the mainstay of treatment. Additionally, intralesional steroids may be used. The corticosteroids function by suppressing the proinflammatory chemokines and cytokines involved in immune responses and granuloma formation.

Additionally, the use of a flashlamp-pumped pulsed dye laser has been reported to successfully treat lesions of nodular cutaneous sarcoidosis in one case.

In systemic sarcoidosis and severe, refractory cutaneous cases, systemic agents such as systemic corticosteroids, hydroxychloroquine, azathioprine, tetracycline derivatives, isotretinoin, and methotrexate may be used. Drugs such as pentoxifylline and thalidomide, through their ability to block tumor necrosis factor (TNF)-alpha, are effective in some cases. Emerging therapeutic options include biologic TNF inhibitors such as infliximab and etanercept.

Suggested Readings

Chong WS, Tan HH, Tan SH. Cutaneous sarcoidosis in Asians: A report of 25 patients from Singapore. *Clin Exp Dermatol.* 2005;30:120–124.

Fernandez-Faith E, McDonnell J. Cutaneous sarcoidosis: Differential diagnosis. *Clin Dermatol.* 2007;25:276–287.

Iannuzzi MC, Rybicki BA, Teirstein AS. Sarcoidosis. *N Engl J Med.* 2007;357:2153–2165.

Khaled A, Souissi A, Zeglaoui F, et al. Cutaneous sarcoidosis in Tunisia. *Giornale Italiano Di Dermatologia E Venereologia.* 2008;143:181–185.

Lodha S, Sanchez M, Prystowsky S. Sarcoidosis of the skin: A review for the pulmonologist. *Chest.* 2009;136:583–596.

Mutlu GM, Rubinstein I. Clinical manifestations of sarcoidosis among inner-city African-American dwellers. *J Natl Med Assoc.* 2006;98:1140–1143.

Roos S, Raulin C, Ockenfels HM, et al. Successful treatment of cutaneous sarcoidosis lesions with the flashlight pumped pulsed dye laser: A case report. *Dermatol Surg.* 2009;35:1139–1140.

Santoro F, Sloan SB. Nail dystrophy and bony involvement in chronic sarcoidosis. *J Am Acad Dermatol.* 2009;60:1050–1052.

Tchernev G, Patterson JW, Nenoff P, et al. Sarcoidosis of the skin—A dermatological puzzle: Important differential diagnostic aspects and guidelines for clinical and histopathological recognition. *J Eur Acad Dermatol Venereol.* 2010;24:125–137.

Tchernev G. Cutaneous sarcoidosis: The 'Great Imitator'. *Am J Clin Dermatol.* 2006;7:375–382.

Westney GE, Judson MA. Racial and ethnic disparities in sarcoidosis: From genetics to socioeconomics. *Clin Chest Med.* 2006;27:453–462.

Leprosy (Hansen Disease)

Donna Culton

Diagnosis Synopsis

Leprosy, or Hansen disease, is a chronic infectious disease caused by *Mycobacterium leprae* that primarily affects the skin and peripheral nervous system. Leprosy is classified into six disease types based on clinical, immunologic, and pathologic criteria: indeterminate leprosy (IL), tuberculoid leprosy (TL), borderline tuberculoid leprosy (BT), midborderline leprosy (BB), borderline lepromatous leprosy (BL), and lepromatous leprosy (LL). Disease manifestations occur along this continuum with clinical features dependent upon mycobacterial load and host immune response. On one end of the spectrum is TL, characterized by a low mycobacterial load (paucibacillary) and a strong cell-mediated immune response. On the opposite end of the disease spectrum is LL, characterized by a high mycobacterial load (multibacillary) and a poor cell-mediated immune response. These polar forms are clinically stable; however, disease states between the poles may change depending on the host response.

Leprosy is most commonly seen in immigrants from endemic areas such as India, Brazil, Africa, Mexico, Indonesia, and Madagascar. Within the United States, sporadic cases have been reported in the south, with Texas and Louisiana identified as endemic foci. Indeed, risk factors for development of disease include birth or residence in an endemic area and having a blood relative with leprosy. Leprosy in returning travelers is exceedingly rare.

Disease transmission is not fully understood, but it is thought to be spread via droplets from nasal secretions of infected and untreated individuals. Given their high mycobacterial burden, patients with LL are most contagious. Following exposure, the average incubation period is 5 years (range 2 to 30 years) with an average age of onset <35.

Signs and symptoms vary greatly depending on the type of leprosy. IL presents as a solitary ill-defined, hypopigmented macule or patch. TL is characterized by a single annular, erythematous, scaly plaque that is often hypopigmented, hairless, hypoesthetic, and anhidrotic. LL is characterized by multiple infiltrated papules symmetrically distributed on the face with a predilection for the alar rim and earlobes, as the mycobacteria grow best in cooler parts of the body. These patients can progress to a leonine facies. Many of the borderline forms show a clinical pattern between these polar forms.

Aside from the skin, peripheral nerve involvement is common and is characterized by nerve enlargement (visible as nerves run close to the skin), anesthesia of skin lesions, stocking and glove neuropathy, and anhidrosis of palms and soles.

Patients with leprosy can also experience exacerbations or adverse events due to the host immune response, which may occur before, during, or after therapy. Such adverse events can be characterized by fevers, arthralgias, neuritic pain, uveitis, and orchitis as well as interesting cutaneous manifestations.

Look For

Indeterminate Leprosy

Solitary ill-defined, hypopigmented macule or patch. Normal sensation.

Tuberculoid Leprosy

Patients will have a solitary hypopigmented macule or slightly infiltrated plaque a few centimeters in diameter (Fig. 4-239). May be anesthetic.

Borderline Tuberculoid Leprosy

Look for a few lesions, discrete macules, or infiltrated plaques scattered over the body. An annular appearance with central clearing is common. Peripheral nerves are often enlarged with the greater auricular, radial cutaneous, medial, lateral popliteal, and posterior tibial nerves most commonly involved.

Midborderline Leprosy

Look for annular plaques as above. This state is not often seen, as it is transitional and unstable.

Borderline Lepromatous Leprosy

Patients will have numerous symmetric lesions smaller than lesions in tuberculoid forms. Lesions may have poorly defined borders with islands of sparing ("Swiss cheese appearance") or poorly defined papules and nodules.

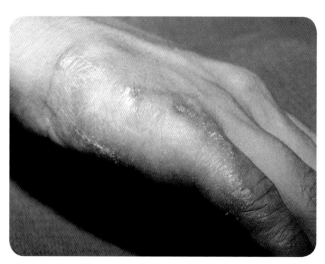

Figure 4-239 Plaque of TL in a 17-year-old Vietnamese patient.

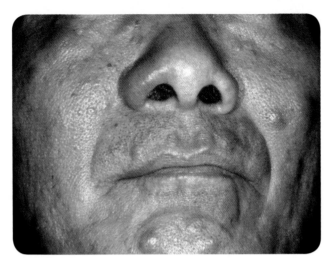

Figure 4-240 Nodules of LL in a Malaysian male.

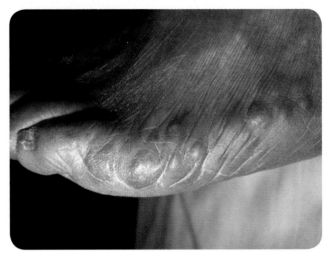

Figure 4-242 Infiltrated papules and nodules of LL.

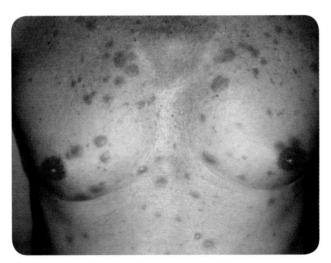

Figure 4-241 Multiple papules and plaques on the chest in LL (same patient as Fig. 4-240).

Lepromatous Leprosy

Look for numerous infiltrated papules and plaques symmetrically distributed over the body (Figs. 4-240–4-242). Lesions are most prominent on cooler parts of the body, with a predilection for lesions over the nasal ala and earlobes that progress to a leonine facies. Other specific findings can include saddle nose deformity, septal perforation, loss of lateral eyebrows, and oral and ocular lepromas. Nerve damage results in anesthesia and typically occurs in a glove and stocking distribution. Thickening of peripheral nerves is also common.

Reactive States

These reactions occur during host immune responses. Type 1 reactions are characterized by previously quiescent plaques becoming indurated with the appearance of papules and nodules on previously normal skin. Type 2 reactions are characterized by tender pink nodules on the extremities accompanied by systemic symptoms such as fevers and arthralgias. This type of reaction is seen in BL and LL patients.

 Diagnostic Pearls

Be sure to ask about country of origin and family history when the diagnosis of leprosy is being considered. Sensory neuropathy (numbness) is often the first clinical sign; therefore, leprosy must be ruled out in any patient with cutaneous findings and unexplained neuropathy.

 Differential Diagnosis and Pitfalls

Indeterminate Leprosy

- Pityriasis alba
- Tinea versicolor
- Pinta

Tuberculoid Leprosy and Borderline Tuberculoid Leprosy

- Mycosis fungoides
- Tinea corporis
- Psoriasis
- Seborrheic dermatitis
- Nummular eczema
- Syphilis
- Granuloma annulare

Lepromatous Leprosy and Borderline Lepromatous Leprosy

- Sarcoidosis
- Eruptive histiocytomas
- Lymphoma

- Mycosis fungoides
- Keloid
- Dermatofibroma
- Yaws
- Tuberculosis
- Syphilis
- Erythema nodosum

Best Tests

Diagnosis of leprosy requires classic skin findings in conjunction with a consistent peripheral nerve abnormality or identification of acid-fast bacilli in tissue. Biopsy is indicated and should reveal acid-fast bacilli by Fite or Ziehl-Neelsen stains. The slit skin smear can also be performed: a small slit is made in an infiltrated lesion, and a smear of the contents is examined for acid-fast bacilli. Earlobe lesions typically have the highest mycobacterial load and, thus, are the optimal site when performing these tests. PCR of tissue samples is also available in some areas. Of note, *M. leprae* cannot be grown in culture, and no serological tests are available.

Lepromin test is a cutaneous delayed hypersensitivity test similar to the tuberculin test. It can be useful to measure immunological status because the test is positive only in the tuberculoid pole and is negative as the disease progresses to the lepromatous pole.

Management Pearls

- Immune reactions in leprosy are considered medical emergencies, and appropriate therapy should begin immediately. These can occur before, during, or after therapy.
- The stigma of leprosy is sometimes worse than the disease itself. It is important to reassure the patient that the disease is curable and that when being treated they can maintain a normal life. Patients do not need to be isolated, and even LL patients become noninfectious within 72 hours after beginning therapy.
- Consultation with an infectious disease specialist is recommended for suspected leprosy cases outside endemic areas.

Precautions: Standard, contact, droplet. (Isolate patient, wear a mask, and limit patient transport.)

Therapy

Treatment consists of multidrug therapy (MDT), which is customized to the subtype of disease in terms of duration of therapy and particular drugs used. MDT is available free of charge to any patient diagnosed with leprosy throughout the world, through the World Health Organization (WHO). Treatment significantly decreases infectivity within 72 hours.

Treatment for this disease benefits when an expert has been consulted.

Paucibacillary disease (duration of treatment 6 months by WHO guidelines):

- Rifampin 600 mg/mo, supervised
- Dapsone 100 mg daily, self-administered

Multibacillary disease (duration of treatment 1 year by WHO guidelines):

- Rifampin 600 mg/mo, supervised
- Dapsone 100 mg daily, self-administered
- Clofazimine 300 mg/mo, supervised and 50 mg daily, self-administered

Type 1 Reversal Reaction
- Prednisolone 40 to 60 mg daily up to 1 mg/kg body weight
- Analgesics
- Taper over 2 to 3 months

Type 2 Reversal Reaction (Erythema Nodosum Leprosum)
- Thalidomide 100 mg four times daily. Taper to the minimal effective dose.
- High doses should be closely monitored, sometimes as inpatients. Clofazimine may be increased to 200 to 300 mg daily. Because thalidomide can be used only in males and nonfertile females, prednisone can be used as an alternative, as above.

Early detection and treatment of nerve involvement is critical to prevent morbidity and deformity. Patients who have sensory loss or new muscle weakness should receive a course of prednisolone, starting at 30 to 40 mg daily. Monitoring with nylon monofilaments for neurological deficits is helpful.

Children may be treated as above with reduced doses.

Suggested Readings

Anderson H, Stryjewska B, Boyanton BL, et al. Hansen disease in the United States in the 21st century; a review of the literature. *Arch Pathol Lab Med.* 2007;131(6):982–986.

Goulart IM, Goulart LR. Leprosy: diagnostic and control challenges for a worldwide disease. *Arch Dermatol Res.* 2008;300(6):269–290.

Parkash O. Classification of leprosy into multibacillary and paucibacillary groups: an analysis. *FEMS Immunol Med Microbiol.* 2009;55:1–5.

Sehgal VN, Sardana K, Dogra S. Management of complications following leprosy: An evolving scenario. *J Dermatolog Treat.* 2007;18(6):366–374.

Lymphomatoid Papulosis

Chris G. Adigun

▪▪ Diagnosis Synopsis

Lymphomatoid papulosis (LyP), also known as Macaulay disease, is a primary cutaneous CD30+ lymphoproliferative disorder. It forms one end of a spectrum of disorders, with cutaneous anaplastic large cell lymphoma (cALCL) being at the other end of the spectrum. It is uncommon and is characterized by recurrent, self-healing papules that typically occur in crops. Large-population analyses have found that it is slightly more prevalent in males, in those aged 50 to 60 years, and has a relative prominence in whites. It is an often chronic condition, and only symptomatic therapy is available. The characteristic papules often evolve to have central necrosis and are typically asymptomatic, although some patients find them pruritic. They tend to occur in crops, and lesions in various stages will occur concurrently. Histologically, LyP has features suggesting malignant lymphoma. The cells tend to present one or more T-cell antigens as well as CD30, a lymphoid activation antigen in the TNF (tumor necrosis factor) receptor family. One subtype of LyP is CD30–, which closely mimics cutaneous T-cell lymphoma (CTCL).

The etiology and mechanisms involved in the development of primary cutaneous CD30+ lymphoproliferative disorders are unknown. However, evidence has suggested that LyP is a precursor lesion to the subsequent development of lymphoma, although most patients do not progress to malignancy. Prognosis is excellent, with 10-year survival near 100%.

The course of disease varies from months to >40 years. Most patients have a long-standing, chronic course without malignant transformation.

◉ Look For

Reddish-brown papules and nodules on the trunk and extremities that evolve with central hemorrhagic crust and necrosis over days to weeks (Figs. 4-243–4-245). Each lesion spontaneously heals within 3 to 8 weeks. It is characteristic for crops of lesions in different stages of evolution to coexist. The distribution of lesions may be generalized or localized to well-defined areas. Patients may have as few as several lesions to as many as 100, which may coalesce to form plaques. The face, palms, soles, genitalia, or scalp may also be involved, although this is less typical.

Older lesions may heal with hypopigmentation or hyperpigmentation. In some patients, lesions leave atrophic (varioliform), disfiguring scars, whereas other patients have

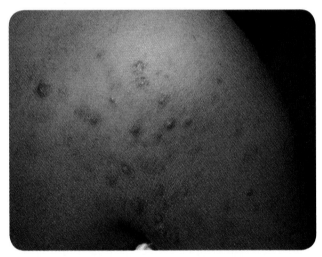

Figure 4-244 Irregular papules of lymphomatoid papulosis.

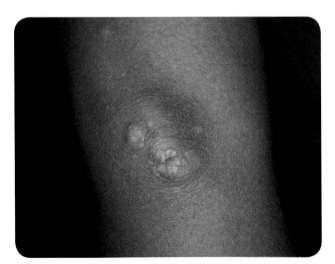

Figure 4-243 Inflammatory papules of lymphomatoid papulosis.

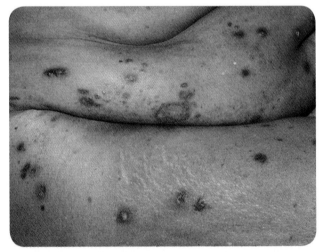

Figure 4-245 Inflammatory and necrotic papules of lymphomatoid papulosis.

lesions that disappear without necrosis or scarring. In patients with darker skin, the pigmentation change is typically more pronounced, persistent, and distressing to patients.

Diagnostic Pearls

- In adults, 10% to 20% of patients with LyP develop lymphoma. Lesions of LyP may precede, coexist, or even follow malignant lymphoma, with the most common associated lymphomas being CTCL, Hodgkin lymphoma, or nodal anaplastic large cell lymphoma (ALCL).
- In patients with darkly pigmented skin, the finding of poikiloderma atrophicans vasculare (telangiectasia, pigmentation, capillary dilation, atrophy) should prompt further investigation into CTCL, whereas a background of poikiloderma in white persons is a common incidental finding.
- In large studies of cutaneous lymphomas in both Singapore and Japan, patients with the diagnosis of LyP presented with the typical papulonecrotic findings typically seen in white patients.
- LyP is primarily a disease of adulthood, although it does rarely occur in children.
- An important clinical finding that distinguishes LyP from cALCL is that in cALCL, patients typically present with solitary nodules—and less commonly papules—that almost uniformly ulcerate. Additionally, these lesions do not typically wax and wane as those in LyP do.
- Primary cALCL has a very good prognosis. This is an important distinction from systemic ALCL with secondary cutaneous involvement, which tends to have a poor prognosis.

?? Differential Diagnosis and Pitfalls

- CD30-negative large T- and B-cell lymphomas
- Other cutaneous lymphomas that are CD30+
- Lymphomas with secondary cutaneous involvement
- Pityriasis lichenoides et varioliformis acuta (PLEVA)
- Pityriasis lichenoides chronica (PLC)
- Folliculitis
- Insect bites
- Langerhans cell histiocytosis
- Lymphocytoma cutis
- Herpes simplex virus (HSV)
- Scabies
- Atopic dermatitis
- HIV-associated cutaneous eruptions
- Kaposi sarcoma

In patients with darkly pigmented skin, prurigo nodularis secondary to atopic dermatitis or other contact dermatitis more commonly occurs, and, thus, these diseases may mimic the presentation of LyP. In addition, in darkly pigmented skin, lesions of Kaposi sarcoma should also be included in the differential, as violaceous lesions may be difficult to differentiate from hyperpigmented lesions in these patients.

Pediatric Patient Differential Diagnosis

In pediatric patients, PLEVA or PLC can have very similar clinical presentations and are much more common than LyP in this age group.

There have been three reported cases of Japanese children diagnosed with LyP that actually presented with typical lesions of hydroa vacciniforme, with recurrent, necrotic, scarring papules limited to the face.

Best Tests

Skin biopsy is mandatory, and biopsies of two or more nonnecrotic, nonexcoriated papules should be obtained if possible. Gene rearrangement studies will usually show no clonality to the lymphocytes in the lesions. In patients with typical LyP, no further staging is required, and meticulous full-skin examination is sufficient.

Management Pearls

No curative therapy is available, and symptomatic treatment options need to be weighed against potential risk, given that therapies do not alter the natural course of the disease. Regardless of treatment, patients require long-term observation for the development of lymphoma.

Therapy

Systemic or mid- to high-potency topical steroids are typically ineffective, and little evidence shows that they hasten resolution. Systemic or topical antibiotics are also ineffective.

Aggressive therapeutic modalities—that alone garner risk, such as systemic chemotherapy or total skin electron beam irradiation—have reportedly induced complete remission of skin lesions. However, lesions almost uniformly recur after several weeks to months, and disease continues along its natural course.

(Continued)

Considering treatment options are not curative, patients with few nonscarring lesions should not be treated. However, for those patients with many lesions or with lesions that leave disfiguring scars, the current recommendation is low-dose oral methotrexate (5 to 10 mg/wk). This has been shown to be the most effective treatment to suppress the development of new lesions. Psoralen plus UVA (PUVA) has shown variable effectiveness, with similar inconsistent findings with topical mechlorethamine and carmustine.

The necessity for long-term follow-up of these patients cannot be overemphasized, as these patients are at increased risk for developing systemic lymphoma.

Suggested Readings

Bradford PT. Skin cancer in skin of color. *Dermatol Nurs.* 2009;21(4): 170–177, 206; quiz 178.

Hong IS, Johnson G, Kovi J. Cutaneous T cell lymphoma (mycosis fungoides) in blacks. *J Natl Med Assoc.* 1981;73(9):859–862.

Nagasawa T, Miwa H, Nakatsuka S, et al. Characteristics of cutaneous lymphomas in Osaka, Japan (1988–1999) based on the European Organization for Research and Treatment of Cancer classification. *Am J Dermatopathol.* 2000;22(6):510–514.

Tabata N, Aiba S, Ichinohazama R, et al. Hydroa vacciniforme-like lymphomatoid papulosis in a Japanese child: a new subset. *J Am Acad Dermatol.* 1995;32(2 Pt 2):378–381.

Tan SH, Sim CS, Ong BH. Cutaneous lymphomas other than mycosis fungoides in Singapore: a clinicopathological analysis using recent classification systems. *Br J Dermatol.* 2003;149(3):542–553.

Willemze R, Meijer CJ. Primary cutaneous CD30-positive lymphoproliferative disorders. *Hematol Oncol Clin North Am.* 2003;17(6):1319–1332, vii–viii.

Yu JB, Blitzblau RC, Decker RH, et al. Analysis of primary CD30 + cutaneous lymphoproliferative disease and survival from the Surveillance, Epidemiology, and End Results database. *J Clin Oncol.* 2008;26(9):1483–1488. [Erratum in: *J Clin Oncol.* 2008;26(13):2238.]

Tuberous Sclerosis

Donna Culton

■■ Diagnosis Synopsis

Tuberous sclerosis complex (TSC), also known as tuberous sclerosis, Bourneville disease, or epiloia, is an autosomal dominantly inherited genetic disorder characterized by the development of hamartomas in multiple organ systems including the skin, central nervous system, kidneys, heart, eyes, and gastrointestinal tract, among others. Hamartomas represent the benign overgrowth of normal tissue components. Their development within various organs alters normal architecture and leads to the clinical findings of TSC, including the classic triad of seizures, mental retardation, and cutaneous hamartomas.

Patients with TSC carry a mutation in one of two genes, *TSC1* (which encodes the protein hamartin) or *TSC2* (which encodes the protein tuberin). Hamartin and tuberin act together as tumor suppressor genes, and, therefore, mutations within either of these genes allow for uncontrolled cell division and hamartoma formation. While unique mutations within these genes have been reported in different ethnic groups, there are no differences in clinical manifestations among these patients.

TSC is inherited in an autosomal dominant fashion, with nearly complete penetrance but variable expressivity. However, approximately 65% of cases are caused by a spontaneous mutation. Prevalence is estimated at 1/6,000 to 1/10,000. There is no predilection in any ethnicity or either sex, with prevalence being equal among whites and individuals of African and Asian descent.

Of the many clinical manifestations, the cutaneous manifestations are the most easily detected and can aid in diagnosis. Hypomelanotic macules, also known as ash leaf spots, are the most common cutaneous finding, occurring in over 90% of patients with TSC. They are present at birth or shortly thereafter and are often the first cutaneous manifestation of TSC. Facial angiofibromas, also known as adenoma sebaceum, are small cutaneous hamartomas found in over 75% of patients with TSC and are typically present by the age of 5 years. Collagenomas, also termed "shagreen patches," are found in approximately 30% of patients with TSC and develop within the first decade of life. Periungual fibromas, or Koenen tumors, are found in 20% of patients with TSC. Oral manifestations include dental pitting and gingival fibromas (seen in 50% of patients).

Other organ systems are typically involved. Neurologic manifestations most commonly include mental retardation (50% of patients) and seizures (75% to 90% of patients). Autism, attention deficit and hyperactivity disorders, and behavioral problems are often seen in association with TSC. Renal manifestations include angiomyolipomas (found in approximately 75% of patients with TSC, more commonly found in females), renal cysts, and renal carcinomas. Cardiac rhabdomyomas are present in 66% of newborns and are typically asymptomatic,

regressing over the first few years of life. Retinal hamartomas are present in approximately 50% of patients with TSC. They are typically asymptomatic but can lead to visual impairment in some cases. Pulmonary findings are seen in 1% of patients with TSC. Lymphangioleiomyomatosis is a progressive lung disease most often seen in adult females. Other less common findings seen in the bone (cysts, sclerotic lesions) and gastrointestinal tract (rectal hamartomatous polyps) have been reported and are usually asymptomatic.

Diagnostic criteria have been developed according to the National Institutes of Health consensus guidelines. Diagnosis can be made when two major OR one major and two minor features are observed.

Major criteria include facial angiofibromas/forehead plaque, periungual/ungual fibromas, ash leaf spots (more than three), shagreen patch, cortical tuber, subependymal nodule, subependymal giant cell astrocytoma, multiple retinal hamartomas, cardiac rhabdomyoma, lymphangiomyomatosis, and renal angiomyolipoma.

Minor criteria include dental pitting, hamartomatous rectal polyps, bone cysts, cerebral white matter migration tracts, gingival fibromas, nonrenal hamartomas, retinal achromic patch, confetti macules, and multiple renal cysts.

◉ Look For

- Hypomelanotic macules—Look for well-demarcated, hypopigmented macules that are tapered or rounded at the ends (Fig. 4-246). Dark-skinned individuals may present with a variant consisting of a vertical hypopigmented patch over the sternum associated with round, oval, or linear hypopigmented macules in the infraclavicular and periareolar areas.

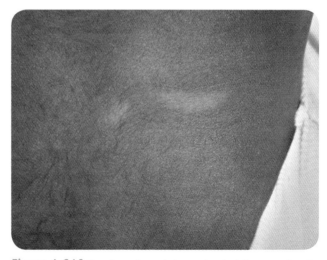

Figure 4-246 Two hypopigmented macules in tuberous sclerosis, one in the shape of an ash leaf.

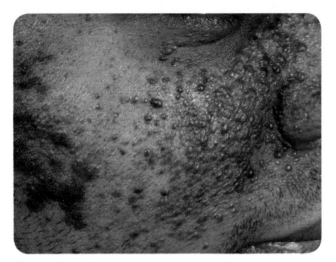

Figure 4-247 Upper cheek and nose with many smooth angiofibromas of tuberous sclerosis.

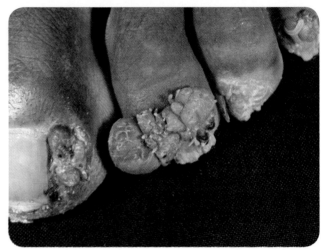

Figure 4-249 Very large periungual fibromas in tuberous sclerosis.

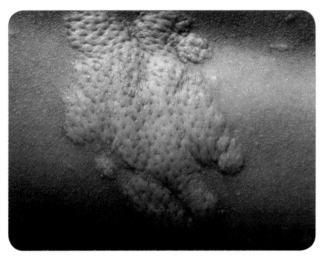

Figure 4-248 Shagreen plaque of tuberous sclerosis.

forehead, and/or a white patch of hair along the frontal hairline (poliosis).

Look for tooth pitting, more commonly seen in permanent teeth.

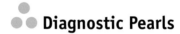

Diagnostic Pearls

Think of TSC when the triad of mental retardation, seizures, and cutaneous findings is present.

Pediatric Patient Considerations

Many of the cutaneous manifestations are seen early (at birth or within the first 5 years of life) and should prompt further workup.

?? Differential Diagnosis and Pitfalls

Angiofibromas

- Fibrous papules (unassociated with TSC)
- Acne vulgaris
- Rosacea
- Trichoepitheliomas
- Sarcoidosis
- Syringomas
- Sebaceous hyperplasia

Hypomelanotic Macules

- Pigmentary mosaicism
- Nevus anemicus

- Facial angiofibromas—Look for skin-colored; yellow, pink, or red; waxy; smooth papules ranging in size from 2 to 5 mm over the forehead, cheeks, nose (especially melolabial folds), and chin (Fig. 4-247). A larger plaque-type variant can be found on the forehead in 20% of patients.
- Collagenoma—Look for an irregular skin-colored or tan, rubbery plaque in the lumbosacral area ranging in size from one to several centimeters (Fig. 4-248). There may be depressions at follicular orifices, giving them an orange peel-like texture.
- Periungual fibromas—Look for smooth, firm, red papules along the nail folds or under the nails (Fig. 4-249). Lesions are more often found on the toes compared to the fingers and may be associated with deep grooves along the nail.

Look for other less common cutaneous manifestations such as tan macules (café au lait spots), stippled hypopigmentation (confetti macules), depigmented macule on the

- Nevus depigmentosus
- Vitiligo

Periungual/Ungual Fibroma

- Acral fibrokeratoma
- Wart
- Subungual exostosis

Connective Tissue Nevi (Shagreen Patch)

- Isolated connective tissue nevus
- Smooth muscle hamartoma
- Leiomyoma
- Elastoma
- Plexiform neurofibroma

 Best Tests

The diagnosis of TSC is based on multiple major and minor criteria, as above. Cutaneous findings are often obvious, and biopsy is not typically necessary but can be helpful to confirm angiofibromas. Further workup should be performed when the diagnosis is suspected. Additional tests to be considered include echocardiography, electrocardiogram, MRI or CT of the brain, electroencephalogram, renal ultrasound, and funduscopy. Molecular genetic studies can be performed in both patients and family members.

 Management Pearls

Management should be multidisciplinary and should include referral to a dermatologist, neurologist, cardiologist, nephrologist, and ophthalmologist.

Tuberous Sclerosis Consensus Conference Guidelines for the Ongoing Evaluation of Established Patients:

- Cranial imaging (CT or MRI)—every 1 to 3 years
- Neurodevelopmental testing—at the time the child enters school and periodically if there are educational or behavioral concerns
- EEG—as indicated for seizure management
- Renal ultrasonography—every 1 to 3 years
- Chest CT—only women upon reaching adulthood
- Dermatologic exam—yearly in patients who may benefit from laser surgery for angiofibromas

Therapy

Treatment should be organ specific and based on symptomatology. While this synopsis focuses on the treatment of the cutaneous findings of TSC, patients with TSC may require treatment for systemic manifestations (epilepsy, renal disease, etc.). Treatments for cutaneous findings are limited. Facial angiofibromas are often the most distressing to patients and are the most common lesion for which the patient and families request treatment. Treatment options include cryosurgery, curettage, dermabrasion, chemical peels, excision, and laser surgery, with laser surgery becoming the most popular treatment. Argon and pulsed-dye lasers can have beneficial results when used on more vascular-appearing red lesions, while CO_2 laser is more useful for fibrous lesions and for improving the texture of the skin. Multiple treatments are often necessary.

All of these modalities have the risk of posttreatment pigmentary alteration when used in darkly pigmented patients. However, reports of treatment with shave excision followed by dermabrasion in darkly pigmented patients have shown little to no posttreatment pigmentary alteration.

Suggested Readings

Darling T. Tuberous sclerosis complex. In: Wolff K, Goldsmith LA, Katz SI, et al., eds. *Fitzpatrick's Dermatology in General Medicine.* 7th Ed. New York, NY: McGraw-Hill; 2008:1325–1331.

Fischer K, Blain B, Zhang F, et al. Treatment of facial angiofibromas of tuberous sclerosis by shave excision and dermabrasion in a dark-skinned patient. *Ann Plast Surg.* 2001;46(3):332–335.

Kumar A, Kandt RS, Wolpert C, et al. Mutation analysis of the TSC2 gene in an African-American family. *Hum Mol Genet.* 1995;4(12):2295–2298.

Leung AK, Robson WL. Tuberous sclerosis complex: a review. *J Pediatr Health Care.* 2007;21(2):108–114.

Zhao XY, Yang S, Zhou HL, et al. Two novel TSC2 mutations in Chinese patients with tuberous sclerosis complex and a literature review of 20 patients reported in China. *Br J Dermatol.* 2006;155(5):1070–1073.

Pseudoxanthoma Elasticum

Chris G. Adigun

■■ Diagnosis Synopsis

Pseudoxanthoma elasticum (PXE) is an inherited disorder of calcification of elastic fibers in the dermis, retina, and cardiovascular system. PXE is inherited in autosomal recessive fashion. The basic defect is in the *ABCC6* gene, which codes for a cellular transport protein. However, the exact relationship between the genetic defect and the phenotype is unknown.

Cutaneous lesions often begin in childhood as "leathery" or "plucked chicken" skin at flexural sites but may not be noted until adolescence because of their asymptomatic nature. The disorder is frequently undiagnosed until the third or fourth decade. A retinal elastic lamina change, called the angioid streak, is characteristic of the condition. It appears later than the skin changes but is present in nearly 100% of patients by age 30. Retinal hemorrhages, leading to central vision loss, and GI hemorrhages are potential complications of the disease. Patients may also have hypertension, mitral valve prolapse, and accelerated atherosclerosis. For unknown reasons, PXE is more common in women. PXE may also be precipitated by long-term D-penicillamine used to treat cystinuria or Wilson disease. Twenty percent of patients with sickle cell disease and thalassemias have eye findings similar to PXE.

Perforating PXE is an uncommon benign entity that presents primarily in overweight, multiparous African American women. It possesses histologic characteristics akin to those of classical PXE but lacks systemic involvement.

The estimated prevalence is 1/100,000. There is no known predilection for any ethnicity. A recent study conducted in South Africa found that there are more genetic variations resulting in PXE among sub-Saharan Africans than among Afrikaners (European-origin descent). Furthermore, a report of genetic analysis of Japanese PXE patients has revealed mutations in the *ABCC6* gene not previously described in this population.

◉ Look For

Small yellowish papules and plaques that cover the sides of the neck, axillae, and the antecubital and popliteal spaces as well as the inguinal and periumbilical areas in a linear or reticular pattern; these papules frequently clinically resemble "plucked chicken skin" (Fig. 4-250). Lesions tend to be symmetrical. Mucous membranes, such as the inner lip, rectum, and vagina, may demonstrate yellowish papules. Yellowish discoloration may be imperceptible in deeply pigmented skin. Late laxity of skin is typical, especially in flexural areas. Retinal angioid

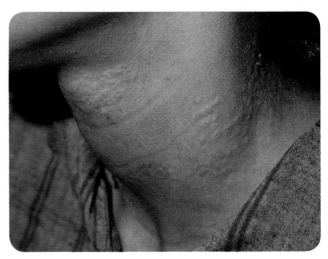

Figure 4-250 Parallel rows of white-yellow papules on the neck in PXE.

streaks can be seen as slate-gray to reddish-brown curved bands radiating from the optic disk on funduscopic exam.

●● Diagnostic Pearls

As the disease process progresses, the skin of the neck, axillae, and groin may become soft, lax, and wrinkled and may hang in folds. Horizontal and oblique mental creases are highly specific for PXE and characteristically occur before the age of 30. Other possible findings include chronic granulomatous nodules, brown reticulate macules, and acneiform papules.

?? Differential Diagnosis and Pitfalls

- Xanthomas—may have the color and figuration of PXE
- Solar elastosis
- Severe photo damage
- Poikiloderma
- Cutis laxa
- Ehlers-Danlos syndrome
- Elastosis perforans serpiginosa
- Dermatofibrosis lenticularis (Buschke-Ollendorff syndrome)
- Marfan syndrome
- Acquired PXE
- Focal dermal elastosis
- Elastoderma
- White fibrous papulosis of the neck
- Granulomatous slack skin/cutaneous T-cell lymphoma

✓ Best Tests

A skin biopsy for histopathology with an elastic stain is the gold standard for diagnosis. A biopsy of a scar or normal-appearing skin may be diagnostic in patients without typical skin findings. If a patient is diagnosed with PXE, an extensive workup is necessary and preventative measures are implemented, including the following:

- Blood pressure assessment and monitoring
- Hematology and complete fasting lipid profile
- Fecal occult blood test
- Serum chemistries, including complete liver and kidney profiles
- Funduscopic exam with retinal photos. Patients should regularly test themselves using an Amsler grid. Repeat funduscopic exam annually or biannually.
- Doppler ankle-brachial index measurements are indicated in patients with claudication.
- Perform echocardiography for patients with a heart murmur.

▲▲ Management Pearls

Because of the eye involvement, contact sports and heavy lifting/straining are not recommended. PXE patients *must* be routinely followed up by an ophthalmologist. The viewing of wavy lines on an Amsler grid should prompt immediate ophthalmologic evaluation.

Therapy

There is no specific treatment for the skin findings of PXE. Plastic surgery to remove lax skin often achieves good cosmetic results. There is anecdotal evidence that certain vitamin and mineral supplements may be advantageous in retinal disease (vitamins A, C, and E; zinc; selenium; and copper).

Suggested Readings

Ramsay M, Greenberg T, Lombard Z, et al. Spectrum of genetic variation at the ABCC6 locus in South Africans: Pseudoxanthoma elasticum patients and healthy individuals. *J Dermatol Sci.* 2009;54(3):198–204. Epub 2009 Mar 31.

Sato N, Nakayama T, Mizutani Y, et al. Novel mutations of ABCC6 gene in Japanese patients with angioid streaks. *Biochem Biophys Res Commun.* 2009;380(3):548–553. Epub 2009 Jan 25.

Uitto J, Li Q, Jiang Q. Pseudoxanthoma elasticum: Molecular genetics and putative pathomechanisms. *J Investig Dermatol.* 2009;130:661–670.

Appendageal Tumors

Mat Davey • Lowell A. Goldsmith

■■ Diagnosis Synopsis

Benign appendageal tumors comprise a wide spectrum of cutaneous lesions arising from adnexal structures or their embryonic precursors. Common examples include tumors with hair follicle differentiation, including angiofibromas and trichoepitheliomas; tumors with sweat (eccrine) duct differentiation, such as syringomas; and localized sites of hyperplasia with one prominent appendage (sebaceous hyperplasia). While these tumors are benign, they are occasionally associated with genetic conditions, and when widespread, they are associated with significant cosmetic and psychosocial distress. Malignant transformation of these lesions is rare, and treatment is primarily cosmetic.

Angiofibroma

Angiofibroma is a term encompassing lesions described as fibrous papules of the nose, facial lesions of tuberous sclerosis (TS), pearly penile papules, oral fibromas, and perifollicular fibromas. Angiofibromas of the face seen with TS consist of several papules and nodules commonly seen in a butterfly distribution and within the nasolabial grooves. These typically develop in childhood and are often the presenting sign of TS. Acral fibrokeratomas include acquired digital fibrokeratoma and periungual fibrokeratoma as well as the periungual fibromas (Koenen tumors) of TS. Pearly penile papules are chronic, asymptomatic, tiny (1 to 3 mm), white papules found on the coronal margin and sulcus of the penis in some 10% of young adult males.

Trichoepithelioma

Trichoepitheliomas are benign neoplasms derived from the hair follicles. They usually present as asymptomatic, smooth, skin-colored papules or small nodules on the face or the trunk. They may occur singly and sporadically, but multiple trichoepitheliomas are often inherited as an autosomal dominant trait. This heritable form (multiple familial trichoepithelioma) may be caused by a mutation in a tumor suppressor gene on chromosome 9. Lesions are more common in women and arise most often during childhood or early adolescence. They are sometimes associated with scalp cylindromas (turban tumors).

Syringomas

Syringomas are benign skin-adnexal tumors that present as small, dome-shaped papules, often in a periorbital distribution; they may, however, occur at any site on the body. They arise from luminal cells of eccrine sweat ducts. The tumors are asymptomatic but do persist over time. They are more common in women. They occur with increased frequency in Down syndrome patients.

Sebaceous Gland Hyperplasia

Sebaceous gland hyperplasia, sometimes known as sebaceous adenoma, is a localized hypertrophy of the sebaceous glands, usually on the central face and forehead. Generally, this hyperplasia does not appear until after 40 years of age, but it may arise in immunocompromised patients, typically those treated with cyclosporine. The condition is benign, and treatment is for cosmetic purposes, though in rare cases eruptions can be severe and disfiguring.

Sebaceous Gland Hyperplasia of the Newborn

Sebaceous gland hyperplasia of the newborn is most prominent around the nose and upper lip, where the density of sebaceous glands is highest. In the newborn, circulating maternal hormones can stimulate sebaceous gland growth and activity leading to sebaceous hyperplasia. Premature infants are less affected, but sebaceous hyperplasia occurs in nearly one half of term newborns. The most common differential diagnosis will be milia and neonatal acne.

◉ Look For

Angiofibroma

Angiofibromas present as small, nontender, 1 mm to 1 cm flesh-colored lesions on the face, under the nail beds, or around the junction of the shaft and the coronal margin of the penis in boys and young adults (Figs. 4-251 and 4-252).

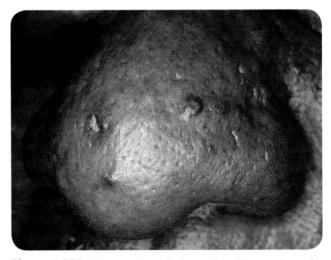

Figure 4-251 Sebaceous hyperplasia papules with some hyperpigmentation on the nose.

Trichoepithelioma

Trichoepitheliomas most often appear as multiple smooth, rounded papules on the face, scalp, neck, and upper trunk, though solitary lesions may appear on any hair-bearing part of the body (Figs. 4-253–4-256). The lesions can be skin-colored or slightly red in color. In the heritable form, they are often symmetrical and occur in a grouped distribution when multiple. The density is often greatest in the midface with a particular predilection for the nose and nasolabial folds.

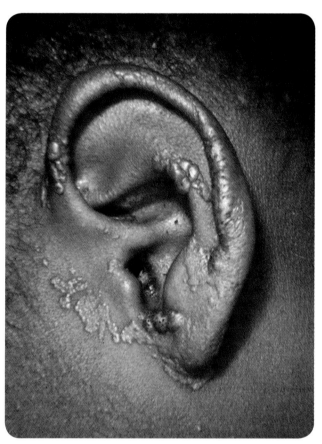

Figure 4-252 Multiple skin-colored angiofibromas on the face and ear in tuberous sclerosis.

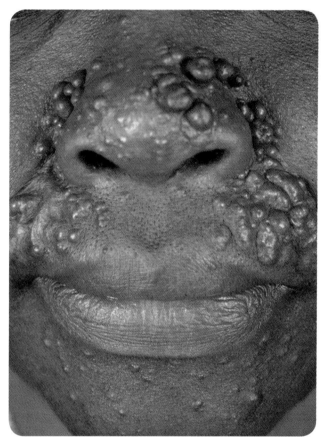

Figure 4-253 Trichoepitheliomas with multiple-sized papules in a typical location.

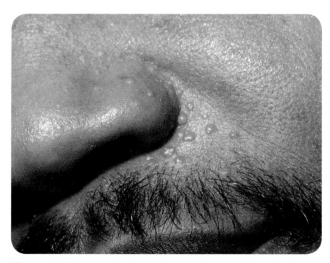

Figure 4-254 Small, slightly lighter than skin-colored trichoepitheliomas near nasal alae.

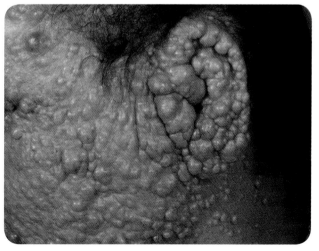

Figure 4-255 Extensive plaques on confluent trichoepitheliomas involving the face, including the ear.

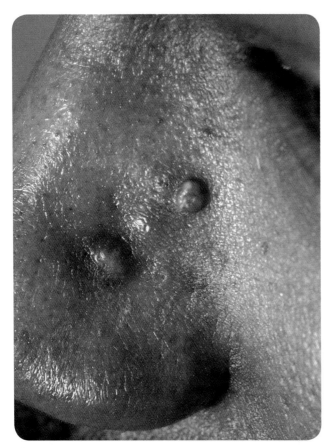

Figure 4-256 Scattered trichoepitheliomas may occur in the common location for these lesions.

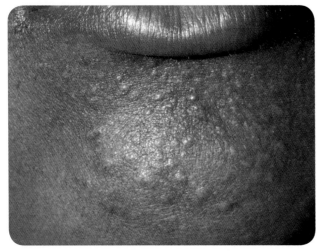

Figure 4-257 Multiple small, slightly hypopigmented papules anywhere on the face may be syringomas.

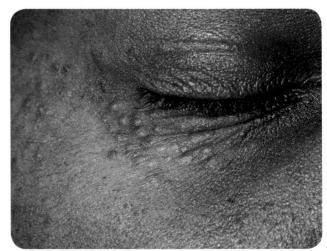

Figure 4-258 Syringomas in a typical location around the eyes.

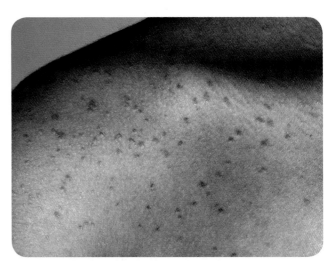

Figure 4-259 Syringomas with multiple regular, slightly pigmented papules on the trunk.

Syringomas

Syringomas often present as multiple discrete, skin-colored papules, 2 to 4 mm in diameter, distributed periorbitally (Figs. 4-257–4-259). They are more common on the lower eyelid and are asymptomatic. The firm papules may be skin colored, yellow, brown, or pink and have also been found to occur on the cheeks, axilla, abdomen, forehead, penis, and vulva. In eruptive syringoma, multiple lesions appear in childhood or early adulthood on the anterior neck, chest, shoulders, abdomen, and pubic area and may regress spontaneously later in life.

Sebaceous Gland Hyperplasia

Small (a few mm but usually <1 cm) yellow papules, often with a central depression (umbilication) and a telangiectatic vessel, that tend to localize on the forehead, temples, and below the eyes. There may be one or two prominent dilated blood vessels that may suggest a basal cell carcinoma. Less commonly, they may also be seen on the chest, areolae, mouth, and genitals. Lesions may be solitary, grouped, annular, or linearly arrayed.

262

Diagnostic Pearls

Angiofibroma

Facial angiofibromas typically have tiny telangiectatic vessels associated with the skin-colored papule, mimicking basal cell carcinomas.

Trichoepithelioma

Trichoepitheliomas are sometimes associated with cylindromas, which are large turban tumors on the scalp.

Syringomas

Clear cell syringomas may be associated with diabetes.

Sebaceous Gland Hyperplasia

The yellow color of sebaceous hyperplasia may be muted and difficult to appreciate on darkly pigmented skin.

?? Differential Diagnosis and Pitfalls

- Acne
- Basal cell carcinoma
- Microcystic adnexal carcinoma
- Verruca vulgaris/verruca planus
- Steatocystoma multiplex
- Sarcoidosis
- Molluscum contagiosum
- Milia
- Xanthelasma

✓ Best Tests

- A skin biopsy is often necessary to exclude malignancies such as basal cell carcinoma.
- Ask for family history of similar lesions.

▲▲ Management Pearls

- While these tumors are benign, when widespread, they are associated with significant cosmetic and psychosocial distress. Cosmetic removal and ablative therapy may be pursued; patients should be warned that treatment may result in scarring and that more lesions often develop over time.
- All of these appendageal lesions may appear as solitary lesions, and biopsy will be required.

Therapy

Appendageal tumors respond to excision (often impractical with many lesions). Ablative therapy with electrosurgery and ablative laser therapy have proven effective in case reports.

The following techniques are useful:

- Simple excision with primary closure (best reserved for those with few lesions or larger lesions)—a punch excision is often sufficient
- Snip excision with healing by secondary intention
- Electrocautery
- Cryotherapy—caution with the possible hypopigmentation left by this treatment modality
- Dermabrasion

In addition, ablative laser therapy may be pursued:

- CO_2 laser
- Erbium:YAG laser
- Fractional laser resurfacing

Suggested Readings

Bader RS, Scarborough DA. Surgical pearl: intralesional electrodesiccation of sebaceous hyperplasia. *J Am Acad Dermatol.* 2000;42(1 Pt 1):127–128.

Camprubí M, Balaguer A, Azon Masoliver A, et al. Unilateral facial angiofibromas; a review of the literature. *Pediatr Dermatol.* 2006;23(3):303–305.

Lane JE, Peterson CM, Ratz JL. Treatment of pearly penile papules with CO2 laser. *Dermatol Surg.* 2002;28(7):617–618.

Langbein L, Cribier B, Schirmacher P, et al. New concepts on the histogenesis of eccrine neoplasa from keratin expression in the normal eccrine gland, syringoma and poroma. *Br J Dermatol.* 2008;159(3):633–645.

Mallory SB. Neonatal skin disorders. *Pediatr Clin North Am.* 1991;38(4):745–761.

Oh ST, Kwon HJ. Premature sebaceous hyperplasia in a neonate. *Pediatr Dermatol.* 2007;24(4):443–445.

Park HJ, Lee DY, Lee JH, et al. The treatment of syringomas by CO(2) laser using a multiple-drilling method. *Dermatol Surg.* 2007;33(3):310–313.

Salim A, Reece SM, Smith AG, et al. Sebaceous hyperplasia and skin cancer in patients undergoing renal transplant. *J Am Acad Dermatol.* 2006;55(5):878–881.

Short KA, Williams A, Creamer D, et al. Sebaceous gland hyperplasia, human immunodeficiency virus and highly active anti-retroviral therapy. *Clin Exp Dermatol.* 2008;33(3):354–355.

Taylor RS, Perone JB, Kaddu S, et al. Appendage tumors and hamartomas of the skin. In: Fitzpatrick TB, Wolff K, eds. *Fitzpatrick's Dermatology in General Medicine.* 7th Ed. New York, NY: McGraw-Hill; 2008:1068–1087.

Terrell S, Wetter R, Fraga G, et al. Penile sebaceous adenoma. *J Am Acad Dermatol.* 2007;57(2 Suppl):S42–S43.

Flat Warts

Lynn McKinley-Grant

■■ Diagnosis Synopsis

Flat warts (plane warts, verruca plana) are benign skin growths caused by human papillomavirus (HPV) types 3, 10, and 28. As the name implies, flat warts are flatter and smoother than common warts. They may be numerous and arranged in groups. Flat warts may be transmitted by direct or indirect contact; autoinoculation is common. Warts can be spread from person to person via contact or within an individual via trauma (Koebnerization) or via shaving. They are most frequently observed in young adults, children, and immunosuppressed patients. They often spontaneously regress, and treatment is, therefore, mainly for cosmetic purposes.

Immunocompromised Patient Considerations

Widespread or extensive warts are often a presenting sign of an immunocompromised state. Warts, in general, tend to be more numerous in immunosuppressed patients and have a higher potential for malignant transformation.

◉ Look For

Minimally elevated, flat-topped papules that may be skin colored or hypopigmented or hyperpigmented, with a tendency to occur in groups or in a linear distribution secondary to trauma (Koebnerization) (Figs. 4-260 and 4-261). Warts are most commonly seen on the face, neck, wrists, and legs.

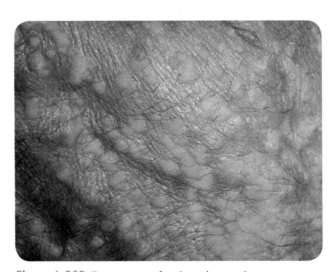

Figure 4-260 Flat warts are often hypopigmented.

264

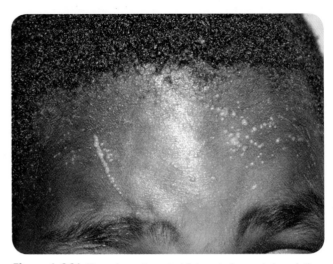

Figure 4-261 Linear hypopigmented flat warts from autoinoculation.

●● Diagnostic Pearls

Flat warts can be both discrete and confluent and have a flat surface. The warts may occur in a linear distribution.

?? Differential Diagnosis and Pitfalls

- Dermatosis papulosa nigrans and small seborrheic keratoses of the face may be confused with flat warts.
- Lichen planus also presents with flat lesions, which are typically more violaceous and pruritic.
- Epidermodysplasia verruciformis is a genetic disease characterized by diffuse flat warts and a high potential for squamous cell carcinoma transformation. Common warts have a more verrucous surface.
- Lichen nitidus is characterized by discrete, dome-shaped papules.
- Molluscum contagiosum lesions are smooth, dome-shaped papules with a central umbilication.
- Follicular eczema or keratosis pilaris is located over the posterior arms and thighs.

✓ Best Tests

This is largely a clinical diagnosis. However, a skin biopsy is diagnostic, when in doubt.

▲▲ Management Pearls

- Flat warts typically remit spontaneously. Therefore, medical intervention is usually instituted for cosmetic reasons when the warts are located on the face or hands, or in immunosuppressed patients to decrease the spread of new lesions.

- Aggressive home therapy with 40% salicylic acid plaster available over the counter (OTC) applied daily or twice daily and taped on with strong adhesive tape (e.g., duct tape). Have the patient pare the wart down with a file or pumice stone between applications of each patch.
- Use caution with liquid nitrogen treatment in darkly pigmented individuals, as there is a risk of hyperpigmentation and hypopigmentation.

Immunocompromised Patient Considerations

Warts in immunosuppressed patients can be quite resistant to traditional therapies.

Therapy

Warts are benign and usually self-limited. Therefore, it is reasonable to not treat them. Any destructive therapy has the possibility of hypopigmentation. Destructive therapies should be used judiciously by those with experience with these procedures. Consider a "test" area before treating numerous lesions or large surface areas. Patients often request treatment, however, in which case therapeutic options include the following:

- Destructive therapy: Cryotherapy using liquid nitrogen applied for 3 to 5 seconds with one to three freeze/ thaw cycles; trichloroacetic acid (TCA) applied topically; electrodesiccation (with caution to avoid scarring); CO_2 laser therapy in extreme cases.
- Topical medications: 5-fluorouracil (1% or 5% cream) applied daily or twice daily; or imiquimod 5% cream can be applied three to five times per week for 6 weeks or longer until lesions disappear. Irritation of the

lesions is expected. Tretinoin 0.1% cream or gel daily or twice daily as tolerated. Tretinoin can be combined with imiquimod as well.

- Intralesional immunotherapy: Topical diphenylcyclopropenone, topical squaric acid, intralesional candida antigen, mumps antigen, and trichophyton antigens can sensitize patients to HPV. This is normally reserved for extreme cases.
- Salicylic acid plasters/ointments (OTC) with therapy as described above. Alternatives include silver nitrate and glutaraldehyde solution.

Immunocompromised Patient Considerations

All therapies for warts can be used in immunosuppressed patients.

Suggested Readings

Androphy EJ, Lowy DR. Warts. In: Fitzpatrick TB, Wolff K, eds. *Fitzpatrick's Dermatology in General Medicine.* 7th Ed. New York, NY: McGraw-Hill; 2008:1914–1923.

Gibbs S, Harvey I. Topical treatments for cutaneous warts. *Cochrane Database Syst Rev.* 2006;3:CD001781.

Gibbs S, Harvey I, Sterling J, et al. Local treatments for cutaneous warts: Systematic review. *BMJ.* 2002;325(7362):461.

Kirnbauer R, Lenz P, Okun MM. Human papillomavirus. In: Bolognia J, Jorizzo JL, Rapini RP, eds. *Dermatology.* 2nd Ed. St. Louis, MO: Mosby/ Elsevier; 2008:1183–1198.

Lipke MM. An armamentarium of wart treatments. *Clin Med Res.* 2006;4(4):273–293.

Micali G, Dall'Oglio F, Nasca MR, et al. Management of cutaneous warts: an evidence-based approach. *Am J Clin Dermatol.* 2004;5(5):311–317.

Prose NS, von Knebel-Doeberitz C, Miller S, et al. Widespread flat warts associated with human papillomavirus type 5: A cutaneous manifestation of human immunodeficiency virus infection. *J Am Acad Dermatol.* 1990;23(5 Pt 2):978–981.

Miliaria Rubra

Saurabh Singh

◨ Diagnosis Synopsis

Miliaria is a common disorder caused by the occlusion of eccrine sweat ducts. There are different clinical patterns of miliaria depending on the level of occlusion.

Miliaria rubra, also known as heat rash or prickly heat, consists of erythematous papules caused by blockage of the eccrine sweat duct. The resultant sweat retention and the escape of sweat into the dermis evoke an inflammatory response with papules. The pathogenesis is often related to conditions of high fever and/or heavy sweating, and it is more prevalent in hot, humid conditions and tropical climates. Predisposing factors also include occlusive clothing, dressings, or ointments.

The lesions can appear within days of exposure to a humid climate but tend to appear months after exposure. Resident bacteria (staphylococci) on the skin may also play a role.

Unlike miliaria crystalline, which is generally asymptomatic, miliaria rubra is a benign disease characterized by intense pruritus and a stinging or "prickly"-type sensation. Anhidrosis develops in affected areas and can last up to weeks. It is a common phenomenon postoperatively and in bedridden and/or febrile patients. Secondary infection is a complication of miliaria rubra that can manifest as either impetigo or multiple discrete abscesses known as periporitis staphylogenes.

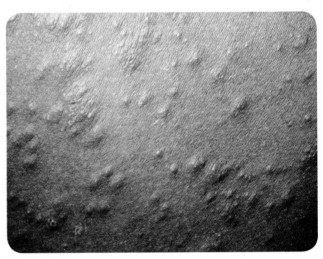

Figure 4-262 Red skin papules of miliaria rubra in type IV skin.

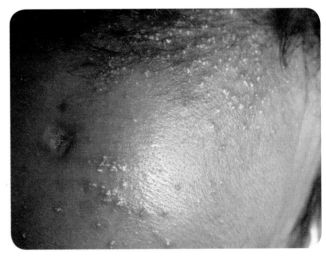

Figure 4-263 Miliaria pustulosa with opaque vesicles.

Pediatric Patient Considerations

While miliaria rubra can occur in people of any age, the disease is most common in infants. This form of miliaria typically affects neonates between 1 and 3 weeks of age.

◉ Look For

Small erythematous and uniform papulovesicles are present and can be widely distributed with background erythema (Fig. 4-262). Miliaria rubra is most prominent in occluded areas, such as the back of hospitalized or bedridden patients. Other sites of predilection in adults include intertriginous and flexural areas and elsewhere on the trunk.

Miliaria pustulosa is a variant of miliaria rubra that consists of superficial (nonfollicular) pustules (Fig. 4-263).

Pediatric Patient Considerations

Miliaria rubra is usually most prominent in occluded areas, such as the back of a nonambulatory child.

◉◉ Diagnostic Pearls

The palms, soles, and acral areas are spared. There is often anhidrosis of the affected site(s).

?? Differential Diagnosis and Pitfalls

- Besides hot climates including incubators, neonatal nurseries, and febrile illnesses, there have been two cases of miliaria rubra triggered by type Ib pseudohypoaldosteronism. This disorder of mineralocorticoid resistance causes excessive loss of salt through eccrine secretions and can be associated with episodes of pustular miliaria rubra. The clinical course was characterized by flares of miliaria rubra, most likely due to abnormal levels of sodium in the sweat. It has also been linked to Morvan syndrome, a rare autoimmune disorder characterized by neuromyotonia, insomnia, hallucinations, pain, weight loss, hyperhidrosis, and miliaria rubra.
- Miliaria rubra is often mistaken for a drug eruption, especially after a new antibiotic is started in a febrile patient.
- Candidiasis often has some pustules.
- Scabies, unlike miliaria, often involves acral sites, especially the presence of burrows in the finger web spaces.
- Varicella manifests as vesicles on an erythematous base ("dewdrops on a rose petal") and presents in different stages of development.
- Folliculitis has follicular-based pustules.
- Acne can also be worsened by occlusion but usually lacks pruritus and is less acute.
- Acute generalized exanthematous pustulosis is more diffuse with widespread pustules.

Pediatric Patient Differential Diagnosis and Pitfalls

The differential also includes the following:

- Herpes simplex virus infection—characteristic grouped vesicles on an erythematous base
- Erythema toxicum neonatorum

✓ Best Tests

- This condition is a clinical diagnosis that could be confirmed by skin biopsy if absolutely necessary.
- Consider bacterial or fungal culture if there is concern for infection.

▲▲ Management Pearls

Patient should be placed in a cool, dry environment. Reassure the patient that the problem is self-limited. Lesions rarely become infected.

Therapy

- Instruct the patient to avoid conditions of excessive heat and sweating. Place the patient in a cool environment if possible, and encourage him/her to wear loose-fitting clothing. Exertion in hot weather should be minimized.
- Treat the underlying cause of any fever and administer antipyretics. Talcum powder or cornstarch may be applied to the skin, but patients should avoid heavy emollients.
- Symptomatic relief may be achieved with cool oatmeal baths or showers, cool compresses, and the application of calamine lotion. Mid-potency steroid lotions can reduce inflammation.

Mid-Potency Topical Corticosteroids (Classes 3 and 4):
- Triamcinolone cream, ointment: apply twice daily (15, 30, 60, 120, 240 g)
- Mometasone cream, ointment: apply twice daily (15, 45 g)
- Fluocinolone ointment, cream: apply twice daily (15, 30, 60 g)

Pediatric Patient Considerations

Avoidance of heat, humidity, occlusive clothing, and ointments.

Suggested Readings

Sato K, Kang WH, Saga K, et al. Biology of the eccrine and apocrine sweat glands. II. Disorders of sweat gland functions. *J Am Acad Dermatol.* 1989;20:713–726.

Tabanelli M, Passarini B, Liguori R, et al. Erythematous papules on the parasternal region in a 76-year-old man. *Clin Exp Dermatol.* 2008; 33(3):369–370.

Granuloma Annulare

Stephanie Diamantis

◼ Diagnosis Synopsis

Granuloma annulare is a benign granulomatous inflammatory disorder of the dermis or subcutis. Its cause is unknown. Small papules may present in isolation or coalesce to form smooth annular plaques, often on the extremities. Lesions are typically asymptomatic or only mildly pruritic, but the appearance may cause patients distress. The disease is more common in women (female-to-male ratio of 2:1), and two-thirds of patients are aged younger than 30. Incidence in people of dark skin color is not reported in the literature.

A small amount of evidence points to granuloma annulare as being associated with certain systemic diseases, such as thyroid disease, diabetes mellitus, malignancy, and infections. "Actinic granuloma" presents with similar lesions but is regarded by many as a separate pathologic entity.

There are three principal variants of granuloma annulare: localized (75% of cases), disseminated (or generalized), and subcutaneous. A fourth variant—perforating granuloma annulare—refers to rare lesions that demonstrate histologic evidence of transepidermal extrusion of degraded collagen.

Granuloma annulare is self-limited. More than 50% of patients with the localized form have spontaneous resolution within 2 months to 2 years, but the eruption may recur. The generalized form tends to persist longer, up to 10 years in some reports.

◉ Look For

In the localized form, patients present with ring-shaped (annular) or arclike (arcuate), nonscaly, reddish-brown plaques or papules (Figs. 4-264–4-266). In dark skin, lesions can appear more hyperpigmented, and the erythema may be less noticeable. Plaque centers are often less pigmented than the edges. They are commonly localized on the fingers, hands, elbows, dorsal feet, or ankles.

Patients with generalized or disseminated granuloma annulare typically have numerous smaller lesions (at least 10) in a widespread distribution that may include extremities, the trunk, and the neck.

Subcutaneous granuloma annulare presents with a firm, skin-colored to slightly erythematous nodule, usually on the lower extremities (Fig. 4-267). It is more common in young children.

The lesions of perforating granuloma annulare also present as grouped 1 to 4 mm papules that may form annular plaques; in some patients, these papules evolve into vesicular or pustular lesions that may umbilicate, ulcerate, or crust, leaving behind a scar as they heal.

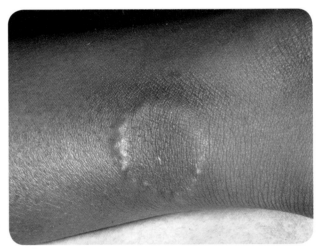

Figure 4-265 Granuloma annulare with typical uniform papules in the annular border.

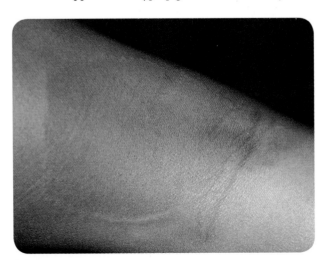

Figure 4-264 Large annular nonscaling hyperpigmented plaque of granuloma annulare.

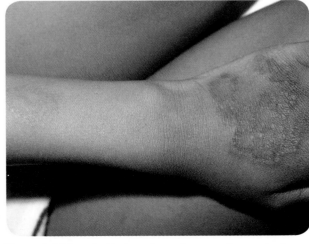

Figure 4-266 Typical lesions of granuloma annulare on the dorsa of the hands in a child.

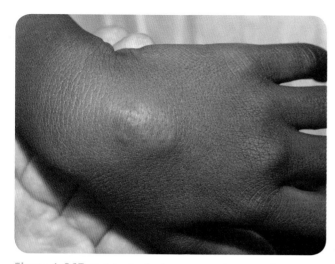

Figure 4-267 Nodule of subcutaneous granuloma annulare.

 Diagnostic Pearls

The annular or arcuate lesions do not have scale. The absence of scale or surface change is a crucial finding in differentiating granuloma annulare from other annular eruptions such as tinea corporis. When stretched, larger lesions show individual papules in a ring, and smaller annular lesions have a small central dell, or depression.

?? Differential Diagnosis and Pitfalls

- Dermatophyte infection (tinea corporis, or "ringworm")—presence of definite scale
- Sarcoidosis
- Erythema annulare centrifugum
- Lichen planus (especially the annular variant)—usually pruritic
- Urticaria—evanescent nature
- Leprosy—anesthetic lesions, in endemic countries
- Erythema elevatum diutinum—over extensor areas, pruritic
- Actinic granuloma
- Necrobiosis lipoidica diabeticorum—atrophic plaques on shins
- Perforating collagenosis
- Elastosis perforans serpiginosa
- Erythema chronicum migrans (Lyme disease)—slow growing, more erythematous
- Erythema gyratum repens
- Sweet syndrome
- Subacute cutaneous lupus erythematosus
- Syphilis
- Annular elastolytic giant cell granuloma
- Pseudolymphoma

- Alopecia mucinosa
- Interstitial granulomatous neutrophilic dermatitis—usually in patients with rheumatoid arthritis

 Best Tests

Skin biopsy will confirm the diagnosis, but a clinical diagnosis is often made by lesional morphology and distribution.

 Management Pearls

There are no clear-cut successful therapies, and large well-designed trials are lacking. The plaques often resolve spontaneously, especially in localized disease; generalized granuloma annulare may prove more persistent. Patient reassurance and education about the benign nature of this disease is essential. Share images of the diagnosis with your patient to reinforce that this is a common process.

Therapy

For localized disease, some treatment success has been achieved with cryotherapy, topical corticosteroids (with or without occlusion), topical calcineurin inhibitors, and careful use of intralesional corticosteroids (triamcinolone 2.5 to 5 mg/mL) injected into the elevated border of a lesion. Smaller therapeutically resistant lesions may be excised. *Note:* Skin atrophy and hypopigmentation are potential side effects with topical or intralesional steroids. High-potency steroids are not recommended for use on the face or body folds. Cryotherapy can also result in hypopigmentation, especially in darker skin.

High-Potency Topical Corticosteroids (Classes 1 and 2)
- Clobetasol cream, ointment—apply twice daily
- Halobetasol cream, ointment—apply twice daily
- Fluocinonide cream, ointment—apply twice daily
- Desoximetasone cream, ointment—apply twice daily

Mid-Potency Topical Corticosteroids (Classes 3 and 4)
- Triamcinolone cream, ointment—apply twice daily
- Mometasone cream, ointment—apply twice daily
- Fluocinolone cream, ointment—apply twice daily

Topical Calcineurin Inhibitors
- Tacrolimus ointment 0.1%—apply twice daily
- Pimecrolimus cream 1%—apply twice daily

(Continued)

For generalized disease, psoralen plus UVA (PUVA), isotretinoin, dapsone, and hydroxychloroquine have been used:

- Isotretinoin—40 mg p.o. daily for 3 months
- Dapsone—100 mg p.o. daily for 8 weeks
- Hydroxychloroquine—200 mg p.o. twice daily for 3 months

Caution: Systemic therapies require careful patient screening and monitoring, and consultation with a dermatologist is recommended.

Other therapies: Other therapies include intralesional interferon (for localized disease), cyclosporin, niacinamide, infliximab, and fumaric acid esters.

Suggested Readings

Cyr PR. Diagnosis and management of granuloma annulare. *Am Fam Physician.* 2006;74:1729–1734.

Hertl MS, Haendle I, Schuler G, et al. Rapid improvement of recalcitrant disseminated granuloma annulare upon treatment with the tumor necrosis factor-alpha inhibitor, infliximab. *Br J Dermatol.* 2005;152(3):552–555.

Prendiville JS. Granuloma annulare. In: Wolff K, Goldsmith LA, Katz SI, et al., eds. *Fitzpatrick's Dermatology in General Medicine.* 7th Ed. New York, NY: McGraw Hill; 2008:369–373.

Requena L, Fernandez-Figueras MT. Subcutaneous granuloma annulare. *Semin Cutan Med Surg.* 2007;26:96–99.

Steiner A, Pehamberger H, Wolff K. Sulfone treatment of granuloma annulare. *J Am Acad Dermatol.* 1985;13:1004–1008.

Histiocytosis

Tess Nasabzadeh

▞▚ Diagnosis Synopsis

Langerhans cell histiocytosis (LCH), or histiocytosis-X, encompasses a rare group of disorders, historically referred to as Letterer-Siwe disease, Hand-Schüller-Christian disease, and eosinophilic granuloma, in which Langerhans cells clonally proliferate and accumulate in organs. Langerhans cells are dendritic histiocytes derived from the bone marrow that normally reside in the epidermis where they play a role in antigen presentation and immune activation. It is unclear if LCH represents a dysfunctional immune response to an antigen or a neoplastic process. The current classification system of LCH is based on the number of organ systems involved, for example, single-system or multisystem LCH. The skin, bone, bone marrow, lungs, liver, spleen, gastrointestinal tract, lymph nodes, and central nervous system may be affected. Skin involvement is seen in 50% to 80% of cases.

LCH occurs in all age groups with a peak in children 1 to 4 years of age. The annual incidence is approximately 0.5 to 5.4 per million persons with males being affected slightly more frequently than females. LCH has no known racial predilection. However, the pattern of disease may vary among different ethnic groups. For example, lung disease is reportedly common among LCH patients in China, and lymph node involvement was the most common presentation in a study of patients in Northeast Egypt.

The spectrum of LCH ranges from spontaneously resolving localized disease to multisystem disease with organ failure and death. Poor prognostic factors include involvement of the spleen, liver, lung, and bone marrow and no response to chemotherapy within the first 6 weeks of treatment. A majority of patients with multisystem LCH have long-term complications such as hypothalamic-pituitary dysfunction, cognitive dysfunction, cerebellar involvement, and growth retardation. Patients with single-system disease are also at risk of long-term sequelae, relapses, and progression to systemic disease.

Pediatric Patient Considerations

Congenital self-healing Langerhans cell histiocytosis (CSHLCH), also known as Hashimoto-Pritzker disease, is a rare, benign variant of LCH. It presents at birth or within the first few weeks of life with generalized papules, vesicles, or nodules and spontaneously resolves within 3 to 4 months. Internal organs are usually not affected.

◉ Look For

LCH typically affects the scalp and skin folds with subtle erythematous to brown papules and plaques that become scaly, crusted, or petechial (Figs. 4-268–4-270). With further progression, they may appear verrucous and waxy, become ulcerative and weeping, and develop hemorrhagic crusts. In an Indian patient, multisystem LCH presented with hypopigmented macules.

Systemic involvement in LCH may be asymptomatic or manifest with signs of organ dysfunction (Fig. 4-271). Organ-specific symptoms include painful swelling with bone involvement; lymphadenopathy with lymph node involvement; hepatosplenomegaly, jaundice, and prolonged prothrombin time with liver and spleen involvement; tachypnea and retractions with lung involvement; malabsorption and diarrhea with gastrointestinal involvement; and diabetes insipidus and progressive encephalopathy with central nervous system involvement.

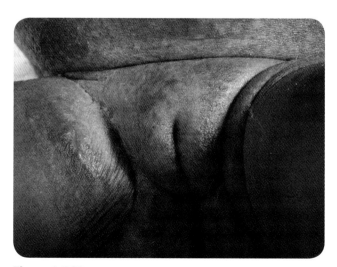

Figure 4-268 Langerhans cell histiocytosis with diffuse infiltration of the groin.

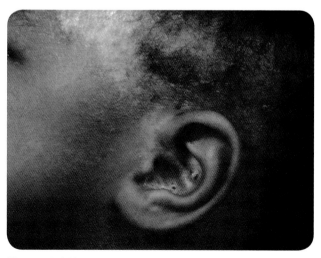

Figure 4-269 Scalp and ear papules and hypopigmentation in Langerhans cell histiocytosis.

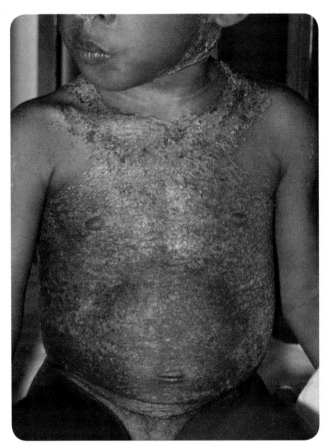

Figure 4-270 Diffuse infiltrated plaques of Langerhans cell histio-cytosis.

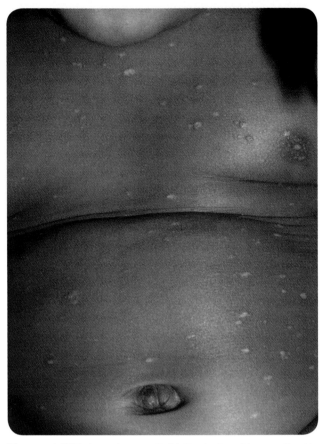

Figure 4-271 Langerhans cell histiocytosis with smooth skin papules and abdominal distention from hepatosplenomegaly.

Pediatric Patient Considerations

The skin lesions in CSHLCH consist of generalized firm, red to brown painless papules and nodules. The face, scalp, extremities, and trunk are most often affected. In two Tunisian children with CSHLCH, the lesions were described as "brown-red papulonodules" and "yellow papules" with ulcerations and scabs. CSHLCH may present as a "blueberry muffin" baby with disseminated purpura. Systemic signs are absent except for mild hepatomegaly in some cases.

 Diagnostic Pearls

You should consider LCH in a child who has been diag-nosed with seborrheic or diaper dermatitis that is resistant to

therapy, has underlying petechiae, or has progressive oozing and crusting.

?? Differential Diagnosis and Pitfalls

- Benign cephalic histiocytosis—a non–Langerhans cell histiocytosis that presents as a self-healing papular erup-tion in children <3 years of age. It is differentiated from LCH with immunohistochemistry.
- Seborrheic dermatitis—It lacks distinct papules.
- Scabies—It may resemble LCH clinically and histologi-cally. Ask about affected family members.
- Atopic dermatitis—It is much more pruritic and respon-sive to steroids.
- Diaper dermatitis—It is localized to the diaper area and is responsive to topical steroids.

Pediatric Patient Differential Diagnosis

In pediatric patients suspected of having CSHLCH, the differential diagnosis includes the following:

- Neonatal pustular melanosis
- Perinatal herpes simplex
- *Listeria monocytogenes*
- Congenital candidiasis
- Neonatal varicella
- Syphilis
- Erythema toxicum

 Best Tests

In LCH and CSHLCH, skin biopsy for histology and immunohistochemistry reveals an infiltrate of CD1a-positive and S100-positive histiocytic cells. An evaluation to rule out extracutaneous involvement is required. This evaluation should include complete blood count, liver function tests, abdominal ultrasound, skeletal survey, and bone marrow aspiration.

 Management Pearls

Patients with LCH and CSHLCH should be followed up long-term by an oncologist, given the unpredictable course of the disease and the risk of relapse.

Therapy

Treatment may not be needed for isolated skin disease. For symptomatic cutaneous lesions, topical steroids are first-line therapy, while second-line therapies include topical nitrogen mustard and psoralen plus UVA (PUVA) therapy. Multiorgan involvement requires administration of chemotherapy by an oncologist.

Suggested Readings

Al-Tonbary YA, Sarhan MM, Mansour AK, et al. Histiocytosis disorders in Northeast Egypt: Epidemiology and survival studies (a 5-year study). *Hematology.* 2009;14(5):271–275.

Belhadjali H, Mohamed M, Mahmoudi H, et al. Self-healing Langerhans cell histiocytosis (Hashimoto-Pritzker disease): Two Tunisian cases. *Acta Dermatoven APA.* 2008;17(4):188–191.

Boradbent V, Egeler RM, Nesbit ME. Langerhans cell histiocytosis—clinical and epidemiological aspects. *Br J Cancer.* 1994;70(Suppl XXIII):S11–S16.

Feroze K, Unni M, Jayasree M, et al. Langerhans cell histiocytosis presenting with hypopigmented macules. *Indian J Dermatol Venereol Leprol.* 2008;74(6):670–671.

Satter EK, High WA. Langerhans cell histiocytosis: A case report and summary of current recommendations of the Histiocyte Society. *Dermatol Online J.* 2008;14(3):3.

Shaffer MP, Walling HW, Stone MS. Langerhans cell histiocytosis presenting as blueberry muffin baby. *J Am Acad Dermatol.* 2005;53:S143–S146.

Walia M, Paul P, Mishra S, et al. Congenital Langherans cell histiocytosis: The self-healing variety. *J Pediatr Hematol Oncol.* 2004;26(6):398–402.

Polymorphous Light Eruption

Randa Khoury

▪▪ Diagnosis Synopsis

Polymorphous light eruption (PMLE), or polymorphic light eruption, is a common acquired cutaneous disorder that is characterized by a pathologic response to ultraviolet (UV) radiation. Erythematous papules, vesicles, and plaques (hence the name "polymorphous") develop minutes to hours after exposure to sunlight or a tanning bed. The lesions are often pruritic, nonscarring, and always restricted to sun-exposed areas. Systemic symptoms such as fever, malaise, headache, myalgias, and arthralgias are usually absent. While lesions can last up to several weeks, most resolve within several days' time.

PMLE has been underreported in the V and VI skin types, because many of these patients and their physicians think that it is normal to break out with the first exposure to the sun. PMLE is most commonly seen in fair-skinned women aged 20 to 30, but it can occur in either sex, in all ages, and in all ethnicities. Attacks most commonly occur during the spring and early summer months and disappear during the winter. While the etiology is not well-defined, investigations support a type IV delayed-type hypersensitivity reaction.

Although the condition frequently recurs, the tendency toward the development of PMLE and the severity of the eruption diminish with repeated sunlight exposure. This key concept in the management of PMLE is termed "hardening." As the summer proceeds, it has been observed that the incidence of new eruptions decreases. Prophylactic phototherapy supports this concept of hardening, or tolerance.

Of note, despite the variability of presentations, individual patients tend to experience the same clinical manifestations with each episode.

PMLEs are more common in fair-skinned individuals (Fitzpatrick skin types I to IV), but one recent study found that the overall incidence of photodermatoses in African Americans is similar to that in whites.

Actinic Prurigo

Recognition of a pinpoint papular variant of PMLE is important for diagnosis and treatment. Formerly thought to be PMLE but now recognized as a distinct entity, actinic prurigo occurs in persons of all skin types, but its prevalence in the general population is unknown. It is known to occur more frequently in Native Americans and is familial in Latin Americans. In this condition, lesions appear hours or days after UV exposure, and there is frequent association with cheilitis and conjunctivitis. No systemic or local photosensitizer is known.

◉ Look For

As the name suggests, there are a variety of morphologic types. The most common are the papular and papulovesicular forms (Figs. 4-272 and 4-273). These are small erythematous to sandpaper-like papules and vesicles distributed in

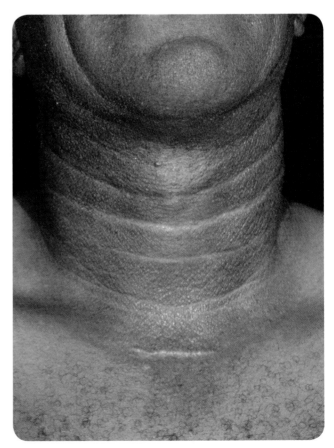

Figure 4-273 Thickened skin with sparing of the upper medial neck, where the skin is shielded from the sun by the chin, is characteristic of chronic and acute photosensitivity diseases.

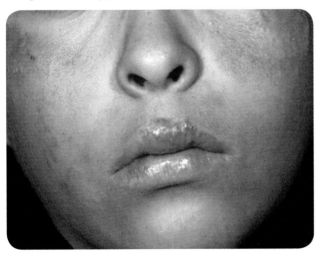

Figure 4-272 Facial papules are common in polymorphous light eruptions; lip lesions are less common.

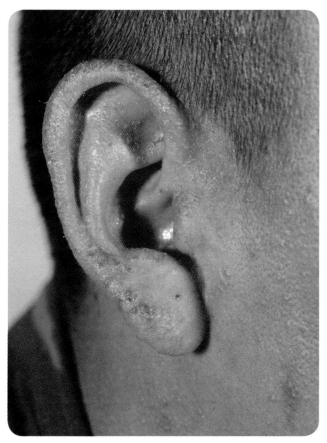

Figure 4-274 Polymorphous light eruption may appear eczematous and be confused with an airborne contact dermatitis to an allergen such as ragweed pollen.

sun-exposed areas (Fig. 4-274). Variants include an eczematouslike form as well as a vesiculobullous form. Some lesions may be difficult to distinguish from erythema multiforme.

Diagnostic Pearls

- Ten percent of the population has this reaction, often with the first episode of sun exposure each season (particularly those from a northern climate who visit a sunny vacation spot). The distribution of lesions is more useful in suggesting this diagnosis than the morphology.
- PMLE may occasionally occur in the winter as the result of the reflection of UV rays off the snow (more common in those who participate in winter sports).
- As a distinction from the ordinary sunburn eruption, people sensitive to longer wavelengths (UVA) can erupt when light goes through window glass (e.g., a bus or car window).

Differential Diagnosis and Pitfalls

- Systemic lupus erythematosus—Check for circulating ANA and other associated lupus antibodies. Direct immunofluorescence will be positive, and skin lesions can be located on sun-exposed and sun-protected areas (in contrast to PMLE, which is primarily in sun-exposed sites).
- Sunburn
- Contact dermatitis to sunscreen, fragrances, or oil of bergamot used in hair preparations
- Solar urticaria—shorter time course with urticarial lesions lasting 1 to 2 hours
- Erythema multiforme—characteristic target lesions; systemic symptoms are prominent (in contrast to PMLE, where fever, malaise, nausea, and headache are rare)
- Hydroa vacciniforme
- Transient acantholytic dermatosis (Grover disease)—peak incidence in winter months; lesions are frequently crusted over, and there is more trunk involvement than extremities and face
- Porphyria cutanea tarda—It will have abnormal porphyrin profile (elevated urine uroporphyrin and stool isocoproporphyrin).
- Erythropoietic protoporphyria—Lesions are very painful, and there is an elevated red blood cell protoporphyrin concentration.
- Photoallergic drug reaction—Investigate for drug history. Not seasonally associated and does not improve over time.
- Phototoxic drug reaction
- Airborne contact dermatitis

✓ Best Tests

- Skin biopsy is suggestive of the diagnosis but is not always necessary.
- Laboratory investigations may be done to rule out other diagnoses. Obtaining ANA, SS-A, and SS-B titers and urine, stool, and serum porphyrin levels will rule out lupus erythematosus and porphyria. In addition, a direct immunofluorescence will be positive in lupus and negative in PMLE.
- Note, however, that previous studies have shown that up to 19% of patients with PMLE can be ANA positive. A recent long-term follow-up study of patients with PMLE demonstrated that although ANA positive, these patients did not have clinical, histopathologic, or laboratory abnormalities suggestive of lupus erythematosus. An ANA alone may not be sufficient in differentiating PMLE from lupus. Skin biopsy may not definitively distinguish PMLE from lupus erythematosus.
- Phototesting with UVA, UVB, and visible light sources may be helpful. Photopatch testing can rule out photoallergic or airborne contact dermatitis.
- Adults with photosensitivity should consider HIV testing, as photosensitivity may be an early sign of HIV infection.

▲▲ Management Pearls

- Prevention is often the best treatment. Instruct patients to limit their sunlight exposure, especially in the early morning and late afternoon hours. The use of tanning beds should be stopped. Patients should also be encouraged to wear protective clothing and use a sunscreen that blocks both UVA and UVB rays, as UVB blocking alone may exacerbate the rash.
- Sunscreens that have high sun protection factor have not demonstrated efficacy in protecting against UVA-induced PMLE. A recent randomized, placebo-controlled trial demonstrated that the addition of a potent antioxidant (such as vitamin E) to a broad-spectrum sunscreen may be much more effective than the sunscreen alone.
- Refer severe and/or recalcitrant cases to a dermatologist.

Therapy

Preventative measures as stated above should be instituted.

Phototherapy
Prophylactic phototherapy two to three times per week for an average of 5 weeks in early spring with the following:

- Psoralen plus UVA (PUVA) 0.5 to 0.6 mg/kg of 8-methoxypsoralen 1 hour prior to UVA exposure
- Narrow-band (311 nm) UVB phototherapy can be efficacious.

In both forms of phototherapy, oral prednisone (1 mg/kg) can be administered for the first week of treatment to minimize erythema and photoexacerbation.

Corticosteroids
- Topical corticosteroids may provide some symptomatic relief (classes 6 and 7 for face and classes 2 and 4 for trunk and arms).

High-Potency Topical Corticosteroids (Class 2)
- Fluocinonide cream, ointment—apply twice daily (15, 30, 60, 120 g)
- Desoximetasone cream, ointment—apply twice daily (15, 60, 120 g)
- Halcinonide cream, ointment—apply twice daily (15, 60, 240 g)
- Amcinonide ointment—apply twice daily (15, 30, 60 g)

Mid-Potency Topical Corticosteroids (Classes 3 and 4)
- Triamcinolone cream, ointment—apply twice daily (15, 30, 60, 120, 240 g)

- Mometasone cream, ointment—apply twice daily (15, 45 g)
- Fluocinolone ointment, cream—apply twice daily (15, 30, 60 g)

Mild-Potency Topical Corticosteroids (Class 6 or 7)
- Desonide cream, lotion—apply twice daily (15, 30, 60 g)
- Hydrocortisone cream 2.5%—apply twice daily (1, 2 oz)

Note: antihistamines are helpful for pruritus.

Systemic Corticosteroids
Systemic corticosteroids may be needed to suppress severe, generalized eruptions:

- Prednisone 0.5 to 2 mg/kg p.o. daily divided twice daily, taper over 1 to 2 weeks

Antimalarials
A course of antimalarials may also be helpful in the treatment and prevention of severe cases:

- Hydroxychloroquine 200 mg p.o. twice daily for 2 to 3 months in early springtime

Vitamins
- Beta-carotene 30 to 300 mg p.o. daily
- Nicotinamide 1 g p.o. three times daily

Immunomodulators
- Thalidomide 50 to 200 mg p.o. nightly

Suggested Readings

Bernal JE, Duran de Rueda MM, Ordonez CP, et al. Actinic prurigo among the Chimila Indians in Colombia: HLA studies. *J Am Acad Dermatol.* 1990;22(6 Pt 1):1049–1051.

Drummer R, Ivanova K, Scheidegger EP, et al. Clinical and therapeutic aspects of polymorphous light eruption. *Dermatology.* 2003;207(1):93–95.

Fesq H, Ring J, Abeck D. management of polymorphous light eruption: clinical course, pathogenesis, diagnosis, and intervention. *Am J Clin Dermatol.* 2003;4(6):399–406.

Honigsmann H. Polymorphous light eruption. *Photodermatol Photoimmunol Photomed.* 2008;24(3):155–161.

Kerr HA, Lim HW. Photodermatoses in African Americans: a retrospective analysis of 135 patients over a 7-year period. *J Am Acad Dermatol.* 2007;57(4):638–643.

Kontos AP, Cusack CA, Chaffins M, et al. Polymorphous light eruption in African Americans: pinpoint papular variant. *Photodermatol Photoimmunol Photomed.* 2002;18(6):303–306.

Ling TC, Gibbs NK, Rhodes LE. Treatment of polymorphic light eruption. *Photodermatol Photoimmunol Photomed.* 2003;19(5):217–227.

Naleway AL, Greenlee RT, Melski JW. Characteristics of diagnosed polymorphous light eruption. *Photodermatol Photoimmunil Photomed.* 2006;22(4):205–207.

Sheridan DP, Lane PR, Irvine J, et al. HLA typing in actinic prurigo. *J Am Acad Dermatol.* 1990;22(6 Pt 1):1019–1023.

Tzaneva S, Volc-Platzer B, Kittler H, et al. Antinuclear antibodies in patients with polymorphic light eruption: a long-term follow-up study. *Br J Dermatol.* 2008;158(5):1050–1054.

Neurofibromatosis

Lowell A. Goldsmith

■■ Diagnosis Synopsis

Neurofibromatosis Type 1

Neurofibromatosis type 1 (von Recklinghausen disease or NF1) is a multisystem genetic disorder with hallmark cutaneous findings, including café au lait macules, neurofibromas, and axillary freckling. NF1 may affect the skin, nervous system, eyes, bone, and soft tissue. It is the most common autosomal dominant genetic disorder, affecting approximately 1 in 3,000 human beings and occurring either as an inherited defect or, frequently, as a spontaneous (i.e., *de novo*) mutation.

NF1 occurs equally in all ethnicities and both sexes and is often first identified in childhood with the appearance of café au lait macules.

The genetic defect is in a tumor suppressor gene on chromosome 17, which codes for neurofibromin, a Ras GTPase activating protein. Patients are at increased risk of developing benign and malignant neoplasms. Benign neoplasms include neurofibromas—complex tumors of admixed Schwann cells, fibroblasts, myelinated and unmyelinated nerve axons, endothelial cells, and mast cells—that occur in one of four forms: cutaneous, subcutaneous, nodular, and deep. Plexiform neurofibromas (present in 25% of patients) are a variant of neurofibroma that are typically deeper, more anatomically complex, and more likely to be symptomatic. Deep plexiform neurofibromas may develop into malignant peripheral nerve sheath tumors. Other malignancies and tumors associated with neurofibromatosis include gliomas (especially optic pathway gliomas in 10% to 15% of patients and especially in early disease stage), pheochromocytomas, meningiomas, sarcomas, gastrointestinal tumors of neuroendocrine origin such as duodenal carcinoid tumors, and juvenile myelomonocytic leukemia. In addition to tumors and skin findings, patients may also have learning disabilities (30% to 50%), skeletal anomalies, vasculopathies, and endocrinologic abnormalities.

The diagnosis of NF1 is made on clinical grounds, based on two or more of the following criteria, initially developed at an NIH consensus conference:

- Six or more café au lait macules >5 mm in diameter in prepubertal individuals and >15 mm in diameter in postpubertal patients
- Two or more Lisch nodules (iris hamartomas) in older patients
- Sphenoid dysplasia or thinning of a long bone's cortex, with or without pseudoarthrosis
- Two or more neurofibromas of any type or a single plexiform neurofibroma
- Freckling in the axillary or inguinal region
- Optic glioma (in early childhood)
- First-degree relative with NF1 (although new mutations are frequent)

Special Infant Considerations

When evaluating an infant, it is important to remember that several of the cardinal features of NF1 have age-related penetrance, and, therefore, many young children will need to be followed over time to make a clinical diagnosis. By age 11, 95% of children can be diagnosed by clinical criteria alone.

Neurofibromatosis Type 2

Patients with neurofibromatosis type 2 (NF2) present primarily with acoustic neuromas (schwannomas of the eighth cranial nerve). NF2, which is ten times less common than NF1, is associated with mutation of a different tumor suppressor gene that is located on chromosome 22 and codes for a protein called merlin. Patients have fewer café au lait macules than those with NF1, and they do not form Lisch nodules in the iris.

◉ Look For

Multiple (six or more) café au lait macules (flat, uniformly darker patches with sharp borders) in postpubertal patients (Figs. 4-275 and 4-276). It is important to note that at least one café au lait macule has been found in 0.3% of white and 18.3% of black infants and in 13% of white and 27% of black older children, respectively.

Café au lait macules may appear lighter than the surrounding skin in heavily pigmented individuals. The macules are typically larger than 15 mm in diameter. Also look for axillary freckling or freckling in other intertriginous areas. Intertriginous freckling consists of 1- to 4-mm tan to red-brown well-defined macules that are often very subtle in infants.

Neurofibromas will increase with age and appear as skin colored or somewhat lighter than the background skin tumors and nodules (Fig. 4-277). Cutaneous neurofibromas are soft and will descend into the underlying dermis with direct pressure (the "button hole" sign) and may at times be segmental (Fig. 4-278). Subcutaneous neurofibromas are tender (often painful) and can be up to several centimeters in size. Plexiform neurofibromas are deep, sometimes involving all layers of the skin to the fascia. They are thick and irregular and may infiltrate or disfigure

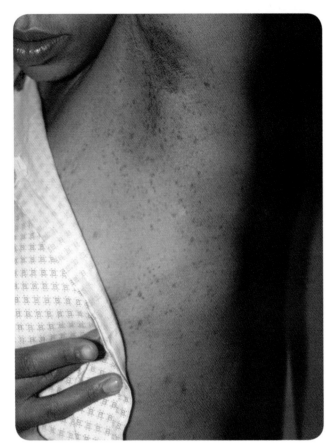

Figure 4-275 Multiple small café au lait macules involving the axillae.

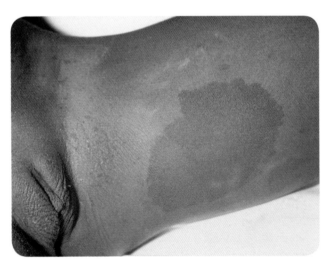

Figure 4-276 Large, flat brown macule (café au lait spot) on the thigh and many small brown macules in the inguinal area in neurofibromatosis.

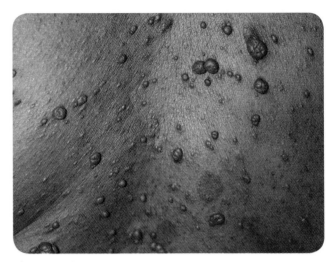

Figure 4-277 Multiple sessile and pedunculated papules in neurofibromatosis.

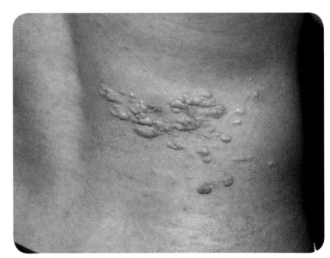

Figure 4-278 Neurofibromas in a segmental distribution.

nearby structures (Fig. 4-279). Plexiform neurofibromas may also cause hyperpigmentation and/or hypertrichosis of overlying skin. Iris hamartomas (Lisch nodules) are also associated with the disease and are ultimately identifiable in 90% of patients.

All children with a high suspicion for NF1 should be evaluated by a dermatologist, ophthalmologist, orthopedic surgeon, neurologist, and pediatrician.

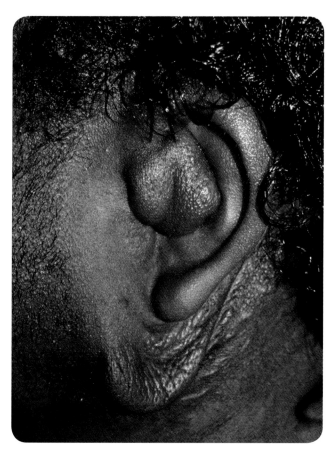

Figure 4-279 Irregular plexiform neurofibroma involving the ear.

Diagnostic Pearls

When applying diagnostic criteria or evaluating a child, it is important to remember the age-related penetrance of manifestations of NF1:

- Sphenoid wing dysplasia—birth
- Long-bone bowing—birth to early childhood
- Optic pathway tumors—birth to early childhood
- Café au lait macules—birth to childhood
- Plexiform neurofibromas—birth to adulthood
- Hypertension—lifelong
- Intertriginous freckling—childhood
- Scoliosis—childhood
- Neurofibromas—late childhood to adolescence
- Nerve sheath tumors—adolescence to adulthood

Special Infant Considerations

Although the NIH diagnostic criteria require café au lait macules to be larger than 5 mm in greatest diameter in prepubescent children, skin lesions present at birth are estimated to grow eight times their size by adulthood; hence, macules smaller than 5 mm in infants may meet criteria for size.

?? Differential Diagnosis and Pitfalls

The differential diagnosis of NF1 includes:

Other Forms of Neurofibromatosis

- Segmental/mosaic NF1
- Watson syndrome
- Autosomal dominant multiple café au lait macules alone (some allelic with NF1)
- Neurofibromatosis type 2
- Schwannomatosis (recently distinguished disorder associated with mutation in the gene INI1)

Other Conditions with Café Au Lait Macules

- McCune-Albright syndrome—premature puberty, bony abnormalities, and a few large café au lait macules with an irregular outline. In NF1, the outline of the café au lait macule is smooth.
- Genetic disorders of DNA repair or chromosomal instability
- Homozygosity for one of the genes causing hereditary nonpolyposis
- Cancer of the colon
- Noonan syndrome

Conditions with Pigmented Macules often Confused with NF1

- LEOPARD syndrome
- Neurocutaneous melanosis
- Peutz-Jeghers syndrome
- Piebaldism

Localized Overgrowth Syndromes

- Klippel-Trenaunay-Weber syndrome
- Proteus syndrome

Conditions Causing Tumors Confused with Those Seen in NF1

- Lipomatosis
- Bannayan-Riley-Ruvalcaba syndrome
- Fibromatosis
- Multiple endocrine neoplasia types 1 and 2B

Isolated neurofibromas without neurofibromatosis are also common (see "Solitary Neurofibroma").

✓ Best Tests

- Examine family members, including those said to have no findings.
- Check for Lisch nodules with a slit-lamp examination.
- If the patient is having neurologic symptoms, obtain an MRI of the brain, orbits, and/or spinal cord. It may also be useful to perform an MRI of any particularly deep or changing plexiform neurofibromas.
- Genetic testing is possible in equivocal cases.

NF1 is a clinical diagnosis. Testing should be individualized and only considered based on symptoms:

- Increased growth velocity or precocious puberty—cranial imaging for optic pathway gliomas
- Painful or rapidly growing mass—MRI and possible biopsy for malignant peripheral nerve sheath tumor or other tumors
- Tibial bowing—X-ray for pseudoarthrosis
- Increased curvature of the spine—spine radiographs for scoliosis
- Dystopia—MRI for plexiform neurofibroma
- Hypertension—abdominal MRI or angiography for renovascular disease or pheochromocytoma; and 24-hour urine catecholamines, homovanillic acid, and vanillylmandelic acid for pheochromocytoma
- Significant weight loss and constitutional symptoms—blood smear and bone marrow evaluation for juvenile chronic myelogenous leukemia

Special Infant Considerations

When an infant does not meet diagnostic criteria but clinical suspicion is high, annual reevaluation of the diagnostic criteria by a physician familiar with NF1 and ophthalmology evaluations should suffice.

▲▲ Management Pearls

Children with NF1 should have the following evaluated annually:

- Height and weight—precocious puberty (optic pathway glioma)
- Blood pressure—hypertension
- Skin exam—dermal and plexiform neurofibromas
- Bone exam—scoliosis
- Neurologic exam—developmental delays and learning disabilities
- Vision screen—optic pathway gliomas

- Sexual maturation—delayed/precocious puberty (optic pathway glioma)
- Psychological/social adjustment—self-esteem problems

Genetic Evaluation

Parents should be carefully examined for any signs of NF so that they may be counseled concerning recurrence rate. Because of the high incidence of de novo mutations, recurrence rates may be difficult to estimate and this counseling should be done by a medical geneticist.

Special Infant Considerations

In addition to an evaluation of the diagnostic criteria for NF1, infants should be screened for other associated manifestations of NF1.

- Neurodevelopmental evaluation—developmental delay
- Head circumference—tumors or hydrocephalus
- Height and weight—precocious puberty
- Blood pressure (at least one forelimb)—renal artery stenosis, pheochromocytoma, coarctation of the aorta
- Cardiovascular evaluation—congenital heart defects

Therapy

- Therapy should be planned by a multispecialist team with experience with this disease.
- Excision of tumors is palliative and should be reserved for symptomatic or grossly disfiguring lesions. Surgery may not be practical for patients with a large burden of disease.
- Simple excision is often performed when there are few or symptomatic neurofibromas. Many small lesions can be treated using monopolar diathermy with a wire loop. Healing is by secondary intention. Vaporization with the carbon dioxide laser has also been used to treat neurofibromas.
- Most plexiform neurofibromas are asymptomatic and require no further treatment other than regular evaluation of growth. Painful or functionally impairing plexiform neurofibromas, however, should be imaged by MRI and considered for excision by a soft tissue tumor oncology team. All orbitotemporal plexiform neurofibromas should be evaluated by a plastic surgeon and/or soft tissue tumor oncology team for possible early excision to prevent future disfiguring and vision-threatening growth.

- Methods for treating plexiform neurofibromas and malignant peripheral nerve sheath tumors with angiogenesis inhibitors and anti-inflammatory agents are largely experimental; thalidomide and 3D planned radiotherapy have also been used.
- Symptomatic or growing optic gliomas in children are treated with a combination of carboplatin and vincristine.
- Ketotifen has been used with success to treat pain and pruritus: 2 to 4 mg p.o. daily. Common antihistamines typically do not work for pruritus in NF1.
- Café au lait macules can be treated cosmetically with the Nd:YAG, ruby, or pulsed dye laser, although it is important to note that laser therapy of café au lait macules has produced mixed results with a recurrence rate of up to 67%.

Special Infant Considerations

Laser therapy of café au lait macules is not recommended in infants.

Suggested Readings

Alper JC, Holmes LB. The incidence and significance of birthmarks in a cohort of 4,641 newborns. *Pediatr Dermatol.* 1983;1(1):58–68.

Boyd KP, Korf BR, Theos A. Neurofibromatosis type 1. *J Am Acad Dermatol.* 2009;61(1):1–14.

DeBella K, Szudek J, Friedman JM. Use of the national institutes of health criteria for diagnosis of neurofibromatosis 1 in children. *Pediatrics.* 2000;105(3 Pt 1):608–614.

Ferner RE, Huson SM, Thomas N, et al. Guidelines for the diagnosis and management of individuals with neurofibromatosis 1. *J Med Genet.* 2007;44(2):81–88.

Hersh JH, American Academy of Pediatrics Committee on Genetics. Health supervision for children with neurofibromatosis. *Pediatrics.* 2008;121(3):633–642.

Needle MN, Cnaan A, Dattilo J, et al. Prognostic signs in the surgical management of plexiform neurofibroma: The Children's Hospital of Philadelphia experience, 1974–1994. *J Pediatr.* 1997;131(5):678–682.

Parsons CM, Canter RJ, Khatri VP. Surgical management of neurofibromatosis. *Surg Oncol Clin N Am.* 2009;18(1):175–196, x.

Xanthomas

Chris G. Adigun

▪▪ Diagnosis Synopsis

Cutaneous xanthomas result from intracellular dermal deposition of lipid, usually related to a disorder of lipoprotein metabolism. Xanthomatous tissue is distinguished by its characteristic yellow to orange hue. Cutaneous xanthomas have a wide variety of morphologies, including macules, papules, plaques, and nodules. The morphologic variants are clues to underlying lipid or lymphoproliferative disorders. The early diagnosis of xanthomas allows for appropriate management of the systemic consequences of their underlying disorder.

Hyperlipidemia is a common underlying abnormality among patients with cutaneous xanthomas. Hyperlipidemia is increasingly common in many countries, but only a small minority of these individuals will go on to develop xanthomas. The exact mechanism of xanthoma development has yet to be elucidated, but lipids found in circulation are the same as those in xanthomas. Therefore, in xanthomas, formation is likely due to the permeation of circulating plasma lipoproteins leaving the dermal capillary vessels that are subsequently phagocytized by dermal macrophages, forming the characteristic "foam" cells seen on histopathological examination.

The major forms of cutaneous xanthomas associated with hyperlipidemia are eruptive, tuberous, tendinous, and plane, including xanthelasma palpebrarum. (*Note:* See entry for "Xanthelasma Palpebrarum" for discussion of this condition). Xanthoma tuberosum and tendinosum tend to occur in familial hypercholesteremia, and eruptive xanthomas (EX) tend to occur in primary or secondary hypertriglyceridemia. Plane xanthomas located in the palmar creases are nearly pathognomonic for familial dysbetalipoproteinemia, whereas plane xanthomas located in intertriginous sites may indicate homozygous familial hypercholesterolemia. Plane xanthomas occurring in a patient who is normolipemic suggest an underlying monoclonal gammopathy. Plane xanthomas also occur with cholestasis resulting from conditions such as biliary atresia or primary biliary cirrhosis. These lesions tend to occur as discrete plaques on the hands and feet, but they may become generalized.

EX are a consequence of severe chylomicronemia and hypertriglyceridemia. These xanthomas are pruritic, small, yellow to orange papules scattered over the trunk and extremities. Hypertriglyceridemia may result from hereditary conditions such as lipoprotein lipase deficiency or familial hyperlipoproteinemia, or from secondary causes such as excessive alcohol intake, diabetes mellitus, or cholestasis. Medications, including systemic retinoids, estrogens, and protease inhibitors for HIV infection, are also common causes of hypertriglyceridemia and subsequent development of EX. Triglyceridemia in the range of 1,500 mg/dL or greater can also lead to pancreatitis. Inherited xanthomas are said to be uncommon in those of African descent. Treatment is aimed at risk factor modification and lowering the triglycerides through pharmacological and behavioral means. The skin lesions usually resolve within 6 months with appropriate treatment.

Necrobiotic xanthogranulomas (NXG) are xanthomatous plaques and nodules to be distinguished from normolipemic and hyperlipemic plane xanthomas. NXG usually occur as firm, yellow-orange plaques or nodules in the periorbital distribution or other areas of the face. These lesions tend to occur in patients with a concurrent monoclonal gammopathy, usually of the IgG-kappa type. Cerebrotendinous xanthomatosis is a rare genetic disease that consists of tendinous xanthomas, cataracts, dementia, and nervous system involvement. This hereditary disorder has been described in various ethnic backgrounds, including those of European, Japanese, and sub-Saharan African descent.

Xanthoma disseminatum (XD) is a rare, potentially progressive mucocutaneous xanthomatosis seen in children and adults that is characterized by the development of brown-to-yellow lipid-containing lesions that form on the skin. XD is classified as a non-Langerhans cell histiocytosis syndrome. It has a predilection for males in childhood or young adulthood. The xanthomatous skin lesions tend to form on the flexor surfaces of the arms and legs and in the periocular region. Involvement has also been seen in the gastrointestinal (GI) tract, respiratory tract, CNS, and optic nerve and can cause significant morbidity and mortality. The most common initial clinical sign of CNS involvement of XD is diabetes insipidus. The skin lesions are typically self-limited, but systemic involvement can have potentially devastating consequences.

◉ Look For

EX—dome-shaped, yellow-orange, firm papules often with an erythematous halo, which can be seen most easily on lightly pigmented skin (**Figs. 4-280–4-282**). In deeply pigmented

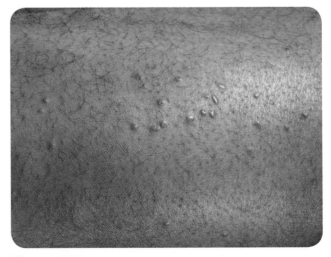

Figure 4-280 Discrete yellow-red papules of eruptive xanthomas.

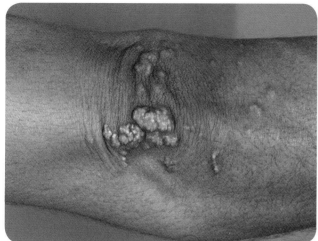

Figure 4-281 Individual and grouped yellow papules in a patient (same patient as Fig. 4-280) with eruptive xanthomas.

skin, however, xanthomas may be tan to dark brown, and the erythema is difficult to detect. Papules are scattered on the trunk, buttocks, and extensor extremities. Frequently, there are several dozen to hundreds of lesions.

Tuberous xanthoma—flat, elevated, or rounded yellowish to orange nodules that are typically located over joints, particularly on the elbows and knees (Figs. 4-283–4-285). Lesions may be solitary, and early lesions may be bright yellow. Older lesions tend to be fibrotic and may lose their color, making them even more difficult to diagnose clinically in deeply pigmented skin.

Tendinous xanthoma—papules or nodules ranging from 5 to 25 mm in diameter, typically located over the tendons of the backs of the hands, dorsal feet, and Achilles tendon.

Plane xanthoma—yellowish-tan to orange flat macules or slightly elevated plaques spread diffusely over large areas of

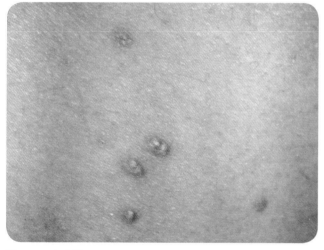

Figure 4-282 Yellow-red papules in a Hispanic man with hyperlipidemia.

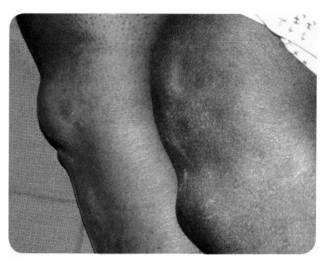

Figure 4-284 Subcutaneous nodules that are tuberous xanthomas around the knees.

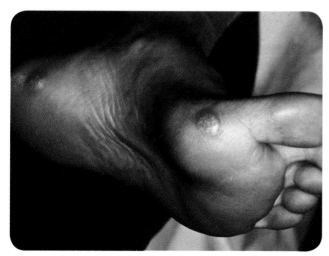

Figure 4-283 Tuberous xanthomas on the foot.

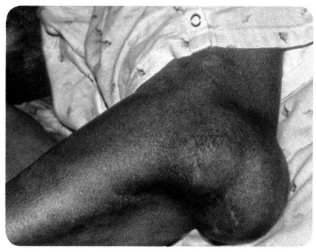

Figure 4-285 Subcutaneous nodule that is a very large tuberous xanthoma around the elbow.

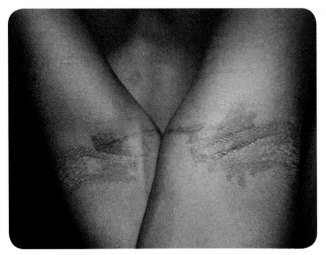

Figure 4-286 Bilateral yellow-brown papules and plaques of planar xanthomas in antecubital spaces.

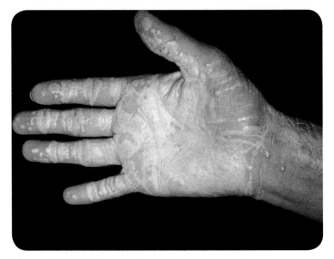

Figure 4-287 Palmar xanthoma.

skin. These tend to occur over the eyelids, neck, trunk, axillae, or shoulders (Fig. 4-286).

Palmar xanthoma—these may present as nodules or yellowish plaques with an irregular border, usually on the palms and flexural surfaces of the digits (Fig. 4-287). Striated xanthomas appear as yellow to yellow-orange streaks that follow the palmar creases. These may also be present on the soles.

NXG—firm, yellow-orange plaques or nodules occurring on the face, most commonly in a periorbital distribution.

XD—small yellowish-red to brown papules on flexor surfaces and often on the eyelids. Lesions may coalesce into plaques as they increase in number and may distort surrounding structures and be disfiguring.

Diagnostic Pearls

- In EX lesions are often in the same stage of development, and onset is rapid. When xanthelasma palpebrarum is present, be careful to check for other visible signs of hyperlipidemia, such as cutaneous xanthomas over joints and in intertriginous locations, as well as arcus senilis in the cornea.
- Tendinous xanthomas tend to occur in association with tuberous xanthomas and xanthelasma, as all three of these morphological forms are associated with primary hyperlipoproteinemias with elevated cholesterol levels. These may also occur in obstructive liver disease, diabetes, myxedema, and normocholesterolemic dysbetalipoproteinemia.
- Plane xanthomas may be seen in individuals with monoclonal gammopathy.
- XD is a very rare disorder. A complete physical exam is indicated, as XD can involve organ systems. There is mucous membrane involvement in 50% of cases, and when

involving the oropharynx, patients may present with dysphagia. If the larynx is involved, patients may have dysphonia and airway obstruction. If lesions are present on the conjunctiva, cornea, or optic nerve, visual disturbance or blindness may occur.

?? Differential Diagnosis and Pitfalls

Eruptive Xanthomas

- XD
- Papular xanthoma
- Eruptive histiocytomas
- Granuloma annulare
- Juvenile xanthogranuloma
- Sarcoidosis
- Leukemia cutis
- Langerhans cell histiocytosis
- Multicentric reticulohistiocytosis
- Lichen myxedematosus
- Erythema elevatum diutinum

Tendinous Xanthoma

Giant cell tumor of the tendon sheath

Tuberous Xanthoma

Erythema elevatum diutinum

Xanthoma Disseminatum

- EX
- Xanthelasma
- Langerhans cell histiocytosis

Plane Xanthomas

- Nevus sebaceus
- Pseudoxanthoma elasticum
- Amyloidosis
- Sarcoidosis

 Best Tests

Skin biopsy of all varieties of xanthoma will reveal similar histopathologic features. This includes numerous foam cells, which are lipid-laden macrophages. In addition, Touton giant cells and cholesterol clefts are also frequently present.

In XD, biopsy of an early lesion will show nonfoamy, scalloped macrophages. Later, lesions will show foam cells, Touton giant cells, and often a mixed inflammatory infiltrate. CT or MRI of the CNS should be performed to rule out CNS involvement in XD. A complete physical exam is also necessary to rule out systemic involvement. Lipid levels are normal in XD. Forty percent of patients will develop diabetes insipidus, and proper investigation of this disorder should be implemented.

In NXG, skin biopsy will reveal distinctive histopathology characterized by granulomas composed of foam cells, lymphocytes, foreign body giant cells, and Touton giant cells alternating with collagen necrobiosis.

▲▲▲ Management Pearls

- For patients with xanthomas that have an underlying lipid abnormality, reduction of the fat content of the diet is critical. It is recommended to keep total triglyceride levels under 1,500 mg/dL. Medium-chain triglycerides (MCTs) can be substituted for dietary fat. In addition, exercise and dietary modifications should be recommended to all patients with lipid abnormalities.
- For patients seeking mechanical removal of their xanthomas, they should be adequately counseled that recurrence is common after surgical or other mechanical removal. An exception is xanthelasma, where recurrence is not as common.
- In XD, the cutaneous lesions may be self-limited and may spontaneously resolve. A small percentage, however, will go on to progressively develop more and more lesions. In this case, either systemic and/or mechanical means may be attempted to treat the lesions.

Therapy

Eruptive Xanthomas
Patients will require dietary modifications and exercise in addition to systemic therapy. Fibrates and niacin work best to lower triglycerides. Avoid bile acid sequestrants, as these drugs may actually worsen hypertriglyceridemia.

Fibrates:

- Clofibrate—1 g p.o. twice daily
- Fenofibrate—48 to 145 mg p.o. daily
- Gemfibrozil—600 mg p.o. twice daily 30 minutes prior to morning and evening meals

Niacin:

- Sustained-release niacin—Begin 500 mg p.o. nightly, which may be increased by 500 mg/d every 8 weeks up to a maximum dose of 2,000 mg/d.

For hyperlipemic patients, dietary modifications and exercise should be implemented. Many will need systemic lipid-lowering therapy in the form of statins, fibrates, nicotinic acid, or bile acid–binding resins. While these measures are important in the treatment of hyperlipidemia, they typically do not cure the cutaneous xanthomas.

XD is a potentially progressive disease. If it does progress, significant morbidity may develop, and mortality may occur. Aggressive treatment may, therefore, be indicated. A case of an African woman from Nigeria with progressive disease has been reported, and she had significant improvement of her skin lesions and symptoms of diabetes insipidus with oral prednisolone, 20 mg twice daily for 22 weeks. Her dysphonia had only mild improvement. In addition, a case of a 15-year-old African American female with disfiguring cutaneous XD has been reported. She was treated with carbon dioxide laser with excellent cosmetic results. She had only minimal, transient postinflammatory hyperpigmentation, despite ablative laser treatment with phototype VI skin. Antineoplastic agents, including Vinca alkaloids, antimetabolites, and alkylating agents, have demonstrated variable responses in few reported cases.

Suggested Readings

Berger GM, Deppe WM, Marais AD, et al. Phytosterolaemia in three unrelated South African families. *Postgrad Med J.* 1994;70(827):631–637.

Carpo BG, Grevelink SV, Brady S, et al. Treatment of cutaneous lesions of xanthoma disseminatum with a CO_2 laser. *Dermatol Surg.* 1999;25(10):751–754.

Jialal I, Omar MA, Bredenkamp B, et al. Type III hyperlipoproteinaemia in a black patient. A case report. *S Afr Med J.* 1981;59(8):267–268.

Shamley DJ, Heckmann JM, Mendelsohn D, et al. Cerebrotendinous xanthomatosis. A case report. *S Afr Med J.* 1988;74(2):79–80.

Spicknall KE, Mehregan DA. Necrobiotic xanthogranuloma. *Int J Dermatol.* 2009;48(1):1–10.

Yusuf SM, Mijinyawa MS, Musa BM, et al. Xanthoma disseminatum in a black African woman. *Int J Dermatol.* 2008;47(11):1145–1147.

Epidermal Nevus

Arden Fredeking

■■ Diagnosis Synopsis

Epidermal nevi (nevi verrucosus) affect 0.1% of the population and are usually recognized at birth but may not appear until childhood when they are seen as a linear array of smooth, dark brown or pinkish-brown, thin plaques or rough skin-colored papules and plaques. Epidermal nevi are hamartomas of ectodermal origin; the term encompasses a variety of lesions with various histologic and clinical patterns. The most typical presentation is as a linear verrucous epidermal nevus. Most develop sporadically, although familial cases have been reported.

Occasionally, epidermal nevi may be associated with other cutaneous, CNS, skeletal, and ocular abnormalities previously known as epidermal nevus syndrome. This entity is now thought to include many distinct genetic diseases, all sharing a phenotype reflecting genetic mosaicism. Some such syndromes include the nevus sebaceus syndrome, Proteus syndrome, CHILD syndrome (congenital hemidysplasia, ichthyosiform erythroderma, and limb defects), Becker nevus syndrome, nevus comedonicus syndrome, and phakomatosis pigmentokeratotica.

◉ Look For

Linear, verrucous, thin plaques that gradually enlarge and become warty in appearance. The lesions tend to be oriented along the lines of Blaschko (Fig. 4-288). The pattern is linear and whorled with a midline demarcation. In pigmented skin, the papules or plaques can appear slightly orange, pink, hypopigmented or tan, or even dark brown.

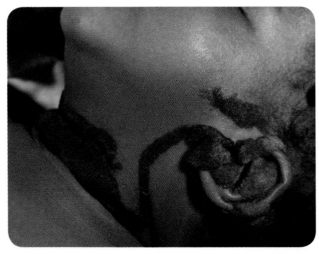

Figure 4-288 Whorled hyperkeratotic lesions of an epidermal nevus.

●● Diagnostic Pearls

There is a tendency for epidermal nevi to assume a more verrucous appearance with age, particularly at puberty.

?? Differential Diagnosis and Pitfalls

- Verruca vulgaris—Verrucous papules and plaques do not tend to assume a whorled pattern and do not respect the midline.
- Epidermal nevi may reflect a somatic mosaicism for K1/K10 mutations as seen in epidermolytic hyperkeratosis (EHK). If these patients have gonadal mosaicism, offspring may have full-blown EHK. Mosaicism for ATP2A2 mutations can cause segmental Darier disease. As in EHK, if these patients have gonadal mosaicism, offspring may have full-blown Darier disease.
- Nevus sebaceus—papillomatous, yellow-orange, linear plaque on the scalp or face
- Psoriasis—may present in a segmental fashion (nevoid psoriasis) but responds to topical steroids
- Inflammatory linear verrucous epidermal nevus (ILVEN)—congenital pruritic, linear, psoriasiform plaque
- Lichen striatus—presents in childhood as asymptomatic linearly arranged, small, flat-topped, pink to skin-colored papules within the lines of Blaschko, usually on an extremity. These lesions spontaneously resolve over months to a few years.
- Mosaic EHK—Skin biopsy reveals reticulate degeneration of the epidermis.
- Mosaic Darier disease—Skin biopsy reveals acantholytic dyskeratosis.

✓ Best Tests

Skin biopsy reveals hyperkeratosis, papillomatosis, and acanthosis.

▲▲ Management Pearls

Epidermal nevi are benign. Biopsy should be considered to rule out mosaic EHK. Those patients bearing epidermal nevi with histopathologic features of EHK should receive genetic counseling for possible mutations in sperm or egg leading to a child with generalized EHK. Symptom-directed screening should be performed in patients with widespread epidermal nevi, and an interdisciplinary team of neurologists, orthopedists, cardiologists, ophthalmologists, oncologists, and rehabilitation specialists should be employed as indicated.

Therapy

Epidermal nevi can be a cosmetic problem. Excisional surgery can be used for small lesions. However, this results in scarring, and extension can still occur even after excision. Carbon dioxide laser has been used to ablate lesions with variable success but also results in scarring. A case report has shown success in treatment with etanercept therapy.

Suggested Readings

Bogle MA, Sobell JM, Dover JS. Successful treatment of a widespread inflammatory verrucous epidermal nevus with etanercept. *Arch Dermatol.* 2006;142:401–402.

Sugarman JL. Epidermal nevus syndromes. *Semin Cutan Med Surg.* 2007;26(4):221–230.

Nummular Dermatitis

Nasir Aziz

Diagnosis Synopsis

Nummular dermatitis (nummular eczema) is an inflammatory skin disease characterized by pruritic, coin-shaped, scaly plaques. Of uncertain etiology, its onset is associated with frequent bathing, irritating and drying soaps, skin trauma, interferon therapy for hepatitis C, and exposure to irritating fabrics such as wool. Venous stasis may be a predisposing factor to developing lesions on the legs. Nummular dermatitis is commonly present in young women with typical atopic dermatitis. It also frequently occurs in middle-aged to older men. Nummular dermatitis seems more common among Asians, especially those who engage in manual labor. Factors contributing to this may be less frequent use of moisturizers in the winter, the cultural habit of taking hot and long showers to "treat" itchy skin, and constant exposure to water for many who work in restaurants.

Look For

Nummular dermatitis can present with round or coin-shaped, red and/or brown scaly plaques, often with minute fissures or erosions (Figs. 4-289–4-292). These plaques are found on the trunk and/or extremities. Erythema may be less prominent in darker-skinned patients.

Diagnostic Pearls

Compared with nummular dermatitis, the scale of psoriasis is thicker and more silvery, and Auspitz sign (bleeding with scale removal) is present. Tinea corporis usually has leading scale (scale on the outside of the plaque). Atopic dermatitis may have more lichenification.

Differential Diagnosis and Pitfalls

- Tinea corporis
- Psoriasis
- Hailey-Hailey disease
- Mycosis fungoides (especially when lesions are on the buttocks of adults)
- Sarcoidosis
- Eczema craquelé
- Contact dermatitis

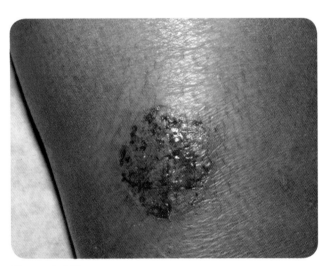

Figure 4-289 Typical circular lesion of nummular dermatitis with scale, crust, and erosions.

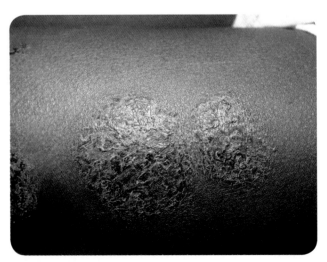

Figure 4-290 Well-delimited plaques of nummular eczema with thick adherent scale/crust.

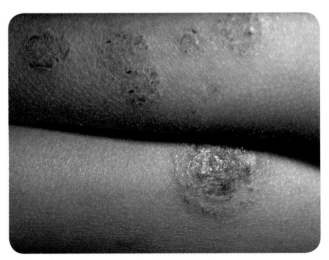

Figure 4-291 Multiple lesions of nummular eczema in several stages of development.

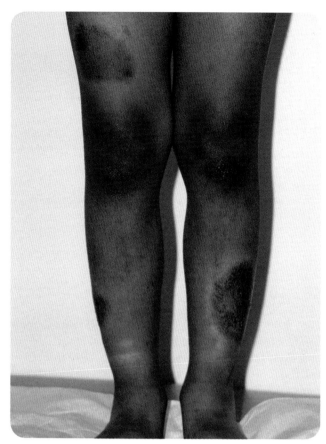

Figure 4-292 Chronic state of nummular eczema with scaling and hyperpigmentation.

- Small plaque parapsoriasis
- Pityriasis rosea
- Seborrheic dermatitis

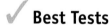 **Best Tests**

Swab crusted plaques for bacterial culture. A skin biopsy will confirm a clinical diagnosis.

 Management Pearls

Look for signs of secondary bacterial infection and treat with antistaphylococcal antibiotics if necessary. Moisturizing creams and ointments are key. If pruritus is severe, use systemic antihistamines.

Therapy

Instruct the patient to apply thick emollients, such as Aquaphor or petroleum jelly (which is more cost-effective), at least twice daily. Patients should take short (5 minutes or less) lukewarm baths or showers, use mild soaps (e.g., Dove, Tone, Purpose) in axillary and groin areas, and apply emollients while the skin is still damp. Use a mid- to high-potency (classes 2 to 5) topical corticosteroid applied directly to the lesions twice daily. The topical steroid should be applied prior to the emollient. For disseminated lesions, Derma-Smoothe/FS offers the most coverage for the least amount of medication. Many dark-skinned patients with dermatitis prefer topicals with an oily base. UVB phototherapy plus emollients may also be considered for widespread disease. Systemic corticosteroids and other immunosuppressants have also been used to treat extensive disease. Once these medications are under consideration, the patient requires evaluation and treatment by a dermatologist.

Suggested Readings

Dalgard F, Holm J, Svensson A, et al. Self reported skin morbidity and ethnicity: a population-based study in a Western community. *BMC Dermatol.* 2007;7:4.

Krupa Shankar DS, Shrestha S. Relevance of patch testing in patients with nummular dermatitis. *Ind J Dermatol Venearol.* 2005;71(6):406–408.

Lee CS, Lim HW. Cutaneous diseases in Asians. *Dermatol Clin.* 2003;21(4): 669–677.

Common Warts

Jennifer Alston DeSimone

▪▪ Diagnosis Synopsis

Common warts (verruca vulgaris) are benign skin proliferations caused by infection of the epidermis with human papillomavirus (HPV), most frequently types 1, 2, and 4. Verruca vulgaris lesions may be acquired from direct contact with HPV-infected skin or, less commonly, from contact with HPV-carrying fomites. Autoinoculation is very common. Warts are frequent at locations that are traumatized. HPV types 2 and 4 may infect virtually any epidermal surface, including mucosal surfaces, but common warts are most often seen on the hands, feet, and knees. Verrucae manifest as skin-colored hyperkeratotic papules. They may be pruritic, and scratching can produce a linear array of lesions via autoinoculation. Verruca vulgaris lesions are more prevalent in children and in immunocompromised patients; widespread, persistent lesions may be a clue to underlying inherited or acquired immunodeficiency.

For unknown reasons, the incidence of common warts is approximately twice as high in whites as in individuals of African descent and ten times more common in Hispanics than those of African descent. In individuals of African descent, the majority of warts are solitary, whereas with Hispanics, most patients present with multiple warts.

Pediatric Patient Considerations

Verruca vulgaris lesions are more prevalent in children aged 4 to 12. The HPV virus is often passed between siblings and may be observed as cyclical infections.

Type 2 can be found in children as condyloma acuminata from diaper changing.

Immunocompromised Patient Considerations

Immunocompromised patients are predisposed to viral infection and are also less able to mount an immune response to adequately clear the HPV (Fig. 4-293). They often demonstrate larger, confluent verrucae that are more resistant to standard therapies.

The presence of warts *per se* is not a reason for expensive immunological testing.

◉ Look For

Look for 2- to 6-mm verrucous hyperkeratotic papules most commonly located on the dorsal hands, distal fingers, subungual skin, and feet (Figs. 4-294–4-297). Close inspection will usually reveal tiny black dots that represent thrombosed capillaries. Confluent verrucous plaques may form in sites of long-standing lesions.

Pediatric Patient Considerations

Scratching often leads to a linear array of papules due to autoinoculation. Perianal and genital warts are often a sign of sexual abuse and must be investigated appropriately (Fig. 4-298).

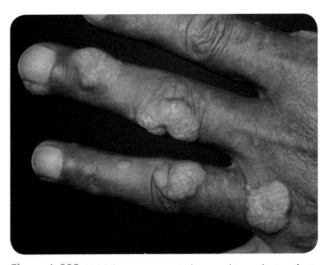

Figure 4-293 Multiple common warts in a renal transplant patient.

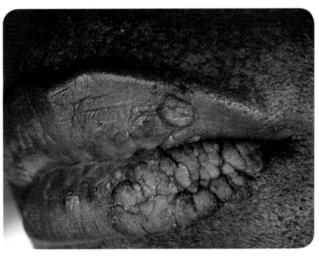

Figure 4-294 Multiple hyperkeratotic lesions on the lips.

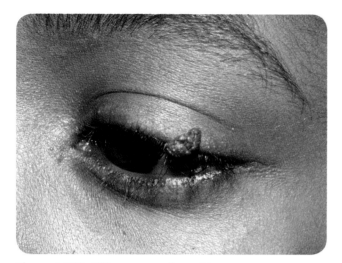

Figure 4-295 Filiform wart on the eyelid.

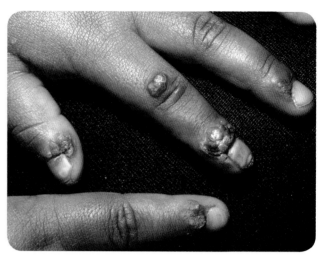

Figure 4-297 Multiple periungual warts.

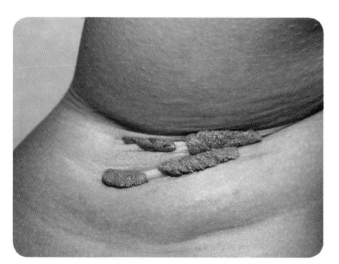

Figure 4-296 Intertriginous warts.

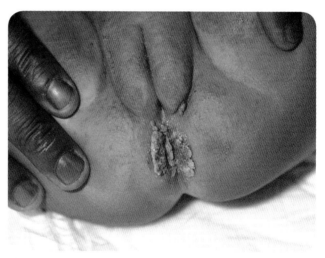

Figure 4-298 Perianal and labial warts in a child must be investigated as a potential sign of sexual abuse.

Immunocompromised Patient Considerations

Lesions may present as confluent verrucous plaques up to 8 cm in diameter.

Diagnostic Pearls

Tiny black or red dots within the lesion are characteristic of common warts and represent thrombosed capillaries. These are best visualized by removing the surface of the wart with a No. 15 surgical blade. Common warts also cause an interruption in the normal skin lines (dermatoglyphics).

?? Differential Diagnosis and Pitfalls

- Keratoacanthomas—These have a central keratin crater.
- Squamous cell carcinoma (SCC)—It can arise in preexisting warts and may be recalcitrant to therapy.
- Prurigo nodularis—It is characterized by pruritic papules and nodules.
- Perforating disorders—These tend to be follicularly based with a central core.
- Seborrheic keratoses—These have a characteristic "stuck-on," waxy appearance.
- Lichen planus—These lesions are typically more planar, violaceous, and pruritic.
- Cutaneous horns—These can arise from warts, hypertrophic actinic keratoses, seborrheic keratoses, and SCCs.

- Actinic keratoses—These tend to be scaly erythematous papules in sun-exposed areas of elderly individuals.
- Lichen nitidus—It is characterized by discrete, dome-shaped papules.
- A clavus, or corn—A painful hyperkeratotic lesion with a central core that lacks the pinpoint thrombosed capillaries and retains normal skin dermatoglyphics. Clavi occur in sites of pressure and repeated friction.
- Foreign body reactions—These may have a history of trauma or inoculation.
- Molluscum contagiosum lesions—These are smooth, dome-shaped papules with a central umbilication.

✓ Best Tests

Verruca vulgaris is a clinical diagnosis. In long-standing, recalcitrant lesions, a skin biopsy to rule out SCC is indicated.

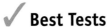 Management Pearls

Be sure to pare the wart down before cryosurgery or application of any topical therapy to improve the chance of treatment success.

Warts are benign and usually self-limited. Therefore, it is reasonable to not treat them. Patients often request treatment, however, in which case therapeutic options include the following:

- Destructive therapy—40% salicylic acid plasters/ointments (OTC) with strong adhesive tape as described above. Can leave on for 2 to 4 days, followed by paring or pumice stone. Alternatives include silver nitrate and glutaraldehyde solution.
- Cryotherapy using liquid nitrogen applied for 5 seconds with 1 to 3 freeze/thaw cycles. Trichloroacetic acid (TCA) or monochloroacetic acid (MCA) under occlusion for 48 to 72 hours. Electrodesiccation and CO_2 laser therapy should be used with caution to avoid scarring.
- Topical medications—5-fluorouracil (1% or 5% cream) applied daily or twice daily or imiquimod 5% cream can be applied three to five times per week for 6 weeks or longer until lesions disappear. Irritation of the lesions is expected. Tretinoin 0.1% cream or gel daily or twice daily as tolerated. Tretinoin can be combined with imiquimod as well.
- Intralesional immunotherapy—Topical diphenylcyclopropenone, topical squaric acid, intralesional candida antigen, mumps antigen, and trichophyton antigens can sensitize patients to HPV. Intralesional interferon alfa 2b 1 mL of 1 million IU three times a week for 3 weeks.
- Intralesional chemotherapy—Intralesional bleomycin 0.5 U/mL with no more than 3 mL injected at one time. (Use with caution as scarring and neuropathy can result.)

Pediatric Patient Considerations

Cantharidin ("beetle juice") is safe and effective when applied to warts without occlusion for 4 to 6 hours every 3 weeks till clear. This treatment is less painful and traumatic and is a good option in the pediatric population.

Immunocompromised Patient Considerations

Imiquimod is less likely to be effective in the immunocompromised patient as it requires a functioning immune system to assert its mechanism of action.

Therapy

- Paring of hyperkeratotic debris, followed by application of liquid nitrogen, either via cotton swab or use of a spray canister, is an effective treatment. Three to four treatments 3 to 4 weeks apart is often curative. Pain is a limiting factor in some patients.
- Multiple over-the-counter salicylic acid–containing products are available for home use in the form of liquid that can be painted onto lesions or impregnated adhesive plaster. Soaking of lesions followed by paring in between daily applications improves response. Increased effectiveness is seen when combined with cryotherapy.
- Topical 5-fluorouracil 5% cream applied one to two times daily until resolution has more recently been described as an effective treatment option. This treatment may also be combined with in-office cryotherapy.
- Pulsed dye laser is another treatment option for recalcitrant warts.
- Non–FDA-approved therapies include intralesional candida antigen and treatment with contact sensitizers. Intralesional candida antigen is often successful in eliciting a host immune response directed at the wart. One to ten lesions are injected with 0.1 mL each of *Candida albicans* skin test antigen. Avoid treatment of lesions on the digits, as a painful compartment syndrome–like response has been reported with use at these sites.
- Contact immunotherapy with squaric acid dibutylester has been used with good results in patients with lesions resistant to other treatments. This treatment requires access to a compounding pharmacy and is best prescribed by a dermatologist familiar with its use.
- In skin of color, it is important to recognize that many treatments for warts will result in hyperpigmentation or hypopigmentation of the treatment field. These changes are usually transient; however, the duration of pigmentary change may be 1 to 2 years.

Suggested Readings

Adalatkhah H, Khalilollahi H, Amini N, et al. Compared therapeutic efficacy between intralesional bleomycin and cryotherapy for common warts: a randomized clinical trial. *Dermatol Online J.* 2007;13(3):4.

Dhar SB, Rashid MM, Islam A, et al. Intralesional bleomycin in the treatment of cutaneous warts: a randomized clinical trial comparing it with cryotherapy. *Ind J Dermatol Venereol Leprol.* 2009;75(3):262–267.

Hama N, Hatamochi A, Hayashi S, et al. Usefulness of topical immunotherapy with squaric acid dibutylester for refractory common warts on the face and neck. *J Dermatol.* 2009;36(12):660–662.

Kartal Durmazlar SP, Atacan D, Eskioglu F. Cantharidin treatment for recalcitrant facial flat warts: a preliminary study. *J Dermatol Treat.* 2009;20(2):114–119.

Micali G, Dall'Oglio F, Nasca MR. An open label evaluation of the efficacy of imiquimod 5% cream in the treatment of recalcitrant subungual and periungual cutaneous warts. *J Dermatol Treat.* 2003;14(4):233–236.

Schellhaas U, Gerber W, Hammes S, et al. Pulsed dye laser treatment is effective in the treatment of recalcitrant viral warts. *Dermatol Surg.* 2008;34(1):67–72; Epub 2007 Dec 5.

Sethuraman G, Richards KA, Hiremagalore RN, et al. Effectiveness of pulsed dye laser in the treatment of recalcitrant warts in children. *Dermatol Surg.* 2010;36(1):58–65.

Pediculosis Corporis (Body Lice)

Aída Lugo-Somolinos

▪▪ Diagnosis Synopsis

Pediculosis is the term used to describe infestations by lice on the skin. Lice are parasitic insects that live in humans and survive by feeding on human blood. Three types of lice live on humans:

- *Pediculus humanus capitis* (head louse)
- *Pediculus humanus corporis* (body louse, clothes louse)
- *Phthirus pubis* ("crab" louse, pubic louse)

Pediculosis corporis, or body louse, is seen most commonly in persons living in crowded, unsanitary conditions or in homeless persons. It is seen in all ethnicities in equal distribution. It presents with intense itching, and sometimes crusted papules can be seen in the abdominal area. Body lice may be vectors for other diseases.

For information specific to pediculosis capitis and pediculosis pubis, see the "Pediculosis Capitis (Head Lice)" and "Pediculosis Pubis (Pubic Lice)" chapters, respectively.

(•) Look For

Look for eggs or lice in the inseams of the clothes. Skin lesions may be excoriations and by themselves are not diagnostic (Fig. 4-299).

•• Diagnostic Pearls

- Itching is the main symptom.
- Nits fluoresce under a Wood light.

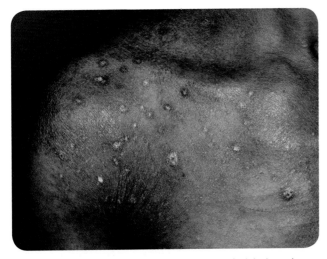

Figure 4-299 Multiple excoriated and lichenified lesions due to pediculosis corporis.

?? Differential Diagnosis and Pitfalls

- Impetigo
- Folliculitis
- Other arthropod bites/stings
- Acne
- Neurotic excoriations
- Delusions of parasitosis
- Irritant contact dermatitis
- Bedbug bites
- Scabies
- Contact dermatitis

✓ Best Tests

Demonstration of the insect or the nit (from a hair visually or under the microscope) is diagnostic. A magnification glass or a Wood lamp may facilitate the diagnosis.

▲▲ Management Pearls

Improving hygiene and the use of clean or new clothes may be the only treatment necessary. In severe cases, permethrin may be used.

Precautions: Standard and contact. (Isolate patient, wear gloves and a gown, limit patient transport, and avoid sharing patient-care equipment.)

Therapy

Educate the patient about the importance of proper hygiene.

Treat clothing and fomites—All clothing and bed linens should be washed with hot water and dried using high heat. Discard or avoid using heavily infested items for 2 weeks (seal in plastic bags), if feasible. Iron the seams of furniture with a hot iron.

For heavy infestation or in situations where regular bathing and changing are not feasible, application of 5% permethrin cream or lotion head to toe for 8 to 14 hours is advisable.

Suggested Reading

Stone SP, Goldfarb JN, Bacelieri RE. Scabies, other mites, and pediculosis. In: Wolff K, Goldsmith LA, et al., eds. *Fitzpatrick's Dermatology in General Medicine.* 7th Ed. New York, NY: McGraw Hill; 2008:2029–2037.

Lichen Simplex Chronicus

Stephanie Diamantis

Diagnosis Synopsis

Lichen simplex chronicus (LSC) is the cutaneous manifestation of chronic rubbing and/or scratching of the skin from any source.

Clinically, lesions of LSC appear as well-defined plaques of lichenification and occasional scaling. Lichenification refers to thickened skin with enhanced skin markings as the result of friction from excessive scratching and rubbing. Individual papules may also be observed (prurigo nodules), as may excoriations, which can become secondarily infected. As these lesions are self-induced, LSC is almost always distributed to areas of the body within hand's reach. LSC was originally thought to be more common in women but affects both sexes. There are no data regarding any ethnic predilection.

The underlying precipitating factors inducing the patients to chronically scratch or rub their skin (causing lesions of LSC) are either known or unknown. LSC is commonly observed in uncontrolled atopic dermatitis and other dermatoses that have pruritus as a feature (e.g., insect bites, scabies). When LSC is observed on relatively normal skin with no obvious underlying precipitants, psychological factors are thought to play a significant role. In either case, an itch-scratch cycle is initiated, and if allowed to continue unabated, plaques of LSC inevitably develop.

Look For

Leathery plaques of thickened skin in which the normal texture is exaggerated (Fig. 4-300). Plaques may be slightly erythematous or hyperpigmented and are often scaly and well demarcated. Excoriations may be apparent as well. Common locations include the scalp, lateral and posterior neck, wrists, elbows, vulva or scrotum, knees, lower legs, and ankles (Fig. 4-301). Postinflammatory hyperpigmentation or hypopigmentation is commonly seen in both treated and untreated plaques of LSC in darkly pigmented patients. These lesions are distinguished from the nodules and erosions that are typical of prurigo nodularis (Fig. 4-302).

Diagnostic Pearls

Accentuation of skin markings is usually evident even when lesions are partially treated or regressing. Postinflammatory hyperpigmentation or hypopigmentation is common, especially in more deeply pigmented skin. LSC is found only at locations where the patient can reach.

?? Differential Diagnosis and Pitfalls

- Psoriasis—characteristic distribution, significant silvery scale present
- Mycosis fungoides

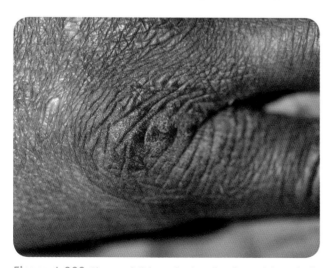

Figure 4-300 Plaque of lichen simplex chronicus with markedly accentuated skin markings.

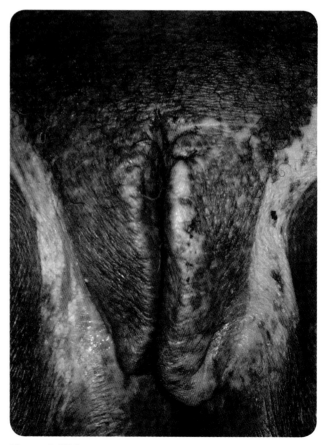

Figure 4-301 Lichen simplex chronicus of the vulva with erosions and hyperpigmentation and hypopigmentation.

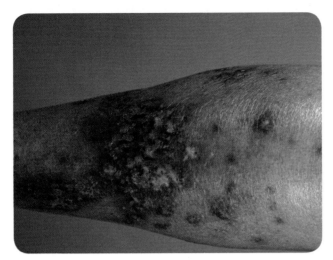

Figure 4-302 Papules and nodules with erosions are typical of prurigo nodularis.

- Contact dermatitis
- Stasis dermatitis
- Atopic dermatitis
- Acanthosis nigricans
- Extramammary Paget disease
- Acne keloidalis nuchae
- Notalgia paresthetica—localized pruritic area at one side of the midscapula area
- Squamous cell carcinoma
- Pretibial myxedema
- Lichen amyloidosis

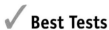 **Best Tests**

Often a clinical diagnosis. Skin biopsy is nonspecific but can rule out other diagnoses (such as mycosis fungoides). Patch testing can be used to rule out allergic contact dermatitis.

▲▲ **Management Pearls**

- The goal of treatment is to eliminate environmental triggers and break the itch-scratch-rash-itch cycle. Most importantly, patients should be encouraged to avoid scratching, since it perpetuates the process. Using barriers to cover plaques of LSC can eliminate scratching and lead to resolution. Maximize the treatment of any underlying skin disease. Use oral antihistamines to lessen pruritus. Keep skin well lubricated with liberal use of emollients. If the itching is generalized, consider systemic causes of pruritus such as medications and renal, thyroid, hematologic, and hepatic abnormalities.
- Psychological evaluation and treatment, including psychoactive medications, behavioral therapy, and alternative treatments, such as hypnosis, have benefited some patients. In select cases, consider consultation with a mental health professional.

Therapy

The goal of therapy for LCS is to relieve pruritus and stop the itch-scratch cycle. Topical steroids applied twice daily with or without occlusion are the first-line therapy. Also consider flurandrenolide (Cordran) tape, a corticosteroid-impregnated tape (60, 200 cm² rolls) that can serve as a reminder for the patient not to rub and also deliver the topical steroid under occlusion. Change the tape once daily.

In general, start with a high-potency topical steroid (class 2 or 3) or a superpotent topical corticosteroid (class 1) if the condition is severe. Schedule close (i.e., 2-week) follow-up when using such agents. Decrease the potency and/or the frequency of application of the corticosteroid preparation as the lesions resolve to avoid inducing skin atrophy. Applying these agents under occlusion may increase potency.

Superpotent Topical Corticosteroids (Class 1)
- Clobetasol 0.05% cream—apply twice daily (15, 30, 45 g)
- Betamethasone dipropionate 0.05% cream—apply twice daily (15, 30, 45 g)
- Diflorasone 0.05% cream—apply twice daily (15, 30, 60 g)
- Halobetasol cream—apply twice daily (15, 50 g)

High-Potency Topical Corticosteroids (Class 2)
- Fluocinonide cream, ointment—apply twice daily (15, 30, 60, 120 g)
- Desoximetasone cream, ointment—apply twice daily (15, 60, 120 g)
- Halcinonide cream, ointment—apply twice daily (15, 60, 240 g)
- Amcinonide ointment—apply twice daily (15, 30, 60 g)

Mid-Potency Topical Corticosteroids (Classes 3 and 4)
- Triamcinolone acetonide cream, ointment—apply twice daily (15, 30, 60, 120, 240 g)
- Mometasone cream, ointment—apply twice daily (15, 45 g)
- Fluocinolone ointment, cream—apply twice daily (15, 30, 60 g)

Alternatively, intralesional injection with triamcinolone acetonide at 3 to 5 mg/mL to the thickened plaque (5 to 10 mg/mL for thickened nodules) may be effective. Repeated injections rarely have the potential to cause hypopigmentation, especially in darker skin.

For pruritus, the following antihistamines often provide relief:

- Diphenhydramine hydrochloride (25, 50 mg tablets or capsules): 25 to 50 mg nightly or every 6 hours, as needed
- Hydroxyzine (10, 25 mg tablets): 10 to 25 mg every 6 hours, as needed
- Cetirizine hydrochloride (5, 10 mg tablets): 5 to 10 mg/d

Additional measures to control itch include use of soothing emollients (containing menthol, pramoxine, camphor), capsaicin cream (0.025% to 0.3%, applied four to six times daily), and 5% doxepin cream. Skin lubrication is essential. Occlusive dressings such as an Unna boot may be helpful to increase the potency of topical steroids and also discourage the patient from picking/scratching.

A topical antibiotic ointment (e.g., mupirocin) can be applied to impetiginized lesions.

Psychiatric interventions also represent a major component of therapy in many patients. Antianxiety (doxepin) and antidepressant medications are beneficial for a significant number of patients. Biofeedback, journaling, and counseling are also helpful in breaking the itch-scratch cycle for many patients.

Suggested Readings

James WD, Berger TG, Elston DM, eds. Pruritus and neurocutaneous dermatoses. In: *Andrews' Diseases of the Skin Clinical Dermatology*. 10th Ed. Philadelphia, PA: Elsevier; 2006:58–59.

Lotti T, Buggiani G, Prignano F. Prurigo nodularis and lichen simplex chronicus. *Dermatol Ther*. 2008;21:42–46.

Nanda V, Parwaz MA, Handa S. Linear hypopigmentation after triamcinolone injection: a rare complication of a common procedure. *Aesthetic Plast Surg*. 2006;30(1):118–119.

Lichen Striatus

Arden Fredeking

Diagnosis Synopsis

Lichen striatus is an uncommon, self-limited skin disorder of younger children of unknown etiology. It has been reported in children as young as 3 months. When it occurs in adults, it tends to be more extensive and pruritic. It presents with linear bands of slightly scaly, pinpoint, and lichenoid papules that follow the lines of Blaschko. Lesions are usually on an extremity; however, lichen striatus can occur anywhere, including the face. Lichen striatus is typically asymptomatic in pediatric patients.

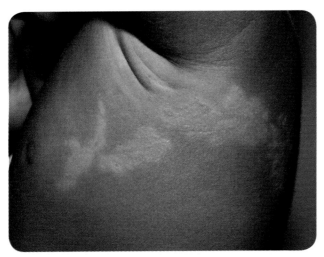

Figure 4-303 Lichen striatus with slightly elevated red and hypopigmented papules.

Look For

Uniform; red, pink, or skin-colored; slightly scaly; pinpoint; flat-topped papules in a curvilinear configuration distributed along the lines of Blaschko (Figs. 4-303 and 4-304). It is most commonly seen on the extremities, though involvement of the trunk and face may occur. The band of involvement may be one continuous band, or it may be interrupted. Papules and plaques are linear and can involve the entire length of an extremity, including the nail (Fig. 4-305). Involvement of the nail can occur without any other cutaneous involvement. The lesions are often subtle and resolve leaving hypopigmentation or hyperpigmentation.

Diagnostic Pearls

The onset is usually fairly rapid and may reach maximal involvement within a few days to weeks.

Differential Diagnosis and Pitfalls

- Linear epidermal nevus
- Linear porokeratosis
- Incontinentia pigmenti
- Linear lichen planus

✓ Best Tests

This is generally a clinical diagnosis. A punch biopsy may be helpful if the diagnosis is in question.

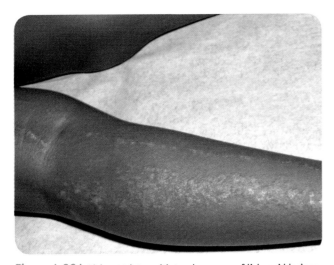

Figure 4-304 Lichen striatus with two long rows of lichenoid lesions.

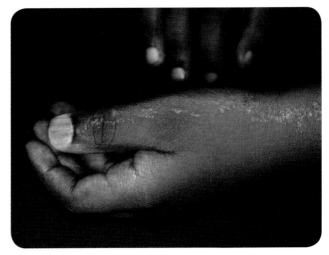

Figure 4-305 Atrophic white papules of lichen striatus on the arm and hand, also causing a thin irregular nail plate on the thumb.

Management Pearls

The disease is self-limited, so aggressive treatment is not indicated. It typically resolves spontaneously within 1 to 2 years.

Therapy

Mid-strength topical corticosteroids may hasten resolution and can be helpful if pruritus is present. In adults, studies have shown promise using pimecrolimus as well as tacrolimus when there is symptomatic pruritus.

Suggested Readings

Campanati A, Brandozzi G, Giangiacomi M, et al. Lichen striatus in adults and pimecrolimus: open, off-label clinical study. *Int J Dermatol.* 2008;47:732–736.

Fujimoto N, Tajima S, Ishibashi A. Facial lichen striatus: successful treatment with tacrolimus ointment. *Br J Dermatol.* 2003;148:587–590.

Sorgentini C, Allevato MA, Dahbar M, et al. Lichen striatus in an adult: successful treatment with tacrolimus. *Br J Dermatol.* 2004;150:776–777.

Discoid Lupus Erythematosus

Stephanie Diamantis

Diagnosis Synopsis

Lupus erythematosus is an autoimmune multisystem disease that has several cutaneous variants. Specific cutaneous lesions of lupus erythematous can be classified based on the location of the inflammation within the skin: acute cutaneous, subacute cutaneous, chronic cutaneous, tumid lupus, and lupus panniculitis. Epidemiologic studies have shown that people of Hispanic, Asian, African American, and African Caribbean descent have an increased incidence of lupus in addition to excess morbidity.

Chronic cutaneous lupus erythematosus (CCLE), also known as discoid lupus erythematosus (DLE), is the most common manifestation of cutaneous lupus and is characterized by chronic lesions that result in permanent, disfiguring scars. Lesions are initially red, scaly plaques that evolve into depigmented atrophic plaques with surrounding hyperpigmentation. Common locations include the face and scalp. Approximately 5% to 10% of patients go on to develop systemic findings. DLE most commonly afflicts women in the third and fourth decades of life, though it may occur at any age. Patients of African and Hispanic descent are at increased risk. Squamous cell carcinoma may develop in chronic DLE scars, especially in sun-exposed areas.

Tumid lupus describes a variant of lupus erythematosus that presents with urticariallike lesions and occurs most commonly on the face and trunk. Lupus panniculitis, also known as lupus profundus, presents with indurated plaques, usually on the face, upper arms, upper trunk, buttocks, and thighs.

Look For

Initially, well-demarcated, erythematous, scaly plaques followed by atrophy, scarring, and depigmentation in the center of the lesion with a peripheral rim of hyperpigmentation (Fig. 4-306). In darkly pigmented skin, lesions can be deeply violaceous, especially at the periphery. In the localized variant, only areas above the neck, such as the scalp, bridge of the nose, cheeks, lower lip, and ears, are affected. In individuals of African descent, the conchal bowl of the ear is a common location. More generalized disease may affect the torso and upper extremities as well. Scarring alopecia may be seen (Fig. 4-307). Mucosal lesions and nail involvement may also be seen.

Diagnostic Pearls

- Only 5% to 10% of patients with DLE will progress to systemic lupus erythematosus (SLE). However, discoid rash is one of the 11 diagnostic criteria for SLE, and 20% of patients with SLE will manifest discoid lesions.
- There may be a positive family history of lupus or connective tissue disease.
- It is unusual to see DLE below the neck if there is no disease above the neck. Patients with disease above and below the neck are said to have generalized DLE and may be at increased risk of developing SLE.
- Peeling back scale in lesions of DLE may reveal follicle-based keratotic spikes known as "the carpet tack sign."
- Alopecia associated with DLE is considered to be scarring, and patients should be advised that there is little chance of hair regrowth.

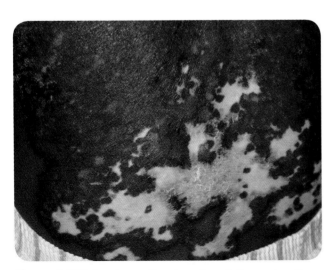

Figure 4-306 Scarring, scaling, hypopigmentation, and erythema in DLE.

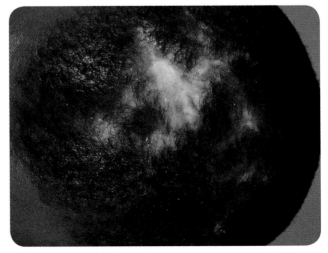

Figure 4-307 Multiple atrophic and inflammatory plaques of DLE.

?? Differential Diagnosis and Pitfalls

- *Trichophyton tonsurans* (tinea capitis) infections of the scalp can be very inflammatory and should be ruled out.
- Acute early lesions may resemble polymorphous light eruptions.
- DLE lesions have been associated with chronic granulomatous disease. In familial cases, check for complement deficiency.
- Other forms of scarring alopecia, such as the follicular degeneration syndrome
- Lichen planus
- Lichen planopilaris
- Burn scar
- Chronic radiation dermatitis
- Subacute CCLE
- Rosacea
- Granuloma faciale
- Dermatomyositis
- Syphilis
- Porphyria
- Sarcoidosis
- Vitiligo
- Scleroderma

✓ Best Tests

- Skin biopsy—In addition to typical findings on hematoxylin and eosin (H&E)–stained sections, direct immunofluorescence on biopsy specimens may show a "lupus band."
- Autoantibody studies (ANA, anti-Ro [SSA] and anti-La [SSB]) may be helpful, especially in cases where systemic signs and symptoms are present.
- Other routine laboratory tests that may demonstrate findings in the case of systemic involvement include CBC with differential, erythrocyte sedimentation, chemistry panel, and urinalysis.

▲▲ Management Pearls

- Avoid sunlight exposure. Sunscreens with both UVB and UVA blockers (avobenzone with octocrylene, titanium dioxide, zinc oxide) are recommended. Excessive heat, excessive cold, and trauma to the affected regions have been shown to worsen the condition. Smoking worsens cutaneous lupus.
- The alopecia is considered to be scarring, and patients should be advised that there is little chance of hair regrowth.
- Camouflage cosmetics may be employed.
- Patients with systemic involvement may require referral to a rheumatologist and/or a nephrologist.

Therapy

The main goals of treatment are to improve the patient's appearance and to prevent additional lesions from developing. Sunscreens, sun-protective clothing, and sun avoidance are essential components of therapy. Topical corticosteroids and antimalarials are first-line therapy.

High-potency topical steroids, flurandrenolide-impregnated tape, and/or intralesional corticosteroids (triamcinolone 3 to 10 mg/mL infiltrated into the dermal plaque) are the mainstay of therapy for cutaneous forms of lupus. Patient use of topical steroids should be monitored closely due to the risk of atrophy. Special care should be taken with facial skin. Often, potent topical steroids are required to get a response, even on the face. Intralesional triamcinolone (4 to 5 mg/mL) can be effective in active lesions, with injections repeated every month while the lesions are active.

High-potency Topical Corticosteroids (Classes 1 and 2)
- Clobetasol cream, ointment—apply twice daily
- Fluocinonide cream, ointment—apply twice daily
- Desoximetasone cream, ointment—apply twice daily
- Halcinonide cream, ointment—apply twice daily
- Amcinonide ointment—apply twice daily

Systemic therapies targeting prevention of progression require knowledge of the drugs and specific monitoring.

Antimalarials (hydroxychloroquine 200 mg twice daily alone or in combination with quinacrine 100 mg/d) can be employed for cases not adequately treated with topical or local agents. **Note:** Before starting these agents, liver and renal function tests should be obtained. Ophthalmologic baseline exam should be performed at or near the time these agents are started. Patients on antimalarials should be seen for ophthalmologic testing every 6 to 12 months.

Systemic retinoids—Acitretin 25 to 50 mg p.o. daily, or isotretinoin 40 to 80 mg p.o. daily for 4 months should be considered as second-line therapy.

Dapsone (100 to 200 mg p.o. daily), methotrexate, mycophenolate mofetil, and other immunosuppressives have also been used. Oral gold has also been reported to be helpful.

Recent studies have shown thalidomide (50 to 100 mg p.o. daily) to be an effective therapy, but it should be reserved for severe cases that are unresponsive to other measures. Caution is advised due to the potential teratogenic and neurologic side effects.

Suggested Readings

Cooper GS, Parks CG, Treadwell EL, et al. Differences by race, sex, and age in the clinical and immunologic features of recently diagnosed systemic lupus erythematosus patients in the southeastern United States. *Lupus.* 2002;11:161–167.

Halder RM, Roberts CI, Nootheti PK. Cutaneous diseases in black races. *Dermatol Clin.* 2003;21:679–687.

James WD, Berger TG, Elston DM, eds. Cutaneous vascular diseases. In: *Andrews' Diseases of the Skin Clinical Dermatology.* 10th Ed. Philadelphia, PA: Elsevier; 2006:816–817.

Jessop S, Whitelaw DA, Delamere FM. Drugs for discoid lupus erythematosus. *Cochrane Database Syst Rev.* 2009;7(4):CD002954.

Lau CS, Yin G, Mok MY. Ethnic and geographical differences in systemic lupus erythematosus: an overview. *Lupus.* 2006;15:715–719.

Lee LA. Lupus erythematosus. In: Bolognia JL, Jorizzo JL, Rapini RP, eds. *Dermatology.* 1st Ed. Philadelphia, PA: Elsevier; 2003:601–613.

Squamous Cell Carcinoma

Erin Luxenberg

Introduction

Many forms of skin cancer occur much less frequently in deeply pigmented skin, and one form, squamous cell carcinoma (SCC), is discussed in detail in this chapter. Melanomas are discussed in another chapter, and other tumors, including Merkel cell carcinoma, keratoacanthoma, Paget disease, and Bowen disease, are briefly discussed in this chapter, with a full discussion online. If you are a first-time user, go to www.essentialdermatology.com/pigmented; go to www.visualdx.com/visualdx if you have already set your password.

■■ Diagnosis Synopsis

SCC is a malignancy of cutaneous epithelial cells occurring most frequently on sun-exposed areas of the skin, particularly the face and dorsal hands. Actinic keratosis may be a precursor lesion. The clinical presentation is highly variable among different demographic groups and tumor subtypes. SCC can involve the oral mucosa and lip, and when it does, it carries a much greater risk of metastases. Risk factors for the development of SCC include chronic sun exposure, fair skin and blue eyes, family history of skin cancer, scarring processes (chronic ulcers, burns, hidradenitis suppurativa, and the scars of discoid lupus erythematosus), ionizing radiation, immunosuppression, certain subtypes of human papillomavirus, and chemical carcinogens. Several genetic syndromes are associated with an increased risk of SCC as well. These include xeroderma pigmentosum, oculocutaneous albinism, epidermodysplasia verruciformis, epidermolysis bullosa, and KID syndrome (keratitis-ichthyosis-deafness). In Africa, patients with albinism are at a very high risk for SCC.

In darker-skinned individuals, SCC has also been found to frequently occur in scars and has been known to occur in non–sun-exposed areas. SCC is about 80 times less likely to occur in heavily pigmented individuals than those with fairer skin types, and its incidence has been observed to be 3.4 per 100,000 among African Americans. Nevertheless, it is the most common skin cancer in African Americans. Also, dark-skinned patients with SCC tend to have a higher mortality rate than white patients. This may be due to either a later diagnosis of the disease or a more highly aggressive form of the disease.

SCC *in situ* (SCCIS) is confined to the epidermis and includes other specific clinical entities such as Bowen disease and erythroplasia of Queyrat (on the male genitalia) (Fig. 4-308). As in invasive disease, SCCIS is more frequent and more aggressive in immunosuppressed individuals.

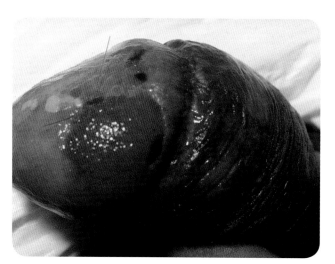

Figure 4-308 Well-demarcated red plaque on the glans that was SCC.

◉ Look For

The majority of SCC lesions appear on chronically sun-damaged skin of the head, neck, forearms, and dorsal hands. The clinical presentation may be variable. SCC often presents as an erythematous, hyperkeratotic papule or nodule that may ulcerate, but it may also be skin colored and/or smooth (Figs. 4-309 and 4-310). In darker-skinned individuals, the tumors may simply appear as erythematous macules with overlying crusts and scales. Over time, the tumor often develops a depressed center, and the growth becomes fixed to the underlying structures. New masses appearing within scars such as burn scars or chronic ulcers should be considered highly suspicious for SCC (Fig. 4-311).

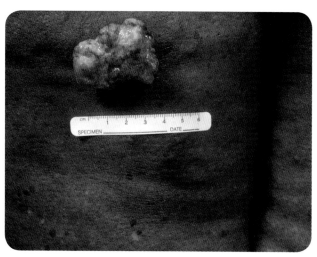

Figure 4-309 Pedunculated ulcerated SCC.

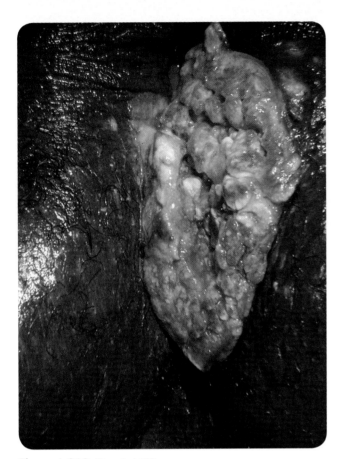

Figure 4-310 Ulcerated SCC.

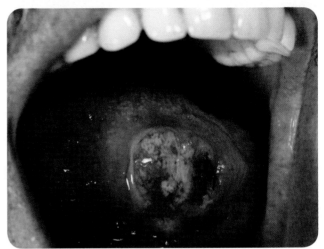

Figure 4-312 Ulcerated SCC of the tongue.

Diagnostic Pearls

- Important predisposing factors and locations include old burn scars, chronic cutaneous ulcers, and inflammation (especially those causing atrophic lesions), previous sites of irradiation or occupational trauma, chronic lymphedema, and areas of venous stasis.
- The lightly pigmented skin of patients with SCC will often display other evidence of sun exposure (e.g., solar elastosis, actinic keratoses, solar lentigines).
- Because SCC in more darkly pigmented patients may occur in non–sun-exposed areas, a higher index of suspicion for irregular lesions in those areas is warranted.
- Careful examination of regional lymph nodes is essential when SCC is considered and especially after it is diagnosed.

?? Differential Diagnosis and Pitfalls

- Rapidly growing nodules should always be biopsied before any destructive procedure, even in a patient who has had multiple skin malignancies. Two mimics for SCC are Merkel cell tumors and metastatic cancers.
- Merkel cell carcinoma—It is a rapidly growing malignancy in sun-exposed regions, most often the face. It may present as a red nodule and may seem cystic. It is twice as common in men as in women and 23 times as common in whites as in African Americans. Cytokeratin 20 is a very useful histologic marker for this malignancy, and polyoma virus is frequently in the lesions.
- Metastatic carcinoma—It can be anywhere on the skin and can be the first sign of an internal malignancy (Fig. 4-313). In women, the usual primary lesions are in the breast, colon, and skin melanoma; in men, lung, colon, and skin melanomas are the most common primary sites.

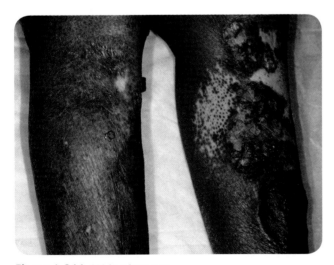

Figure 4-311 SCC in a burn scar.

Verrucous carcinoma is a rare, well-differentiated variety of SCC that presents as a glassy or shiny nodular growth. Oral, anogenital, foot, and subungual variants exist.

Oral SCCs are often related to tobacco usage and papillomavirus infection (Fig. 4-312).

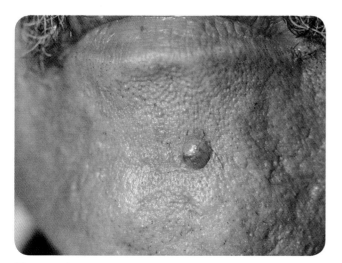

Figure 4-313 Metastatic carcinoma resembling a basal cell carcinoma because of prominent vessels.

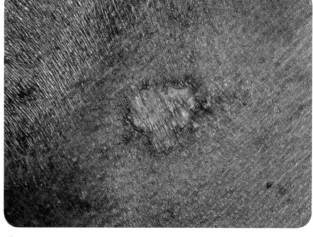

Figure 4-314 Atrophic plaque of carcinoma *in situ* (Bowen disease).

- Actinic keratosis—This condition is rare in deeply pigmented skin.
- Bowen disease—It usually presents as a single or a few persistent plaques of carcinoma *in situ* (Fig. 4-314). When on the glans penis, lesions are called erythroplasia of Queyrat.
- Keratoacanthoma—It is a neoplasm that may be a low-grade SCC. It is a rapidly growing, well-differentiated neoplasm that assumes a distinct crater-shaped appearance and usually occurs as a solitary lesion on the sun-exposed skin of the middle-aged and elderly population. Men are more commonly affected than women, and fair-skinned individuals are at greater risk than those with dark skin. Keratoacanthomas are rarely seen in African American patients. More deeply pigmented individuals at risk include those who are immunocompromised, and the lesions in these individuals will often occur in areas of previous trauma, surgical scars, or irradiation.
- Eccrine poroma—a neoplasm limited to the feet, often the sole
- Amelanotic melanoma
- Lymphomas—may present as single nodules on the head and neck
- Basal cell carcinoma
- Extramammary Paget disease—this is a rare neoplastic condition of apocrine gland-bearing skin that may be associated with internal malignancy. It is clinically and histologically similar to Paget disease of the nipple, appearing as pruritic, erythematous, scaling plaques, but the location is usually genital or perianal skin. It is more common in middle-aged to elderly white women. However, men of Asian descent are affected twice as often as women of the same ethnic group. These men are also more prone to extramammary Paget disease in more than one location. Extramammary Paget disease often goes

undiagnosed because, clinically, it can appear similar to chronic dermatitis.

A variety of diseases that are not malignancies may mimic SCCs:

- Verruca vulgaris
- Sporotrichosis
- Mycobacterium marinum
- Nummular dermatitis
- Atypical fibroxanthoma
- Irritated seborrheic keratosis
- Chronic draining or ulcerative lesions
- Hypertrophic discoid lupus erythematosus
- Hypertrophic lichen planus
- Prurigo nodularis
- Pyogenic granuloma

✓ Best Tests

- A thorough history and physical exam is the most effective means of detection. Biopsy of the lesion will demonstrate characteristic histopathology.
- Palpate for regional lymphadenopathy, and perform a complete skin exam in any patient with a suspicious lesion. Imaging studies may be indicated when a biopsy shows malignancy.

▲▲ Management Pearls

SCC of the head and neck (including the oral mucosa), particularly in African American patients, has a higher likelihood of metastasis and a worse prognosis for disease-free survival. Refer these patients to a specialist.

Therapy

Both Mohs micrographic surgery and standard surgical excision with 3- to 4-mm margins are first-line treatments. In high-risk SCC in which Mohs surgery is not performed, 6-mm margins are typically required. In cases of known or suspected nodal metastases, sentinel or formal lymph node dissection is often indicated.

For patients who are not surgical candidates, a number of therapeutic modalities are available. For superficial SCCs, electrodesiccation and curettage (times 3) with margins of 3 to 4 mm may be used. Radiation therapy is another reasonable alternative for poor surgical candidates.

Several treatments may be tried as second-line or third-line options, particularly in patients who are not amenable to surgery or those with an extensive burden of disease. These include the following:

- Topical imiquimod
- Topical or intralesional 5-fluorouracil
- Electrochemotherapy with intralesional bleomycin
- Intralesional interferon alpha
- Photodynamic therapy

Suggested Readings

Abe S, Kabashima K, Nichio D, et al. Quadruple Extra-mammary Pagets disease. *Acta Derm Venerol.* 2006;86:80–81.

Cox NH, Eeedy DJ, Morton CA. Therapy Guidelines and Audit Subcommittee, British Association of Dermatologists. Guidelines for Management of Bowen's Disease: 2006 Update. *Br J Dermatol.* 2007;156(1):11–21.

Drake AL, Walling HW. Variations in presentation of squamous cell carcinoma in situ (Bowen's disease) in immunocompromised patients. *J Am Acad Dermatol.* 2008;59(1):68–71.

Foo CI, Lee JS, Guilanno V, et al. Squamous cell carcinoma and Bowen's disease of the skin in Singapore. *Ann Acad Med Singapore.* 2007;36(3) 189–193.

Karaa A, Khachemoune A. Keratoacanthoma: A Tumor in search of a classification. *Int J Dermatol.* 2007;46(7):671–678.

Kim M, Boone SL, West DP, et al. Perception of skin cancer risk by those with ethnic skin. *Arch Dermatol.* 2009;45(2):207–208.

Rigel DS, Cockerell CJ, Carucci J, et al. Actinic keratosis, basal cell carcinoma and squamous cell carcinoma. In: Bolognia JL, Jorizzo JL, Rapini RP, eds. *Dermatology.* 2nd Ed. Philadelphia, PA: Elsevier; 2007: chap 108.

Settle K, Taylor R, Wolf J, et al. Race impacts outcome in Stage III/IV squamous cell carcinomas of the head and neck after concurrent chemoradiation therapy. *Cancer.* 2009;115(8):1744–1752.

Shepherd V, Davidson EJ, Davies-Humphreys J. Extramammary Paget's disease. *BJOG.* 2005;112(3):273–279.

Tinea Corporis

Meaghan Canton Feder

Diagnosis Synopsis

Tinea corporis, also known as ringworm of the body, is a skin rash caused by an inflammatory or hypersensitivity reaction to dermatophyte infection of the stratum corneum. The three dermatophyte species of fungus are *Trichophyton* (this is the most common and can infect skin, hair, and nails), *Microsporum* (infects skin and hair), and *Epidermophyton* (infects skin and nails). Anthropophilic fungi are spread from humans to humans, and zoophilic fungi are spread from animals to humans. Fungal organisms are spread through direct contact with those infected or through fomites.

The lesions of tinea corporis usually take the form of annular, erythematous, scaly plaques. The plaques grow slowly and heal in the center, causing a ring formation, which is how it got the name ringworm. Sometimes there is no inflammation, and the only sign of infection is scaling patches.

Tinea corporis is more prevalent in warm, humid climates and may also occur as a result of the spread of infection from other body locations. See separate descriptions for discussions of tinea capitis (scalp), tinea faciale (face), tinea pedis (foot), and tinea cruris (groin). Majocchi granuloma, a variant presentation, is also discussed separately.

Tinea imbricata is a distinct form of tinea corporis caused by *Trichophyton concentricum* that consists of scaly plaques distinctly arranged in concentric rings (Fig. 4-315). It is more prevalent in tropical climates such as southwest Polynesia, Melanesia, Southeast Asia, India, and Central America.

Pediatric Patient Considerations

Fungal organisms spread easily among children by direct contact and through fomites.

Immunocompromised Patient Considerations

Immunocompromised patients are more susceptible to fungal organisms, and widespread tinea corporis can be an early sign of AIDS.

Look For

Tinea corporis presents as annular, red, scaly patches that can appear anywhere on the body (Figs. 4-316 and 4-317). The borders are often raised, scale is prominent, and lesions can sometimes be papules, vesicles, or crusts. As the plaques spread, the lesions heal in the center, giving them a ring shape. On darker skin, tinea corporis appears as annular plaques with abundant scale, and the erythema is less noticeable.

Immunocompromised Patient Considerations

In HIV patients, the annular, erythematous, scaly patches of tinea are larger and more extensive.

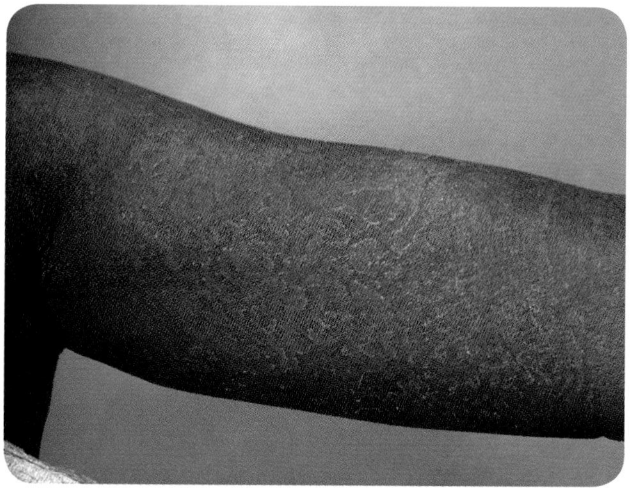

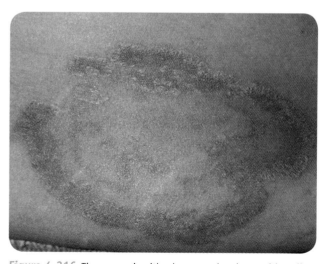

Figure 4-315 Wood-grain–like concentric scaling in a variant of tinea corporis that is often called tinea imbricata and can be seen in temperate climates.

Figure 4-316 Tinea corporis with a large annular plaque with scaling.

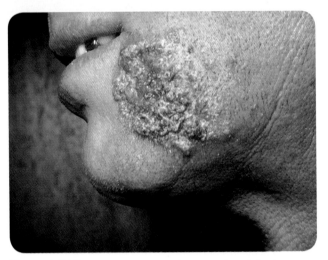

Figure 4-317 Red crusted plaque of dermatophyte infection.

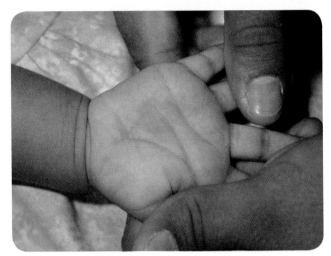

Figure 4-318 Tinea nigra can occur in infancy and childhood; it is less common in adults.

 Diagnostic Pearls

If a dermatophyte infection is already being treated with topical steroids, there could be an absence of redness and minimal scaling despite the lesion being loaded with fungi. A KOH preparation should be performed.

Pediatric Patient Considerations

All pediatric patients presenting with pruritic, scaly plaques should be thought to have a dermatophyte infection, and a KOH preparation should be performed. Topical steroids can mask scale and inflammation. Usually the centers of tinea lesions are clear, but they can be hyperpigmented.

?? **Differential Diagnosis and Pitfalls**

- Seborrheic dermatitis
- Psoriasis
- Parapsoriasis
- Candidiasis
- Erythrasma
- Impetigo
- Subacute cutaneous lupus erythematosus
- Tinea versicolor
- Granuloma annulare
- Mycosis fungoides
- Nummular dermatitis—If it continues to spread with topical steroid treatment, then consider tinea.
- Secondary syphilis
- Pityriasis rosea

- Tinea nigra—areas of brown scaling, usually limited to the palms, caused by *Hortaea werneckii* (Fig. 4-318)
- Erythema annulare centrifugum

 Best Tests

- KOH—Scrape the scaly, active border with a scalpel blade, small curette, or the edge of a glass slide. Collect scale on a slide and cover with a cover slip. Direct a drop of 10% KOH solution to the edge of the cover slip. Under the microscope, observe for branching or curving fungal hyphae.
- Fungal culture—A fungal culture will allow species identification, but it will take several weeks.
- Wood lamp—This is an ultraviolet light that will illuminate *Microsporum* dermatophytes as a green fluorescence. However, the most common fungus, *Trichophyton*, does not fluoresce under a Wood lamp.

Pediatric Patient Considerations

A KOH should be performed in all patients in whom tinea is suspected. If Majocchi granuloma is suspected, a biopsy is necessary.

 Management Pearls

- Topical steroids should be avoided because they have the potential to worsen the infection.

- Small, localized lesions should be treated topically; extend 2 cm outside the border of the lesion. More extensive disease will require 3 to 4 weeks of oral antifungal agents.

Therapy

Limited

Use topical antifungals for 2 to 6 weeks, based on clinical response:

- Terbinafine 1% cream—apply once to twice daily (over the counter)
- Clotrimazole 1% cream—apply twice daily (over the counter)
- Econazole cream—apply once to twice daily
- Oxiconazole cream—apply twice daily
- Ciclopiroxolamine cream, lotion—apply twice daily
- Ketoconazole cream—apply twice daily

Extensive Disease or Disease Unresponsive to Topicals

- Terbinafine—250 mg daily for 2 weeks
- Itraconazole—100 to 200 mg daily for 2 to 4 weeks or 200 mg twice daily for 1 week
- Griseofulvin ultramicrosize—330 to 375 mg daily for 4 to 8 weeks

Most cases can be treated with topical antifungal creams. Twice-daily application for 2 to 4 weeks is usually sufficient. Patients should be instructed to apply the cream to the lesion as well as a 2-cm area surrounding it for 1 to 2 weeks after clinical resolution.

For more extensive involvement or Majocchi granuloma, oral griseofulvin or terbinafine can be used. Griseofulvin is dosed at 20 mg/kg/d for 4 to 6 weeks; terbinafine is dosed at 6 mg/kg/d for 2 weeks.

Suggested Readings

Das S, Goyal R, Bhattacharya SN. Laboratory-based epidemiological study of superficial fungal infections. *J Dermatol.* 2007;34(4):248–253.

James WD, Berger TG, Elston DM, eds. Tinea corporis (tinea circinata). In: *Andrews' Diseases of the Skin: Clinical Dermatology.* 10th Ed. Philadelphia, PA: Saunders Elsevier; 2006:302–303.

Lohoue Petmy J, Lando AJ, Kaptue L, et al. Superficial mycoses and HIV infection in Yaounde. *J Eur Acad Venereol.* 2004;18(3):301–304.

Neji S, Makni F, Cheikhrouhou F, et al. Epidemiology of dermatophytoses in Sfax, Tunisia. *Mycoses.* 2009;52(6):534–538.

Omar AA. Importance of mycological confirmation of clinically suspected cases of tinea corporis, tinea pedis and tinea cruris. *J Egypt Publ Health Assoc.* 2004;79(1-2):43–58.

Ozkutuk A, Ergon C, Yulug N. Species distribution and antifungal susceptibilities of dermatophytes during a one year period at a university hospital in Turkey. *Mycoses.* 2007;50(2):125–129.

Sellami A, Sellami H, Makni F, et al. Childhood dermatomycoses study in Sfax Hospital, Tunisia. *Mycoses.* 2008;51(5):451–454.

Nonbullous Impetigo
Meaghan Canton Feder

▪ Diagnosis Synopsis

Nonbullous impetigo, or impetigo contagiosa, is a highly contagious superficial skin infection primarily caused by *Staphylococcus aureus* in industrialized countries and group A *Streptococcus* (*Streptococcus pyogenes*) in developing countries. It is the most common bacterial infection in children and affects adults who have extensive, close contact with infected children. Adults are also at risk if they have a minor trauma, atopic dermatitis, or an infestation, such as scabies, because these dermatologic conditions predispose them to infection. Small epidemics of impetigo can occur in crowded environments such as army barracks.

Clinically, impetigo presents as small, discrete erythematous vesicles and/or pustules that quickly transition into superficial erosions with a characteristic honey-colored crust. Lesions are usually located in exposed areas of the body and most commonly present on the face, around the nose and mouth, and on extremities. There are usually no systemic symptoms associated with impetigo, with the exception of regional mild lymphadenopathy.

Impetigo occurs more frequently in warmer, humid climates.

Although methicillin-resistant *S. aureus* (MRSA) infection of the skin usually presents as recurrent furunculosis or skin abscesses, MRSA has been shown to cause impetigo. Culture and sensitivities should always be performed in patients with lesions suspicious for cutaneous infection, and empirical coverage for MRSA should be instituted if clinical suspicion is high.

Pediatric Patient Considerations

Nonbullous impetigo is more commonly seen in young children. It is caused by *S. aureus* or group A *Streptococcus* (*S. pyogenes*) as in adults. In children, constitutional symptoms and fevers are minimal. Usually, impetigo develops at the site of minor trauma such as insect bites or abrasions. It can also result from infection of lesions of atopic dermatitis, scabies, herpes simplex virus (HSV), or poison ivy, where children are scratching. Children can also develop impetigo from pets, unwashed hands, direct contact with other children, and crowded living situations.

In infants, it has been suggested but not proven that boys develop impetigo more frequently in the diaper area and lower abdomen, while girls develop impetigo more frequently on the face.

◉ Look For

Look for small, discrete vesicles or pustules that quickly rupture, draining golden-yellow discharge. The lesions crust over, forming classic honey-colored thickened papules and plaques (**Figs. 4-319–4-321**). The lesions are usually

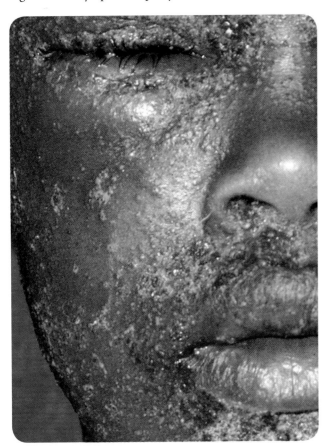

Figure 4-319 Diffuse staphylococcal impetigo with swelling and crusting.

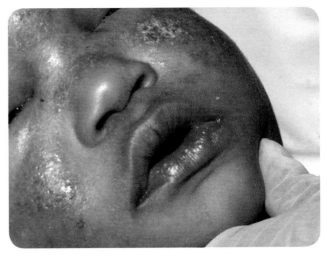

Figure 4-320 Crusting and edema due to impetigo.

310

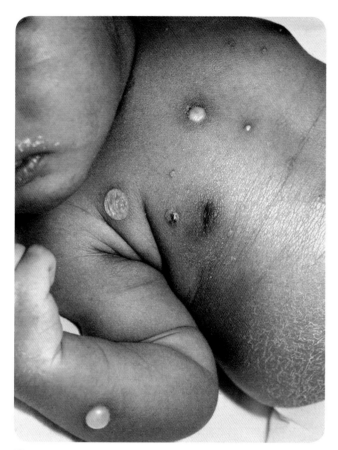

Figure 4-321 Bullous and nonbullous lesions of impetigo.

located in exposed areas, mainly on the face and extremities. If crusts are removed, the skin beneath is red and moist, and the exudate will re-form the honey-colored crusts. Lesions tend to be multiple but in one location. The lesions can be spread to other parts of the body and to others by direct contact or by a contaminated fomite such as a towel.

Impetigo caused by streptococcal infections usually presents with mild regional lymphadenopathy.

 ## Diagnostic Pearls

- Honey-colored or golden-yellow crusted papules and plaques, sometimes with small inflammatory halos. The initial superficial vesicles are rarely seen, as they are fragile and transient.
- The face is the most common location, particularly around the nose.
- Lesions may persist for weeks or months and can develop atrophy under a tightly adherent crust.

Pediatric Patient Considerations

Nonbullous impetigo is very infectious and can easily spread among schoolchildren or those playing contact sports.

?? Differential Diagnosis and Pitfalls

A diagnosis of nonbullous impetigo is often mistakenly disregarded due to the lack of inflammation or induration.

- Superficial fungal infection—perform KOH; also, tinea does not present with weepy, thick, honey-colored crusts.
- Atopic dermatitis—It can appear impetiginized.
- Contact dermatitis—Impetigo has more crusted lesions and tends to involve more of the face. Linear lesions and pruritus are not seen in impetigo but are seen in contact dermatitis from poison ivy.
- Erysipelas
- Cellulitis
- Burns
- Insect bite reaction
- HSV—It can appear impetiginized; take a viral culture.
- Varicella—Discrete lesions of varicella are usually umbilicated and can involve the mouth; neither is seen in impetigo.
- Scabies
- Pediculosis capitis—If a patient has recurrent impetigo on the head and neck, look for head lice.
- Pemphigus foliaceus

✓ Best Tests

- Gram stain of exudate/lesional fluid will reveal Gram-positive cocci.
- Bacterial culture of a skin lesion with antibiotic sensitivity. Sensitivities should be performed on any *S. aureus* isolates to determine antibiotic resistance.
- Bacterial culture of nares to rule out MRSA if there are recurrent impetigo infections.
- Skin biopsy is rarely needed, but if performed would show mild dermal inflammation and more superficial inflammation with scattered cocci and debris of polymorphonuclear leukocytes and epidermal cells.

▲▲ Management Pearls

- Prevention—Those with impetigo should use separate towels and soap. They should wash hands regularly. In the hospital, both standard and contact precautions should be implemented to avoid the spread of impetigo.
- To promote healing, lesions should be soaked in soap and water or Domeboro soaks and crusts gently removed. Topical mupirocin ointment should be applied to the wound twice a day.
- Given the prevalence of MRSA, maintain a high index of suspicion for this diagnosis, and make the initial choice of empiric antibiotic therapy accordingly. It is helpful to be aware of patterns of antimicrobial resistance within your community.

Pediatric Patient Considerations

For children in high-risk categories, such as those in day care or those who play contact sports, mupirocin or bacitracin ointment should be applied to cuts and other superficial skin traumas to avoid infection.

Therapy

Localized Disease

Treat by soaking in warm soap and water for 15 to 20 minutes three times a day and gently removing crusts. Apply mupirocin ointment twice daily. In patients who develop resistance to mupirocin, retapamulin may be used.

Widespread Disease

Treat with systemic antibiotics in combination with topical therapies. Systemic antibiotics include penicillin or first-generation cephalosporin, for at least 7 days. If MRSA is suspected, consult current CDC guidelines, as treatment for MRSA is rapidly changing. If there is colonization of MRSA in the nasal passage, then eradication of MRSA nasal carriage may be attempted with application of 2% mupirocin ointment to the nares.

- Penicillin 250 mg p.o. four times daily for 7 to 10 days for streptococcal impetigo
- Cephalexin 250 to 500 mg p.o. four times daily for 7 to 10 days
- Erythromycin 250 mg p.o. four times daily for 7 to 10 days
- Dicloxacillin 250 mg p.o. four times daily for 7 to 10 days

Pediatric Patient Considerations

Localized and Limited
Mupirocin ointment or cream for few lesions (three times per day for 7 to 14 days).

Widespread

Cephalexin 25 to 50 mg/kg/d p.o. divided three to four times per day or twice daily

Dicloxacillin—administer 1 hour before a meal or 2 hours after a meal (12.5 to 25 mg/kg/d divided every 6 hours for children <40 kg and 250 to 500 mg every 6 hours for children more than 40 kg)

Erythromycin 3 to 50 mg/kg/d (stearate/base) p.o. divided every 6 to 8 hours.

Standard cephalosporins and penicillins are of no benefit in treating MRSA. Treatment for MRSA is rapidly changing, and current CDC guidelines should be consulted.

Suggested Readings

Koning J. Treatment for impetigo: evidence favours topical treatment with mupirocin, fisidic acid. *Br Med J.* 2004;329(7468):695–696.

Nakaminami H, Noguchi N, Ikeda M, et al. Molecular epidemiology and antimicrobial susceptibilities of 273 exfoliative toxin-encoding-gene-positive *Staphylococcus aureus* isolates from patients with impetigo in Japan. *J Med Microbiol.* 2008;57(10):125.1–1258.

Rayner C, Munckhof WJ. Antibiotics currently used in the treatment of infections caused by *Staphylococcus aureus. Intern Med J.* 2005;36(2):142–143.

Steer AC, Danchin MH, Carapetis JR. Group A Streptococcal infections in children. *J Pediatrics Child Health.* 2007;43(4):203–213.

Steer AC, Tikoduadua LV, Manalac EM, et al. Validation of an integrated management of childhood illness algorithm for managing common skin conditions in Fiji. *Bull Work Health Organ.* 2009;87(3):173–179.

Tan HH, Tay YK, Goh CL. Bacterial skin infections at a tertiary dermatological centre. *Singapore Med J.* 1998;39(8):353–356.

Pityriasis Lichenoides et Varioliformis Acuta

Stephanie Diamantis

:: Diagnosis Synopsis

Pityriasis lichenoides refers to a spectrum of skin diseases that includes pityriasis lichenoides et varioliformis acuta (PLEVA) and its subtype febrile ulceronecrotic Mucha-Habermann disease (FUMHD) as well as pityriasis lichenoides chronica (PLC). Pityriasis lichenoides can occur in either sex and in all ages and has no ethnic predisposition. In the pediatric population, pityriasis lichenoides has a peak onset between ages 5 and 10 and occurs more frequently in boys. The febrile ulceronecrotic variant shows a male predominance and a peak onset in the second decade of life. Etiology is unknown, but theories have centered upon an inflammatory response triggered by infection versus an inflammatory response secondary to a T-cell dyscrasia. At this stage, a T-cell lymphoproliferative etiology is favored.

PLEVA, also known as Mucha-Habermann disease, is a disorder that is characterized by the acute-subacute onset of asymptomatic recurrent crops of erythematous papules and vesicles that spontaneously resolve over weeks to months. Papules become necrotic and then heal with pigmentary change or minor scarring. Because of its recurrent nature, PLEVA demonstrates varying stages of evolution: small ulcers, crusted papules, vesicles, pustules, and varicella-like scarring are present concurrently.

FUMHD is a subtype of PLEVA that presents more explosively with rapid evolution of papules to coalescent ulcers with crusting and hemorrhagic bullae. These lesions are often painful and may become secondarily infected. Systemic symptoms such as high fever, malaise, sore throat, gastrointestinal distress, central nervous system symptoms, anemia, arthritis, interstitial pneumonitis, splenomegaly, and sepsis can accompany the skin eruption. Fatalities have been reported with this subtype of PLEVA, with a mortality rate of up to 25%, especially in elderly or immunocompromised individuals.

PLC is a related but more chronic form of pityriasis lichenoides. PLC is characterized by crops of scaly, erythematous papules that spontaneously regress over months. Darkly pigmented patients can present with multiple widespread hypopigmented macules. The course is more indolent, and pustules, vesicles, and crusts characteristic of PLEVA are absent.

Pityriasis lichenoides is generally viewed as a benign disorder that lasts from 1 to 3 years. However, there are case reports of progression to cutaneous T-cell lymphoma. No guidelines have been established for monitoring this possible progression.

(●) Look For

PLEVA is characterized by crops of 2- to 3-mm erythematous macules that rapidly evolve into scaly papules (Fig. 4-322). The centers of the papules become vesicular, pustular, and then necrotic with an overlying red-to-brown hemorrhagic crust (Fig. 4-323). Lesions are in different stages of evolution, given that they arise in crops, and are usually localized to the trunk, proximal extremities, and flexural surfaces. Lesions may be asymptomatic or mildly pruritic. Fever and malaise are rarely present. Postinflammatory hypopigmentation is common in darkly pigmented skin (Fig. 4-324).

The lesions of FUMHD are typically larger and covered by a black crust. They heal with scarring. High fever and other systemic manifestations are more likely.

PLC tends to present with smaller papules with scale that occur on the trunk and proximal extremities. In darkly pigmented patients, eruptions of hypopigmented macules without scale can occur.

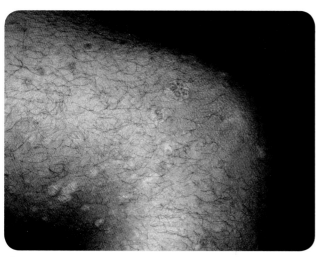

Figure 4-322 PLEVA with multiple papular lesions.

Figure 4-323 PLEVA with pustular lesions with red bases.

313

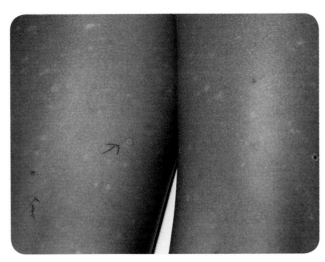

Figure 4-324 PLEVA with hypopigmented and papular lesions.

Diagnostic Pearls

- PLEVA is characterized by scattered lesions in multiple stages of evolution/healing.
- In darkly pigmented individuals, look for numerous, regularly sized, oval, hypopigmented macules of postinflammatory hypopigmentation.

Differential Diagnosis and Pitfalls

- Lymphomatoid papulosis—Predominantly CD30+ cells in the infiltrate. Patient is older. Characterized by more nodular lesions. Active lesions do not spontaneously resolve as quickly as PLEVA.
- Drug eruption—A medication history helps make this diagnosis. Systemic symptoms can be more pronounced, including fever, lymphadenopathy, and facial edema. Eosinophilia on CBC and histology may be helpful if present.
- Vasculitis—Check serologies for RF, ANA, anti-ds DNA, ANCA, cryoglobulins, and C3 and C4 levels. Lesions are mostly purpuric, more monomorphic, and localized to lower extremities in cutaneous small vessel vasculitis.
- Varicella (chickenpox)—Prodrome of mild fever, malaise, and myalgia followed by pruritic erythematous papules. Lesions are pruritic. Recurrent eruptions are not a feature of varicella. VZV viral culture or PCR can exclude this diagnosis.
- Arthropod bites
- Dermatitis herpetiformis—Exquisitely pruritic. Ruled out by direct immunofluorescence on the skin biopsy.
- Pityriasis rosea—Herald patch, scaly papules/plaques. Crusts, vesicles, and bullae are not common findings.

- Lichen planus—Very pruritic, lesions are typically monomorphic and rarely crusted.
- Perforating dermatoses
- Toxoplasmosis
- Erythema multiforme
- Guttate psoriasis
- Cutaneous T-cell lymphoma
- Secondary syphilis
- Gianotti-Crosti syndrome

✓ Best Tests

Skin biopsy is helpful in confirming the diagnosis.

Lab tests to look for underlying disease or rule out diagnoses in the differential diagnosis list include the following:

- Monospot or heterophil antibody test to evaluate for EBV
- RPR or VDRL
- Toxoplasma Sabin-Feldman dye test, ELISA, and indirect immunofluorescence/hemagglutination

▲▲ Management Pearls

- PLEVA is often self-limited and often resolves over a period of weeks to months. Large ulcerations in the ulceronecrotic form of PLEVA require local wound care.
- FUMHD is considered a dermatologic emergency.
- There is evidence to support the fact that the distribution of lesions can predict outcome. Patients with disseminated involvement of the skin have an average clinical course of 11 months, while those with lesions restricted to extremities have demonstrated an average clinical course of 33 months.
- PLC can also occur rarely as a paraneoplastic phenomenon (occurs after the development of a primary tumor or follows a course parallel to that of a primary tumor).

Therapy

Lesions of pityriasis lichenoides tend to spontaneously resolve without treatment. Because of the self-resolving nature, few clinical trials have been performed; treatment options are based on small case series, case reports, and anecdotal evidence. First-line therapies include oral antibiotics, topical corticosteroids or topical immunomodulators (e.g., tacrolimus), and light therapy (especially helpful in PLC). Systemic antibiotics are employed mainly for their anti-inflammatory activity. For more persistent and severe cases, treatment options include methotrexate, acitretin, dapsone, cyclosporine, or a combination of the above.

Commonly used oral antibiotics are as follows:

- Azithromycin 10 mg/kg up to 500 mg on day 1, then 5 mg/kg up to 250 mg daily to complete a 5-day course, given bimonthly until resolution.
- Tetracycline 500 mg three to four times daily for a 2- to 4-week course; maintenance dose of 1 g/d
- Erythromycin 250 mg four times daily

Steroids
- Topical steroids can be applied for mild to moderate disease
- Prednisone 40 to 60 mg p.o. daily for PLEVA with systemic manifestations

Retinoids
- Acitretin 25 to 50 mg p.o. daily

Natural ultraviolet light, narrow-band UVB, or PUVA (psoralen plus UVA) have been reported to be helpful. Narrow-band UVB has achieved complete response in patients with a mean cumulative dose of approximately 20 J/cm^2 over 40 exposures.

Combination therapy (antibiotics plus PUVA or methotrexate plus PUVA) may be superior for the rare ulceronecrotic form.

Pruritus can be treated with antihistamines:

- Diphenhydramine hydrochloride (25, 50 mg tablets or capsules): 25 to 50 mg nightly or every 6 hours as needed
- Hydroxyzine (10, 25 mg tablets): 12.5 to 25 mg, every 6 hours as needed
- Cetirizine hydrochloride (5, 10 mg tablets): 5 to 10 mg/d
- Loratadine: 10 mg once daily

Suggested Readings

Bowers S, Warshaw EM. Pityriasis lichenoides and its subtypes. *J Am Acad Dermatol.* 2006;55:557–572.

Clayton R, Warin A. Pityriasis lichenoides chronic presenting as hypopigmentation. *Br J Dermatol.* 1979;100:297–302.

Helbling I, Chalmers RJ, Yates VM. Febrile ulceronecrotic Mucha-Habermann disease: A rare dermatologic emergency. *Clin Exp Dermatol.* 2009;34(8):e1006–e1007.

Khachemoune A, Blyumin ML. Pityriasis lichenoides pathophysiology, classification and treatment. *Am J Clin Dermatol.* 2007;8(1):29–36.

Wood GS, Hu C, Garrett AL. Parapsoriasis and pityriasis lichenoides. In: Wolff K, Goldsmith LA, Katz SI, et al., eds. *Fitzpatrick's Dermatology in General Medicine.* 7th Ed. New York, NY: McGraw Hill; 2008:240–243.

Xerosis and Eczema Craquelé (Asteatotic Dermatitis)

Nasir Aziz

▪▪ Diagnosis Synopsis

Xerosis

Xerosis (dry skin) is also known as ashy skin, a slang term originating in the African American community. In many individuals, the stratum corneum of the epidermis fails to retain moisture, manifesting clinically as dry, cracked, and powdery skin. Xerosis causing ashiness reduces the skin's shine and presents as white patches in dark skin. Multiple studies have shown that transepidermal water loss is larger in black skin compared with white skin, thereby predisposing the latter to xerosis.

Significant differences in the level of ceramides in the stratum corneum have been found, with the lowest levels in individuals of African descent, followed by whites, Hispanics, and Asians. One study found that ceramide levels were inversely correlated with transepidermal water loss and directly related to water content. While the evidence regarding differences in corneocyte desquamation is scant, some observers have noted that individuals of African descent have a 2.5 times greater spontaneous desquamation rate compared with whites and Asians, which could explain the higher frequency of xerosis seen. Lastly, the difference in sebaceous gland activity between "white" and "black" skin remains disputed. One study measuring sebaceous gland activity in 649 male and female patients, 67 of whom were designated black, found no difference in sebaceous gland activity between the white and black participants. Other studies have found increased sebum production, pore size, and skin microflora in the skin of individuals of African descent.

Eczema Craquelé

Eczema craquelé is also known as winter itch, asteatotic eczema, xerotic eczema, and desiccation dermatitis. These entities represent the extreme end of the spectrum of xerosis.

Xerosis is the predisposing factor to the development of eczema craquelé. It refers to a condition of rough, dry skin texture with fine scale and occasionally fine fissuring. It is often pruritic. The pathogenesis involves a decrease in the amount of lipids in the stratum corneum and a deficiency in the water-binding capacity of this layer. The most common cause of xerosis is aging; however, it can be associated with a number of environmental factors and/or disease states, such as low humidity, frequent bathing, harsh soaps, congenital and acquired ichthyoses, atopic dermatitis, hypothyroidism, Down syndrome, renal failure, malnutrition and malabsorptive states, HIV, lymphoma, liver disease, Sjögren syndrome, carcinomatosis, and certain drugs. Asteatotic dermatitis is a rare presentation of zinc deficiency.

Eczema craquelé begins as dry skin that progresses to superficially fissured, inflamed, and sometimes crusted dermatitis. A generalized dermatitis can develop. The condition is seen mostly in elderly individuals. This may be due to decreased sebaceous/sweat gland activity and keratin synthesis in elderly persons, as well as a host of other factors such as malnutrition, drugs, and underlying illnesses. The condition is exacerbated by low humidity and frequent bathing without moisturizing. Pruritus is frequent, and painful lesions can occur if the fissures are deep.

◉ Look For

Xerosis

For xerosis, look for dry, powdery white scale mostly involving the extremities, though it can be widespread and even involve the face (Fig. 4-325). Xerosis usually has a slow and indolent course, progressing over years. It is characterized by dry, dull, rough skin with fine branlike scales that flake off easily.

Eczema Craquelé

In contrast, eczema craquelé usually has a more acute or subacute onset. It is characterized by redness and tight-appearing, polygonally cracked skin with fine, interconnected horizontal and vertical fissures (Figs. 4-326 and 4-327). This forms an irregular network of fissures and cracks similar to broken window glass. It is most severe on the distal legs and occasionally the arms and trunk. The face, scalp, groin, and axillae are usually spared from the fine, dry scales of the condition. Crusting, oozing, and bleeding fissures may be seen in advanced cases.

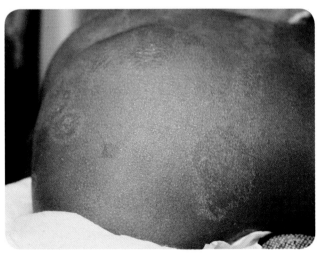

Figure 4-325 Xerotic dry skin with mild annular eczematous plaques.

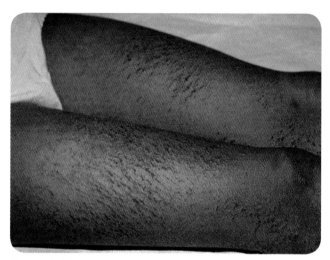

Figure 4-326 Eczema craquelé with red linear areas on xerotic skin on a common location, the legs.

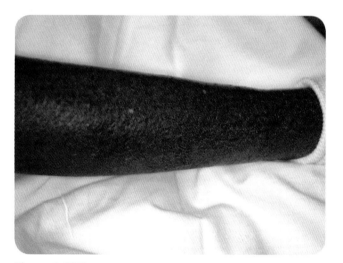

Figure 4-327 Heavy scaling and cracking of eczema craquelé.

Pediatric Patient Considerations

Asteatotic eczema is seen mostly in the elderly but is also reported in atopic children in the winter and in adolescents who bathe frequently without moisturizing, especially in dry climates or winter climates with low humidity.

Pruritus is frequent. Rarely, in children, the lesions can be painful if the fissures are deep.

Diagnostic Pearls

- Patients will often have a history of washing with harsh soaps, taking frequent or very hot showers, a winter climate with low humidity, and/or heating using a wood stove.

- The appearance of this dermatitis has been described as "cracked porcelain," "crazy pavement," and like a "dried-up riverbed."

?? Differential Diagnosis and Pitfalls

- In ichthyosis, the extremities have a fish-scale appearance.
- Atopic dermatitis has a characteristic flexural distribution.
- Psoriasis is usually localized with sharply demarcated plaques.
- Hypothyroidism causes very dry skin and may increase one's tendency to get eczema craquelé.

✓ Best Tests

This is usually a clinical diagnosis. Further testing may reveal a systemic cause. Check for thyroid function, renal function, liver function, HIV, zinc level, malabsorption, cancer, or Sjögren syndrome if clinical suspicion warrants (lesions are widespread or fail to respond to therapy).

▲▲ Management Pearls

- Look for signs of secondary dermatitis. If there are signs of dermatitis (redness, inflammation), consider a mild topical corticosteroid ointment such as triamcinolone 0.1% ointment twice daily for a short course of 1 week.
- Treat superficial crusts and signs of impetiginization with oral antibiotics for 7 to 10 days. Tell patients to avoid too frequent and too hot baths or showers. Encourage patients to use mild soaps (e.g., Dove, Tone, Purpose, or Cetaphil cleanser) and invest in a humidifier.

Therapy

- Use a mild- to mid-potency topical steroid on inflamed areas.
- Use ointments (these have fewer preservatives in them) if the condition seems to be flaring with multiple topical medications.
- Avoid the use of neomycin, as this can be a potent contact allergen.

Xerosis

For xerosis without signs of inflammation, instruct the patient to frequently apply a thick moisturizing cream or ointment such as petroleum jelly or Aquaphor ointment to wet skin. Eucerin, Cetaphil creams, and Vanicream are excellent moisturizing agents.

(Continued)

317

Eczema Craquelé

Eczema craquelé is best treated with heavy emollients after bathing. Immediate application of a moisturizing cream to the damp skin following bathing will "hold in" moisture.

Suggested Readings

Berardesca E, Maibach H. Ethnic skin: Overview of structure and function. *J Am Acad Dermatol.* 2003;48(6 Suppl):S139–S142.

Pochi PE, Strauss JS. Sebaceous gland activity in black skin. *Dermatol Clin.* 1988;6(3):349–351.

Rawlings AV. Ethnic skin types: Are there differences in skin structure and function? *Int J Cosmet Sci.* 2006;28(2):79–93.

Uhoda E, Pierard-Franchimont C, Petit L, et al. Skin weathering and ashiness in black Africans. *Eur J Dermatol.* 2003;13(6):574–578.

Wesley NO, Maibach HI. Racial (ethnic) differences in skin properties: The objective data. *Am J Clin Dermatol.* 2003;4(12):843–860.

Ichthyoses

Tess Nasabzadeh

Lifelong scaling of the skin is seen in a number of diseases. A few of the more common forms are discussed in this chapter, and others (erythrokeratodermia variabilis, Netherton syndrome, and congenital hemidysplasia, ichthyosiform nevus, and limb defects [CHILD] syndrome) are available on VisualDx online. (If you are a first-time online user, go to www.essentialdermatology.com/pigmented; if you already have your password set up, go directly to www.visualdx.com/visualdx.)

Diagnosis Synopsis

Ichthyosis Vulgaris

Ichthyosis vulgaris, an autosomal dominant disease, is the result of a filaggrin gene mutation and occurs in approximately 1 in 250 to 1,000 children. Specific filaggrin gene mutations are unique to a given population such as the Europeans, Chinese, or Japanese. Patients with ichthyosis vulgaris have extremely dry skin and a fine, fish-skin–like scale. The condition first begins in childhood between 3 and 12 months of age and patients often have decreased scaling by adulthood. Adult-onset ichthyosis vulgaris is associated with systemic disease including malignancy, HIV, and autoimmune diseases. There is no known race/ethnicity or gender predilection. The disease is exacerbated by low humidity and alkaline skin care products such as soap and detergent.

Darier Disease

Darier disease, also known as keratosis follicularis and Darier-White disease, is an autosomal dominant disorder with an overall estimated prevalence of 1 in 30,000 to 100,000. In Saudi Arabia there is a greater prevalence of 1 in 10,000. It is caused by over 150 different mutations in the ATP2A2 gene, which encodes a sarcoplasmic/endoplasmic reticulum calcium-ATPase pump (SERCA2). Darier disease presents in early adolescence to mid-adult life with greasy, hyperkeratotic papules. Exacerbating factors include heat, perspiration, mechanical pressure such as under collars of sweaters or shirts, UV light, menstruation, and some medications. In North American and European populations, men and women are equally affected, but a study of Asian patients in Singapore found a male predominance.

X-Linked Ichthyosis

X-linked ichthyosis is a disorder due to a deficiency of the steroid sulfatase enzyme that affects 1 in 6,000 males. During the first few weeks of life, there is desquamation of large, loosely adherent, translucent scales followed by the development of tightly adherent, dark-brown scales. There is no known racial, ethnic, or geographic predilection.

Lamellar Ichthyosis

Lamellar ichthyosis is a lifelong disorder beginning usually as a collodion baby. Ectropion is a prominent characteristic. There will be lifelong temperature intolerance, secondary dermatophyte infection, and scarring alopecia. There is genetic heterogeneity, but most cases are due to mutations in an epidermal transglutaminase.

Collodion Baby

Collodion baby refers to the presentation of a newborn encased in a taut, shiny, thickened stratum corneum. This phenotype is the result of a number of different congenital disorders of keratinization such as lamellar ichthyosis and nonbullous congenital ichthyosiform erythroderma. In about 10% to 20% of cases, termed self-healing collodion baby, there is spontaneous resolution after the membrane is shed.

Epidermolytic Hyperkeratosis

Epidermolytic hyperkeratosis, also known as bullous congenital ichthyosiform erythroderma of Brocq, is a congenital disorder due to a mutation in the gene encoding keratin 1 or keratin 10 with a prevalence of 1 in 200,000 to 300,000. It is transmitted in an autosomal dominant manner with frequent spontaneous mutations and manifests with erythroderma and blistering at birth and then with hyperkeratosis later in life. The two main clinical categories of this disease are based on the presence or absence of palm and sole involvement.

◉ Look For

Ichthyosis Vulgaris

Ichthyosis vulgaris presents with small, fine, polygonal scales, most apparent on the extensor extremities (Figs. 4-328–4-330). The color of the scales may be white, "dirty" gray, or brown, with darker scales being more common in dark-skinned patients.

Darier Disease

In Darier disease there are small, symmetrical, skin-colored or yellow-brown, greasy papules in a seborrheic distribution on the chest, face, scalp, and retroauricular folds (Fig. 4-331). In patients with dark skin, the lesions often have a dirty gray coloration. Intertriginous areas are also affected, and there may be, even more rarely, pits of hemorrhagic lesions on the palms and soles. Lesions may be pruritic and malodorous. Nail involvement is often seen with thin nail plates and chipped, cracked nail margins with

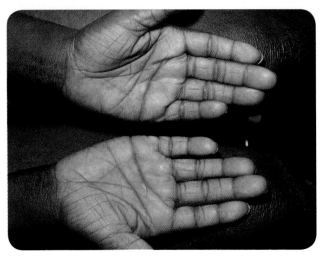

Figure 4-328 Hyperlinear palms are characteristic of ichthyosis vulgaris.

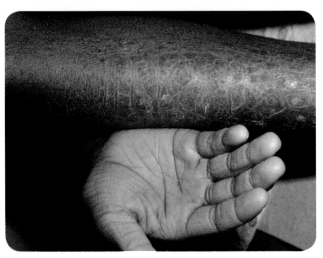

Figure 4-329 Ichthyosis vulgaris with adherent scales and hyperlinear palms.

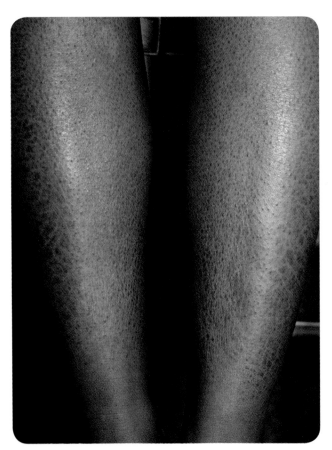

Figure 4-330 Mild to moderate scaling of ichthyosis vulgaris.

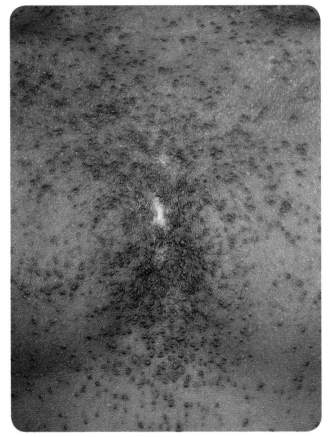

Figure 4-331 Darier disease is a disorder of keratinization with rough scaling papules on chest, face, and scalp and frequent nail thinning with red- and white-striped bands.

parallel white or red bands in the nail bed. A characteristic nail finding is a V-shaped notch in the free edge of the nail. Oral lesions on the hard palate are sometimes seen. In dark-skinned individuals, specifically those of African and Asian descent, Darier disease has been reported to be associated with white hypopigmented macules (guttate leucoderma).

X-Linked Ichthyosis

X-linked ichthyosis results in dirty yellow to brown, polygonal, adherent scales that are widespread and worsen with age. In early childhood the face looks "dirty" due to the involvement of the scalp, preauricular, and posterior cervical regions (Fig. 4-332). The palms, soles, hair, and nails are normal. With age, the trunk and extremity lesions worsen, while the head and neck lesions improve. Corneal opacities may be seen in 50% of patients and abnormal testicular descent occurs in almost one-third of cases.

Lamellar Ichthyosis

Large platelike scales and a prominent ectropion. Very red and scaling (Figs. 4-333 and 4-334).

Collodion Baby

A collodion baby is covered in a tight, shiny, parchmentlike membrane (Fig. 4-335). Absence of eyebrows, eyelashes,

and scalp hair is common in these newborn babies. There may be underlying erythema and the skin often undergoes cracking and fissuring. The newborn may also have ectropion, eclabium, and contracture of joints and digits.

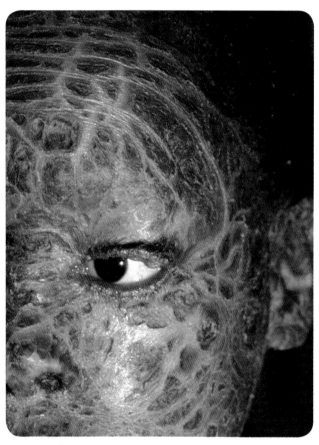

Figure 4-334 Lamellar ichthyosis with prominent ectropion and large black scales.

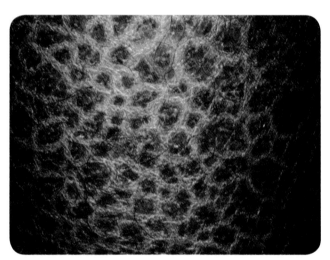

Figure 4-332 Skin in X-linked ichthyosis can be very dark and well delineated for adjacent scales.

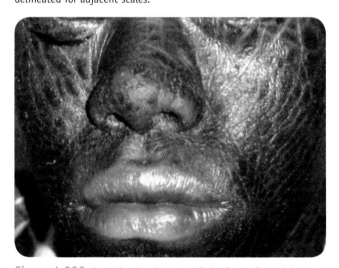

Figure 4-333 Extensive involvement of the face, often with ectropion, is characteristic of lamellar ichthyosis.

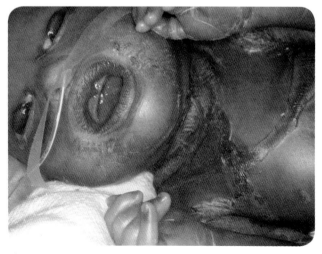

Figure 4-335 Ectropion, eclabium, and cracked skin strongly suggest a collodion baby. Thicker and yellower plates of skin would be more suggestive of a harlequin fetus.

321

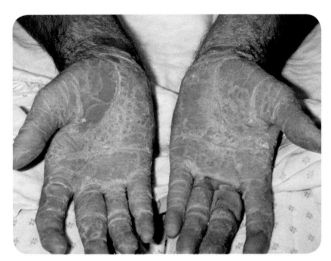

Figure 4-336 Epidermolytic hyperkeratosis may have massive irregular thickening of the palms and soles.

Epidermolytic Hyperkeratosis

Epidermolytic hyperkeratosis presents at birth with widespread erythroderma (Fig. 4-336). The fragile skin is susceptible to blisters and peeling. By a few months of age, the erythroderma and blisters begin to resolve and hyperkeratotic plaques develop, mostly in the flexor extremities. About 60% of patients have a diffuse palmoplantar keratoderma. A very rare, localized variant involving the external genitalia has been reported, one case of which involved an African American woman.

 Diagnostic Pearls

Ichthyosis Vulgaris

Ichthyosis vulgaris is often associated with accentuated palmar creases and hyperkeratosis of the palms and soles. An atopic diathesis is seen in 50% of patients. A test called "palpable dryness" was reported by a group in South India as detecting even mild forms of ichthyosis vulgaris and consists of gently palpating the outstretched palm of a patient from the distal wrist crease to the tips of the fingers. If the patient has ichthyosis vulgaris, a "peculiar" roughness will be appreciated.

Darier Disease

The skin lesions in Darier disease have a rough surface that feels similar to very coarse sandpaper or a fine grater.

X-Linked Ichthyosis

X-linked ichthyosis is characterized by a boy with a "dirty face." Scale is dark, and the popliteal and antecubital fossae are often involved. There is a spring-summer "molt" and the scale improves during the humid summer months. Since this disease only manifests in male patients, diagnosis can be facilitated by a good family history that is consistent with an X-linked recessive inheritance pattern.

Lamellar Ichthyosis and Collodion Baby

A collodion baby appears to be encased in a thick plastic wrap or cellophane wrap. This is a common presentation of lamellar ichthyosis. Harlequin fetus has larger plaques of scales, massive ectropion, and eclabium and may be fatal from fluid loss and systemic infections.

Epidermolytic Hyperkeratosis

Epidermolytic hyperkeratosis can be difficult to diagnosis in the neonatal period since the blistering may resemble epidermolysis bullosa and staphylococcal scalded skin syndrome. The presence of mild hyperkeratosis in a newborn with epidermolytic hyperkeratosis can aid in correct diagnosis.

?? Differential Diagnosis and Pitfalls

- Eczema craquelé—usually adults
- Atopic dermatitis
- Ichthyosiform presentation of sarcoidosis—usually adults
- Seborrheic dermatitis
- Pemphigus foliaceous—usually adults
- Acanthosis nigricans and confluent reticulate papillomatosis
- Grover disease—a histologic mimic of Darier disease but with older age of onset (e.g., 4th or 5th decade)
- Pityriasis rubra pilaris, which has hereditary forms, must be considered.
- Staphylococcal scalded skin syndrome
- Progressive symmetric erythroderma (Gottron syndrome)—plaques are fixed
- Epidermal nevi (related to CHILD syndrome, epidermolytic hyperkeratosis, and erythrokeratoderma variabilis)—Localized or even half body lesions sometimes with bony defects should be biopsied for specific pathology, which influences prognosis and genetic counseling.

✓ Best Tests

- Biopsy can be helpful and sometimes diagnostic (e.g., epidermolytic hyperkeratosis and Darier disease).
- Carefully examine all members of the family for mild forms of the disease.
- In X-linked ichthyosis, serum protein electrophoresis shows increased mobility of the beta-lipoprotein fraction due to increased cholesterol sulfate level.
- Netherton syndrome may have markedly elevated serum IgE levels.
- Testing for specific mutations should be done in consultation with a medical geneticist.

▲▲ Management Pearls

- All topicals may have increased absorption through the incomplete skin barrier in patients with these diseases. There can be increased systemic toxicity from salicylic acid and retinoic acid—these agents should be used with extreme caution.
- Useful for the management of ichthyosis are topical therapy and bathing with mechanical scale removal. Occlusive emollients such as petrolatum ointment prevent water loss from the skin while topical humectants and moisturizers work in a similar manner but bring some moisture to the skin as well. Keratolytics such as lactic acid, glycolic acid, salicylic acid (in concentrations of 0.5% to 10%), and urea (in concentrations of 5% to 10%) can be useful. Daily bathing with gentle rubbing of a sponge or loofah will help to remove scales and hyperkeratosis. Moisturizing bath oils can also be useful, and adding two handfuls of sodium bicarbonate to the bath water can aid in scale removal. Patients should be instructed to use only nondrying soaps such as Dove or nonsoap cleansers such as Cetaphil. Humidification of the environment, especially during the winter, is also important in managing the ichthyoses.
- Neonates with collodion membrane, Netherton syndrome, and epidermolytic hyperkeratosis with erythroderma and blistering need to be closely monitored in the NICU setting for fluid, temperature, and electrolyte imbalances and skin infections. Babies with Netherton syndrome are particularly susceptible to hypernatremia. Those cases with severe ectropion warrant consultation with an ophthalmologist.
- Genetic counseling should be offered to patients and family members to help explain the natural history of the disorder, the inheritance pattern, and the risk of having a child with the condition. Prenatal diagnostic testing is available for many of the ichthyoses.
- In Darier disease, superinfection with herpes simplex virus needs to be treated with antiviral agents if the clinical suspicion is high, even in the presence of negative viral cultures. In addition, sun protection and the use of cool, loose, cotton clothing can help prevent exacerbations in Darier disease.

Therapy

All topical drugs may be absorbed and may have systemic side effects. Many of these have been reported in these disorders when large areas of skin have been treated with topical agents.

Treatment of the ichthyoses is based on the management principles discussed earlier. In addition, topical retinoids (tretinoin 0.025 to 0.1%, adapalene 0.1%, or tazarotene 0.05% gel) applied once daily for weeks to months have been used with success in Darier disease and X-linked ichthyosis. Asian patients with Darier disease may have poor responses to topical retinoids.

Systemic retinoids are teratogenic, can affect bony growth, and should only be administered by those familiar with the use of these drugs. Systemic retinoids such as acitretin and isotretinoin (0.5 to 1 mg/kg/d) and retinoic acid metabolism blocking agents such as liarozole (1 to 2 mg/kg/d) can also be utilized in severe cases of ichthyosis and are usually effective in lamellar ichthyosis but must be continued for life. It is important to note that since these medications increase skin fragility, they should be used carefully and at low doses in epidermolytic hyperkeratosis where the fragile skin is already blistering. In Netherton syndrome, topical retinoids are relatively contraindicated, but varied success has been reported with topical and low-dose systemic corticosteroids, psoralen plus UVA (PUVA) therapy, cyclosporine, and topical tacrolimus and pimecrolimus.

Strategies for treating epidermal nevi (related to CHILD syndrome, epidermolytic hyperkeratosis, and erythrokeratoderma variabilis), which can pose a cosmetic concern for the patient, include surgical excision of small lesions and carbon dioxide laser, although both result in scarring, and laser therapy can lead to abnormal pigmentation in dark-skinned individuals.

Suggested Readings

Achar A, Naskar B, Laha R, et al. Epidermolytic hyperkeratosis: A case report. *J Indian Med Assoc.* 2009;107(3):171–172.

Akiyama M. FLG mutations in ichthyosis vulgaris and atopic eczema: Spectrum of mutations and population genetics. *Br J Dermatol.* 2010;162: 472–477.

Al-Zoman AY, Al-Asmari AK. Pattern of skin diseases at Riyadi Military Hospital. *Egypt Dermatol Online J.* 2008;4(2):1–10.

Cardoso CL, Freitas P, Assis Taveira LA, et al. Darier disease: Case report with oral manifestations. *Med Oral Patol Oral Cir Bucal.* 2006;11:E404–E406.

Cserhalmi-Friedman PB, Squeo R, Garzon GM, et al. Epidermolytic hyperkeratosis in a Hispanic family resulting from a mutation in the keratin 1 gene. *Clin Exp Dermatol.* 2005;25:241–243.

Fernandes NF, Janniger CK, Schwartz RA. X-linked ichthyosis: An oculocutaneous genodermatosis. *J Am Acad Dermatol.* 2010;62:480–485.

Goh BK, Ang P, Goh CL. Darier's disease in Singapore. *Br J Dermatol.* 2005;152:284–288.

Hazan C, Orlow SJ, Schaffer JV. X-linked recessive ichthyosis. *Dermatol Online J.* 2005;11(4):12.

Krupashankar DS. Standard guidelines of care: CO$_2$ laser for removal of benign skin lesions and resurfacing. *Indian J Dermatol Venereol Leprol.* 2008;74:S61–S67.

Kwak J, Maverakis E. Epidermolytic hyperkeratosis. *Dermatol Online J.* 2006;12(5):6.

Oji V, Traupe H. Ichthyosis: Clinical manifestations and practical treatment options. *Am J Clin Dermatol.* 2009;10(6):351–364.

Okulicz JF, Schwartz RA. Hereditary and acquired ichthyosis vulgaris. *Int J Dermatol.* 2003;42:95–98.

Song J, Li M, Yang LJ, et al. Identification a novel missense mutation p.R761L in Chinese patients with Darier's disease. *Arch Dermatol Res.* 2010;302:311–314.

Sugathan P, Riyaz N. Palpable dryness: A useful clinical sign in ichthyosis vulgaris. *Indian J Dermatol Venereol Leprol.* 1991;57:314.

Swann MH, Pujals JS, Pillow J, et al. Localized epidermolytic hyperkeratosis of the female external genitalia. *J Cutan Pathol.* 2003;30:379–381.

Theiler M, Mann C, Weibel L. Self-healing collodion baby. *J Pediatrics.* 2010;PMID: 20334876.

Zeller TA, Karel DJ. A newborn with peeling skin. *J Fam Pract.* 2009; 58(6):317–319.

Seborrheic Dermatitis

Kristina L. Demas • Lowell A. Goldsmith

▪▪ Diagnosis Synopsis

Seborrheic dermatitis is a chronic, relapsing inflammatory skin condition with a predilection for sebaceous glands of the body, face, scalp, and chest. This condition has an estimated prevalence of 3% to 5% and affects more men than women. Although the etiology is unknown, the pathogenesis is most likely related to an abnormal immune response to *Malassezia furfur* (*Pityrosporum ovale*), a species of yeast that commonly colonizes the skin. Although there is no apparent racial or ethnic predilection, seborrheic dermatitis does commonly affect darker skin and may manifest differently than in lighter skin.

There are two main clinical presentations: infantile and adult.

Infantile Seborrheic Dermatitis

Infantile seborrheic dermatitis is an inflammatory disease of the scalp, face, postauricular, presternal, and intertriginous areas ("seborrheic areas") of infants. Characteristically, the rash begins within the first month of life and gradually resolves by 4 months of age. It is hypothesized that increased activity of the sebaceous glands in response to elevated infantile hormones plays an important role in its pathogenesis.

Adult Seborrheic Dermatitis

In adults, the disorder is characterized by dryness, erythema, scaling, pruritus, and fine greasy scaling in specific sites including the scalp, face (especially the eyebrows and nasolabial folds), anterior chest, external ear canal, posterior ears, eyelid margins (blepharitis), groin (scrotum or labia minora), and perianal area. Large variations may exist in the severity and morphology of the scale, depending on the body location involved.

In individuals with lighter shades of brown skin, redness may be seen along with the flaking. Most often, however, the areas that are involved are either hypopigmented or hyperpigmented compared to the normal skin tone, possibly due to inflammation. The longer the condition is left untreated, the greater the hypopigmentation or hyperpigmentation. Hypopigmentation and hyperpigmentation usually resolve when the condition is treated.

Certain medications such as gold compounds, phenothiazines, lithium, methyldopa, griseofulvin, psoralens, stanozolol, and interferon alpha exacerbate the condition. Stress and neurological conditions (e.g., Parkinson disease and stroke) commonly increase the severity of the disorder.

Even with treatment, seborrhea tends to be chronic and relapsing. Expect remissions and exacerbations. Seborrheic dermatitis may improve during the summer months and is often worse in winter months.

Immunocompromised Patient Considerations

Seborrheic dermatitis is more common and more severe in persons infected with the human immunodeficiency virus (HIV), and so this disorder is increased in populations with a higher prevalence of HIV. It may regress with highly active antiretroviral therapy, but remissions and exacerbations can be expected.

◉ Look For

Infantile Seborrheic Dermatitis

Well-defined, erythematous macules and plaques with varying degrees of greasy, yellow scale. The scale adheres to the skin and may be confluent. Common sites of involvement include the scalp, face, skin folds, postauricular, presternal, and intertriginous areas (Figs. 4-337 and 4-338). Scalp disease tends to be minimally inflamed, whereas the skin folds often display significant erythema and maceration. In darkly pigmented infants, the rash may be associated with postinflammatory hypopigmentation.

Adult Seborrheic Dermatitis

Symptoms may vary and can range from mild scaling, classically referred to as "dandruff," to severe scaling.

Look for dandruff which appears as a fine, powdery white scale on the scalp extending to the forehead. This is often accompanied by mild itching. More severe seborrheic dermatitis is characterized by greasy scales within

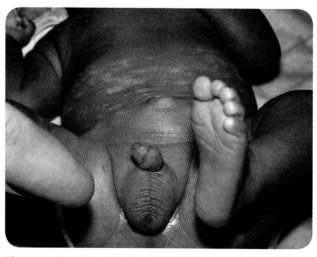

Figure 4-337 Seborrheic dermatitis in diaper area and on abdomen.

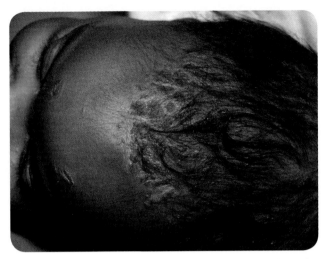

Figure 4-338 Seborrheic dermatitis with thick crusts on the scalp.

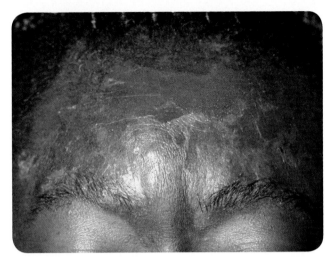

Figure 4-339 Sebopsoriasis of forehead.

erythematous plaques. Distribution is normally symmetrical. The scales may also involve the scalp, eyebrows, eyelids, lips, ears, skin folds, anterior chest, and the umbilicus (Figs. 4-339 and 4-340). Besides an itchy scalp, patients with more severe seborrheic dermatitis may also complain of a burning sensation in other affected areas.

In darker skin types, look for arcuate facial lesions with discrete papules resulting in either moderate hypopigmentation or hyperpigmentation. Plaques may sometimes appear crusted and grayish in color.

Diagnostic Pearls

Infantile Seborrheic Dermatitis

- Maceration and erosions in the diaper area often signify *Candida albicans* superinfection.
- If acutely weeping with superficial erosions, consider secondary infection with group A streptococcal species.
- Severe or generalized seborrheic dermatitis requires consideration of immunodeficiency.

Adult Seborrheic Dermatitis

- Rosacea and seborrheic dermatitis occur in the same area, and both have redness with telangiectases. All redness in the midface is not rosacea, which typically has acneform papules.
- Many patients report improvement of symptoms during the summer.

Differential Diagnosis and Pitfalls

Infantile Seborrheic Dermatitis

- The most difficult diagnoses to separate from infantile seborrheic dermatitis are psoriasis and atopic dermatitis.

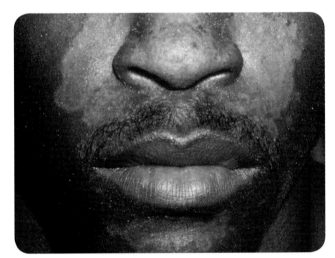

Figure 4-340 Seborrheic dermatitis with symmetrical scaling, redness, and hypopigmentation of the face.

Both psoriasis and atopic dermatitis, however, have dry rather than greasy scale. Additionally, psoriasis more commonly affects the lower abdomen and umbilicus than seborrheic dermatitis, and atopic dermatitis more commonly affects the shins and forearms than seborrheic dermatitis. Occasionally, it is impossible to distinguish between these diagnoses, and one must follow the patient clinically for more specific signs to develop.

- "Cradle cap" may be caused by seborrheic dermatitis or atopic dermatitis. Atopic dermatitis is much more pruritic, and the scale of atopic dermatitis is dry rather than waxy.
- When localized in the diaper area, dermatoses to consider include the following:
  - Candidiasis
  - Psoriasis—Consider in those with particularly difficult-to-remove scales; examine the patient in locations characteristic for psoriasis.

- Allergic contact dermatitis
- Irritant contact dermatitis
- Tinea cruris
- Intertrigo
- Langerhans cell histiocytosis
- Scabies
- Kawasaki disease
- Sexual abuse
- Acrodermatitis enteropathica
- Lichen sclerosus
- Perianal streptococcal infection
- Congenital syphilis

Adult Seborrheic Dermatitis

By region:

- Scalp—psoriasis, dandruff, dermatitis, impetigo, atopic dermatitis, Langerhans cell histiocytosis
- Ear canal—psoriasis or contact dermatitis (irritant or allergic)
- Face—rosacea, contact dermatitis, psoriasis, impetigo
- Chest and back—pityriasis versicolor, pityriasis rosea, Darier disease, tinea, atopic dermatitis
- Eyelids—atopic dermatitis, psoriasis, contact dermatitis
- Intertriginous areas—inverse psoriasis, candidiasis, tinea

Note:

- Tinea capitis usually presents with scaling of scalp in the absence of alopecia.
- In psoriasis, plaques tend to be thicker with silvery-white scales and less pruritic. There is an overlap disorder between psoriasis and seborrheic dermatitis termed "sebopsoriasis."

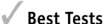

Best Tests

Infantile Seborrheic Dermatitis

This is usually a clinical diagnosis. A skin biopsy can be suggestive but not diagnostic of the disease.

Adult Seborrheic Dermatitis

- Diagnosis rests largely on the history and clinical examination. A skin biopsy can be suggestive of disease but is not diagnostic.
- Consider skin scraping with KOH preparation to rule out tinea.
- Consider HIV testing if there are risk factors or the patient is sexually active.
- Zinc deficiency may lead to a seborrhealike eruption; consider obtaining zinc level, especially in patients with poor nutritional health.

▲▲ Management Pearls

Infantile Seborrheic Dermatitis

- Lesions of seborrheic dermatitis on the body should respond within 2 weeks of starting therapy, and one should consider alternative diagnoses if lesions are persistent.
- Avoid salicylic acid preparations, as they may cause salicylism or irritation.

Adult Seborrheic Dermatitis

- It is essential for the patient to understand that this is a disease in which relapses are common, and that there is no cure.
- Ask patients if they oil their scalp because of dryness; this is a clue to the diagnosis as patients often do not mention this spontaneously.
- The patient may be weaned off therapy if the lesions are controlled but should restart therapy at the first sign of recurrence. Patients should avoid harsh deodorant soaps and use soap substitutes such as Cetaphil. Treatment of seborrheic dermatitis and healing of hyperpigmented and hypopigmented areas may take months.

Therapy

Infantile Seborrheic Dermatitis
Scalp
- For mild disease, wash the scalp with a mild shampoo ("no tears" shampoo) daily. If not responsive, wash daily with a selenium sulfide shampoo.
- For thick scale, massage olive, mineral, or baby oil into the scalp daily prior to bathing.
- For inflammatory lesions, apply a mild topical steroid daily (Derma-Smoothe/FS oil, hydrocortisone 2.5% ointment).

Body
- Mild class 6 or 7 topical steroid creams or ointments (desonide or hydrocortisone 2.5% twice daily) are usually sufficient.
- Topical antiyeast creams (e.g., ketoconazole 2% cream) may also be applied once to twice daily to increase efficacy. *Candida* diaper dermatitis is also usually present.

Adult Seborrheic Dermatitis
Treat dandruff with medicated shampoos. For African Americans, daily shampooing may not be needed. In people of color with either tight curly hair or a

(Continued)

chemically processed hair style, daily shampooing is not feasible. If the style of hair is curly or natural, patients of African descent prefer oils on the scalp to help with dryness of the hair.

Scalp

Apply topical steroid to scalp daily as needed. Prior to washing hair, apply medicated shampoo to dry scalp for 30 minutes, wash hair, and then apply conditioner.

- Ketoconazole 2% shampoo—apply to wet scalp and rinse. Use twice a week. Lather should also be used to cleanse the face and any other involved areas.
- 2% Pyrithione zinc shampoo
- 1% Ciclopirox shampoo
- Fluocinolone acetonide 0.01% in peanut oil (Derma-Smoothe F/S) can be applied to the hair, left on overnight, and washed out the next day.
  - With topical corticosteroids, long-term use should be avoided, so that potential side effects such as thinning of the skin and blood vessel growth are prevented.

- Also consider overnight applications of coal tar solution; apply every night at bedtime and shampoo out in the morning.
- Tar- and salicylic acid–based preparations (e.g., Neutrogena T/Gel, T/Sal)
- Tea tree oil and tea tree oil shampoo

Facial

- Use any of the above shampoos as facial cleanser or zinc pyrithione bar soap (ZNP) daily
- Nizoral cream twice daily (15, 30 g) until clear
- Nonfluorinated topical steroids twice daily
- Desonide cream, lotion
- Hydrocortisone cream 2.5% apply twice daily
- Tea tree oil
- Sunlight

Suggested Readings

Johnson BA, Nunley JR. Treatment of seborrheic dermatitis. *Am Fam Physician.* 2000;61(9):2703–2710, 2713–2714.

Luigi N, Rebora A. Seborrheic dermatitis. *N Engl J Med.* 2009;360:387–396.

■■ Diagnosis Synopsis

Lichen Planus

Lichen planus (LP) is an inflammatory disease of unknown etiology affecting the skin, hair follicles, nail unit, and mucous membranes. LP is most common in adults in the fourth to sixth decades of life. There is no known gender predilection. LP is considered rare in children, although it seems to be more prevalent in children from the Indian subcontinent.

Classic LP presents with pruritic, small, flat-topped, red to purple papules most commonly seen on the volar wrists. Papules can be widespread and involve the trunk, inner thighs, shins, hands, oral mucosa, and genitalia (e.g., erosive or annular lesions on the glans penis or vulvovaginal LP). Oral LP often presents as lacy, netlike, white plaques, though a variety of morphologies can be seen in the mouth, the second most common being the ulcerative form. Oral lesions may accompany skin lesions or present in isolation, and oral LP may have a protracted or chronic course compared with cutaneous LP. Lichen planopilaris (LPP), the variant of LP affecting hair follicles, is typified by erythema and scale around hair follicles and scarring hair loss, most commonly on the scalp. Graham-Little-Piccardi-Lassueur syndrome describes patients with LPP of the scalp and alopecia/LPP-like lesions involving the eyebrows, axillae, and pubic area.

Nail changes occur in approximately 10% of patients with skin or mucosal LP and are often found in the absence of cutaneous disease. Nail LP changes can include fissuring, longitudinal ridging, and lateral thinning. The most specific nail finding is a dorsal pterygium, indicating scarring of the nail matrix.

While LP shows no ethnic predilection in adults, postinflammatory hyperpigmentation is typically prominent and lasting in patients with darker skin types. With resolution of erosive LP, hyperpigmented scars remain in areas previously involved by persistent violaceous erythema. A silvery white or gray lacelike appearance of the surface of the oral mucosa is commonly encountered in dark-skinned patients. The actinic variant of LP may stem from significant long-term sun exposure and preferentially affects African American patients.

Certain medications cause an LP-like eruption (lichenoid drug eruption). More common drugs include antihypertensives such as ACE inhibitors, beta-blockers, and thiazide diuretics; antimalarials; penicillamine; nonsteroidal anti-inflammatory drugs; gold; griseofulvin; tetracycline; and antiepileptics.

LP can spontaneously resolve, usually after a year, or follow a remitting or chronic course. There is an association with hepatitis C, predominantly in certain geographical areas (Japan and Mediterranean regions). LP has also been inconsistently linked to hepatitis B vaccination and primary biliary cirrhosis.

Lichen Nitidus

Lichen nitidus is a benign skin eruption of unknown etiology characterized by very small, flat-topped, monomorphic, flesh-colored papules. At times, a linear distribution may be evident secondary to the Koebner phenomenon. Common locations include the flexor aspects of the wrists and forearms, lower abdomen, inner thighs, and penis. Pruritus may occur but is generally absent. The course is typically chronic, and lesions can last for months to years.

Actinic lichen nitidus, a variant of lichen nitidus, has been reported in darkly pigmented patients (especially those in the Middle East and the Indian subcontinent) with a history of significant sun exposure.

◉ Look For

Lichen Planus

Classic lesions of LP are characterized by the five Ps: purple, planar, polygonal, pruritic, and papules (Figs. 4-341–4-343). The most common locations are the volar wrists and flexural surfaces. Papules can also be widespread and involve the trunk, inner thighs, shins, hands, and genitalia. As the lesions become older, their surfaces develop adherent scales that form fine, grayish-white streaks called Wickham striae. Lesions in patients with dark skin are often dark violet or slate-blue in color with prominent postinflammatory pigment change. Additional morphologies of LP include hypertrophic, atrophic, erosive, follicular (LPP), annular, linear, guttate, actinic (in sun-exposed areas), bullous, and ulcerative. Koebnerization (linear groups of lesions related to trauma) is not uncommon.

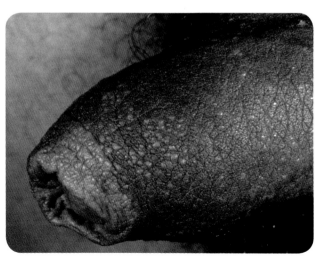

Figure 4-341 Multiple small shiny papules of lichen nitidus in a typical location.

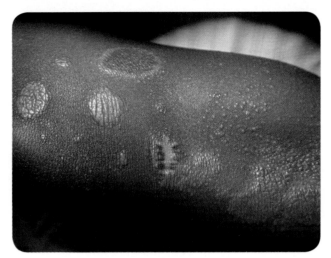

Figure 4-342 Multiple plaques of lichen planus with a red annular border and hyperpigmented centers.

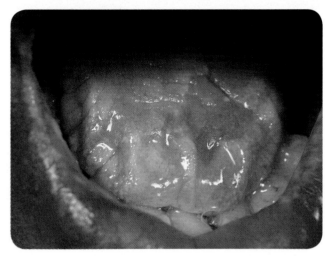

Figure 4-344 Lichen planus of the mouth with erosions and hyperkeratosis.

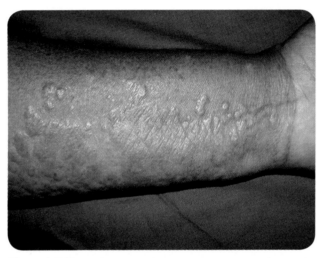

Figure 4-343 Purple polygonal nonscaling papules in a characteristic location, usually including the wrist.

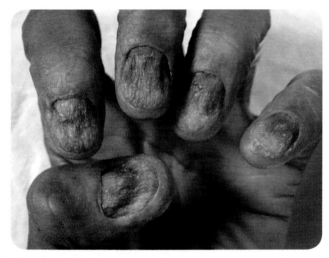

Figure 4-345 Lichen planus with complete destruction of the nail plates and abnormal keratinization of the nail bed.

Mucous membrane involvement may consist of lacy, net-like, white plaques with a violaceous base, most often found on the buccal mucosa or tongue but also found on the genitals and throughout the gastrointestinal tract (Fig. 4-344). Painful erosions and ulcers may occur in these locations, as well as the atrophic, bullous, pigmented, and papular forms.

Nails are frequently involved with a variety of lesions (Fig. 4-345). Dorsal pterygium involving the proximal nail fold is characteristic of LP and describes the V-shaped extension of the proximal nail fold distally.

The hypertrophic variant of LP commonly involves the shins, and the annular variant favors the penis.

Lichen Nitidus

Uniform clusters of pinhead-sized, flat-topped, skin-colored papules with a shiny surface, commonly located on

the glans penis, upper extremities, chest, and/or abdomen (Fig. 4-341). Single rows of minute papules in a linear distribution are common on the extremities. Rarely does scale accompany the lesions. Rarely, the lesions may scale and be generalized.

●● Diagnostic Pearls

Lichen Planus

- If LP is suspected on the glabrous skin or nails, carefully examine the oral mucosa for a reticular, lacy network of papules or plaques.
- Wickham striae on lesion surface are highly diagnostic of LP.
- Linear lesions may result from trauma (Koebner phenomenon).

Lichen Nitidus

Pruritus is generally absent. Lesions are often located on the glans of the penis.

Differential Diagnosis and Pitfalls

Lichen Planus

- Lichenoid drug eruption
- Psoriasis
- Subacute cutaneous lupus erythematosus
- Chronic graft versus host disease
- Granuloma annulare
- Sarcoidosis
- Warts
- Pityriasis rosea
- Secondary syphilis (palm and sole lesions)
- Lichen simplex chronicus
- Prurigo nodularis
- Amyloidosis
- Kaposi sarcoma
- Lichen nitidus
- Lichen spinulosus
- LP-like keratosis—usually solitary
- Erythema dyschromicum perstans
- Mycosis fungoides
- Pityriasis lichenoides et varioliformis acuta (PLEVA)

Differential Diagnosis of Oral and Mucosal LP

- Oral candidiasis
- Leukoplakia
- Pemphigus vulgaris
- Seborrheic dermatitis (genital lesions)
- Lichen sclerosus (vulvar lesions)
- Contact dermatitis to metals—Eruption is adjacent to a filling.

Differential Diagnosis of LPP

- Alopecia areata—lack of erythema
- Seborrheic dermatitis
- Discoid lupus erythematosus
- Pseudopelade of Brocq
- Frontal fibrosing alopecia

Differential Diagnosis of Nail Apparatus LP

- Onychomycosis
- Psoriasis

Lichen Nitidus

- Lichen spinulosus
- Keratosis pilaris

- LP
- Psoriasis
- Flat warts

Best Tests

Lichen Planus

- Skin biopsy will confirm the diagnosis, although it can often be made clinically. Direct and indirect immunofluorescence can rule out autoimmune diseases such as pemphigus and pemphigoid.
- Practitioners in geographic locales in which LP is associated with hepatitis virus infections should consider obtaining serologic tests for hepatitis B and C as well as a liver function panel.

Lichen Nitidus

Skin biopsy will confirm the diagnosis.

▲▲ Management Pearls

Lichen Planus

- Oral LP needs to be followed and managed carefully. Patients with persistent, severe oral LP are at higher risk for oral squamous cell carcinoma (SCC). Approximately 0.4% to 5% of patients with oral erosive LP develop oral SCC.
- Consultation with a dermatologist is recommended. Consider a dental consultation for severe oral LP.

Lichen Nitidus

Educate the patient regarding the benign nature.

Therapy

Lichen Planus

First-line therapies for limited lesions include topical and intralesional corticosteroids. As pruritus is usually significant, oral antihistamines may be of added benefit. If a drug-induced eruption is considered, withdraw any potential offending medication.

Topical corticosteroids, in cream or ointment formulations, should be applied twice daily to only the lesions. Initially, use a high- or mid-potency topical steroid (class 2 or 3).

(Continued)

High-Potency Topical Corticosteroids (Class 2)

- Twice daily

Midpotency Topical Corticosteroids (Classes 3 and 4)

- Twice daily

Superpotent Topical Corticosteroids (Class 1)

- For severe disease, a superpotent topical steroid can be tried for a short 2-week course, with close follow-up.
- Twice daily
- Triamcinolone acetonide (3 to 10 mg/mL and in some cases up to 20 mg/mL) may be infiltrated into thicker papules and plaques at 1-month intervals. Be wary of skin atrophy.

For more severe or widespread disease, systemic steroids may be of benefit. Referral to a dermatologist is recommended. Other effective modalities for widespread disease include phototherapy (UVB, UVA1 and PUVA [psoralen plus UVA]), systemic retinoids (especially in the hypertrophic variant), and other immune-suppressing medications (mycophenolate mofetil, cyclosporine).

Control of pruritus may be achieved with the use of oral antihistamines or topical antipruritic agents such as lotions containing menthol, camphor, pramoxine, phenol, or doxepin hydrochloride.

Antihistamines

- Diphenhydramine 25 to 50 mg nightly or every 6 hours, as needed
- Hydroxyzine 12.5 to 25 mg every 6 hours, as needed
- Cetirizine hydrochloride 5 to 10 mg/d
- Loratadine 10 mg daily

Oral LP

Care should be taken to maintain impeccable oral hygiene and prevent overgrowth of *Candida*. Avoid mechanical injury from dentures or other irritative or caustic foods/tobacco, as this can exacerbate oral LP. Potent topical steroids in a gel or Orabase formulation are well tolerated.

Palliative mouthwashes can be used for symptom control. Consider a cocktail of diphenhydramine elixir, aluminum/magnesium hydroxide antacid, and viscous lidocaine in a 1:1:1 ratio (sometimes called "magic mouthwash"). Swish and spit several times daily, as needed, for oral discomfort.

Vulvovaginal LP

Most commonly treated with superpotent topical steroids or topical calcineurin inhibitors (e.g., tacrolimus ointment). Permanent scarring complications and malignancy have been identified as risks in vulvovaginal LP.

Lichen Planopilaris

First-line treatment for mild to moderate disease (involving <10% of the scalp) is intralesional injection of triamcinolone acetonide at 10 mg/mL administered every 4 to 6 weeks. Rapidly progressive or severely symptomatic disease may be arrested with oral prednisone at 1 mg/kg daily tapered over 2 to 4 months. Cases refractory to intralesional therapy may warrant treatment with oral immunomodulators, which require careful patient screening and monitoring.

Other treatments reported for LPP include oral retinoids, thalidomide, topical tacrolimus, and oral antimicrobials such as griseofulvin, dapsone, and tetracyclines. Topical minoxidil may have an adjunctive role.

Lichen Nitidus

Low-dose topical corticosteroids may be helpful if pruritus is prominent. Phototherapy and systemic retinoids have also been tried with some success.

Suggested Readings

Abdel-Naser MB, Verma SB, Abdallah MA. Common dermatoses in moderately pigmented skin: Uncommon presentations. *Clin Dermatol.* 2005;23:446–456.

Glorioso S, Jackson SC, Kopel AJ, et al. Actinic lichen nitidus in 3 African American patients. *J Am Acad Dermatol.* 2006;54(2 Suppl):S48–S49.

Ismail SB, Kumar SK, Zain RB. Oral lichen planus and lichenoid reactions: Etiopathogenesis, diagnosis, management, and malignant transformation. *J Oral Sci.* 2007;49(2):89–106.

James WD, Berger TG, Elston DM, eds. Lichen planus and related conditions. In: *Andrews' Diseases of the Skin: Clinical Dermatology.* 10th Ed. Philadelphia, PA: Elsevier; 2006:217–226.

Kanwar AJ, De D. Lichen planus in children. *Indian J Dermatol Venereol Leprol.* 2010;76(4):366–372.

Scher RK, Daniel CR III. Lichen planus. In: *Nails: Diagnosis, Therapy, Surgery.* 3th Ed. Philadelphia, PA: Elsevier; 2005:112–116.

Shengyuan L, Songpo Y, Wen W, et al. Hepatitis C virus and lichen planus: A reciprocal association determined by a meta-analysis. *Arch Dermatol.* 2009;145(9):1040–1047.

Subacute Cutaneous Lupus Erythematosus

Stephanie Diamantis

⬛⬛ Diagnosis Synopsis

Lupus erythematosus is an autoimmune multisystem disease that has several cutaneous variants. Specific cutaneous lesions of lupus erythematous can be classified based on the location of the inflammation within the skin: acute cutaneous, subacute cutaneous, chronic cutaneous, tumid lupus, and lupus panniculitis. Epidemiologic studies have shown that people of Hispanic, Asian, African American, and African Caribbean descent have an increased incidence of lupus in addition to excess morbidity.

Acute cutaneous lupus erythematosus (ACLE) is characterized by transient malar erythema without scarring. This type is strongly associated with systemic findings. The inflammatory infiltrate is seen in the superficial dermis on biopsy.

Subacute cutaneous lupus erythematosus (SCLE) is characterized by a photosensitive cutaneous eruption lasting longer than ACLE that resolves without scarring. SCLE is characterized by annular plaques with raised borders and central clearing or papulosquamous lesions that are restricted to sun-exposed skin. The sides of the face, the lower neck, and the extensor surfaces of the arms are the most commonly affected sites. Scarring is not characteristic, but dyspigmentation can occur. While the etiology remains poorly understood, there is a strong association with anti-Ro antibodies and SCLE. In addition, anti-Ro antibodies are also seen in Sjögren syndrome, and some patients can have both SCLE and Sjögren syndrome. Risk factors for developing cutaneous lesions include sex (increased female-to-male ratio, especially during childbearing years) and ethnicity, with individuals of African descent demonstrating a higher incidence when compared to whites. Approximately 10% to 15% of patients can evolve to have systemic manifestations of lupus.

Of note, certain drugs—such as hydrochlorothiazide, terbinafine, and other antihypertensives (e.g., calcium channel blockers and ACE inhibitors) and nonsteroidal anti-inflammatory drugs—have been reported to trigger SCLE. These drug-induced SCLE lesions run an unpredictable course, and they may not clear after discontinuing the offending drug.

◉ Look For

Lesions are nonscarring and nonindurated (secondary to inflammatory infiltrate being confined to superficial dermis) and are characterized as follows:

- Annular type—photodistributed annular or polycyclic plaques with a raised, erythematous border and central clearing, commonly on the back (Fig. 4-346)
- Papulosquamous type—photodistributed erythematous, scaly papules and plaques that may look eczematous in nature

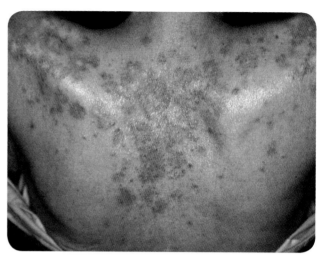

Figure 4-346 Annular lesions on the upper back are characteristic of lupus erythematosus.

⬤⬤ Diagnostic Pearls

SCLE is more common in sun-exposed areas of the neck, shoulders, upper extremities, and trunk, whereas ACLE is more frequent on the cheeks.

?? Differential Diagnosis and Pitfalls

Annular Variant

- Granuloma annulare—mainly in children and young adults, biopsy will help differentiate granuloma annulare and SCLE; facial lesions are extremely rare
- Tinea corporis—usually has scale at the leading edge; check KOH.
- Erythema marginatum—seen more commonly in children; cutaneous feature of acute rheumatic fever
- Polymorphic light eruption—Most lesions resolve within several days.
- Erythema multiforme—characteristic targetoid lesions; tends to involve the palms
- Annular psoriasis—Biopsy will assist in differentiating psoriasis from SCLE.
- Annular urticaria—wheals that are characteristically pruritic
- Polymorphic light eruption

Papulosquamous Variant

- Erythema annulare centrifugum (EAC)—mostly seen on hips and thighs in patients in their fifties; biopsy can help differentiate EAC from SCLE; usually has scale trailing the leading edge

- Sarcoidosis—more infiltrative plaques
- Lichen planus—pruritic, scaly papules that involve the wrists, forearms, genitalia, and presacral area; biopsy will assist in differentiating lichen planus from SCLE
- Syphilis—Check RPR.

✓ Best Tests

- Most patients demonstrate positive titers of antinuclear antibodies (ANA) as well as anti-Ro (SS-A) and, to a lesser extent, anti-La (SS-B) cytoplasmic antibodies. Antibodies to double-stranded DNA (anti-dsDNA) are more commonly found in SLE.
- Lesional skin biopsies are positive (60% of the time) for basement membrane zone bound immunoglobulin using direct immunofluorescence techniques.
- Be sure to take a thorough medication exposure history. Patients with SCLE merit a full evaluation to exclude systemic disease, including a CBC, urinalysis, electrolytes, BUN and creatinine, ESR, complement levels, and, often, a chest X-ray and ECG.

▲▲ Management Pearls

- Withdraw any potential inciting medication and employ sun-protective measures given the extreme sensitivity to ultraviolet light.
- Systemic manifestations, such as renal and central nervous system disease, are present in 10% to 15% of patients, and patients must be followed with these potential complications in mind. Consultation with rheumatology, nephrology, neurology, and/or dermatology is recommended.

Therapy

The main goals of treatment are to improve the patient's appearance and to prevent additional lesions from developing. Sunscreens, sun-protective clothing, and sun avoidance are essential components of therapy. Topical corticosteroids and antimalarials are first-line therapy.

High-potency topical steroids, flurandrenolide-impregnated tape, and/or intralesional corticosteroids (triamcinolone 3 to 10 mg/mL infiltrated into the dermal plaque) are the mainstay of therapy for cutaneous forms of lupus. Patients' use of topical steroids should be monitored closely due to the risk of atrophy. Special care should be taken with facial skin. Often, potent topical steroids are required to get a response, even on the face. Intralesional triamcinolone

(4 to 5 mg/mL) can be effective in active lesions, with injections repeated every month while lesion is active.

High-Potency Topical Corticosteroids (Classes 1 and 2)
- Clobetasol cream, ointment—Apply twice daily.
- Fluocinonide cream, ointment—Apply twice daily.
- Desoximetasone cream, ointment—Apply twice daily.
- Halcinonide cream, ointment—Apply twice daily.
- Amcinonide ointment—Apply twice daily.

Systemic therapies targeting prevention of progression require knowledge of the drugs and specific monitoring.

Antimalarials (hydroxychloroquine 200 mg twice daily alone or in combination with quinacrine 100 mg/d) can be employed for cases not adequately treated with topical or local agents. *Note*: Before starting these agents, liver and renal function tests should be obtained. Ophthalmologic baseline exam should be performed at or near the time these agents are started. Patients on antimalarials should be seen for ophthalmologic testing every 6 to 12 months.

Systemic retinoids—Acitretin 25 to 50 mg p.o. daily, or isotretinoin 40 to 80 mg p.o. daily for 4 months should be considered as second-line therapy.

Dapsone (100 to 200 mg p.o. daily), methotrexate, mycophenolate mofetil, and other immunosuppressives have also been used. Oral gold has also been reported to be helpful.

Recent studies have shown thalidomide (50 to 100 mg p.o. daily) to be an effective therapy, but it should be reserved for severe cases that are unresponsive to other measures. Caution is advised due to the potential teratogenic and neurologic side effects.

Suggested Readings

Cooper GS, Parks CG, Treadwell EL, et al. Differences by race, sex, and age in the clinical and immunologic features of recently diagnosed systemic lupus erythematosus patients in the southeastern United States. *Lupus*. 2002;11:161–167.

Halder RM, Roberts CI, Nootheti PK. Cutaneous diseases in black races. *Dermatol Clin*. 2003;21:679–687.

James WD, Berger TG, Elston DM, eds. Cutaneous vascular diseases. In: *Andrews' Diseases of the Skin: Clinical Dermatology*. 10th Ed. Philadelphia, PA: Elsevier; 2006:816–817.

Lau CS, Yin G, Mok MY. Ethnic and geographical differences in systemic lupus erythematosus: An overview. *Lupus*. 2006;15:715–719.

Lee LA. Lupus erythematosus. In: Bolognia JL, Jorizzo JL, Rapini RP, eds. *Dermatology*. 2nd Ed. St. Louis, MO: Mosby/Elsevier; 2008:601–613.

Psoriasis and Pustular Psoriasis

Kimberly Capers Arrington

■■ Diagnosis Synopsis

Psoriasis

Psoriasis is a chronic, intermittently relapsing inflammatory disease that is classically characterized by sharply demarcated erythematous, silvery, scaly plaques most often seen on the scalp, elbows, and knees. Additional sites of involvement include the nails, hands, feet, and trunk. Approximately 2% of the world's population suffers from psoriasis, and its prevalence varies from country to country and among ethnic groups. The disease has been reported in North America, Middle and Central America, the Caribbean Islands, South America, Africa, Central and Southeast Asia, and Australia.

Psoriasis can develop at any age, in either sex, and in all ethnicities, but it occurs most frequently in whites. Psoriasis is about three times more common in whites compared with African Americans. Using population-based methods, one study found the prevalence of psoriasis to be 2.5% and 1.3% in whites and African Americans, respectively. In both groups, the disease carried a substantial burden. Also, psoriasis is more common in Asians and individuals of African descent than in American and Latin American Indians. Psoriasis is often of the small plaque variant in Asians versus large plaques in North Americans. As a result, the small plaques may be confused for guttate in these patients. There are no published data on the severity of psoriasis in different ethnic groups.

Psoriasis is a polygenic disease where genetically susceptible individuals with certain HLA types (HLA-Cw6, HLA-B13, HLA-B17, HLA-B37, and HLA-Bw16) mount aberrant immune responses after exposure to infection, drug ingestion, hypocalcemia, psychogenic stress, and/or external injury to the skin. Aberrant T-cell function and keratinocyte responses are believed to be major culprits in the pathogenesis of psoriasis. Diet has also been proposed as an explanation for the low incidence of psoriasis in West Africa. The staple maize, which is prominent in Africa, is high in omega-6 linoleic acid, a PGE2 precursor that may decrease the cellular immune response underlying psoriasis. High dietary intake of omega-3 fatty acids has also been proposed as a protective factor.

Chronic plaque psoriasis is the most common variant, and disease burden can range from 1% to 2% (mild disease) to >90% (erythrodermic psoriasis) of the total body surface area (BSA). Classic findings include well-demarcated; circular, oval, or polycyclic; erythematous; silvery; scaly plaques that are often symmetrical in distribution. Lesions are often mildly pruritic and resolve with postinflammatory hyperpigmentation or hypopigmentation. Scarring is not a feature of resolution. During exacerbations, erythematous papules usually surround existing plaques, and a ring of intense erythema surrounds the plaques. During resolution, plaques will have a decreased amount of scale and central clearing, creating annular psoriatic lesions. Lesions can last from months to years in the same location.

Other variants include guttate psoriasis, pustular psoriasis, psoriatic arthritis, erythrodermic psoriasis, palmar plantar psoriasis, and inverse psoriasis. Some variants coexist.

Guttate psoriasis—Guttate psoriasis is characterized by an acute, generalized eruption of small, discreet, raindroplike (hence the name guttate) papules with fine scale that occurs 2 to 3 weeks after an upper respiratory infection. It most commonly occurs in children and is associated with an elevated antistreptolysin O, anti-DNase B, or streptozyme titer. Guttate psoriasis can be pruritic, and postinflammatory pigmentary changes can follow. However, scarring and systemic symptoms such as fever, malaise, lymphadenopathy, myalgias, and arthralgias are usually absent. Guttate psoriasis occurs in all ethnicities and both sexes and is most commonly seen in children and adults younger than 30 years. The clinical course is unpredictable. In children, spontaneous remission over weeks to months is common, while in young adults, it may represent the first stage in the development of chronic plaque psoriasis. In cases where a streptococcal infection cannot be identified, viruses such as rubella, roseola, and varicella have also been implicated as inciting factors. HIV-1 infection is thought to be a possible trigger factor. Medications have been cited as causative agents as well.

Psoriatic arthritis—Up to 30% of psoriatic patients may have erosive psoriatic arthritis requiring systemic therapies.

The clinician should be aware of several key points in patients with psoriasis:

- Cardiovascular disease—The presence of psoriasis may have an impact on other organ systems. Psoriatic patients have an increased relative risk for cardiovascular disease, including cerebrovascular accidents, pulmonary emboli, and myocardial infarctions. Additional risk factors for cardiac disease (diabetes, cholesterol, hypertension, obesity, smoking, etc.) should be appropriately screened for and addressed.
- While research-oriented severity scales exist (Psoriasis Area and Severity Index), the BSA is generally used clinically as a reference for evaluating response to treatment.
- Oral or IM steroids—Only in rare cases, such as erythroderma or severe pustular psoriasis, should oral steroids be considered. This is because the use of systemic steroids will lead to severe psoriasis rebound after steroid discontinuation.

Pediatric Patient Considerations

Psoriasis is fairly common in childhood, but it is rare in infancy; it is seen in <1% of infants by age 1 and in 2% of children by age 2. Infantile psoriasis resembles adult psoriasis, presenting with discrete, oval, erythematous plaques with white scale and often involving the trunk, extremities, and face. There is usually less white scale on the plaques of infants compared to adults. Lesions may be pruritic. Psoriasis in infancy typically involves the diaper area and face. Nail findings of pitting, onycholysis, oil spots, and subungual hyperkeratosis are present in 10% of affected infants.

Immunocompromised Patient Considerations

The prevalence of psoriasis in patients with HIV is approximately 5% and is associated with a more severe clinical course. Psoriasis may pre-exist in the HIV patient or manifest as a progression of the virus.

Pustular Psoriasis

Pustular psoriasis is characterized by the presence of widespread, erythematous, sterile pustules on clinical examination and a predominantly neutrophilic infiltrate on a cellular level. Pustular psoriasis can be a severe inflammatory disease that requires hospitalization and aggressive therapy. Untreated disease can also progress to erythroderma. While many cases are idiopathic, risk factors that can trigger an episode include hypocalcemia, infection, a rapid withdrawal of corticosteroids (or weeks after an IM injection), pregnancy, medications (salicylates, lithium, iodine, trazodone, penicillin, interferon, hydroxychloroquine), and topical irritants such as tar and anthralin. Only a small number of patients have a preceding history of plaque-type psoriasis. There are four subtypes of pustular psoriasis: von Zumbusch, exanthematic, annular, and localized pattern. There may be an inflammatory polyarthritis. Relapses and remissions may occur over a period of years. Postinflammatory pigmentary changes can be quite prominent in darkly pigmented skin.

Pregnancy—Approximately 50% of pregnant patients with psoriasis report improvement of disease burden. However, there are many reports that show the development of pustular psoriasis in pregnant patients who are hypocalcemic. Pustular psoriasis that occurs during pregnancy is termed impetigo herpetiformis.

(●) Look For

Psoriasis

Sharply demarcated, erythematous, silver-scaled plaques of the scalp, elbows, and knees (Figs. 4-347–4-349). Additional

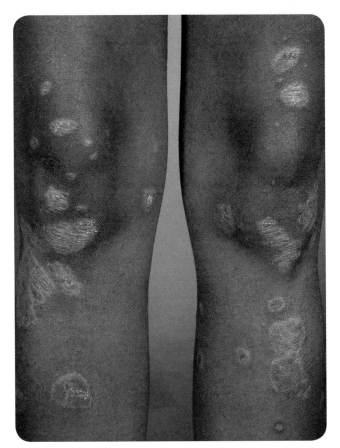

Figure 4-347 Red scaly psoriatic plaques distributed symmetrically on both legs.

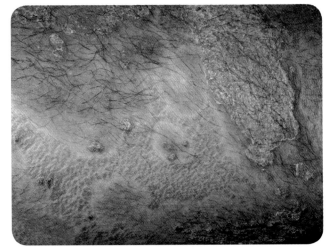

Figure 4-348 Plaque psoriasis with hyperpigmentation and hypopigmentation where lesions have resolved.

sites of involvement include the hands, feet, and trunk. In dark skin, the plaques may look violaceous to bluish-black. Most plaques will have overlying grayish scales, although the typical silvery scale may be absent. Rings of blanched skin called Woronoff rings may surround individual plaques.

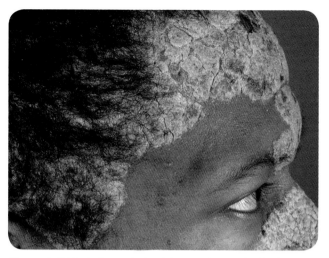

Figure 4-349 Scalp psoriasis with extension to the forehead and the nose.

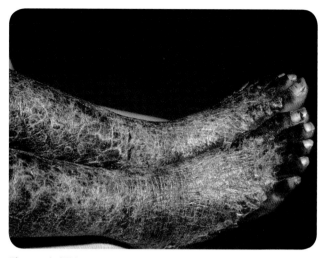

Figure 4-351 Extensive psoriasis with erythroderma.

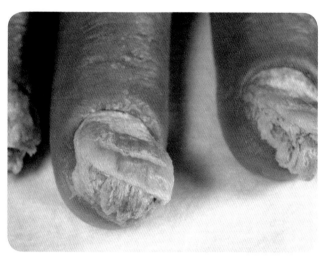

Figure 4-350 Psoriatic nails with destruction of the nail plates and hyperkeratosis of the nail beds.

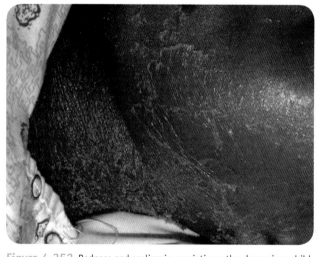

Figure 4-352 Redness and scaling in psoriatic erythroderma in a child.

- Nails—Fingernails are affected more often than toenails. Nail pitting, onycholysis ("oil spots"), splinter hemorrhages, subungual hyperkeratosis, and leukonychia may be seen (Fig. 4-350).
- Joints—In psoriatic arthritis, look for distal and proximal interphalangeal arthritis; "sausage digits" can be monoarticular or asymmetric oligoarthritis.
- Axilla, groin, intergluteal cleft—These are locations for inverse psoriasis. Look for shiny, erythematous, sharply demarcated plaques. Fissuring can be noted. Localized dermatophyte infections as well as *Candida* can trigger psoriasis in these areas. Because of the moist environment and occlusion, heavy scale is not seen in these areas.

Erythroderma in psoriasis—Psoriasis can become generalized and involve the entire skin (Figs. 4-351 and 4-352).

There can be increased water loss through the skin, abnormalities in temperature regulation with associated chills and shivering, increased cardiac output, and in some patients cardiac failure. Erythroderma has other causes besides psoriasis, including drug eruptions and mycosis fungoides (cutaneous T-cell lymphoma).

Guttate psoriasis—Look for hundreds of small, droplike (guttate), inflammatory, scaly papules concentrated on the trunk and proximal extremities (Fig. 4-353). In darkly pigmented skin, the lesions often appear gray in color, and sometimes the scales are silvery-white. Infrequently, pustules may arise after acute relapses. The lesions can be extensive and may also be seen on the scalp, neck, face, and extremities. Postinflammatory pigmentary changes can be quite prominent in dark skin.

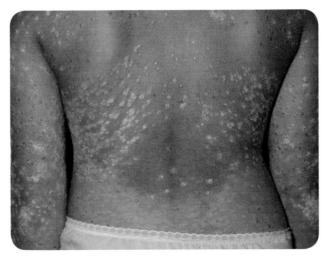

Figure 4-353 Extensive guttate psoriasis with papules and scaling papules.

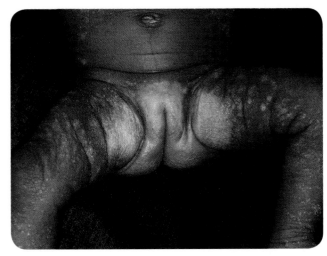

Figure 4-355 Generalized psoriasiform lesions often starting underneath the diaper region are characteristic of infantile psoriasis.

Pediatric Patient Considerations

Red or salmon-red plaques, often with silvery-white or grayish-white scale (Figs. 4-354 and 4-355). The plaques are usually symmetrical and well demarcated. In infants, the diaper area will often have bright red plaques with no scale. The scalp, palms, and soles may have diffuse erythema and scale. Psoriasis of the scalp may cause hair loss as noted by a study of children in southeast Nigeria; compared with other conditions, psoriasis was a less common cause of hair loss in this group.

Pustular Psoriasis

- von Zumbusch—Look for clusters of sterile 2- to 3-mm pustules on a background of erythema. Pustules may become confluent, forming large plaques of pus

(Fig. 4-356). Flexures and the anogenital area are most commonly affected, but the palms, soles, and oral mucosa may also be involved. Pustules may form on the nail matrix, with subsequent loss of the nail plate (Fig. 4-357). Fingertips can show atrophy with long-standing disease.

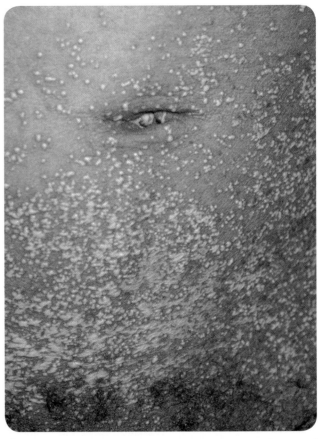

Figure 4-356 Pustular psoriasis with multiple confluent and discrete inflammatory pustules.

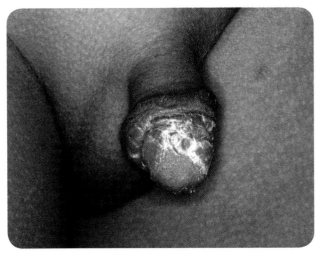

Figure 4-354 Psoriasis of the glans in a child.

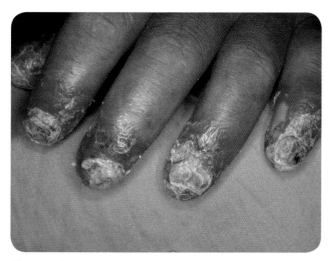

Figure 4-357 Pustular psoriasis with destruction of the nail plates and deep large pustules near the tip of the digits.

Only rarely do other forms of psoriasis coexist with lesions of von Zumbusch type.

- Annular—Look for pustules at the periphery of erythematous annular lesions, located most commonly on the trunk. The lesions expand peripherally, with healing occurring in the center.
- Exanthematic—Look for acute onset of small, sterile pustules without significant systemic symptoms. It is believed to have clinical and histological overlap with acute generalized exanthematous pustulosis (AGEP).

Localized Types

- Pustulosis palmaris et plantaris—Look for palmar and/or plantar 2- to 4-mm pustules, often located on the medial aspect of the foot and misdiagnosed as a bacterial or fungal infection.
- Acrodermatitis continua—Look for pustules on the fingertips and nail bed, often with subsequent nail dystrophy and loss.
- Chronic subcorneal pustulosis with vasculitis—It is a rare variant of generalized pustular psoriasis with a predilection for the neck, trunk, and shins. It has been described in black South Africans

Diagnostic Pearls

- Very thick, silvery scale favors the diagnosis of psoriasis. Involvement of plaques in the navel and the gluteal cleft also favor a diagnosis of psoriasis. When in doubt, nail involvement favors psoriasis as well.
- Removal of scale will result in pinpoint bleeding (Auspitz sign), suggesting the diagnosis. Appearance of plaques at sites of cutaneous trauma (Koebner phenomenon) at some time over the lifetime of the disease is seen in 30% to 50% of patients, especially in those with more active

disease. Beta-blockers may induce psoriasis even in the small amounts found in some eye preparations. A careful history addressing drugs should be obtained.

Guttate psoriasis—Sore throat is the most common associated factor in patients aged 20 to 30 years. History should try to ascertain a precipitating infection. Note that plaque psoriasis in Asians may be of the small plaque variant; the small plaques, therefore, may easily be mistaken for guttate psoriasis.

Pustular psoriasis—Frequent spiking fevers and discomfort may be suggestive of an alternative diagnosis such as a systemic infectious disease.

Pediatric Patient Considerations

- Areas of increased friction in the diaper area (e.g., under elastic bands) are involved first with subsequent spread to the face, trunk, and body folds. Infantile psoriasis is rarely generalized.
- Infantile psoriasis is rarely pruritic. There is often a strong family history of psoriasis.

?? Differential Diagnosis and Pitfalls

- Lichen planus—Very pruritic; associated with hepatitis C. Lichen planus may mimic and coexist with psoriasis in a given patient. Biopsy will differentiate psoriasis from lichen planus. The typical colors of psoriasis and lichen planus (erythematous and violaceous, respectively) may be underappreciated in darker skin types.
- Subacute cutaneous lupus erythematosus (SCLE)—Check ANA; it will be positive in most lupus patients. SCLE is characterized by annular plaques with raised borders and central clearing or papulosquamous lesions that are restricted to sun-exposed skin.
- Pityriasis rubra pilaris (PRP)—Look for orange-red, waxylike keratoderma of the palms and soles (Fig. 4-358). Islands of normal skin within larger plaques are characteristically seen in PRP. PRP and psoriasis are histologically different, and a biopsy will aid in the diagnosis. A family history of psoriasis is often noted in psoriatic patients.
- Mycosis fungoides—generalized lymphadenopathy; circulating malignant lymphocytes as determined by flow cytometry; leonine facies; a CD4/CD8 ratio >10 as determined by flow cytometry
- Secondary syphilis—Check RPR, and check for history of primary chancre and systemic symptoms.
- Chronic atopic dermatitis—Patients are often aware of their atopic history, which commonly starts in childhood. Mild to moderate spongiosis is seen on histology. Look for lichenified plaques on the flexural surfaces and neck. It is more pruritic than psoriasis.
- Seborrheic dermatitis—sebaceous distribution

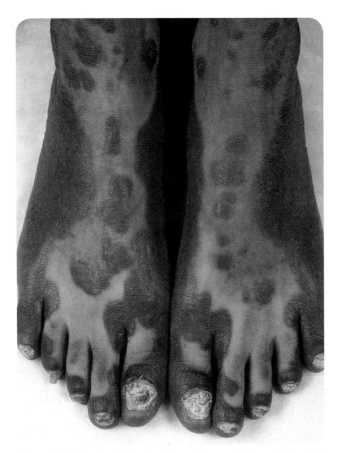

Figure 4-358 Sharply bordered hyperpigmented lesions of pityriasis rubra pilaris on the feet. Nail plate destruction is very common.

- Pityriasis rosea—Look for herald patch, collarette of scale, and orientation of lesions (fir-tree pattern in skin tension lines). It is does not follow an intermittently relapsing course.
- Tinea corporis—scale at leading edge of erythema with central clearing. Check KOH.
- Drug eruption—Drug eruptions are often present with urticarial, exanthematous, or vesicular/bullous lesions. In addition, systemic symptoms are more pronounced than in classic psoriasis, including fever, lymphadenopathy, and facial edema. Eosinophilia on CBC and histology are often seen (but not an invariable finding). Look for nonsteroidal anti-inflammatory drugs, sulfonamides, and penicillin.

Pediatric Patient Differential Diagnosis

- Juvenile PRP is a chronic disorder of cornification, with onset in early childhood. PRP is usually acquired, but there are heritable forms. It can present in three forms, type III (acute), type IV (localized), and type V (atypical). In type III, there is fairly rapid onset of extensive, confluent, scaling plaques in association with thick keratoderma of the hands and feet. It often

begins in the scalp and rapidly involves the trunk and extremities. Type IV is usually limited to the knees and elbows. Type V is present from birth.
- Seborrheic dermatitis—favors intertriginous areas and has a greasy rather than dry, flaky scale
- Atopic dermatitis—usually spares the diaper area and more commonly affects the shins and forearms
- Cutaneous candidiasis—responds to antifungal therapy; has satellite pustules; KOH preparation demonstrates pseudohyphae
- Acrodermatitis enteropathica—initially vesicular or bullous; periorificial and acral preference; often associated with diarrhea, alopecia, and failure to thrive
- Irritant diaper dermatitis—spares skin folds and limited to diaper area
- Pityriasis rosea
- Mycosis fungoides
- Lichen planus
- Chronic atopic dermatitis
- Seborrheic dermatitis
- Tinea corporis
- Drug eruption

✓ Best Tests

- This diagnosis is most often made clinically. If there is doubt, perform a skin biopsy.
- Consider plain films or bone scans in patients with joint complaints.

Guttate psoriasis—Often, this diagnosis can be made clinically based on history and its characteristic clinical appearance. Bacterial cultures of the throat or perianal area may help to isolate an organism in certain cases. The presence of antibodies to streptolysin O, anti-DNase B, or streptozyme can confirm previous infection. Perform a skin biopsy if the diagnosis is in doubt and a urinalysis if there is concern for post-streptococcal glomerulonephritis.

Pustular psoriasis—Biopsy for histology. Culture a pustule to rule out secondary Gram-positive superinfection. Some abnormalities that have been described include neutrophilia with WBC up to 30,000, absolute lymphopenia, elevated sedimentation rate, hypoalbuminemia, anemia, elevated transaminases, elevated alkaline phosphatase and bilirubin, and hypocalcemia. A decreased creatinine clearance has been observed.

Pediatric Patient Considerations

A skin biopsy may help to differentiate psoriasis from seborrheic dermatitis, but because the treatment is similar, empiric therapy is reasonable before biopsy. KOH preparation may help distinguish from *Candida*.

Management Pearls

Ultraviolet light is one of the best therapies to treat extensive or widespread disease. Consider narrow-band UVB 3 times weekly, or recommend natural sun exposure, if possible. Some cases of psoriasis are light-induced, and this should be determined first by careful history.

The National Psoriasis Foundation is an excellent resource for patients: http://www.psoriasis.org/home/.

Therapy

Note that psoriasis is often too widespread to practically treat with topical agents or recalcitrant to topical therapy alone. However, this should be evaluated on a case-by-case basis because systemic treatments often require monitoring and carry a potential risk of systemic side effects. In addition, potent corticosteroids should not be used in the intertriginous areas because of skin thinning and striae formation.

Topical Treatments
Most patients with darker skin prefer ointments and gels over creams and lotions. Also, the patient should hydrate his/her skin prior to applying corticosteroids.

High-Potency Topical Corticosteroids (Classes 1 and 2)
- Fluocinonide cream, ointment—Apply twice daily (15, 30, 60, 120 g).
- Desoximetasone cream, ointment—Apply twice daily (15, 60, 120 g).
- Halcinonide cream, ointment—Apply twice daily (15, 60, 240 g).
- Amcinonide ointment—Apply twice daily (15, 30, 60 g).
- Clobetasol cream, ointment—Apply twice daily.

Mid-Potency Topical Corticosteroids (Classes 3 and 4)
- Triamcinolone cream, ointment—Apply twice daily (15, 30, 60, 120, 240 g).
- Mometasone cream, ointment—Apply twice daily (15, 45 g).
- Fluocinolone cream, ointment—Apply twice daily (15, 30, 60 g).

Vitamin D Analog
- Calcipotriene cream, ointment—Apply twice daily to affected areas (30-, 60-, 100-g tubes; 60-mL scalp solution). Therapy can be rotated with steroid treatment.

Tar-Based Therapy
- 10% Liquor carbonis detergens (LCD) in ointment—Apply daily (compound 440-g jar).
- Anthralin 0.1, 0.25, 0.5% cream—Begin with lowest strength, and apply short contact (e.g., 10 minutes); advance as tolerated.
- Tar bath oils, 2.5% coal tar (240, 180, 240 mL)

Scalp Therapy
Thick, scaly plaques within the scalp can be a difficult management problem. Consider loosening scale with an oil-based treatment such as Baker P&S applied nightly (120 mL) or treating with fluocinolone peanut oil formulation applied nightly (supplied 120 mL). For patients of African descent with a lot of periocular lesions and especially scalp lesions, Derma-Smoothe FS is an excellent product. Have the patient shampoo with tar-based shampoos.

Systemic Therapy
- Methotrexate 10 to 20 mg p.o. weekly
- Mycophenolate mofetil 1 g p.o. twice daily
- Cyclosporine 2 to 3 mg/kg p.o. daily
- Tacrolimus 1 to 3 mg p.o. daily
- Acitretin 25 to 50 mg p.o. daily

Systemic therapies and TNF-alpha inhibitors are generally prescribed by dermatologists or rheumatologists for moderate to severe plaque psoriasis and/or psoriatic arthritis (use as directed). Be sure to check PPD prior to use.

- Etanercept—50 mg SC twice weekly for 3 months, then once weekly maintenance dosage of 50 mg
- Alefacept—IM injection of 15 mg once weekly for 12 weeks
- Infliximab—5 mg/kg IV initial infusion followed by 5 mg/kg at 2 and 6 weeks after the first infusion, then every 6 to 8 weeks
- Adalimumab—80 mg SC initially, followed by 40 mg every other week starting 1 week after the initial dose

The biologics and their effectiveness in different ethnic groups have been documented. Hogan documented the favorable response of infliximab in an African American woman with severe psoriasis and psoriatic arthritis over the course of 6 years. Furthermore, a study of admixed Hispanic patients with Crohn disease found that the effectiveness and safety profile of infliximab was similar to the global response; they note that ethnicity does not seem to influence the response rate. Similarly, low-dose etanercept was found to be a valuable treatment in Asians

(Continued)

with moderate to severe psoriasis; the drug was generally well tolerated, and side effects such as reactivation of tuberculosis were not seen. Finally, in a study that compared the pharmacokinetics of etanercept between healthy Japanese and American patients with rheumatoid arthritis, no difference in efficacy at similar doses was noted. Although the biologics are effective medications, serious central nervous system disease including progressive multifocal leukoencephalopathy led to the eventual withdrawal of efalizumab from the US market in 2009.

UV Light

UV light can be used alone or in combination with acitretin systemically.

- UVB radiation (295 to 320 nm)—Perform three times weekly until remission is induced, followed by maintenance doses. It can be used alone or in conjunction with topical tar.
- Narrow-band UVB (311 nm)—Use three times weekly until remission is induced.
- Photochemotherapy (psoralen plus UVA; PUVA)—increased risk of skin cancer over prolonged usage
  1. Patients ingest 8-methoxypsoralen, with exposure to UVA within 2 hours of ingestion. Perform three times weekly in increasing doses until remission, then twice or once weekly as a maintenance dose.
  2. Bath PUVA involves dissolving the psoralen capsules in water, and soaking affected skin for 15 to 30 minutes prior to UVA exposure.

Referral to dermatology is indicated for management with systemic medications.

Pediatric Patient Considerations

Note: To avoid striae, be sure to warn parents to not use potent corticosteroids in intertriginous areas (1% hydrocortisone should be used in these areas).

   Note: While useful in older patients, the topical calcineurin inhibitors, tacrolimus and pimecrolimus, are not approved for use in patients aged younger than 2 years.

Localized Disease (Topical Treatments)
Midpotency Topical Corticosteroids (Classes 3 and 4)
Midpotency topical corticosteroid treatment needs supervision with scheduled follow-up to observe for steroid atrophy.

- Triamcinolone cream, ointment—Apply twice daily (15, 30, 60, 120, 240 g).

- Mometasone cream, ointment—Apply twice daily (15, 45 g).
- Fluocinolone cream, ointment—Apply twice daily (15, 30, 60 g).

High-Potency Topical Corticosteroids (Class 2)
High-potency topical corticosteroids should be limited to the thickest plaques and used for only short periods of time (do not write for numerous refills).

- Fluocinonide cream, ointment—Apply twice daily (15, 30, 60, 120 g).
- Desoximetasone cream, ointment 0.25%—Apply twice daily (15, 60, 120 g).
- Halcinonide cream, ointment—Apply twice daily (15, 60, 240 g).
- Amcinonide ointment—Apply twice daily (15, 30, 60 g).

Vitamin D Analog
Calcipotriol cream, ointment—Apply twice daily to affected areas (30-, 60-, 100-g tubes; 60-mL scalp solution). Therapy can be rotated with steroid treatment, eg, steroid cream Saturday and Sunday twice daily and calcipotriol Monday through Friday twice daily.

Intertriginous and Facial Therapy
Use low-potency topical steroids on thinner-skinned areas of the face and on intertriginous areas.

- Desonide or alclometasone ointment or cream 30 g twice daily.
- Tacrolimus ointment 0.03%, 0.1% twice daily or pimecrolimus cream 1% twice daily.

Tar-based Therapy
- 10% coal tar solution (LCD) in Aquaphor ointment—Apply daily (compound 440-g jar of Aquaphor)
- Anthralin cream 0.1%, 0.25%, 0.5%—Begin with lowest strength, and apply short contact (e.g., 10 minutes); advance as tolerated.
- Tar bath oils, Balnetar 2.5% coal tar (240 mL), Zetar (180 mL), Doak Tar Oil (240 mL)

Scalp Therapy
Thick, scaly plaques within the scalp can be a difficult management problem. Consider loosening scale with an oil-based treatment such as Baker P&S applied nightly (120 mL) or treating with fluocinolone peanut oil formulation applied nightly (supplied 120 mL). Have patient shampoo with tar-based shampoos such as Neutrogena T/Gel.

   Tazarotene gel (0.05% or 0.1%) applied to lesions nightly; may be better tolerated when used with a topical corticosteroid

Systemic Therapy

- Phototherapy, either UVB or physician-administered PUVA, can be a wonderful therapy, providing bodywide clearing. If plaques are extensive, referral for phototherapy should be considered.
- Oral systemic therapy includes acitretin (25 mg/d). A retinoid and methotrexate (10 to 20 mg/wk) are alternatives in the most severe cases.

Because these agents have a variety of acute and chronic consequences, referral to a dermatologist or others skilled in the use of these agents is indicated for management with these medications or other systemic therapies.

Immunocompromised Patient Considerations

HIV-associated psoriasis is often severe and refractory to treatment. This is interesting, because HIV is a disease of T-lymphocyte depletion and psoriasis is a disease of cytokine-mediated T-lymphocyte proliferation. Psoriasis, however, is nonetheless exacerbated by HIV. Treatment for mild cases consists of topical preparations such as calcipotriol, tazarotene, and corticosteroids. Moderate to severe cases should be treated with first-line agents such as UV therapy or antiretrovirals; second-line therapy is oral retinoids. Judicious use of systemic immunosuppressants is recommended for refractory cases; clinicians should remain vigilant for the appearance of opportunistic infection.

Suggested Readings

Barlow RJ, Schulz EJ. Chronic subcorneal pustulosis with vasculitis: A variant of generalized pustular psoriasis in black South Africans. *Br J Dermatol.* 1991;124(5):470–474.

Farber EM, Grauer F, Zaruba F. Racial incidence of psoriasis. *Cesk Dermatol.* 1965;40(5):289–297.

Farber EM, Nall L. Psoriasis in the tropics. Epidemiologic, genetic, clinical, and therapeutic aspects. *Dermatol Clin.* 1994;12(4):805–816.

Food and Drug Administration. FDA Statement on the Voluntary Withdrawal of Raptiva From the U.S. Market. http://www.fda.gov/Drugs/DrugSafety/PostmarketDrugSafetyInformationforPatientsandProviders/ucm143347.htm Accessed January 30, 2010.

Gelfand JM, Stern RS, Nijsten T, et al. The prevalence of psoriasis in African Americans: Results from a population-based study. *J Am Acad Dermatol.* 2005;52(1):23–26.

Jacyk WK. Pityriasis rubra pilaris in black South Africans. *Clin Exp Dermatol* 1999;24(3):160–163.

Kawai S, Sekino H, Yamashita N, et al. The comparability of etanercept pharmacokinetics in healthy Japanese and American subjects. *J Clin Pharmacol.* 2006;46(4):418–423.

Lee CS, Lim HW. Cutaneous diseases in Asians. *Dermatol Clin.* 2003;21(4):669–677.

Lew W, Lee E, Krueger JG. Psoriasis genomics: Analysis of proinflammatory (type 1) gene expression in large plaque (Western) and small plaque (Asian) psoriasis vulgaris. *Br J Dermatol.* 2004;150(4):668–676.

Mamkin I, Mamkin A, Ramanan SV. HIV-associated psoriasis. *Lancet Infect Dis.* 2007;7(7):496.

May J, Hogan D. Severe psoriasis in an African American woman treated with infliximab therapy for 6 years. *Int J Dermatol.* 2007;46(12):1312.

Menon K, Van Voorhees AS, Bebo BF Jr, et al; for the National Psoriasis Foundation. Psoriasis in patients with HIV infection: From the Medical Board of the National Psoriasis Foundation. *J Am Acad Dermatol.* 2009;62:291–299.

Na JI, Kim JH, Park KC, Youn SW. Low-dose etanercept therapy in moderate to severe psoriasis in Korean. *J Dermatol* 2008;35(8):484–490.

Nnoruka EN, Obiagboso I, Maduechesi C. Hair loss in children in South-East Nigeria: common and uncommon cases. *Int J Dermatol.* 2007;46(Suppl 1):18–22.

Sánchez JM, Maldonado JC, Torres EA, et al. Infliximab in Hispanics: Characterization of response to infliximab in an ethnic minority with Crohn's disease. *P R Health Sci J.* 2005;24(1):11–17.

Tinea Versicolor

Donna Culton

▣ Diagnosis Synopsis

Tinea versicolor, also known as pityriasis versicolor, is a common benign superficial fungal infection of the skin resulting from infection with yeast from the *Malassezia* genus—*M. globosa*, *M. sympodialis*, *M. furfur*, and possibly others. The yeast forms of these organisms are part of the normal skin flora and ubiquitous in the environment. Tinea versicolor occurs when the organisms convert to their hyphal form under conditions of high temperature and humidity. Endogenous host factors also contribute to clinical disease.

Clinically, the infection manifests as macules, patches, and thin plaques with fine scale and varying pigmentation. Given the lipophilic nature of the fungus, the disease typically occurs in a seborrheic distribution including the face, neck, upper chest, and upper back. In most patients, the condition is non-pruritic, and the primary concern is over its appearance.

The condition occurs equally in men and women. Young adults and teenagers appear to be affected more frequently than older adults and young children, which is attributable to increased activity of sebaceous glands in this age range. The distribution is worldwide, but there is an increased prevalence in tropical areas with high humidity and temperatures. The true prevalence among different ethnicities is not clear, but there is an increased frequency of visits for African American and American Indian populations compared to whites, Asians, and Hispanics. It is unclear whether there is an increased susceptibility among these patients (perhaps due to increased lipid content in the skin or increased activity of the sebaceous glands) or if they seek care more often given the more noticeable pigment change that accompanies the condition in these groups of patients.

Risk factors other than high heat and humidity include oily skin, excessive sweating, pregnancy, poor nutrition, corticosteroid use, and some immunodeficiency states.

The condition is not contagious. It is often recurrent in susceptible individuals.

Pediatric Patient Considerations

In prepubertal children, the most common distribution is on the face, as oil glands in the classic seborrheic distribution are less active before puberty.

Immunocompromised Patient Considerations

Immunosuppression due to medications (as seen in transplant patients) is also a known risk factor for tinea versicolor, with cyclosporine and azathioprine use having frequent associations with the condition.

◉ Look For

Hyperpigmented or hypopigmented macules and patches or barely elevated papules/plaques, usually on the chest, back, and upper arms in a seborrheic distribution (Figs. 4-359–4-361). The macules may coalesce to form irregular patches. Most cases have a fine, dusty-appearing scale, but in some cases, the scale may be so fine that it is imperceptible. Whereas tinea versicolor often presents as tan lesions in light-skinned patients, these are infrequent

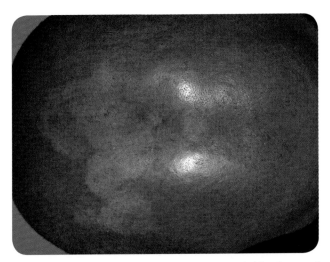

Figure 4-359 Glabrous scalp with hypopigmented thin plaques of tinea versicolor.

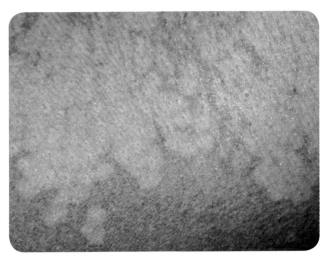

Figure 4-360 Hypopigmentation is commonly seen in tinea versicolor in deeply pigmented skin and is often the patient's chief complaint.

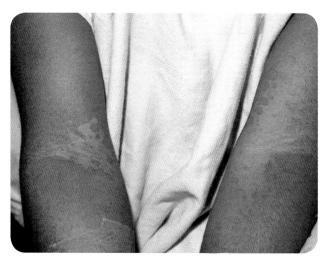

Figure 4-361 Extensive antecubital hypopigmentation with tinea versicolor.

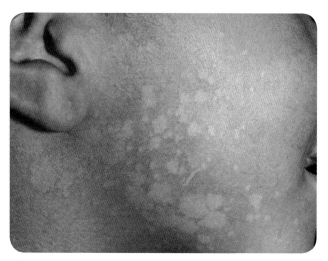

Figure 4-362 Children will frequently have tinea versicolor on the face, unlike adults.

in patients with more heavily pigmented skin where hypopigmented macules and patches predominate. The involvement of the face may be more common in African American patients, especially in children (Fig. 4-362).

Distinctly follicular forms may also occur with 2 to 3 mm follicularly based superficial papules and pustules typically appearing on the back, chest, and sometimes the extremities. Pruritus is more common than with typical tinea versicolor. Only by appropriate culture and potassium hydroxide (KOH) examination can it be distinguished from a bacterial folliculitis.

Pediatric Patient Considerations

Facial involvement can occur and is more frequent in infants.

Diagnostic Pearls

Examination with a Wood lamp accentuates the pigmentary findings, and an orange fluorescence may be seen. The scale can be difficult to see at first glance; however, stretching of the involved skin will accentuate the fine scale of tinea versicolor.

Differential Diagnosis and Pitfalls

- Confluent and reticulated papillomatosis of Gougerot and Carteaud
- Seborrheic dermatitis
- Erythema dyschromicum perstans
- Atopic dermatitis—will often be more pruritic
- Pityriasis rosea—not limited to seborrheic distribution

- Pityriasis alba—ill defined and typically limited to the face and upper arms
- Guttate psoriasis
- Nummular eczema
- Vitiligo—will have depigmented macules and patches that lack scale
- Erythrasma
- Tinea corporis—typically not as widespread in distribution, KOH will show long, branching hyphae and no yeast
- Patch stage mycosis fungoides (cutaneous T-cell lymphoma)
- Indeterminate leprosy—only in patients living in endemic areas, not a consideration in travelers
- Secondary syphilis
- Progressive macular hypopigmentation

Best Tests

Lightly scrape the scaling edge of a lesion onto a glass slide, and cover with a coverslip. Add a small drop of 10% to 20% KOH to the edge of the coverslip. The capillary action will be enough to wet the specimen. Heat over an open flame for 1 to 3 seconds, and examine under the microscope. Look for short, nonbranching hyphae and spores. Grapelike clusters of spores are often described as "meatballs," and the hyphae are described as having a "spaghetti" appearance.

Management Pearls

- Inform patients that skin color changes will typically resolve within 1 to 2 months of treatment (but sometimes will take much longer).

- Recurrence of tinea versicolor is very common, and most patients prone to it will require a preventive regimen in addition to a primary treatment regimen.
- Tinea versicolor is not contagious and is not due to poor hygiene.

Therapy

The condition typically responds to short courses of topical or oral antifungals. Prophylactic treatments are usually necessary to prevent relapse.

Systemic Treatment for Adults
- Ketoconazole 200 mg p.o. daily for 10 days or a single 400 mg dose
- Fluconazole 150 to 300 mg p.o. once weekly for 2 to 4 weeks or 300 mg p.o. repeated after 2 weeks
- Itraconazole 200 mg p.o. daily for 5 to 7 days

Oral ketoconazole and fluconazole have similar efficacy.

Topically, for Large Skin Areas
- Selenium sulfide 2.5% lotion—Apply for 10 minutes daily for 7 days; repeat the same regimen in 1 month.
- Pyrithione zinc 2% shampoo—Apply for 10 minutes daily for 7 days; repeat the same regimen in 1 month.
- Propylene glycol 50% in water—Apply twice daily for 2 weeks.
- Bifonazole 1% shampoo—Apply daily for 3 weeks.
- Ketoconazole 2% shampoo—Apply daily to scalp and body for 5 to 10 minutes for 1 to 14 days.

Topically, More Limited Areas
- Clotrimazole 1% cream—Apply twice daily for 2 to 6 weeks.

- Sulconazole 1% cream—Apply daily for 2 weeks.
- Econazole 1% cream—Apply once to twice daily for 2 weeks.
- Ketoconazole 2% cream—Apply once to twice daily for 2 to 4 weeks.
- Ciclopirox 0.77% cream or lotion—Apply once or twice daily for 4 weeks.
- Terbinafine 1% cream or solution—Apply once or twice daily for 1 to 2 weeks.

Prevention of Recurrence
- Selenium sulfide 2.5% lotion—Apply first and third day of the month.
- Ketoconazole 2% shampoo—Lather on scalp and body for 5 to 10 minutes once a week.
- Ketoconazole 400 mg p.o. once a month
- Fluconazole 300 mg p.o. once a month
- Itraconazole 400 mg p.o. once a month

Note that the use of systemic antifungals carries a small risk of liver toxicity.

Suggested Readings

Halder RM, Roberts CI, Nootheti PK. Cutaneous diseases in the black races. *Dermatol Clin.* 2003;21:679–687.

Janik MP, Heffernan MP. Yeast infections: Candidiasis and tinea (pityriasis) versicolor. In: Wolff K, Goldsmith LA, Katz SI, Gilchrest BA, Paller AS, Leffell DJ, eds. *Fitzpatrick's Dermatology in General Medicine.* 7th Ed. New York, NY: McGraw-Hill; 2008:1822–1830.

Mellen LA, Vallee J, Feldmen SR, Fleischer AB Jr. Treatment of pityriasis versicolor in the United States. *J Dermatol Treat.* 2004;15:189–192.

Mollet I, Ongenae K, Maeyaert JM. Origin, clinical presentation, and diagnosis of hypomelanocytic skin disorders. *Dermatol Clin.* 2007;25: 363–371.

Keratosis Pilaris

Stephanie Diamantis

■■ Diagnosis Synopsis

Keratosis pilaris (KP) is a common benign skin disorder of the follicular orifice characterized by small follicular papules on the extensor lateral extremities due to the retention of keratin at the follicular opening. KP is generally most evident in adolescents and young adults and is rare in the elderly. KP is often worse in the dry winter months. Studies characterizing the frequency of KP in ethnic populations are lacking.

Frequently, there is a family history of the condition, and autosomal dominant inheritance with variable penetrance has been described. KP tends to be refractory to most treatments, with complete cure highly unlikely; however, the condition tends to improve with age.

KP most often occurs as described above but does have three clinical variants, all of which have hyperkeratotic follicular papules with varying degrees of atrophy:

- Keratosis pilaris atrophicans faciei (ulerythema ophryogenes)—Erythematous hyperkeratotic papules distributed on the lateral third of the eyebrows in young children. This condition has a strong association with Noonan syndrome and woolly hair.
- Atrophoderma vermiculatum (honeycomb atrophy)—atrophic pits in a reticulate or worm-eaten array localized to the face of older children
- Keratosis follicularis spinulosa decalvans—widespread KP, scarring alopecia, and eye abnormalities.

KP is seen with increased incidence in several syndromes and disease states, which include the following: atopic dermatitis, ichthyosis vulgaris, erythromelanosis follicularis faciei et colli (erythema, brown pigmentation, and KP), Lassueur-Graham-

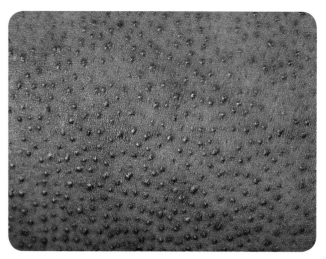

Figure 4-364 Close-up of the skin of the patient in Figure 4-363 shows that the follicles are hyperpigmented but the surrounding skin is not.

Little-Piccardi syndrome (cicatricial alopecia of the scalp, loss of pubic and axillary hairs, and KP), cardiofaciocutaneous syndrome, Noonan syndrome, diabetes, Down syndrome, woolly hair, and obesity.

◉ Look For

Multiple monomorphic 1 to 2 mm follicular papules over the extensor arms, giving the appearance of gooseflesh (Figs. 4-363–4-366). Lateral cheeks, anterior thighs, and buttocks may also be involved. Perifollicular erythema is less apparent in darkly pigmented individuals.

●● Diagnostic Pearls

- The symmetry of follicular papules over the arms and/or legs (most often laterally distributed) is one clue to the diagnosis.
- KP can be widespread in younger years and slowly localizes to the arms and legs as children get older. Parents and siblings are often affected.

?? Differential Diagnosis and Pitfalls

- Folliculitis
- Milia—usually not based around the follicle
- Lichen spinulosus—grouped in annular clusters, preferentially involves the trunk in addition to the extremities
- Acne vulgaris—comedones are usually present
- Atopic dermatitis
- Pityriasis rubra pilaris
- Darier disease

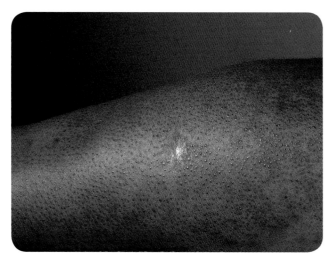

Figure 4-363 Uniform hyperkeratosis of all of the hair follicles on the legs.

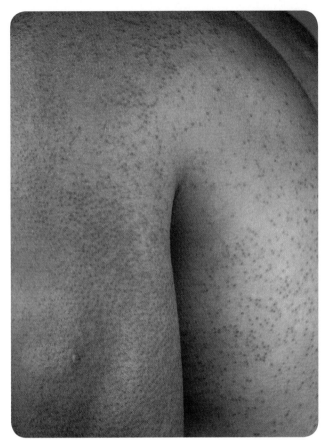

Figure 4-365 The shoulders are frequently involved with keratosis pilaris.

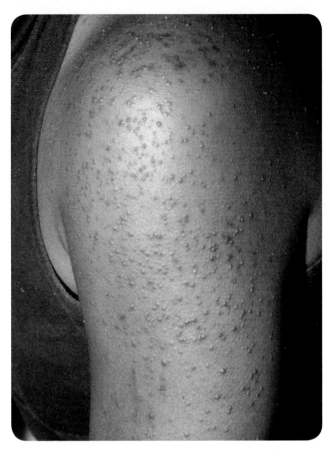

Figure 4-366 Renal transplant patient with very inflammatory keratosis pilaris.

- Kyrle disease
- Phrynoderma (vitamin A deficiency)
- Lichen nitidus—Koebnerization (trauma-induced linear lesions) may be present.
- Lichen planopilaris

Variants of KP (see "Diagnosis Synopsis" above for details):

- Keratosis pilaris atrophicans
- Keratosis follicularis spinulosa decalvans
- Atrophoderma vermiculatum

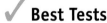 Best Tests

KP is a clinical diagnosis, although a skin biopsy will confirm the diagnosis.

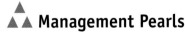 Management Pearls

- Reinforce the chronic nature of the disorder. Facial lesions will improve over time.
- Prevent excessive dryness by using soft soaps or soapless cleansers in conjunction with regular use of emollients after bathing.

Therapy

Therapy is directed at reducing the rough texture or erythema of individual lesions rather than "curing" the patient. Keratolytics such as lactic acid or salicylic acid 4% to 12% lotions or creams applied twice daily may diminish the thickness/roughness of the papules. Alternatively, topical retinoids such as tazarotene cream or tretinoin cream applied daily may improve texture. Topical calcipotriene has been used with limited success.

Suggested Readings

Callaway SR, Lesher JL Jr. Keratosis pilaris atrophicans: case series and review. *Pediatr Dermatol.* 2004;21(1):14–17.

Dunwell P, Rose A. Study of skin disease spectrum occurring in an Afrocaribbean population. *Int J Dermatol.* 2003;42(4):287–289.

Janjua SA, Iftikhar N, Pastar Z, et al. Keratosis follicularis spinulosa decalvans associated with acne keloidalis nuchae and tufted hair folliculitis. *Am J Clin Dermatol.* 2008;9(2):137–140.

Thiers BH. The use of topical calcipotriene/calcipotriol in conditions other than plaque-type psoriasis. *J Am Acad Dermatol.* 1997;37(3 Pt 2): S69–S71.

Prurigo Nodularis

Stephanie Diamantis

■■ Diagnosis Synopsis

Prurigo nodularis is a chronic condition of uncertain etiology. Patients present with multiple, discrete, severely pruritic nodules that mostly appear on the dorsal extremities and anterior areas of the thighs and legs. The lesions are rarely seen on the face. The lesions are brought about by repetitive rubbing or scratching of discrete areas of the skin, and patients often state that they are unable to stop. Prurigo nodularis may be secondary to skin conditions associated with pruritus, such as atopic dermatitis and xerosis, as well as systemic conditions associated with generalized pruritus without a primary skin rash, such as psychiatric conditions, HIV infection, renal or hepatic impairment, malignancies, and others.

Lesions are firm, dome-shaped, smooth-topped or crusted, 1 to 2 cm nodules that enlarge slowly over time. The nodules can be very firm and thick and frequently have a smooth surface. Lichenification of the lesions is often not present.

◉ Look For

Nodules and papules that range in size from 0.5 to 2 cm in diameter and enlarge slowly over time. The nodules can be very firm and thick and are usually limited to the extremities (Fig. 4-367). They may have scaly or crusted centers and appear hyperpigmented or violaceous. Often, central excoriations are present. Bacterial superinfection is not uncommon.

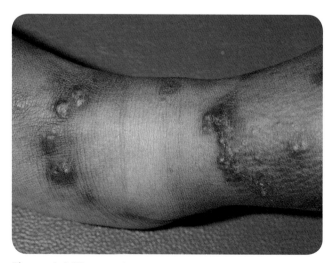

Figure 4-367 Grouped papules and nodules of prurigo nodularis around the ankle and foot.

●● Diagnostic Pearls

Lesions are almost always in areas that can be scratched or rubbed, especially on the extremities.

?? Differential Diagnosis and Pitfalls

- Multiple keratoacanthomas
- Hypertrophic lichen planus
- Hypertrophic discoid lupus
- Pemphigoid nodularis
- Nodular scabies
- Keloid/hypertrophic scar
- Acne keloidalis nuchae
- Hypertrophic actinic keratosis/cutaneous horn
- Lymphoma/pseudolymphoma
- Lymphomatoid papulosis
- Warts
- Molluscum contagiosum
- Mastocytosis
- Cutaneous amyloidosis
- Dermatofibromas
- Pilomatrixomas
- Foreign body reactions
- Xanthomas
- Knuckle pads
- Multicentric reticulohistiocytosis
- Persistent insect bite reaction
- Mycosis fungoides
- Perforating skin disorders

✓ Best Tests

- Skin biopsy will confirm the clinical impression. Other steps may include the following:
  - Culture for bacteria if there is any indication of pyoderma.
  - Consider HIV testing if the patient's HIV status is unknown.
  - Obtain a CBC, liver and thyroid function tests, and a chemistry panel to rule out hematologic malignancies and renal or hepatic disease as a cause of pruritus.
  - An elevated serum IgE may indicate atopy.
- A thorough history and physical exam is often the most important evaluation for underlying causes of prurigo nodularis. If there is any suspicion of lymphoma based on a review of systems, a chest radiograph and/or abdominal CT scan may be obtained.

▲▲ Management Pearls

The very indolent nature of these lesions should be communicated to the patient early in the course so that he/she can develop appropriate expectations. These lesions are very difficult to treat because they are chronically picked at and scratched by the patient. Stopping the itch-scratch cycle is paramount for the patient to improve.

Therapy

The goal of therapy for prurigo nodularis is to relieve pruritus and stop the itch-scratch cycle. Topical steroids applied twice daily with or without occlusion are the first-line therapy. Also consider flurandrenolide (Cordran) tape, a corticosteroid-impregnated tape (60, 200 cm² rolls) that can serve as a reminder for the patient not to rub and also deliver the topical steroid under occlusion. Change the tape once daily.

In general, start with a high-potency topical steroid (class 2 or 3) or a superpotent topical corticosteroid (class 1) if the condition is severe. Schedule close (i.e., 2-week) follow-up when using such agents. Decrease the potency and/or the frequency of application of the corticosteroid preparation as the lesions resolve to avoid inducing skin atrophy. Applying these agents under occlusion may increase potency.

Super-Potent Topical Corticosteroids (Class 1)
- Clobetasol 0.05% cream—apply twice daily (15, 30, 45 g)
- Betamethasone dipropionate 0.05% cream—apply twice daily (15, 30, 45 g)
- Diflorasone 0.05% cream—apply twice daily (15, 30, 60 g)
- Halobetasol cream—apply twice daily (15, 50 g)

High-Potency Topical Corticosteroids (Class 2)
- Fluocinonide cream, ointment—apply twice daily (15, 30, 60, 120 g)
- Desoximetasone cream, ointment—apply twice daily (15, 60, 120 g)
- Halcinonide cream, ointment—apply twice daily (15, 60, 240 g)
- Amcinonide ointment—apply twice daily (15, 30, 60 g)

Mid-Potency Topical Corticosteroids (Classes 3 and 4)
- Triamcinolone acetonide cream, ointment—apply twice daily (15, 30, 60, 120, 240 g)
- Mometasone cream, ointment—apply twice daily (15, 45 g)
- Fluocinolone ointment, cream—apply twice daily (15, 30, 60 g)

Alternatively, intralesional injection with triamcinolone acetonide at 3 to 5 mg/mL to the thickened plaque (5 to 10 mg/mL for thickened nodules) may be effective. Repeated injections rarely have the potential to cause hypopigmentation, especially in darker skin.

For pruritus, the following antihistamines often provide relief:
- Diphenhydramine hydrochloride (25, 50 mg tablets or capsules): 25 to 50 mg nightly or every 6 hours, as needed
- Hydroxyzine (10, 25 mg tablets): 10 to 25 mg every 6 hours, as needed
- Cetirizine hydrochloride (5, 10 mg tablets): 5 to 10 mg/d

Additional measures to control itch include use of soothing emollients (containing menthol, pramoxine, camphor), capsaicin cream (0.025% to 0.3%, applied four to six times daily), and 5% doxepin cream. Skin lubrication is essential. Occlusive dressings such as an Unna boot may be helpful to increase the potency of topical steroids and also discourage the patient from picking/scratching.

A topical antibiotic ointment (e.g., mupirocin) can be applied to impetiginized lesions.

Additional treatments shown to be effective in prurigo nodularis are as follows:
- Phototherapy—PUVA (psoralen plus UVA), UVB, and narrowband UVB phototherapy have successfully been used for more diffuse lesions.
- Cryosurgery should be attempted on only one or a few lesions to prove efficacy. Warn patients about the risk of hypopigmentation or hyperpigmentation and further scarring.
- Naltrexone may also be effective by acting on central and peripheral itch pathways, which are in part mediated by opioid receptors.
- Prednisone (20 to 30 mg/d) and azathioprine (50 mg twice daily) have proven beneficial.
- Severe refractory cases have been treated with thalidomide (100 to 300 mg daily) with excellent results.
- Cyclosporine (3 to 4.5 mg/kg daily)

Referral to a dermatologist is recommended if systemic therapies are a consideration.

Psychiatric interventions also represent a major component of therapy in many patients. Antianxiety (doxepin) and antidepressant medications are beneficial for a significant number of patients. Biofeedback, journaling, and counseling are also helpful in breaking the itch-scratch cycle for many patients.

Suggested Readings

James WD, Berger TG, Elston DM, eds. Pruritus and neurocutaneous dermatoses. In: *Andrews' Diseases of the Skin: Clinical Dermatology*. 10th Ed. Philadelphia, PA: Elsevier; 2006:58–59.

Lee MR, Shumack S. Prurigo nodularis: A review. *Australas J Dermatol* 2005;46:211–220.

Lotti T, Buggiani G, Prignano F. Prurigo nodularis and lichen simplex chronicus. *Dermatol Ther* 2008;21:42–46.

Matthews SN, Cockerell CJ. Prurigo nodularis in HIV-infected individuals. *Int J Dermatol* 1998;37(6):401–409.

Nanda V, Parwaz MA, Handa S. Linear hypopigmentation after triamcinolone injection: A rare complication of a common procedure. *Aesthetic Plast Surg* 2006;30(1):118–119.

Wu JJ, Huang DB, Pang KR, et al. Thalidomide: Dermatological indications, mechanisms of action and side effects. *Br J Dermatol* 2005;153:254–273.

Scabies

Rodolfo E. Chirinos

■ Diagnosis Synopsis

Scabies is a parasitic infestation caused by the itch mite, *Sarcoptes scabiei var. hominis*, and is transmitted via direct skin-to-skin contact and less frequently by fomites (e.g., clothing, towels, and bedding). Human scabies is extremely contagious, spreading between individuals who share close contact or living spaces, which is why transmission among family members is so common. Scabies is very common in children in many countries and is often seen in infants who are being adopted in the United States from orphanages in other countries. Data suggesting a lower prevalence of scabies in African Americans have not been critically substantiated, and the diagnosis of scabies must be considered in all ethnic groups.

The most common predisposing factors are poor hygiene, overcrowding, poor nutritional status, homelessness, dementia, and sexual contact. Certain populations are at particularly high risk of developing severe or crusted scabies (formerly known as Norwegian scabies), including patients receiving systemic or potent topical glucocorticoids, organ transplant recipients, mentally impaired or physically incapacitated individuals, HIV-infected individuals, and individuals with hematologic malignancies. Outbreaks frequently occur in institutions such as hospitals, nursing homes, kindergartens, prisons, and long-term care facilities.

Seasonality trends of scabies have been documented, with some studies suggesting a higher incidence in autumn and winter partly because mites survive longer away from the body in cooler weather, and colder weather encourages overcrowding in humans. In addition, mites may be sensitive to antimicrobial peptides contained in human sweat, leading to reduced infestation in summer.

The scabies mite is an obligate human parasite that completes its entire life cycle on humans. After mating the male mite dies, and the fertilized female burrows itself into the stratum corneum of the epidermis where it lays approximately one to three eggs per day, which hatch in 3 to 4 days and give rise to larvae. The mite remains gravid for life and lives for approximately 30 days. On average, an estimated 10 to 15 adult female mites live on an infected host, but the number can reach millions in humans with crusted scabies, which is therefore far more contagious than normal scabies. Mites in all life cycle stages can penetrate the intact epidermis by the secretion of enzymes that dissolve the skin, which is then ingested by the mite as nutrient. Larvae eventually cut through the roof of the burrow to reach the skin surface and mature into adults in 14 to 17 days. The initial infection is asymptomatic, with symptoms developing after 3 to 6 weeks as a result of the delayed type-IV hypersensitivity reaction to the mite or its saliva, eggs, or excrements (scybala). Reinfestation is associated with a brisk immune response and a rapid onset of symptoms within 24 to 72 hours.

◉ Look For

The telltale diagnostic sign is the burrow, the excavated tunnel in which the mite lives. These burrows are fine, threadlike, serpiginous grayish lines measuring 1 to 10 mm, with a terminal tiny (smaller than a pinhead) black speck representing the mite itself (Fig. 4-368). Look for burrows, typically located on the hands and feet, particularly the interdigital spaces of the hands and thenar and hypothenar eminences, along with small erythematous papules and vesicles on the flexor wrists, elbows, anterior axillary folds,

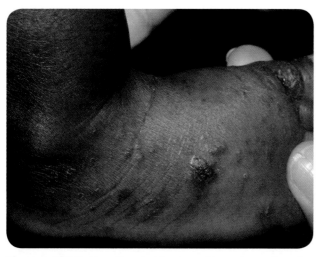
Figure 4-368 Scabies with a short burrow, vesicles, and crusted papules.

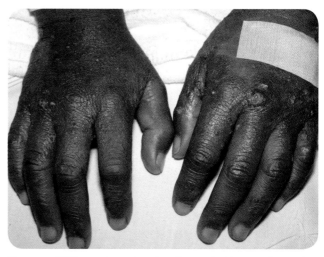
Figure 4-369 Papules and erosions in a typical location for scabies.

areolae, umbilicus, belt line, penile shaft, scrotum, buttocks, thighs, and ankles (Figs. 4-369 and 4-370). On the wrists, discrete burrows are barely visible to the naked eye and are often dismissed as excoriations or impetiginized skin. Scabies typically spares the head and neck areas in adults. Pruritic lesions of the areola in women or the penis and scrotum of men are highly suggestive of scabies (Fig. 4-371). Classic scabies is typically described as an intense, intractable, generalized pruritus, especially at night and after a hot shower. Occasionally, patients are asymptomatic.

Secondary lesions are due to scratching and include excoriations, impetiginized lesions with crusts, and prurigolike nodules. Often, they are more prominent than burrows, especially when the infestation has been present for some time. Poststreptococcal glomerulonephritis has been reported to complicate infection, especially in tropical countries.

Crusted scabies, as the name implies, consists of thick, gray, scaly, hyperkeratotic or crusted plaques and carries a high mortality related to secondary sepsis. Pruritus is less intense or absent. Any site can be involved, but the most common sites are the hands, feet, knees, elbows, genitalia, buttocks, and scalp. Patients may present with generalized erythema (erythroderma) and scaling. Infection usually also involves the subungual area and may cause thickened dystrophic nails and longitudinal nail splitting.

Scabies may also present with scattered reddish to brown nodules, typically on the glans penis, scrotum, thighs, and axillary regions.

In patients with type IV to VI skin types, small white papules are typically seen in the interdigital spaces, and the mite is seen as a tan to reddish pinpoint-sized object at the end of the burrow in contrast to the dark point in lighter-skinned patients. Mites can often be detected within penile burrows.

Pediatric Patient Considerations

In infants and young children, the scalp, face, and neck are frequently affected.

Involvement of the palms and soles, including the development of acral pustules, is unique to infantile scabies.

Diagnostic Pearls

- Look closely for the burrow. Mites can often be isolated from scabies preps of fresh, nonexcoriated burrows and papules. Avoid excoriated lesions for scabies preps. The tiny black dot (or, in skin types IV to VI, tan to reddish point) present at the edge of an intact linear papule represents a mite. Look for and inquire about lesions and symptoms in family members, caretakers, and pets.
- Burrows can be best identified by mineral oil or ink enhancement (Indian ink or gentian violet) or by topical tetracycline followed by fluorescence detection with a Wood lamp.
- Pruritus tends to be more intense at night and when the patient is warm.
- A negative scabies prep does not rule out infection; mites can be infrequent and difficult to isolate in patients with normal immune function.

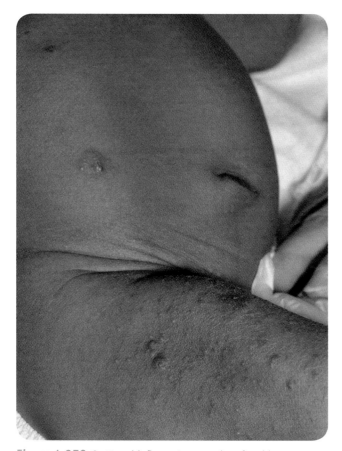

Figure 4-370 Scattered inflammatory papules of scabies.

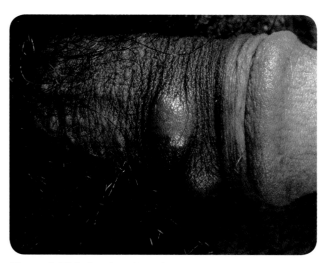

Figure 4-371 Chronic scabies often presents as genital nodules.

- In adults, sexual contact is an important method of transmission, and screening for sexually transmitted diseases may be warranted.

Differential Diagnosis and Pitfalls

- Papular urticaria
- Atopic dermatitis
- Contact dermatitis
- Folliculitis
- Impetigo
- Bites from bedbugs, chiggers, fleas, lice, midges, mosquitoes, or other mites
- Animal scabies—Humans develop excoriated urticarial papules and vesicles in areas of direct contact with infested animals, such as forearms, thighs, abdomen, and chest.
- Nummular eczema
- Viral exanthema (e.g., varicella)
- Dermatitis herpetiformis
- Herpes gestationis
- Eczema herpeticum
- Pruritic urticarial papules and plaques of pregnancy (PUPPP)
- Urticaria pigmentosa (infant)
- Seabather's eruption
- Dyshidrotic dermatitis
- Lichen planus
- Id reaction
- Neurotic excoriations
- Prurigo nodularis
- Syphilis
- Infantile acropustulosis
- Cutaneous larva migrans
- Bullous pemphigoid (usually in the elderly)
- Psoriasis (resembling crusted scabies)
- Langerhans cell histiocytosis (infants and young children)
- Chronic lymphocytic leukemia (nodular scabies)
- B-cell lymphoma (nodular scabies)
- Lymphomatoid papulosis (nodular scabies)

✓ Best Tests

- Perform a scabies prep. Put a small amount of mineral oil on the area to be tested and use a blunt curette to gather material from under the finger nails or a No. 15 blade to gently scrape the terminal end of the burrow where you see the tiny black (or, in skin types IV to VI, tan to reddish) speck. Scrapings are then placed on a glass slide with a cover slip. Examine under the light microscope for the presence of mites, their eggs, or scybala (fecal pellets).
- Burrows may be more easily identified by covering a suspected burrow with the ink from a fountain or marking pen and then wiping away with an alcohol pad after a minute or two. The ink will penetrate the burrow, making it more visible.
- In cases of crusted scabies, add a few drops of 10% potassium hydroxide (KOH) solution to the skin scraping to break down the excess keratin. Scales will typically contain many mites. KOH may dissolve the scybala, which are best seen using saline or mineral oil.

Management Pearls

- Treat the entire family and all close contacts at the same time. Close contacts may be infected but not yet symptomatic and will, therefore, be unaware of the infection. If untreated, they will pass the mite back to others.
- Untreated nails can act as a reservoir of infection, resulting in treatment failure. This is why it is recommended to trim the nails very short, followed by brushing of the fingertips with a topical scabicide on consecutive days in addition to the regular treatment.
- Children, especially in poor countries, frequently present with scabies superinfected by group A streptococci or *Staphylococcus aureus*, which should be treated first.
- Patients should be instructed to launder bed linens, towels, and clothing used in the last 72 hours prior to treatment in hot water and dry on high heat. Items that cannot be laundered can be sealed in airtight plastic bags for 10 to 14 days. All carpets and upholstered furniture should be thoroughly vacuumed, followed by disposal of the vacuum bags or canisters. It is important that such control measures coincide with the pharmacologic treatment of household members.
- Make sure to tell the patient that lesions can take a week or more to clear, as the immune reaction will continue despite killing the mite with the treatment. More importantly, pruritus may persist for up to 4 weeks despite complete eradication of live mites.
- Scabies is very difficult to eradicate from hospital settings once an outbreak has occurred. Prompt identification of affected patients and appropriate isolation is essential. Hospital infection-control teams should be involved at the outset of case identification to help control spread.

Precautions: Standard and Contact. (Isolate patient, wear gloves and a gown, limit patient transport, and avoid sharing patient-care equipment.)

Therapy

CDC-Recommended Regimens
Permethrin 5% cream applied to all areas of the body from the neck down and washed off after 8 to 14 hours. The treatment is repeated again a week later.

OR

Ivermectin 200 μg/kg orally, repeated in 2 weeks, as it might not be effective against all stages of the scabies life cycle (i.e., no ovicidal action).

Permethrin is effective and safe, and it is less expensive than ivermectin. One study demonstrated increased mortality among elderly, debilitated persons who received ivermectin, but this observation has not been confirmed in subsequent reports.

Note that resistance to topical permethrin appears to be on the rise.

CDC-Recommended Alternative Regimen
Lindane (gamma benzene hexachloride) 1% lotion (max 30 mL) or cream (max 30 g) applied in a thin layer to all areas of the body from the neck down and thoroughly washed off after 8 hours. Lindane is not recommended as first-line therapy because of toxicity. It should only be used as an alternative if the patient cannot tolerate other therapies or if other therapies have failed.

Lindane should not be used immediately after a bath or shower, and it should not be used by persons who have extensive dermatitis, women who are pregnant or lactating, or children younger than 2 years of age. Lindane resistance has been reported in some areas of the world, including parts of the United States. Seizures have occurred when lindane was applied after a bath or used by patients who had extensive dermatitis. Aplastic anemia after lindane use has also been reported.

Other Topical Scabicides
Other topical scabicides to consider include benzyl benzoate 10% emulsion, 25% lotion; crotamiton 10% cream, lotion; malathion 0.5% lotion; sulphur precipitate 2% to 10% in petrolatum; monosulfiram 5% soap, 25% solution, emulsion; esdepallethrin 0.63% aerosolized spray; and ivermectin 1.8% cream.

Crusted Scabies
For patients with crusted scabies, an attempt should be made to remove as much of the crusted scale as possible prior to initiating therapy with a topical scabicide. Mechanical debridement can be facilitated with warm soaks followed by the application of a keratolytic agent (e.g., ammonium lactate 12% cream). Such patients may require repeated applications of a topical scabicide and repeated doses of ivermectin.

Pruritus
Antihistamines for pruritus are an important adjunctive treatment:

- Diphenhydramine hydrochloride (25, 50 mg tablets or capsules): 25 to 50 mg nightly or every 6 hours as needed
- Hydroxyzine (10, 25 mg tablets): 10 to 25 mg every 6 hours as needed
- Cetirizine hydrochloride (5, 10 mg tablets): 5 to 10 mg/d
- Loratadine (10 mg tablets and RediTabs): 10 mg tablet or RediTab once daily

Consider a short course of topical or oral corticosteroids for patients in whom the reaction is severe. Intralesional corticosteroids have been used in the treatment of nodular scabies.

Suggested Readings

Hengge UR, Currie BJ, Jäger G, et al. Scabies: a ubiquitous neglected skin disease. *Lancet Infect Dis.* 2006;6(12):769–779.

Hicks MI, Elston DM. Scabies. *Dermatol Ther.* 2009;22(4):279–292.

Karthikeyan K. Scabies in children. *Arch Dis Child Educ Pract Ed.* 2007;92(3):ep65–ep69.

Leone PA. Scabies and pediculosis pubis: An update of treatment regimens and general review. *Clin Infect Dis.* 2007;44(Suppl 3):S153–S159.

Lomholt G. Scabies in blacks. *Arch Dermatol.* 1979;115(6):675.

Mackenzie R. Scabies in negroes. *Br Med J.* 1969;1(5642):513.

Rietschel RL, Lewis CW, Jones HE, et al. Scabies and the role of race. *Arch Dermatol.* 1979;115(1):109–110.

Wilson M, Lountzis N, Ferringer T. Zoonoses of dermatologic interest. *Dermatol Ther.* 2009;22(4):367–378.

Atopic Dermatitis (Eczema)

Erin Luxenberg

Atopic dermatitis is one of the most common skin diseases and will be discussed in detail. A rare complication of the disease with disseminated herpes simplex infection will also be discussed. Discussions on some rare genetic syndromes, Netherton disease, Wiskott-Aldrich syndrome, and the hyper-IgE syndrome, in which patients often have severe atopic dermatitis, can be found on VisualDx online. (If you are a first-time online user, go to www.essentialdermatology.com/pigmented; if you already have your password set up, go directly to www.visualdx.com/visualdx.)

■■ Diagnosis Synopsis

Atopic Dermatitis (Eczema)

Atopic dermatitis (eczema) is a common disorder that more often affects allergy-prone people, especially those with the atopic triad of eczema, asthma, and allergic rhinitis. It is two times more prevalent in patients with pigmented skin and in individuals of lower socioeconomic status. The exact pathophysiologic mechanism causing the disease is unknown, but there is an association with mutation in the filaggrin genes, which leads to defects in the skin's barrier function. Most patients with atopic dermatitis have marked xerosis and an inability to retain epidermal moisture. Known triggers of the disease and its associated itching include heat, humidity, soaps, chemicals, lack of sleep, fabrics with small fibers such as wool, and stress. Scratching, by itself, intensifies the itching. The clinical presentation ranges from pruritus and xerosis, to lichenified papules and plaques, to weeping and crusted areas of dry skin. Infants and children are most frequently affected, but the condition can persist into adulthood.

Pediatric Patient Considerations

Children are affected more frequently than adults. In infants, atopic dermatitis is recognized by one or more of the following principal characteristics: intense pruritus; a screaming, fussy baby; face, scalp, torso, and extensor involvement during infancy; a chronic, relapsing course of lesions; and a family history of the atopic triad of atopic dermatitis, allergic rhinitis, and/or asthma. In children, as in adults, presentation of the atopic lesions is often associated with asthma and allergic rhinitis, and there is frequently a familial history of atopy. In childhood, the disease involves the flexural aspects of extremities as opposed to the extensor areas affected in infants.

Upward of 10% of children in some Asian populations are affected by atopic dermatitis, and the vast majority of these cases are mild. African American children tend to continue to present with the infantile distribution of lesions in the facial/extensor area throughout childhood. Scratching induces lichenification, and lichen planus-like-appearing atopic dermatitis has thus far been reported only in heavily pigmented children.

Eczema Herpeticum (Kaposi Varicelliform Eruption)

Eczema herpeticum is a generalized infection of herpes simplex virus (HSV) in a patient with a preexisting skin disease such as atopic dermatitis. Vesicles, pustules, and erosions appear most prominently in areas of skin involved with the dermatitis. Presentation can range from mild and transient to life threatening. Eczema herpeticum is more commonly seen in patients with atopic dermatitis but may also be seen in cases of Darier disease, pemphigus, burns, mycosis fungoides, pityriasis rubra pilaris, and other forms of dermatitis such as irritant contact and seborrheic dermatitis.

Patients can develop hundreds of lesions over a short period of time; this is often associated with malaise, lymphadenopathy, and fever (Fig. 4-372). Primary infection is usually more severe than recurrent episodes, which are uncommon. The disease is typically self-limited, lasting 2 to 4 weeks, but can be shortened by antiviral therapy. It mostly affects children but can occur in any age group. In healthy patients, mild cases can be self-limited and may only require supportive care. Severe cases may result in systemic viremia, multiorgan involvement, and serious morbidity and mortality, especially in infants.

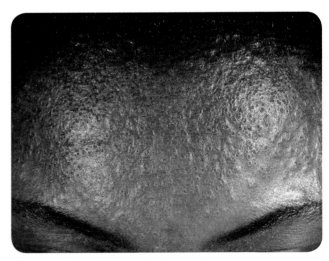

Figure 4-372 Multiple annular lesions of eczema herpeticum on the forehead.

◉ Look For

Atopic Dermatitis (Eczema)

Known as "the itch that rashes," itch will precede the rash, which develops after rubbing or scratching. Look for thickened, scaly, red-brown papules and plaques involving the flexural surfaces in adults. Generally, lesions are most often located on the face (sparing the nose), neck, antecubital fossae, popliteal fossae, and extremities (Fig. 4-373). When infected, plaques can develop thick, oozing, yellow crusts. Chronic papules and plaques can be deeply pigmented, especially in heavily pigmented skin. Dark skin can present with extensive follicular accentuation and shininess without the discrete lichenified plaques often seen in fairer skin tones (Fig. 4-374). These patients also have more postinflammatory hyperpigmentation or hypopigmentation than those with lighter skin.

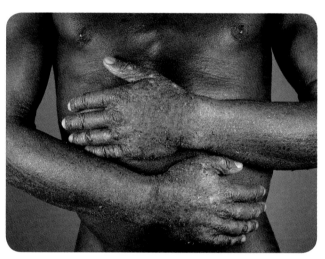

Figure 4-373 Generalized scaling and fine crusted lesions are common in atopic dermatitis.

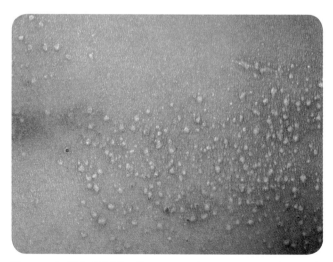

Figure 4-374 Multiple discrete papules are common in atopic dermatitis.

Pediatric Patient Considerations

In neonates and infants, atopic dermatitis consists of pink to red scaly plaques with variable degrees of crusting. They occur most on the face and scalp, with general sparing of the diaper area and nasal tip. Uninvolved skin can be dry, slightly erythematous, and even scaly. Hair loss and an extension of a facial rash can result from the infant rubbing his or her head against a crib sheet to alleviate the itch. These babies usually have poor-quality sleep due to the pruritus. Lesions are frequently impetiginized due to secondary infection (Fig. 4-375).

In later infancy, plaques tend to involve the extensor areas of the legs and arms, and in older children and teenagers, the lesions tend to involve flexural surfaces. As children age, lesions are less likely to be exudative and are most prominent on the posterior neck, antecubital fossae, popliteal fossae, and extremities (Figs. 4-376 and 4-377).

In darkly pigmented children, look for hyperlinear palms and extensive accentuation of the follicles, as these children may not present with the common lichenified pink plaques (Fig. 4-378).

Pityriasis alba, dry, hypopigmented patches, will commonly present on the cheeks in children.

Eczema Herpeticum (Kaposi Varicelliform Eruption)

Look for umbilicated vesicles or pustules. The lesions are usually grouped in a herpetiform pattern, and multiple scattered umbilicated vesicles, pustules, and discrete erosions can often be seen.

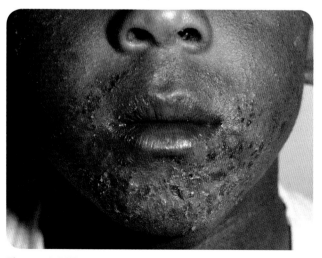

Figure 4-375 Atopic dermatitis with marked erosions and crust suggests secondary bacterial infection.

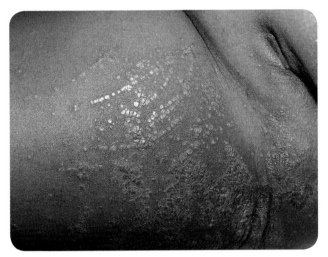

Figure 4-376 Linear shiny papules of atopic dermatitis in the groin of a girl.

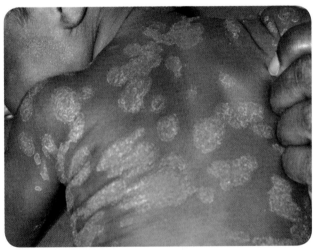

Figure 4-377 Large well-delimited scaly plaques are frequent in atopic dermatitis.

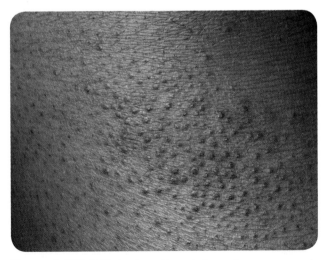

Figure 4-378 Follicular hyperpigmented papules are commonly seen in atopic dermatitis in dark skin.

Diagnostic Pearls

Atopic Dermatitis (Eczema)

- Obtain an adequate childhood and family history of allergies and skin disease.
- In adults, persistent dry skin or eyelid dermatitis is a clue to atopic dermatitis.
- Increased risk of infection by HSV and *Staphylococcus*
- In general, it is rare for an adult without a personal or family history of atopy to develop atopic dermatitis. Such patients should be referred to a dermatologist to rule out other entities, specifically cutaneous T-cell lymphoma and chronic skin allergies.
- Hyperlinearity of the palms and flexor surface of the fingers as well as hair breakage in the temporal area are common.

Pediatric Patient Considerations

- Cutaneous signs of atopic dermatitis in darkly pigmented children include linear transverse folds just below the edge of the lower eyelids (Dennie-Morgan folds), perinasal and periorbital pallor ("headlight sign"), more distinct periorbital hyperpigmentation from chronic rubbing, thinning of the lateral eyebrows (Hertoghe sign), and hyperkeratosis and hyperpigmentation producing the appearance of a "dirty neck."
- In infants, there is usually sparing of the diaper area in atopic dermatitis, in contrast to its involvement in seborrheic dermatitis.

Eczema Herpeticum (Kaposi Varicelliform Eruption)

- Scattered umbilicated vesicles in varying numbers can be concentrated most in skin folds. These lesions may appear as "punched-out" erosions. The patient is generally already affected with an inflammatory dermatitis, and herpetic eruption is frequently concentrated in the affected areas.
- The lesions are often superinfected with bacteria, which may complicate the morphological diagnosis due to the yellow, crusty appearance.

?? Differential Diagnosis and Pitfalls

Atopic Dermatitis (Eczema)

- Seborrheic dermatitis
- Allergic or irritant contact dermatitis
- Lichen simplex chronicus
- Nummular eczema
- Scabies
- HIV-associated dermatitis

- Mycosis fungoides/cutaneous T-cell lymphoma—mainly adults
- Tinea corporis
- Psoriasis
- Pityriasis rosea
- Langerhans cell histiocytosis—mainly children

Pediatric Patient Considerations

- Severe disease in children—Wiskott-Aldrich syndrome, selective IgA deficiency, or hyper-IgE syndrome, Netherton syndrome

Eczema Herpeticum (Kaposi Varicelliform Eruption)

- Primary varicella
- Disseminated zoster in the immunosuppressed host
- Impetigo
- Disseminated molluscum contagiosum
- Erysipelas
- Contact dermatitis
- Dermatitis herpetiformis
- Vesicular drug reaction or viral exanthem

Best Tests

Atopic Dermatitis (Eczema)

- Take a careful history, as atopic dermatitis is primarily a clinical diagnosis. Most patients will have a family history of asthma or atopy, and many will admit to the atopic triad of eczema, asthma, and allergic rhinitis.
- In select cases, the following investigations may help rule out imitators:
  - Skin biopsy—may not be specific for atopic dermatitis
  - Skin scrapings—rule out scabies and tinea
  - Serum immunoglobulin levels (IgE, IgA, IgM, IgG)— though serum IgE level is elevated in 80% of patients, not routinely done or necessary
  - In certain cases—oral food challenges, radioallergosorbent test or skin allergy testing, HIV testing
- Bacterial culture should be sent if lesions appear infected. Impetigo appears with thick, oozing, yellow or red crusts. A Tzanck smear viral culture, and/or viral PCR should be performed if the patient might have eczema herpeticum, consisting of acute onset of an oozing, vesicular eruption or erosions with serpiginous borders.

Eczema Herpeticum (Kaposi Varicelliform Eruption)

- In suspected eczema herpeticum (Kaposi varicelliform eruption—Tzanck preparation of scrapings from the roof of a vesicle to look for multinucleated giant cells and viral culture of PCR for HSV.

Management Pearls

Atopic Dermatitis (Eczema)

- Secondary bacterial infection may exacerbate atopic dermatitis. Treat with a 10-day course of oral antibiotics to cover *Staphylococcus aureus* infection.
- Counsel patients on typical triggers, and encourage their avoidance. Factors that are known to exacerbate atopic dermatitis include the following: stress, certain bathing habits (e.g., prolonged, hot showers), infection, irritants (e.g., detergents, scented soaps, woolen clothing), sweating, environmental allergens, and dry low-humidity air in winter.
- Emollients and moisturizing skin care routines are essential. Nonsoap cleansers and sensitive, fragrancefree soaps are recommended. Have the patient apply emollients such as petroleum jelly to damp skin immediately after bathing and again three or more times during the day.
- Some darkly pigmented patients prefer ointments rather than creams or gels. Narrow-band UVB is also successful. Tacrolimus may also be a first line of treatment.

Pediatric Patient Considerations

- Emphasis on good skin care is important. This includes use of nonsoap cleansers and the use of fragrancefree and dyefree emollients to ease itching and prevent the need for oral antihistamines. Adequate humidification during winter is important.
- In infants, it can be associated with failure to thrive, recurrent infections, hematologic abnormalities, and chronic diarrhea.

Eczema Herpeticum (Kaposi Varicelliform Eruption)

- Patients with eczema herpeticum may pass the HSV infection to others.
- Ophthalmologic evaluation in any patient with facial involvement

Therapy

Atopic Dermatitis (Eczema)
Topical corticosteroids are used to treat active, inflamed plaques. Nonfluorinated topical steroids should be used on the face, and mid- to high-potency preparations can be used on the trunk and extremities. Patients frequently become sensitive to preservatives in topical medications,

(Continued)

so ointments are recommended, as these usually contain fewer irritating and allergy-inducing factors.

For Localized Disease
Darkly pigmented individuals do well with steroid-sparing agents such as tacrolimus, as there is less hypopigmentation. A thin layer of tacrolimus ointment to the affected skin is considered safe and effective. However, this medication should *not* be used with occlusive dressings.

Midpotency topical corticosteroids such as triamcinolone or fluocinolone can also be used effectively; close supervision with scheduled follow-up is needed.

Use low-potency topical steroids such as desonide on the face and intertriginous areas.

For Extensive Disease
Cyclosporin, azathioprine, tacrolimus, and mycophenolate mofetil have all been used to treat extensive, resistant disease in both adults and children with varying degrees of success. Phototherapy—including UVB, PUVA (psoralen plus UVA), and, most recently, narrow-band UVB—has also been used successfully in many patients.

Avoid oral or intramuscular steroids in all patients.

For Pruritus
Antihistamines can be a helpful component of treatment. If pruritus continues after dermatitis is well controlled, physicians may consider using oral antihistamines.

For Infection
Antibiotic therapy is beneficial when there is evidence of overlying infection, characterized by honey-colored crust, denuded skin, or oozing. Treat with a 10-day course of oral antibiotics to cover *S. aureus* infection. As methicillin-resistant *S. aureus* (MRSA) becomes more prevalent in the community, therapy should be appropriately tailored. Dilute bleach baths up to three times weekly may be useful in a patient with multiple open areas due to excoriation or a history of multiple superinfections. Secondary infection due to HSV should be treated with acyclovir.

Eczema Herpeticum (Kaposi Varicelliform Eruption)
While some patients will have a self-limited course of disease and not require treatment, others will require hospitalization and intravenous acyclovir or even intravenous foscarnet in acyclovir-resistant cases. If hospitalized, the patient should be isolated from others, and universal protective precautions should be used. In systemically ill patients, maximize supportive measures. This includes meticulous attention to fluid and electrolyte balance, wound care, pain control, and nutrition.

Monitor for and treat any complicating infection with the appropriate antibiotic therapy. Cool compresses and emollients may provide some symptomatic relief.

Treatment with acyclovir, or its prodrugs valacyclovir or famciclovir, works best to target the virus.

Anti-staphylococcal antibiotics target bacteria of the skin that could cause superinfection by invasion of the open wounds.

Pediatric Patient Considerations

In children, intermittent use of topical corticosteroids is advised to treat the active, inflamed, palpable plaques. Once the areas are smooth, the steroids should be discontinued. In general, use low- to midpotency preparations on the face and mid- to high-potency preparations on the trunk and extremities. The goal of treatment is to quickly clear the dermatitis with the lowest-effective-strength topical steroid. Be careful of atrophy from steroids in skin folds and occluded areas. Try to use ointments, which usually require fewer preservatives and stabilizers. Topical nonsteroidal agents, including tacrolimus and pimecrolimus, are typically less effective than topical corticosteroids in children and frequently elicit a burning sensation with their application. The FDA has placed a black box warning on these in children younger than 2 years because of reported cases of lymphoma.

Studies have shown that these types of medications do not vary in effectiveness depending on ethnicity, so children of all skin types can be treated with the same medications.

Suggested Readings

Brenninkmeijer EE, Schram ME, Leeflang MM, et al. Diagnostic criteria for atopic dermatitis: A systematic review. *Br J Dermatol* 2008;158(4):754–765.

Bussman C, Peng WM, Bieber T, et al. Molecular pathogenesis and clinical implications of eczema herpeticum. *Exp Rev Mol Med* 2008;10:e21.

Eichenfield LF, Lucky AW, Langley RG, et al. Use of pimecrolimus cream 1% (Elidel) in the treatment of atopic dermatitis in infants and children: The effects of ethnic origin and baseline disease severity on treatment outcome. *Int J Dermatol* 2005;44(1):70–75.

Herbert BA, Jones NP, Bowen SE. Lichenoid and other clinical presentations of atopic dermatitis in an inner city practice. *J Am Acad Dermatol* 2008;58(3):503–504.

Kang K, Polster AM, Nedorost ST, et al. Atopic dermatitis. In: Bolognia JL, Jorizzo JL, Rapini RP, eds. *Dermatology*. 2nd Ed. St. Louis, MO: Mosby/Elsevier; 2008:199–214.

Saeki H, et al. Prevalence of atopic dermatitis in japanese elementary school children. *Br J Dermatol* 2005;152(1):110–114.

Willams HC. Clinical practice. Atopic dermatitis. *N Engl J Med*. 2005; 352(22):2314–2324.

Folliculitis

Mat Davey

◼◼ Diagnosis Synopsis

Folliculitis refers broadly to inflammation of the pilosebaceous unit, clinically presenting as folliculocentric papules and pustules. Etiologic factors include infectious pathogens (such as bacteria, viruses, fungi, and yeast), physical irritation, systemic drugs, and underlying disease states.

The most common pathogen associated with bacterial folliculitis is *Staphylococcus*. Both methicillin-sensitive *Staphylococcus aureus* (MSSA) and methicillin-resistant *S. aureus* (MRSA) may cause folliculitis. The incidence of community-acquired MRSA (CA-MRSA) disease has been increasing and is associated with a unique presentation. Whereas MSSA folliculitis is usually localized to the axillae, bearded area, buttocks, and extremities, MRSA folliculitis is oftentimes more widespread, affecting the periumbilical area, chest, flank, and scrotum. Those at increased risk of developing staphylococcal folliculitis include immunocompromised patients or individuals with nasal *Staphylococcus* carriage, hyperhidrosis, skin injury, and preexisting dermatitis.

Less common causes of bacterial folliculitis occur among patients with specific risk factors and are associated with unique presentations. Patients on chronic antibiotic therapy (e.g., those taking tetracycline for acne vulgaris) are at increased risk of developing Gram-negative folliculitis. Commonly associated organisms in this setting are *Klebsiella* species, *Escherichia coli*, *Enterobacter* species, and *Proteus* species. Patients with this subset of folliculitis often display a more chronic and unremitting course. *Pseudomonas* folliculitis, or hot tub folliculitis, is a subset of folliculitis associated with infection of hair follicles with *Pseudomonas* bacteria. Outbreaks occur in people after bathing in a contaminated spa, swimming pool, or hot tub. It is also associated with the use of contaminated loofah sponges (that remain constantly wet in the shower) and contaminated water in the workplace.

Malassezia folliculitis (also known as *Pityrosporum* folliculitis) is an acute, intensely pruritic eruption caused by *Malassezia furfur*, the causative organism of tinea versicolor. The condition frequently manifests as follicular papules and pustules on the upper trunk of young to middle-aged adults. Immunocompromised patients, including those on chronic oral prednisone and diabetics, are at higher risk. High heat, humidity, and occlusive clothing or personal care products predispose to the condition. Recent use of oral antibiotics is also a risk factor.

Less common infectious etiologic factors associated with folliculitis include *Candida* (seen in diabetics, the immunocompromised, and those on antibiotics), herpes simplex virus type 1, and varicella-zoster virus.

Eosinophilic folliculitis, a culture-negative folliculitis, is a unique entity that is not associated with an identified organism at present. It is most commonly seen in HIV-infected or immunologically impaired patients. It is characterized by multiple pruritic pustules and papules on the face, trunk, and extremities, which are often extremely symptomatic and refractory to treatment.

Sterile folliculitis may be secondary to physical irritation or medications. Perspiration, friction, occlusion, shaving, and chemical irritants, particularly mineral oil and tar-based products, may lead to irritation-associated folliculitis (Figs. 4-379 and 4-380). Systemic medications, especially steroids, have been shown to induce a sterile folliculitis. Other medications commonly associated with folliculitislike eruptions include anabolic steroids, phenytoin, lithium, isoniazid, halogenated compounds, and epidermal growth factor receptor inhibitors.

Regardless of the causative agent, individual lesions of folliculitis may be asymptomatic, painful, or pruritic. Lesions often heal spontaneously without scarring, although deep infection and excoriation may lead to scars. Folliculitis occurs in both sexes as well as all ethnicities and age groups (Fig. 4-381).

Fox-Fordyce disease, a rare inflammatory condition of apocrine gland-bearing regions caused by obliteration of the follicular infundibulum with keratin, may present as a folliculitis. The etiology is unknown, although an endocrine role has been postulated. The disease manifests as intensely pruritic, skin-colored, or keratotic papules in the axillary, pubic, and periareolar areas. Heat, humidity, and stress may be exacerbating factors. It is most common in women during adolescence, but it can be seen between puberty and age 35.

◉ Look For

In cases of bacterial folliculitis, look for small, erythematous papules and pustules pierced by a central hair. They may be of varying sizes and will be in a follicular configuration.

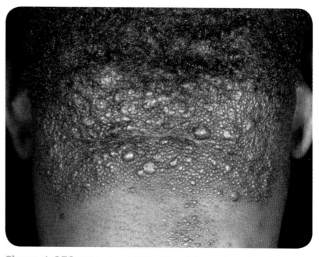

Figure 4-379 Oil-induced folliculitis of the scalp and neck.

Deeper lesions are more nodular and may be fluctuant. Such lesions are frequently tender and may erupt to form crusts on the surface of the skin. Sites of predilection include the face, scalp, axillae, thighs, and inguinal area. CA-MRSA folliculitis can present in an atypical distribution in the periumbilical area, chest, flank, and scrotum.

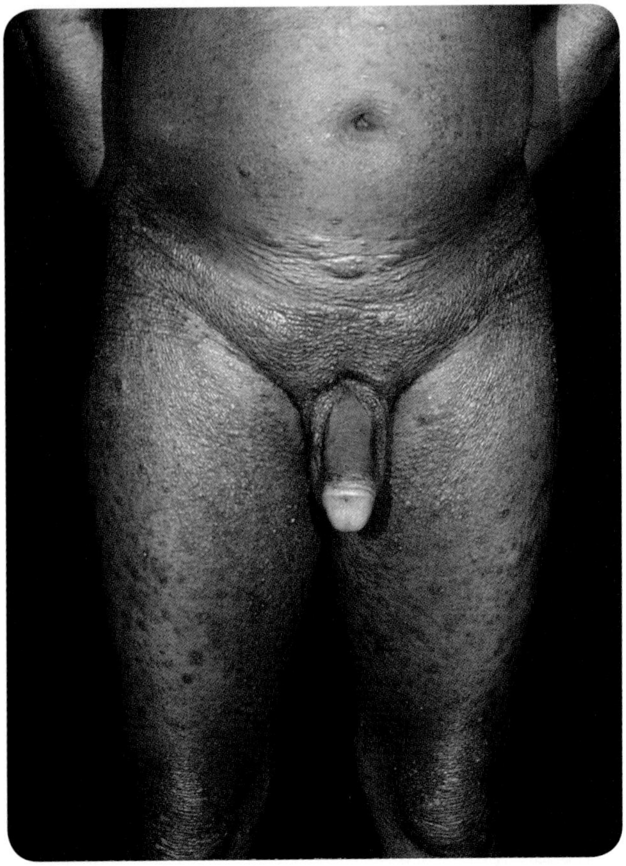

Pseudomonas folliculitis spares the palms, soles, and face. Look for follicular, erythematous papules and pustules that may have crusts and are typically found on the trunk/bathing suit area and in intertriginous areas. There is more peripheral redness than with the usual case of staphylococcal folliculitis.

In *Malassezia* folliculitis, look for monomorphous, erythematous papules and pustules in a follicular pattern on the upper back and neighboring areas near the arms, neck, shoulders, and scalp (Fig. 4-382). It is rarely seen on the face.

In eosinophilic folliculitis, papules and pustules are usually excoriated due to severe pruritus. Lesions predominate on the face, superior chest, and back (Fig. 4-383).

In patients with Fox-Fordyce disease, look for multiple monomorphous, small (2 to 3 mm) skin-colored to light brown to yellow papules in apocrine-dense areas such as the axillae, areolae, and pubic areas (mons pubis and labia

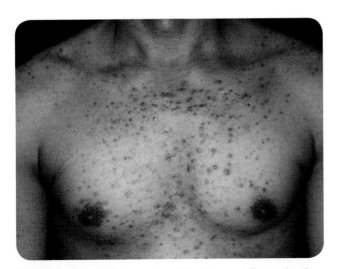

Figure 4-380 Oil-induced folliculitis with intertriginous sparing.

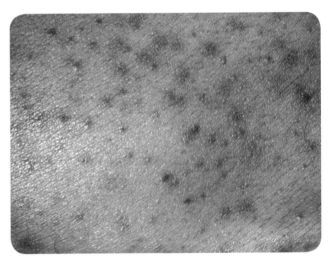

Figure 4-382 *Malassezia* (*Pityrosporum*) folliculitis in a patient with HIV infection.

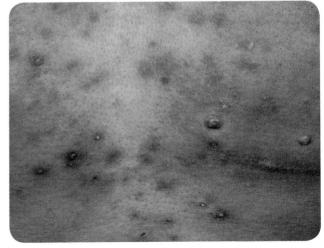

Figure 4-381 Multiple papules with minimum inflammation in a common location for folliculitis.

Figure 4-383 Eosinophilic folliculitis in a characteristic location in a patient with AIDS.

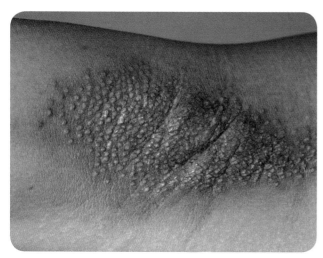

Figure 4-384 Multiple grouped follicular noninflammatory papules in the axillae are characteristic of Fox-Fordyce disease.

majora) (Fig. 4-384). Each papule is perifollicular and has a central punctum. Keratotic material may be expressed. Sometimes the papules may contain a milky fluid.

In all of the above cases, erythema is often less pronounced in darkly pigmented individuals. Look for pigmented brown papules and postinflammatory changes as clues to the underlying disease process.

●● Diagnostic Pearls

- Bacterial folliculitis occurs more frequently among people (especially men) who exercise daily. Shaving, occlusion, and chronic rubbing may incite or exacerbate the disease.
- Gram-negative folliculitis is more common among individuals taking long-term antibiotics (such as for the treatment of acne).
- Down syndrome, seborrheic dermatitis, and anticonvulsant therapy are associated with *Malassezia* folliculitis.
- In Fox-Fordyce disease, the pruritus is extreme and is out of proportion to the degree of redness.

?? Differential Diagnosis and Pitfalls

- Molluscum contagiosum
- Pseudofolliculitis barbae
- Acne keloidalis nuchae
- Acute generalized exanthematous pustulosis
- Keratosis pilaris
- Perforating diseases
- Milia
- Perioral dermatitis
- Acne
- HIV

- Rosacea
- Candidiasis
- Seabather's eruption
- Insect bites
- Miliaria rubra
- Scabies
- Tinea corporis
- Eruptive xanthomas

✓ Best Tests

- Most cases can be diagnosed clinically. Skin biopsy may be needed in cases that prove unresponsive to therapy.
- Perform an aerobic culture of lesions, especially in severe or recalcitrant cases. Sensitivities should be performed on any *S. aureus* isolates to determine antibiotic resistance.
- Perform a KOH preparation if yeast or fungi are under consideration.
- Patients with recurrent bacterial folliculitis should have their anterior nares swabbed to assess for bacterial colonization.
- Any further workup will be dictated by the clinical scenario. Patients suspected of being immunosuppressed or having underlying systemic disease merit additional tests, such as a CBC, HIV testing, etc.

▲▲ Management Pearls

- In patients with bacterial folliculitis, treatment is directed at the underlying infection or avoidance of external irritants. Changing the patient's skin routine is often beneficial. Antibacterial soaps are sometimes helpful. In widespread, recalcitrant, or severely symptomatic cases, systemic antibiotics can shorten the course of the illness.
- Given the prevalence of MRSA, maintain a high index of suspicion for this diagnosis, and make the initial choice of any empiric antibiotic therapy accordingly. Eradication of MRSA nasal carriage may be accomplished by application of mupirocin 2% cream (twice daily for 5 days) to the nares. The combination of rifampin (600 mg daily for 10 days) plus trimethoprim/sulfamethoxazole (TMP-SMX)—one double-strength tablet twice daily for 10 days—has also been shown to eradicate colonization.
- In cases of *Malassezia* folliculitis, topical creams containing imidazole are sometimes effective; however, systemic medications are usually necessary to treat organisms deep in the follicle. Topical agents (i.e., ketoconazole shampoo) may need to be continued for longer periods to prevent relapse.
- Severe cases of eosinophilic folliculitis may respond to narrowband UVB phototherapy.
- In patients with Fox-Fordyce disease, oral contraceptives can be a useful adjuvant to therapy.

Therapy

In cases of mild-to-moderate bacterial folliculitis, topical antibiotics applied twice daily may be beneficial. Possible topical regimens include the following:

- Mupirocin 2% ointment/cream
- Erythromycin 2% solution/gel
- Clindamycin 1% solution/gel/lotion
- Benzoyl peroxide gel/wash can also be used without combination with an antibiotic: 2.5%, 4%, 5%, or 10% gel depending on skin dryness. (Use milder strengths when the skin is dry, and use higher concentrations on very oily skin.)

If there is no response to topical therapy after approximately 1 month or for widespread or deep-seated cases, use an antistaphylococcal oral antibiotic:

- Dicloxacillin or cephalexin 500 mg p.o. four times daily for 10 to 14 days
- Azithromycin 500 mg the first day, then 250 mg daily for 5 days is an alternative

Standard cephalosporins and penicillins are of no benefit in treating CA-MRSA. Refer to current CDC guidelines, as treatment is rapidly changing.

For patients with *Pseudomonas* folliculitis, ciprofloxacin 500 mg p.o. twice daily for 10 days should be prescribed for those who are immunosuppressed and patients with persistent disease.

In *Malassezia* folliculitis, a combination of an oral and a topical agent work best. Topical therapies include:

- Imidazole antifungal creams—clotrimazole, miconazole, econazole, or ketoconazole applied to the involved areas twice daily for 2 to 4 weeks
- Ciclopirox—apply to involved areas twice daily for 4 weeks
- Ketoconazole shampoo—apply twice weekly for 4 weeks

Oral therapy includes:

- Ketoconazole 200 mg daily for 1 to 2 weeks
- Itraconazole 200 mg daily for 1 to 2 weeks
- Fluconazole 300 mg once weekly four to six times.

In patients with eosinophilic folliculitis, use high-potency topical corticosteroids (class 2) on truncal skin, moderate-potency steroids (classes 3 and 4) on other areas, and low-potency steroids (classes 6 and 7) on the face. In addition, oral antihistamines such as hydroxyzine 10, 25 mg p.o. every 6 hours or diphenhydramine 25 mg p.o. every 6 hours as tolerated may help with pruritus.

In Fox-Fordyce disease, use mid-potency topical steroids (classes 3 and 4) and palliative topical antipruritic formulations such as pramoxine with menthol and camphor. Oral contraceptives have also demonstrated efficacy. In addition, topical retinoids such as tretinoin 0.025% cream applied nightly and topical clindamycin 1% solution/lotion applied to affected areas twice daily may be of benefit. Surgical excision is an option for severe cases. Liposuction may offer relief without the morbidity of surgery. For severe cases, oral isotretinoin is effective, but the lesions seem to recur after discontinuing the medication.

Pediatric Patient Considerations

For uncomplicated infections not caused by MRSA, topical mupirocin may be used twice daily. If involvement is more widespread, oral antibiotics should be used. First-generation cephalosporins, penicillin, and amoxicillin/clavulanic acid are good options.

For CA-MRSA, refer to current CDC guidelines, as treatment recommendations are rapidly changing.

Suggested Readings

Boni R, Nehrhoff B. Treatment of Gram-negative folliculitis in patients with acne. *Am J Clin Dermatol.* 2003;4(4):273–276.

Budavari JM, Grayson W. Papular follicular eruptions in human immunodeficiency virus-positive patients in South Africa. *Int J Dermatol.* 2007;46(7):706–710.

Cohen PR. Community-acquired methicillin-resistant *Staphlococcus aureus* skin infection presenting as a periumbical folliculitis. *Cutis.* 2006;77(4):229–232.

Helm TN, Chen PW. Fox-Fordyce disease. *Cutis.* 2002;69(5):335–342.

Luelmo-Aguilar J, Santandreu MS. Folliculitis: Recognition and management. *Am J Clin Dermatol.* 2004;5(5):301–310.

Yu Y, Cheng AS, Wang L, et al. Hot tub folliculitis or hot hand-foot syndrome caused by *Pseudomonas aeruginosa. J Am Acad Dermatol.* 2007;57(4):596–600.

Perforating Diseases

Aída Lugo-Somolinos

■■ Diagnosis Synopsis

Acquired perforating disease or dermatosis (APD) is a term utilized to group several conditions characterized histologically by the transepidermal extrusion of dermal components. The conditions grouped under this term include Kyrle disease, perforating folliculitis, reactive perforating collagenosis, and perforating disorder of renal disease. Elastosis perforans serpiginosa is another perforating disease that is not included under this term because it has unique clinical and histopathologic characteristics.

The etiology of APD is not known, although trauma has always been implicated as a cofactor. The conditions are almost exclusively seen in the setting of diabetes, renal failure, and dialysis. Up to 10% of North Americans receiving hemodialysis may present with APD, and the frequency is increased in patients of African descent.

APD is characterized by umbilicated papules and nodules with central keratotic crusts occurring predominantly on the extremities. The lesions are very itchy, and Koebner phenomenon is common.

Elastosis perforans serpiginosa (EPS) is unique because the keratotic papules are arranged in a serpiginous pattern; the areas of involvement are usually the neck, trunk, and extremities; and it is associated with several inherited disorders such as Down syndrome, osteogenesis imperfecta, Marfan syndrome, and cutis laxa.

EPS has also been associated with treatment with D-penicillamine in patients with Wilson disease. Almost all patients are aged younger than 30, but patient ages in reported cases range from 5 to 89 years. It is more common in men and has been reported in nearly all ethnicities equally.

Pediatric Patient Considerations

EPS may be a marker of an inherited disorder such as Down syndrome, osteogenesis imperfecta, Marfan syndrome, or cutis laxa.

◉ Look For

In APD, look for umbilicated papules and central keratotic crusts in the extremities of hemodialysis patients (Figs. 4-385–4-389). In darkly pigmented patients, these lesions are very hyperpigmented. Itching is always present. Koebner phenomenon is common.

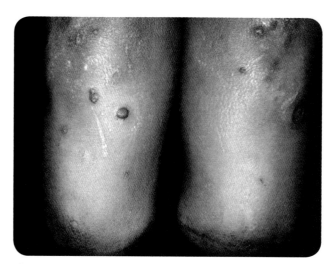

Figure 4-386 Kyrle disease on the extremities.

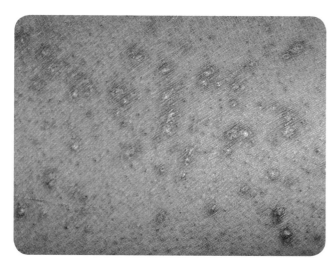

Figure 4-385 Kyrle disease in renal disease associated with diabetes.

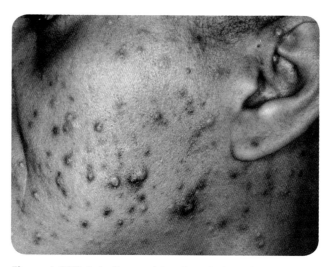

Figure 4-387 Kyrle disease with various-sized papules and nodules (same patient as Fig. 4-386).

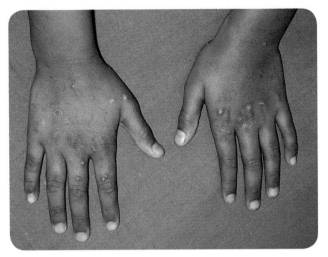

Figure 4-388 Perforating collagenosis in a patient from India.

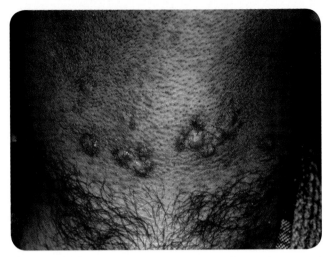

Figure 4-390 Elastosis perforans serpiginosa in a patient treated with penicillamine for 16 years for Wilson disease.

Pediatric Patient Considerations

Look for other signs of inherited disorders.

●● Diagnostic Pearls

- Compressing the papules may express keratin debris or yield hairs or hair fragments. Koebnerization may be present.
- Penicillamine therapy is sometimes associated with perforating diseases, classically EPS.

?? Differential Diagnosis and Pitfalls

Acquired Perforating Disease or Dermatosis

- Acne vulgaris and acneiform eruptions
- Folliculitis
- Keratosis pilaris
- Prurigo nodularis
- Perforating pseudoxanthoma elasticum
- Perforating granuloma annulare
- Flegel disease (hyperkeratosis lenticularis perstans)

Elastosis Perforans Serpiginosa

- Porokeratosis of Mibelli
- Granuloma annulare
- Annular sarcoidosis
- Tinea corporis
- Kyrle disease
- Perforating folliculitis

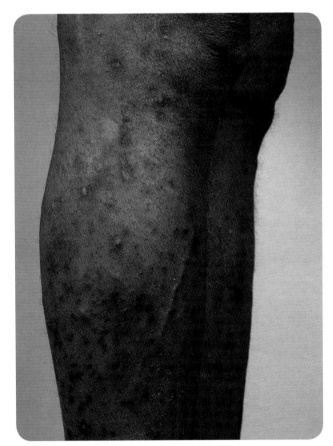

Figure 4-389 Perforating collagenosis, which resembles an eczematous dermatitis in this patient.

In EPS, look for skin-colored to red umbilicated papules often occurring on the extremities and less often on the face and trunk (Fig. 4-390). The lesions are commonly arranged in arcuate or serpiginous patterns. The umbilicated papules have a tightly adherent central crust, which causes bleeding when removed.

✓ Best Tests

- Skin biopsy of APD will show the characteristic extrusion of dermal material through channels traversing an invaginated epidermis. Masson trichrome and Verhoeff-van Gieson stains may help differentiate between the different types of acquired perforating disorders.
- Skin biopsy of EPS will demonstrate dense elastic tissue in the dermis and papillary dermis. A transepidermal channel filled with elastic fibers, degenerated epithelial cells, and granulation tissue is typical.

▲▲ Management Pearls

The association of APD with certain systemic diseases, or their treatments (like penicillamine), is frequent enough such that additional laboratory tests may be indicated if history and/or exam findings are corroborative. These include:

- BUN/creatinine
- Liver function tests
- Uric acid
- Glucose tolerance test
- Thyroid function tests
- Serum parathyroid hormone level

Therapy

Acquired Perforating Disease or Dermatosis

Symptomatic control of pruritus is important. This may be managed with the following:

- Diphenhydramine 25 to 50 mg p.o. three times daily, as necessary
- Hydroxyzine 10 to 25 mg p.o. three times daily, as necessary
- Cetirizine 10 mg p.o. daily
- Doxepin 10 to 25 mg p.o. at night

Soothing lotions containing menthol, phenol, or camphor

Topical corticosteroids or doxepin may also be tried to alleviate itch.

A substantial body of evidence is lacking, but successful treatments have included:

- Oral retinoids (acitretin, isotretinoin)
- Topical retinoids (tretinoin 0.1%, tazarotene)
- Allopurinol 100 mg p.o. daily
- UVB treatment

Elastosis Perforans Serpiginosa

- Discontinuing the D-penicillamine is curative.
- Cryotherapy appears to be effective in eliminating active lesions.
- Intralesional steroids 5 to 10 mg/mL
- Topical retinoids (tretinoin and tazarotene)
- Laser

Suggested Readings

Hodulik S, Carruthers R, Lebwohl MG. Perforating dermatoses. In: *Treatment of Skin Disease, Comprehensive Therapeutic Strategies*. 2nd Ed. St. Louis, MO: Mosby; 2006:478.

Lewis KG, Bercovitch L, Dill SW, et al. Acquired disorders of elastic tissue: Part I. increased elastic tissue and solar elastotic syndromes. *JAAD*. 2004;51(1):1–21.

Neurotic Excoriations

Nasir Aziz

■■ Diagnosis Synopsis

Neurotic excoriation is a skin condition wherein the individual compulsively and habitually scratches and picks at the skin. Unlike patients with dermatitis artefacta, those with neurotic excoriations will usually admit their involvement in creating the lesion. There is a strong relationship between neurotic excoriations and underlying mental illness, most often obsessive compulsive disorder and depression. The disorder is predominantly seen in middle-aged women but can be seen in almost any age. The continued scratching can lead to the itch-scratch-rash cycle, further perpetuating the condition.

◉ Look For

Neurotic excoriators typically produce lesions distributed on the extensor surfaces of the arms and forearms, in addition to the scalp, face, upper back, and buttocks (Figs. 4-391 and 4-392). Lesions can range from millimeters to centimeters and are often in different stages of development or healing. Broken hairs may be seen, and scarring alopecia may develop if the patient picks at the scalp.

●● Diagnostic Pearls

Unlike dermatitis artefacta, patients with neurotic excoriations are more willing to admit their complicity, but cannot stop themselves from producing the lesions. They also do not seek to gain anything from the habit.

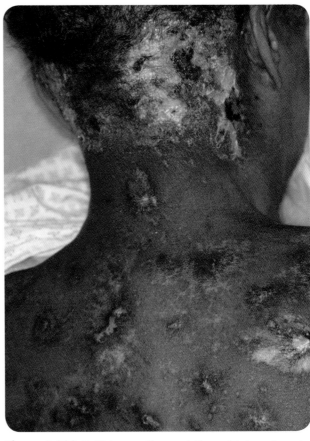

Figure 4-392 Multiple neurotic excoriations with hypopigmentation and hyperpigmentation in a typical location.

?? Differential Diagnosis and Pitfalls

- Evaluate for other causes of pruritus
- Consider neuropathic injury in a localized area of large excoriation
- Systemic disease, including neoplasms
- Delusions of parasitosis
- Scabies

✓ Best Tests

Swab crusted plaques for bacterial culture. A skin biopsy will confirm a clinical diagnosis. If the lesions heal when covered by an occlusive dressing and reappear when exposed, suspect the diagnosis.

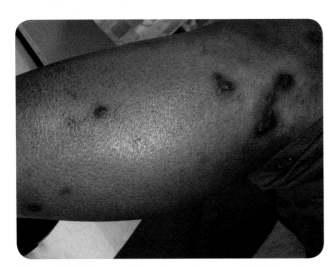

Figure 4-391 Scattered irregular papules, some of which are linear, are suggestive of being self-induced.

Management Pearls

In a nonjudgmental manner, reassure the patient that the problem is a common one and that manipulation may be contributing to continuance of the rash. Some patients scratch and excoriate during sleep and they should be questioned about sleep patterns. Have the patients keep their fingernails clipped very short. Refer the patient to a mental health professional or a drug treatment center, if applicable.

Therapy

Treat neurotic excoriations with occlusive dressings and topical antipruritics. Antihistamines may be effective. Steroid injections may help existing dermatitis but will not prevent the formation of new excoriated plaques. Systemic antibiotics are useful if the lesions are infected, although this is not typical.

Suggested Readings

Arnold LM, Auchenbach MB, McElroy SL. Psychogenic excoriation. Clinical features, proposed diagnostic criteria, epidemiology and approaches to treatment. *CNS Drugs.* 2001;15(5):351–359.

James WD, Berger TG, Elston DM, eds. Pruritus and neurocutaneous dermatoses. In: *Andrews' Diseases of the Skin: Clinical Dermatology.* 10th Ed. Philadelphia, PA: Saunders Elsevier; 2006:61.

Sandoz A, Koenig T, Kusnir D, et al. Psychocutaneoous diseases. In: Fitzpatrick TB, Wolff K, eds. *Fitzpatrick's Dermatology in General Medicine.* 7th Ed. New York, NY: McGraw-Hill; 2008:916.

Infantile Acropustulosis

Alicia Ogram

Diagnosis Synopsis

Infantile acropustulosis (IA) is an uncommon pruritic vesiculopustular disorder of childhood. Some have suggested there is an increased incidence in infants and boys of African descent and during summer months; however, others have disputed this claim.

IA may begin in the neonatal period up to 30 months of age, with most cases beginning by 10 months. IA is a chronic disorder characterized by periodic eruptions of intensely itchy vesicopustules on the acral surfaces. The lesions begin as small red papules, which evolve into vesicles and pustules by 24 hours. The pustules are intensely pruritic, last 7 to 10 days, and appear in crops every 2 to 3 weeks to months. The intervals between each episode lengthen, and the intensity and duration of each eruption decrease until complete resolution occurs, usually by 2 to 3 years of age. The lesions are found on the hands and feet with a predilection for the edges of the palms and soles. They can occasionally be seen on the scalp, trunk, and extremities. Healing can occur with slight hyperpigmentation and scaling. The infant may often have severe pruritus, causing significant irritability, sleeplessness, excoriation, and secondary infection.

The etiology of IA is unknown. Several authors, however, have noted that scabies infestation often precedes IA. It has recently been postulated that there are two forms of IA, a *de novo* or idiopathic form and a form related to prior scabies infestation, which may be a cutaneous hypersensitivity reaction to persistent scabies antigens. Other than clues provided by history, the two forms are clinically indistinguishable.

Look For

The classic lesions of AI are recurrent crops of tense 2- to 4-mm, well-defined pustules on the palms and soles of an infant that last approximately 1 week (Fig. 4-393). However, lesions may appear on any surface of the hands and feet, with additional lesions elsewhere on the body; they may be in any stage of presentation (Fig. 4-394). Early lesions are erythematous pinpoint macules or papules. Late lesions may be 2- to 4-mm hyperpigmented macules (postinflammatory hyperpigmentation). Infants are usually irritable and sleep deprived due to the pruritus; they are otherwise well.

Diagnostic Pearls

Palmar and plantar accentuations are the most important clue to this diagnosis. IA should be diagnosed only after a thorough evaluation—of the patient and family members—excludes scabies.

Differential Diagnosis and Pitfalls

- Scabies infestation—careful examination for a typical burrow or nodular lesions. Family members should also be questioned and examined
- Eosinophilic pustular folliculitis—occurs mainly on the scalp rather than the hands and feet
- Congenital cutaneous candidiasis—less pruritic and usually more widespread

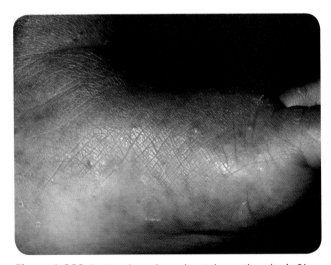

Figure 4-393 Scattered papules and pustules on the soles in IA.

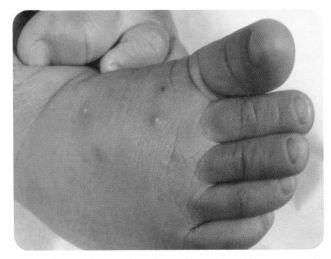

Figure 4-394 Scattered papules and pustules on the dorsum of the foot in IA.

- Erythema toxicum neonatorum—less pruritic and usually more widespread
- Transient neonatal pustular melanosis—less pruritic and usually more widespread. Vesicles and pustules desquamate leaving brown macules on the chin, neck, palms, and soles. Tzanck smear shows abundant neutrophils.
- Hand-foot-and-mouth disease—affects children after age 1, associated with constitutional symptoms and oral lesions. The palmar and plantar vesicles are nonpruritic, more oval shaped, and oriented along dermatoglyphics.
- Impetigo
- Herpes simplex infection—grouped or single vesicles on erythematous bases in crops on skin and mucous membranes. Tzanck smear shows multinucleated giant cells.
- Langerhans cell histiocytosis—generalized papules, vesicles, pustules, or nodules. Biopsy shows Langerhans cells in the dermis with Birbeck granules on electron microscopy.
- Congenital syphilis
- Dyshidrotic eczema
- Pustular psoriasis—Pustules are less well defined and often coalescent.
- Pustular tinea pedis—Pustules are less well defined and often coalescent.

✓ Best Tests

- Skin scrapings for scabies should be performed on any lesion that resembles a burrow.
- Gram stain, Tzanck smear, and potassium hydroxide preparations will rule out bacterial, herpes virus (multinucleated giant cells), or fungal infections, respectively, and show numerous neutrophils, occasional eosinophils, and no bacteria.
- Histopathology varies depending on the stage of the disease, from focal vesiculation in the Malpighian layer in the acute stages to well-circumscribed subcorneal pustules with polymorphic neutrophils and occasional eosinophils in later stages. The dermis is edematous and has a perivascular lymphocytic infiltrate.
- Peripheral blood eosinophilia has been reported.

▲▲▲ Management Pearls

- Always rule out scabies first, as this can present similarly.
- Parents should be instructed that IA is a self-limited disease and that treatment is aimed at controlling symptoms rather than curing the disease.

Therapy

High-potency topical steroids twice daily are highly effective for relieving flares and should be first line. Dapsone has been recommended in the past for severe, recalcitrant cases, but the risks of hemolytic anemia, peripheral neuropathy, hepatitis, and allergic reaction must be weighed. Antihistamines can be used for pruritus in older children but are contraindicated in neonates.

Suggested Readings

Dromy R, Raz A, Metzker A. Infantile acropustulosis. *Pediatric Dermatol.* 1991;8(4):284–287.

Humeau S, Bureau B, Litoux P, et al. Infantile acropustulosis in six immigrant children. *Pediatric Dermatol.* 1995;12(3):211–214.

Laude TA. Skin disorders in black children. *Curr Opin Pediatrics.* 1996;8(4):381–385.

Mancini AJ, Frieden IJ, Paller AS. Infantile acropustulosis revisited: History of scabies and response to topical corticosteroids. *Pediatric Dermatol.* 1998;15(5):337–341.

Mengesha YM, Bennett ML. Pustular skin disorders, diagnosis and treatment. *Am J Clin Dermatol.* 2002;3(6):389–400.

Van Praag MC, Van Rooij RW, Folkers E, et al. Diagnosis and treatment of pustular disorders in the neonate. *Pediatric Dermatol.* 1997;14(2):131–143.

Vicente J, Espana A, Idoate M, et al. Are eosinophilic pustular folliculitis of infancy and infantile acropustulosis the same entity? *Br J Dermatol.* 1996;135(5):807–809.

Wagner A. Distinguishing vesicular and pustular disorders in the neonate. *Curr Opin Pediatrics.* 1997;9:396.

Bullous Disorders

Mat Davey

◼◼ Diagnosis Synopsis

Bullous disorders of the skin encompass a wide range of disease processes that vary both in their clinical presentation and in severity. Clinical manifestations range from benign, localized blisters to fatal, widespread denudation of the skin. The most common acquired autoimmune blistering disorder among those with darkly pigmented skin is bullous pemphigoid (BP). Less common acquired blistering diseases include pemphigus vulgaris (PV) and dermatitis herpetiformis (DH). DH is most common in individuals of Northern European descent and is discussed on VisualDx online. (If you are a first-time online user, go to www.essentialdermatology.com/pigmented; if you already have your password set up, go directly to www.visualdx.com/visualdx.) Inherited disorders include the family of genodermatoses known as epidermolysis bullosa (EB).

Bullous pemphigoid (BP), the most common acquired blistering disorder, is a chronic autoimmune disease usually presenting after the age of 60; the incidence increases with age. IgG autoantibodies bind to antigens on the basement membrane of the skin, activating and releasing inflammatory mediators resulting in localized or at times generalized tense bullae. BP can occur on any body surface, but mucous membrane involvement is rare. Pruritus is common. It can last months to years. There is no predilection in any ethnicity or either sex. BP has been associated with other autoimmune diseases such as diabetes mellitus, thyroiditis, dermatomyositis, lupus erythematosus, rheumatoid arthritis, ulcerative colitis, myasthenia gravis, and multiple sclerosis. Radiation therapy or drugs (furosemide, nonsteroidal anti-inflammatory drugs, captopril, penicillamine, and some antibiotics) have also been associated with BP.

Less common acquired autoimmune blistering disorders include PV and DH. EB acquisita is an autoimmune disorder with autoantibodies to type VII collagen. Its blistering can cause scarring and result in milia (Fig. 4-395).

Cicatricial pemphigoid has antibodies to basement membrane components and has scarring of the skin, conjunctivae, mouth, and other mucous membranes.

Pemphigus vulgaris (PV) is a chronic autoimmune intraepidermal blistering disease involving IgG autoantibodies against the keratinocyte cell surface molecule desmoglein, interfering with cell-cell adhesion (acantholysis) and causing flaccid bullae and erosions on the skin and/or mucous membranes. The disease appears equally in men and women, often in their fifties and sixties. Severe cases can be life threatening. Complications are related to the use of high-dose steroids, secondary infection, loss of the skin barrier, and poor oral intake. PV occurs in all ethnicities but is more common among those of Jewish ancestry. PV is also associated with other autoimmune diseases, especially myasthenia gravis. Another variant of pemphigus is pemphigus foliaceus

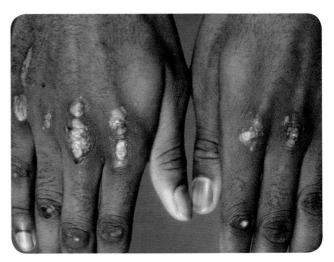

Figure 4-395 Seventeen-year-old patient with EB acquisita with plaquelike scars and a few small milia.

(PF). There are several subtypes of PF, including fogo selvagem and pemphigus erythematosus. Fogo selvagem refers to endemic PF (Brazil and other portions of Latin America, Tunisia), and pemphigus erythematosus is a localized form. Pemphigus erythematosus may coexist with other autoimmune disorders, such as myasthenia gravis or lupus erythematosus.

Linear IgA dermatosis is an immune-mediated disorder that occurs in children and adults. There are idiopathic and medication-induced subtypes of this disease. A number of agents have been reported to cause linear IgA disease, including vancomycin, lithium, diclofenac, captopril, IL-2, IFN-gamma, D-penicillamine, and iodine contrast media. It is most common after the fourth decade of life and presents with a combination of annular or grouped vesicles or bullae, occurring most frequently on the extensor surfaces. Mucosal erosions are common and may be severe at times. Pruritus and burning may be associated with the eruption. The disease is defined by the presence of a homogenous deposition of IgA in a linear band at the epidermal-dermal junction.

Pediatric Patient Considerations

Both BP and PV are rare in children, although a recent rise in infant-onset BP has been noted.

In children, onset of linear IgA dermatosis is usually before age 5, and it appears as clusters or rings of tense bullae in the perioral and perineal regions.

Chronic bullous dermatosis of childhood, also known as chronic bullous disease and linear IgA bullous dermatosis, is an immunobullous dermatosis with IgA autoantibodies against antigens in the skin basement membrane resulting in separation at this layer and blister formation. It has clinical similarities to childhood BP. The onset typically occurs between the ages of 6 months and 6 years, with a 3:2 predominance in girls over boys. It is usually self-limited over several months (up to 2 to 4 years), following a less chronic course than childhood pemphigoid, pemphigus, or DH. Lesions tend to burn or itch, with the blistering becoming less severe with time.

Epidermolysis bullosa (EB) is a group of genetic diseases characterized by blistering in response to minor trauma. It is divided into four major categories based on the depth of skin blistering: (i) EB simplex (intraepidermal skin separation), (ii) junctional EB (skin separation at the lamina lucida), (iii) hemidesmosomal EB (skin separation at the hemidesmosomal level), and (iv) dystrophic EB (sublamina densa skin separation). In milder cases of EB simplex, significant friction or trauma is required to produce blisters, and the first signs may not develop until the patient begins to walk or crawl. In the more severe cases of EB simplex, blistering occurs in response to minimal trauma, and large bullae and erosions are present at birth or within the first days of life. All forms of EB simplex worsen in hot, humid environments and improve with age.

⊙ Look For

BP presents with tense bullae most often seen on the lower abdomen, thighs, and forearms with a flexural predilection (Figs. 4-396 and 4-397). Bullae may be extensive or localized and may appear on normal-looking skin or have an erythematous base. Individual bullae can be filled with either serous or blood-tinged fluid. In addition, fixed urticarial plaques may be heavily pigmented in darkly pigmented patients.

PV presents with flaccid bullae, erosions, and crusts (which can become quite thick). Fluid in the bullae is clear at first but may become hemorrhagic or seropurulent (Fig. 4-398). The vesicles and erosions can affect mucosal surfaces, including conjunctiva and oral mucosa. Large areas of epidermis can denude, creating risk for bacterial infection and sepsis. Look for active vesicles at the margins of plaques. Following successful therapy, cutaneous manifestations of pemphigus tend to resolve in lighter skin types, whereas postinflammatory pigmentary changes often occur in patients with darker skin types. PF presents with crusts and superficial erosions mainly on the scalp, face, and upper trunk (Fig. 4-399). Lesions may be exacerbated by sun and heat and almost never have mucosal involvement.

In linear IgA dermatosis, look for grouped or annular papules, vesicles, or bullae on the elbows, knees, and buttocks (Fig. 4-400).

Diabetics may have large blisters frequently on the legs (Fig. 4-401).

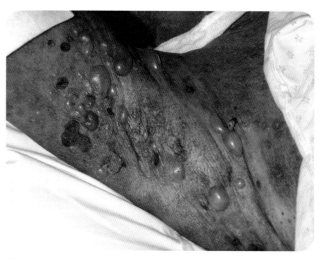

Figure 4-397 Bullae in bullous pemphigoid may be in multiple stages of development.

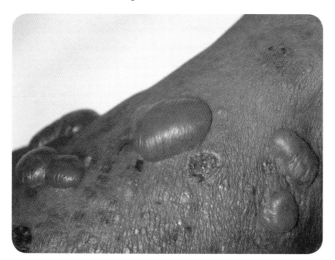

Figure 4-396 Tense bullae without peripheral inflammation are characteristic of bullous pemphigoid.

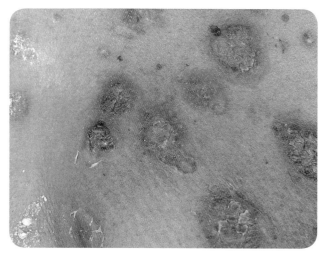

Figure 4-398 Erosions and scaling plaques in PV.

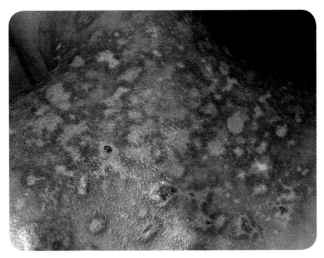

Figure 4-399 Erosions, crusts, and hypopigmented and hyperpigmented lesions of pemphigus foliaceus in a typical location.

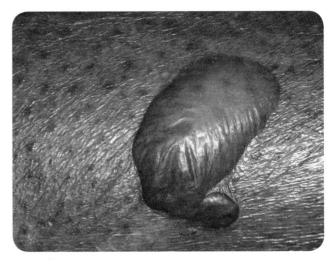

Figure 4-401 Diabetics may have a few bullae on the anterior shin, probably associated with trauma.

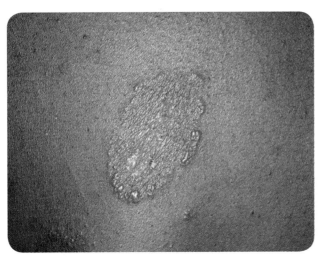

Figure 4-400 Linear IgA disease with a collarette of small vesicles around a central hyperpigmented lesion.

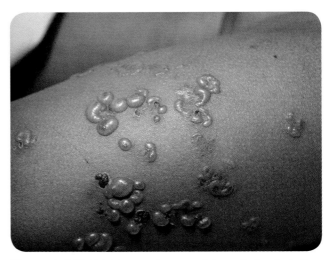

Figure 4-402 Multiple, mostly grouped tense bullae in bullous dermatosis of childhood.

Pediatric Patient Considerations

In children, blisters of linear IgA dermatosis are often tense and sometimes appear at the edge of a previous blister, giving a "collarette" appearance.

Bullous dermatosis of childhood presents with multiple large vesicles and oval or sausage-shaped bullae, which can be serpiginous or annular in configuration (Fig. 4-402). A crust forms around older blisters after they have erupted, and new blisters will form at the periphery to mimic "a string of pearls." Lesions are concentrated on the inferior abdomen, buttocks, legs, and genitalia. Oral, perioral, ocular, and scalp lesions can occur. Some patients may present with abrupt onset accompanied by fever and constitutional symptoms.

In EB, the cutaneous findings vary wildly based on the clinical subtype present. Infants with EB simplex can be divided into three main subtypes: (a) EB simplex Weber-Cockayne (EBS-WC; mildest, with disease limited to the hands and feet) (Fig. 4-403), (b) EB simplex Koebner (EBS-K; intermediate form with generalized blistering) (Fig. 4-404), and (c) EB simplex Dowling-Meara (severe with widespread blistering, possible internal organ involvement, and potential death in the neonatal period). As with EB simplex, infants with junctional EB, hemidesmosomal EB, and dystrophic EB present with large variation in skin findings based on the specific subtype. These range from localized blisters to widespread blistering/denudation of the skin and early death. In the severe form of recessive dystrophic EB, there is atrophy and scarring, and frequent life-threatening squamous cell carcinomas may occur beginning in the second and third decades (Fig. 4-405).

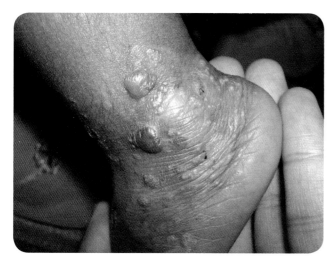

Figure 4-403 EB simplex in an infant, with intact vesicles and healing lesions.

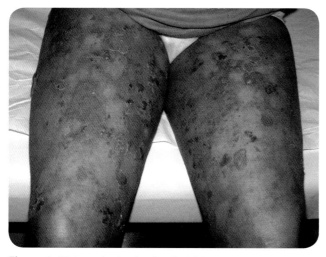

Figure 4-404 EB simplex (Koebner) with intact bullae and erosions.

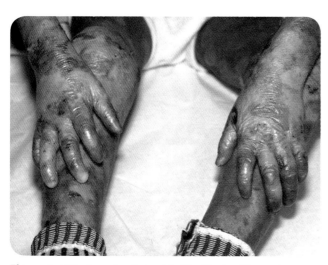

Figure 4-405 Recessive dystrophic EB with atrophic scarring.

 Diagnostic Pearls

- BP should always be considered when tense bullae are present in patients aged more than 60. Nikolsky sign, where slight friction induces an erosion or vesicle, is often absent. BP almost never starts with mucosal lesions; this is a good distinction from PV, which frequently begins with oral erosions.
- In PV, Nikolsky sign will be present in active disease. The Asboe-Hansen sign ("bulla-spread phenomenon"), in which gentle pressure on an intact bulla forces the fluid to spread under the skin, away from the site of the pressure, may also be present.
- In pemphigus erythematosus, antinuclear antibodies may be positive.
- Grouped blisters on the extensor areas should suggest the diagnosis of either linear IgA disease or DH. The presence of blisters in an annular arrangement strongly suggests the presence of linear IgA dermatosis. In the drug-induced form of linear IgA dermatosis, mucosal involvement usually does not occur.
- In chronic bullous disease of childhood, clustering of vesicles and bullae in an annular shape ("string of pearls") is a frequent finding.

?? **Differential Diagnosis and Pitfalls**

Traumatic/Insects/Environmental

- Urticaria/papular urticaria
- Insect bite reactions
- Scabies
- Allergic contact dermatitis

Drugs/Toxins/Infection

- Herpes simplex virus
- Disseminated herpes zoster
- Erythema multiforme
- Toxic epidermal necrolysis or Stevens-Johnson syndrome
- Bullous impetigo

Systemic Illnesses/Genetic/Other

- Bullous lupus erythematosus
- Diabetic bullae
- Porphyria cutanea tarda or pseudoporphyria
- EB acquisita
- Transient acantholytic dermatosis (Grover disease)
- Hailey-Hailey disease
- Eczematous dermatitis

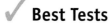 **Best Tests**

- Take a complete history—including medication history—to assess for any aggravating/causative factors.

- Skin biopsy for routine histology is taken at the edge of a blister/vesicle. A second biopsy for direct immunofluorescence (DIF) should be completed on normal-appearing skin adjacent to a lesion. The histopathologic findings of these biopsies are often diagnostic.
- Indirect immunofluorescence (IIF) of serum is oftentimes positive for specific IgG autoantibodies in patients with BP and PV. Patients with DH often display antigliadin, antiendomysial or antireticulin IgA autoantibodies.
- Linear IgA dermatosis—Immunofluorescence of a skin biopsy demonstrates a bandlike deposition of IgA at the epidermal-dermal junction, which is diagnostic for the disorder.
- Bullous dermatosis of childhood—Skin biopsy for histology and immunofluorescence. Histopathology demonstrates subepidermal neutrophil-rich bullae. DIF of uninvolved skin shows a linear deposition of IgA at the basement membrane zone. IIF will demonstrate circulating IgA antibodies in up to 80% of patients.

▲▲ Management Pearls

Management and therapy of these diseases should be done in conjunction with a dermatologist; the details of therapy are discussed on VisualDx online.

- Secondary infection of lesions should be treated aggressively with appropriate systemic antibiotics.
- Blistering conditions such as BP/PV are rarely related to an underlying neoplasm. A thorough history and general physical exam are usually sufficient. However, systemic symptoms or an atypical presentation should warrant further workup of underlying malignancy.
- Patients requiring long-term use of glucocorticoids and/or cytotoxic drugs need to be monitored carefully for side effects.
- Patients should be instructed to minimize trauma to the skin. Patients with oral disease may need dietary modifications (e.g., avoidance of caustic or hard foods).
- Involve a dermatologist in the patient's care. Depending on the extent and severity of disease, consultations with dentistry, ophthalmology, or otolaryngology may be indicated.

Pediatric Patient Considerations

- Infants with EB should be followed closely by a dermatologist. Once EB has been established, all categories of EB (dystrophic, junctional, and simplex) may present identically in the neonatal period, and clinical distinction is often not possible until later in infancy or childhood. Therefore, in the newborn period, genetic counseling and anticipatory guidance should be limited until the exact diagnosis is confirmed by immunofluorescence studies and/or electron microscopy.

Therapy

BP—Localized disease:

- High-potency topical corticosteroids applied twice daily to affected areas on the body.

BP—Extensive disease:

- Prednisone at 0.5 to 1 mg/kg/d, and taper slowly with clearing. Patients taking long-term systemic corticosteroids should receive calcium (at least 1 g daily) and vitamin D supplementation with or without other method(s) of osteoporosis prevention.
- Dapsone (50 to 100 mg/d), azathioprine (75 to 150 mg/d), mycophenolate mofetil (1.0 to 1.5 g twice daily), cyclophosphamide (1 to 3 mg/kg/d), cyclosporine (1 to 5 mg/kg/d), and methotrexate (5 to 10 mg weekly) also serve as important steroid-sparing agents. Their use should be considered if the patient requires several months of systemic corticosteroids in the range of 40 to 60 mg.
- Recently, tetracycline (500 mg four times daily) in combination with nicotinamide (500 mg three times daily) or minocycline (100 mg twice daily) have been used for their anti-inflammatory effects and as steroid-sparing agents, though controlled studies have not yet been done to prove efficacy.
- For resistant cases, plasma exchange, intravenous immunoglobulin (IVIG), or rituximab (anti-CD20) can be attempted.

PV or PF—If PV or PF is limited in distribution and not severe, therapy with potent topical corticosteroids can be attempted. If it is severe, systemic corticosteroids are the primary therapy:

- Initial therapy should be prednisone with a dose of at least 1 mg/kg. Patients will be on steroids for months to years, and all the side effects of corticosteroids must be considered and managed as preventively as possible.
- For their steroid-sparing effects, other therapies should be considered early in the course of disease and include:

1. Methylprednisolone, 10 to 20 mg/kg IV pulse therapy infused over 1 hour for 1 to 5 days
2. Mycophenolate mofetil (1.5 g twice daily)
3. Azathioprine (100 to 300 mg/d)
4. Dapsone (100 to 200 mg/d)
5. Cyclophosphamide (50 to 200 mg/d)
6. Cyclosporine (5 mg/kg/d)
7. High-dose IVIG
8. Tetracycline (1 g twice daily) plus niacinamide (1 g twice daily)

Linear IgA dermatosis—Discontinue the offending medication.

- Prednisone 1 mg/kg/d, with a slow taper with clearing.
- Dapsone (100 to 200 mg/d), azathioprine (75 to 150 mg/d), and mycophenolate mofetil (1.0 to 1.5 g twice daily) also serve as important steroid-sparing agents. Their use should be considered if the patient requires several months of systemic corticosteroids in the range of 40 to 60 mg.

Note: Patients who are on chronic systemic steroid therapy need to supplement their diet with at least 1 g of calcium each day as a preventive to osteoporosis.

Pediatric Patient Considerations

Bullous Dermatosis of Childhood

- Sulfapyridine 100 to 200 mg/kg/d divided four times daily, not to exceed 4 g/d. Once the lesions have improved, the dose can be tapered to keep the skin under control (usually <0.5 g daily). *Note*: The patient should be tested for glucose-6-phosphate dehydrogenase (G6PD) deficiency prior to initiating therapy.
- Dapsone 25 to 50 mg/kg/d, not to exceed 400 mg/d. Once the lesions have improved, the dose can be tapered to keep the skin under control (usually <5 mg daily). *Note*: The patient should be tested for G6PD deficiency prior to initiating therapy.

Be certain to monitor the patient carefully with frequent CBCs and LFTs on either medication.

Prednisone is sometimes added to either of the above therapies to control severe disease (but a long course is not recommended due to adverse effects).

EB—Skin care involves prevention of blisters, blister care, and pain control.

Prevention of blisters:

- Avoid overheating by providing a cool environment and not overdressing.
- Avoid applying tape, bandages, or adhesives to the skin.
- Dress in loose-fitting clothes (elastic leg bands may be cut from disposable diapers to prevent friction).
- Ideal shoes have soft and permeable leather, ample toe room, and few seams.
- Absorbent powders may be applied inside of socks to prevent friction. Ideal socks are superabsorbent cotton sport socks.

- Avoid friction by patting moist areas dry rather than rubbing and by lubricating the skin with generous use of emollients.

Blister care:

- Drain blisters that are larger than a dime or that appear tense. Use a sterile needle or lancet to pierce the blister roof, drain the contents, and leave the remaining blister roof intact.
- Apply topical antibiotic ointment to erosions and drained blisters.
- Cover open areas with nonadherent dressings, and change them daily.
- Watch for signs of infection (e.g., yellow crust, foul-smelling exudate, purulence, induration, increased erythema, severe pain), and culture and treat with appropriate systemic antibiotics.

Pain control with dressing changes:

- Acetaminophen 15 mg/kg orally every 4 to 6 hours
- Ibuprofen 10 mg/kg orally every 6 to 8 hours (in infants older than 6 months)

Opiates may be necessary for more severe pain but can affect feeding/stooling activities of young infants.

Suggested Readings

Di Zenzo G, Marazza G, Borradori L. Bullous pemphigoid: physiopathology, clinical features and management. *Adv Dermatol*. 2007;23:257–288.

Feliciani C, Caldarola G, Kneisel A, et al. IgG autoantibody reactivity against bullous pemphigoid (BP) 180 and BP230 in elderly patients with pruritic dermatoses. *Br J Dermatol*. 2009;161(2):306–312.

Fine JD. Management of acquired bullous skin diseases. *N Engl J Med*. 1995;333(22):1475–1484.

Joly P, Roujeau JC, Benichou J, et al. A comparison of oral and topical corticosteroids in patients with bullous pemphigoid. *N Engl J Med*. 2002;346(5):321–327.

Leighty L, Li N, Diaz LA, et al. Experimental models for the autoimmune and inflammatory blistering disease, Bullous pemphigoid. *Arch Dermatol Res*. 2007;299(9):417–422.

Mao X, Payne AS. Seeking approval: present and future therapies for pemphigus vulgaris. *Curr Opin Investig Drugs*. 2008;9(5):497–504.

Saouli Z, Papadopoulos A, Kaiafa G, et al. A new approach on bullous pemphigoid therapy. *Ann Oncol*. 2008;19(4):825–826.

Stanley JR. Pemphigus. In: Fitzpatrick TB, Wolff K, eds. *Fitzpatrick's Dermatology in General Medicine*. 7th Ed. New York, NY: McGraw-Hill; 2008:459–468.

Stanley JR. Bullous pemphigoid. In: Fitzpatrick TB, Wolff K, eds. *Fitzpatrick's Dermatology in General Medicine*. 7th Ed. New York, NY: McGraw-Hill; 2008:475–480.

Yeh SW, Sami N, Ahmed RA. Treatment of pemphigus vulgaris: current and emerging options. *Am J Clin Dermatol*. 2005;6(5):327–342.

Incontinentia Pigmenti

Chris G. Adigun

■■ Diagnosis Synopsis

Incontinentia pigmenti (IP), also known as Bloch-Sulzberger syndrome, is an uncommon X-linked disease that is lethal in the majority of males. The expressivity in females appears to be variable. The disease first presents at birth or within the first few weeks of life with characteristic skin findings. IP typically progresses through four clinical stages: vesicles and bullae (stage 1, 90% of cases), verrucous lesions (stage 2), linear hyperpigmentation (stage 3), and hypopigmentation and atrophy (stage 4). Within days of birth, erythema, vesicles, and/or pustules develop, typically in a linear pattern. These lesions then evolve into verrucous lesions over the course of several weeks. After several months, hyperpigmented macules appear. The final stage is characterized by hypopigmentation within these same areas of affected skin. Most cases are associated with developmental abnormalities of the eyes, teeth, nails, and musculoskeletal or central nervous systems. Clinical presentations vary widely, ranging from cases with very subtle cutaneous and dental involvement, to cases with incapacitating neurologic and ophthalmologic manifestations.

Ocular findings include both retinal and nonretinal abnormalities, usually related to vascular occlusion. Neurological manifestations occur in 18% to 36% of cases, with seizures, delayed psychomotor development, hemiplegia, hemiparesis, spasticity, and mental retardation. Extensive cutaneous involvement of the scalp and neck skin is associated with more severe cranial impairment.

Recurrence of the vesiculobullous stage after resolution in infancy is rare. This typically occurs in children aged younger than 18 months after a systemic infection. The infection leads to the production of tumor necrosis factor-alpha, which subsequently triggers apoptosis in residual NEMO (NF-kappa B essential modulator) mutated cell lines (the causative mutation in IP). This reproduces cutaneous findings similar to those seen at birth.

More than 700 cases of IP have been reported to date, and most of these cases have been described in whites. However, the disorder has been found to occur in other ethnicities. Furthermore, it is difficult to elucidate whether the predominance in whites is due to reporting bias rather than actual predominance. Males very rarely survive, and in the occasional cases that they do, it is attributed to the presence of an additional X chromosome, such as in Klinefelter syndrome, somatic mosaicism, or hypomorphic alleles.

◉ Look For

Cutaneous findings are the most common first sign of IP. The dermatologic presentation evolves from birth through childhood with four classic clinical stages:

Stage 1: Vesiculobullous or Inflammatory Stage

Ninety-two percent of cases develop by 2 weeks of life. Look for linear vesicles within erythematous plaques, sometimes in a whorled pattern (Fig. 4-406). Pustules may develop. Trunk, extremities, and scalp are frequently affected, with sparing of the face. Vesicles/bullae typically clear by 4 months.

Stage 2: Verrucous Stage

Onset is usually by 2 to 6 weeks of life. Look for warty linear plaques, primarily on the extremities, which may or may not correspond to previous location of vesicular lesions. Typically bilateral, 80% of cases clear by 6 months.

Stage 3: Hyperpigmented Stage

Ninety-eight percent of patients with IP experience this stage, characterized by linear and whorled hyperpigmented and slate-gray areas that follow the lines of Blaschko (Figs. 4-407 and 4-408).

Stage 4: Hypopigmented Stage

Areas of previous hyperpigmentation often lighten to hypopigmented areas with time. These lesions are hairless and may have signs of cutaneous atrophy; they are most commonly distributed on the extremities.

Hair findings include vertex alopecia. Areas of vesiculation may lead to scarring alopecia in their place. Uncommonly, agenesis of eyebrows and eyelashes occurs.

Nail findings occur in up to 40% of patients and include nail plate disruption, ridging, or pitting. These abnormalities

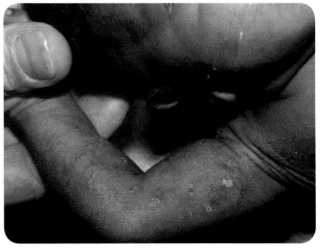

Figure 4-406 Newborn with papular and scaling lesions of incontinentia pigmenti.

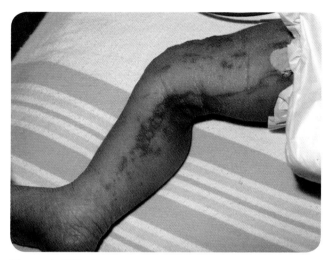

Figure 4-407 Linear hyperpigmentation of incontinentia pigmenti.

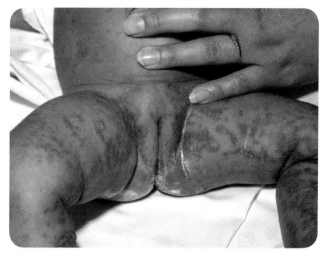

Figure 4-408 Lichenoid and hyperpigmented lesion of incontinentia pigmenti.

may improve over time. In puberty or later, subungual and periungual keratotic tumors may develop.

Dental abnormalities are the second most common clinical sign of IP. Over 65% of patients have severe dental anomalies. Partial anodontia predominates, followed by pegged or conical teeth.

Eye findings are less frequent but are severe, and nearly 20% will experience vision-threatening eye abnormalities. Ocular involvement is associated with neurologic sequelae. These include retinal and nonretinal anomalies.

CNS involvement typically presents with seizures, spastic paralysis, motor retardation, and microcephaly. Thirty percent of patients with IP will have some CNS deficit.

Diagnostic Pearls

- Cutaneous stages may overlap—with both vesicles and verrucous lesions occurring concurrently, or some stages may not occur at all.
- The absence of cutaneous findings does not eliminate the diagnosis of IP, especially in adult women whose lesions may have already resolved. In this circumstance, a negative family history should not rule out a diagnosis of IP. In addition, examining mothers of patients with suspected IP for areas of atrophy, hypopigmentation, or hair loss is warranted. Inquiring about dental abnormalities or premature tooth loss may also be helpful.
- Laboratory findings during the first stage of IP can be dramatic and aid in the diagnosis. These are high-grade leukocytosis and eosinophilia. Levels are highest at 3 to 5 weeks of life.

?? Differential Diagnosis and Pitfalls

Differential diagnosis tends to change depending on the stage, as the clinical findings vary greatly.

Stage 1: Vesiculobullous

- Bullous impetigo
- Herpes simplex virus (HSV)
- Varicella
- Langerhans cell histiocytosis
- Erythema toxicum neonatorum
- Dermatitis herpetiformis
- Epidermolysis bullosa acquisita
- Bullous systemic lupus erythematosus
- Linear IgA bullous dermatosis
- Neonatal pemphigus vulgaris
- Bullous pemphigoid
- Blistering drug eruption
- Heritable epidermolysis bullosa
- Bullous mastocytosis

Stage 2: Verrucous

- Verruca vulgaris
- Linear epidermal nevus—lesions become more verrucous with time and are not preceded by vesicles
- Lichen striatus—uncommon in infants, no preceding vesicles
- Conradi-Hunermann (chondrodysplasia punctata)—no preceding vesicles, has multiple skeletal dysplasias

Stage 3: Hyperpigmented

- Linear and whorled nevoid hypermelanosis—no preceding vesicles/verrucous changes
- Dermatopathia pigmentosa reticularis—no preceding vesicles/verrucous stages
- Naegeli-Franceschetti-Jadassohn—no preceding vesicles/verrucous changes; associated with hypohidrosis, heat intolerance

379

Stage 4: Hypopigmented

- Pigmentary mosaicism (formerly hypomelanosis of Ito)—no preceding vesicles/verrucous changes
- Focal dermal hypoplasia (Goltz syndrome)—initial blistering/desquamation followed by linear areas of severe atrophy with fat herniation

Differential Diagnosis of Cutaneous Lesions Associated With Cerebral Atrophy

- Sturge-Weber syndrome
- Klippel-Trenaunay-Weber syndrome
- Parry-Romberg syndrome

✓ Best Tests

- Bacterial cultures, viral cultures, Gram stain, Tzanck smear to evaluate for viral/bacterial infectious etiologies
- Punch biopsy of vesicular/verrucous lesion will reveal characteristic findings.
- Laboratory examination will reveal significant peripheral blood leukocytosis as well as eosinophilia with counts elevated to 5% or as high as 79%. Highest levels are between 3 and 5 weeks of age.

▲▲ Management Pearls

- It is absolutely critical to perform a thorough examination in the case of suspected IP. Once the diagnosis is confirmed, a multidisciplinary approach to manage the potential sequelae is mandated. Patients will need immediate referrals to ophthalmology and neurology. Swift evaluation by ophthalmology is imperative for the management of retinal pathologies, as delayed intervention may lead to severe ocular deficiency or even blindness. Anticonvulsants may be required early on; thus, neurological examination is also essential. Patients will also ultimately need a dental evaluation, and although this is not urgent, it should be performed prior to the age of 2 years.
- Management of skin lesions is centered on reassurance. Spontaneous resolution is the rule. Vesicles may need sterile dressings to prevent bacterial superinfection.
- Subungual/periungual tumors require surgical excision to prevent development of lytic changes of underlying phalangeal bones.
- Patients and also their families often need to be referred to genetics for proper evaluation and counseling, and prenatal diagnosis is possible in affected families.

Therapy

Short-term management of vesicles is with sterile dressings, but further treatment is not necessary.

Some patients and their parents may be tempted to request laser therapy for the hyperpigmented lesions, but they should be discouraged, as laser intervention in this circumstance has been reported to elicit an extensive vesiculobullous eruption.

Furthermore, laser therapy in darker skin types is frequently associated with cosmetically disfiguring complications, including persistent hyper- or hypopigmentation and scarring. A recent report from Japan with Asian subjects investigated the effectiveness of Q-switched lasers for various pigmentary disorders and concluded that a diagnosis of IP should be suspected if postinflammatory hyperpigmented lesions do not resolve within 1 year after their Q-switched laser intervention.

For persistent hyperpigmentation, bleaching agents such as hydroquinone may be used.

The atrophy and hypopigmentation that characterize the final stage of IP are lifelong and tend not to resolve or improve with time. This skin manifestation is more apparent in patients with darker skin and can be more distressing in these patients as well. Good treatments have not been developed for this condition in this population, and cosmetic cover-ups should be recommended.

Suggested Readings

Berlin AL, Paller AS, Chan LS. Incontinentia pigmenti: A review and update on the molecular basis of pathophysiology. *J Am Acad Dermatol.* 2002;47(2):169–187; quiz 188–190.

Darné S, Carmichael AJ. Isolated recurrence of vesicobullous incontinentia pigmenti in a schoolgirl. *Br J Dermatol.* 2007;156(3):600–602.

Ehrenreich M, Tarlow MM, Godlewska-Janusz E, et al. Incontinentia pigmenti (Bloch-Sulzberger syndrome): A systemic disorder. *Cutis.* 2007;79(5):355–362.

Emre S, Firat Y, Güngör S, et al. Incontinentia pigmenti: A case report and literature review. *Turk J Pediatr.* 2009;51(2):190–194.

Goldberg MF. The skin is not the predominant problem in incontinentia pigmenti. *Arch Dermatol.* 2004;140(6):748–750.

Halder RM, Nootheti PK. Ethnic skin disorders overview. *J Am Acad Dermatol.* 2003;48(6 Suppl):S143–S148.

Nagase T, Takanashi M, Takada H, et al. Extensive vesiculobullous eruption following limited ruby laser treatment for incontinentia pigmenti: A case report. *Australas J Dermatol.* 1997;38(3):155–157.

Watanabe S. Basics of laser application to dermatology. *Arch Dermatol Res.* 2008;300(Suppl 1):S21–S30.

Contact Dermatitis

Aída Lugo-Somolinos

■■ Diagnosis Synopsis

Irritant Contact Dermatitis

Irritant contact dermatitides (ICD) are reactions caused by direct physical or chemical injury to the epidermis. The damage caused by an irritant leads to inflammation, manifested in the skin as erythema, edema, and scaling. ICD should be differentiated from true allergic contact dermatitis, which is a delayed type-IV hypersensitivity (immune) reaction. Patients typically present complaining of a burning or stinging sensation early in the course of ICD. Symptoms and a rash usually follow the exposure in a few hours if the irritant is strong; this is in contrast to allergic contact dermatitis, where symptoms are usually delayed by approximately 2 days following exposure. As the irritation becomes chronic and the skin is continually inflamed, pruritus can become a predominant symptom.

The hands are the most common location for ICD, although any body surface can be involved, including the genitals. Patients with a history of atopic dermatitis are particularly predisposed. Environmental factors include repeated exposure to water or frequent hand washing, soaps and solvents, fiberglass, mild acids, and alkalis. Dry air can also predispose to ICD. Exposures are frequently occupational. High-risk jobs include cleaning, health care, food preparation, and hairdressing. ICD can occur at any age. It is more common in women. Ethnic differences exist, with Asians—especially Japanese—having more irritation than whites and Hispanics. Individuals of African descent have less potential for developing irritant dermatitis, and this is thought to be due to a better skin barrier.

Allergic Contact Dermatitis

Allergic contact dermatitides (ACD) are delayed hypersensitivity reactions (type-IV cell-mediated reactions). The most frequent sensitizers in the general population are nickel, neomycin, fragrances, quaternium-15, gold, formaldehyde, cobalt, and bacitracin. Chromates, rubber chemicals, lanolin, other common environmental chemicals, poison ivy, and other plants are also common sensitizers. It remains unclear whether ACD occurs with the same frequency in different ethnicities, but there is a possible decreased susceptibility in individuals of African descent.

Nickel is found in jewelry, belt buckles, green paints, and metal closures on clothing. Chromates are found in shoe and glove leathers. Rubber chemicals are found in gloves, respirators, balloons, and elastic in garments. Neomycin and bacitracin are common in triple-antibiotic first aid ointments and other combination topical preparations. Eye preparations, eardrops, and some vaccines also cause ACD. Other common allergen-containing products include cosmetics, soaps, and dyes. ACD can occur at any age, but its incidence decreases with increasing age. A detailed allergen exposure history should be elicited.

Poison ivy, poison oak, and poison sumac dermatides are type-IV delayed hypersensitivity immune reactions to an oily resin (urushiol) found on the leaves and in the stems and roots of plants of the *Rhus* genus (poison ivy, oak, and sumac). The reaction occurs either in the course of an initial sensitization or in previously sensitized individuals. Skin lesions usually begin to appear 48 hours after initial exposure, and they usually consist of erythematous, linear plaques and vesicles on the extremities. Pruritus is often severe. If not washed away, the resin may be easily and unwittingly transferred to other body locations, where it will incite the same reaction. Poison ivy, oak, or sumac dermatitis can occur in people of all races and ages, although dark-skinned individuals, the elderly, and very young children may be less susceptible. Scratching does not spread lesions; the lesions with the most antigen appear first and then, as the immune response increases, lesions with less antigen begin to erupt. Symptoms are usually related to severe pruritus.

Phytophotodermatitis

Phytophotodermatitis is a cutaneous phototoxic eruption caused by the interaction of furocoumarins found in some common plants and solar UVA radiation. Approximately 24 hours after plant contact and subsequent exposure to sunlight, a burning erythema develops. Limes, other citrus fruits, celery, wild parsnip, figs, meadow grass, certain weeds, and oil of bergamot are frequently causative. Common scenarios include squeezing limes outdoors, gardening and agricultural work, and hiking in areas of causative plants. There is no predilection for any age or ethnicity or either sex, although phytophotodermatitis may be more noticeable in fair skin types. The condition is benign and self-limited, and treatment is supportive.

The term berloque dermatitis refers to phytophotodermatitis from natural oil of bergamot in perfumes. This eruption is typically seen on the faces and necks of women applying aerosolized fragrances and often has persistent hyperpigmentation (Fig. 4-409). This has become rare since the introduction of artificial oil of bergamot.

Pediatric Patient Considerations

ACD susceptibility in the pediatric population increases with age, so it is rare in very young children. Atopic children may have a superimposed ACD.

Immunocompromised Patient Considerations

Immunocompromised subjects may be at less risk of developing ACD, especially if they are taking immunosuppressive medications.

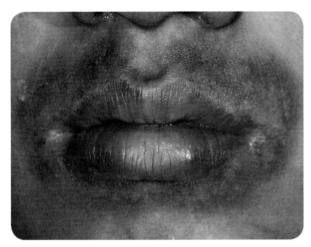

Figure 4-409 Hyperpigmentation after phytophotodermatitis occurring on lips after sucking limes and then sun exposure.

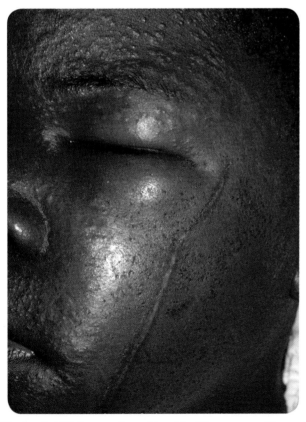

Figure 4-410 Contact dermatitis with diffuse eye swelling and discrete papules on the forehead.

◉ Look For

In acute cases, lesions tend to be vesicular or bullous. Subacute cases are papular, erythematous, and scaly. Look for well-demarcated borders and geometric shapes with straight edges and right angles. Eyelid edema is frequently seen when an allergen is innocently transferred from finger to lid (Fig. 4-410). Affected areas are typically severely pruritic. Contact dermatitis can be found at any body location. When the dermatitis is chronic, thickened plaques develop and secondary bacterial infection is possible (Figs. 4-411–4-414).

With poison ivy, look for linear red and brown-red plaques and vesicles and crusted plaques, vesicles, and bullae (Fig. 4-415). A "black dot variant" has been described (the oil from the plant leaves a black dot on the skin).

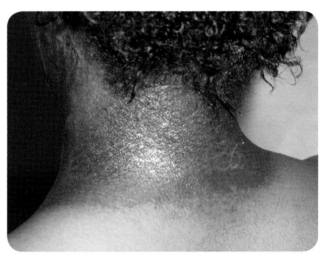

Figure 4-411 Lichenified and hyperpigmented contact dermatitis from a hair straightener.

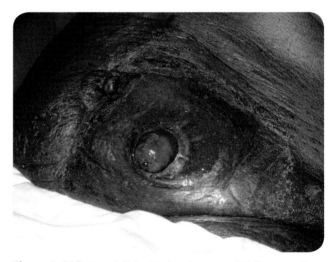

Figure 4-412 Chronic lichenified contact dermatitis from an ostomy adhesive.

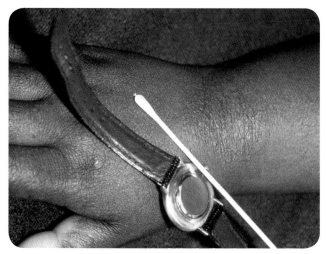

Figure 4-413 Chronic lichenification of contact dermatitis caused by nickel on a watch case.

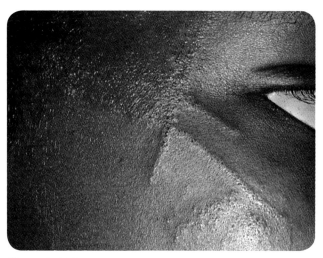

Figure 4-415 Linear lesions of contact dermatitis from poison ivy.

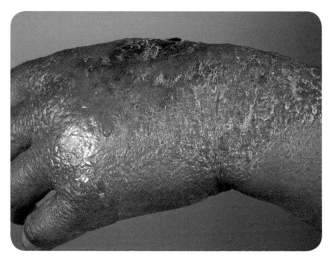

Figure 4-414 Erosions and crusting due to contact dermatitis from formaldehyde.

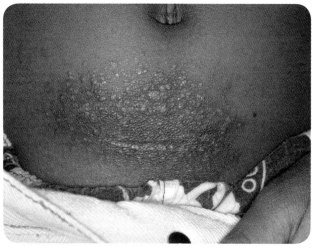

Figure 4-416 Typical chronic contact dermatitis from nickel-containing buttons on blue jeans.

 ## Diagnostic Pearls

- Diagnosis and etiology are often based on clinical exam and history. Individual lesions have well-demarcated borders, often with geometric shapes with straight edges and right angles. The distribution of the rash should drive the examiner's history to possible allergen exposures. Facial distributions often suggest a personal skin care product. Ear lobes suggest nickel allergy from earrings. Hand dermatitis should provoke questions regarding occupation, hobbies, and habits. There are photo-dependent allergic reactions as well.
- ACD may present more commonly with hypopigmentation, hyperpigmentation, and lichenification.
- The lower abdomen is often involved with chronic contact for nickel sensitivity in the buttons of jeans (Fig. 4-416).

?? Differential Diagnosis and Pitfalls

- Erysipelas
- Scabies—look for burrows
- Herpes simplex virus infection—grouped instead of linear vesicles
- Seborrheic dermatitis
- Mycosis fungoides
- Dyshidrotic eczema
- Stasis dermatitis
- Nummular eczema
- Lichen simplex chronicus
- Cellulitis—usually unilateral, look for systemic symptoms
- Atopic dermatitis

✓ Best Tests

- The diagnosis can often be made with a careful history and physical examination. Conduct patch testing to verify the allergen in cases of ACD.
- Skin biopsy, which demonstrates dermatitis, helps confirm an "eczema," but it will not differentiate between different types (allergic contact, atopic, etc.) and does not identify the allergen.
- Patch testing is the gold standard for the diagnosis of ACD.

Pediatric Patient Considerations

Patch testing can be done safely in the pediatric population.

Immunocompromised Patient Considerations

Patch testing should not be done if the subject is taking prednisone or any other immunosuppressant. Consider discontinuing prednisone at least 2 weeks before performing patch testing.

▲▲ Management Pearls

- Identify the inciting allergen, if possible. Treatment is aimed at preventing contact with the allergen and control of symptoms, including antihistamines and topical and oral corticosteroids.
- Recommend the patient avoid common triggers (e.g., fragrance, lanolin, nickel) and buy recommended soaps, cleansers, and cotton gloves (as opposed to latex gloves). Do not disregard preparations that have been used for some time, because over-the-counter preparations often change ingredients or the patient may be newly sensitized. Preservatives in topical corticosteroids are common contactants, as can be the corticosteroid itself. Soap substitutes and emollients are often helpful to minimize irritation and soothe the affected skin.
- For patients needing systemic treatment, do not prescribe a 6-day course of quickly tapering steroids. The delayed hypersensitivity reaction is at least a 2-week process, and shorter courses of oral steroids will result in rebound of the dermatitis.

Therapy

Use high-potency topical corticosteroids on truncal and extremity skin. Use mild-potency topical steroids on thinner skin and classes 6 and 7 steroids on the face and intertriginous areas (desonide cream, lotion, or ointment twice daily). Use steroid ointments with fewer preservatives if there seems to be flaring with multiple topical medications. If the patient's condition is exacerbated with the use of topical steroids, consider an allergy to this agent. This would be an indication for referral to dermatology for patch testing and further management.

High-Potency Topical Corticosteroids (Class 1 or 2)
- Fluocinonide cream, ointment—apply twice daily (15, 30, 60, 120 g)
- Desoximetasone cream, ointment—apply twice daily (15, 60, 120 g)
- Halcinonide cream, ointment—apply twice daily (15, 60, 240 g)
- Amcinonide ointment—apply twice daily (15, 30, 60 g)
- Clobetasol cream, ointment—apply twice daily (15, 60 g)

Mid-Potency Topical Corticosteroids (Classes 3 and 4)
- Triamcinolone cream, ointment—apply twice daily (15, 30, 60, 120, 240 g)
- Mometasone cream, ointment—apply twice daily (15, 45 g)
- Fluocinolone ointment, cream—apply twice daily (15, 30, 60 g)

Topical calcineurin inhibitors (pimecrolimus 1% cream, tacrolimus 0.1% ointment) applied twice daily may be an alternative to topical corticosteroids in the treatment of the inflammatory response, if the patient tolerates them.

Antihistamines
- Diphenhydramine hydrochloride—25 to 50 mg every 6 to 8 hours, as needed
- Hydroxyzine—25 mg every 6 hours, as needed
- Cetirizine hydrochloride—5 to 10 mg daily

In severe cases involving large body areas, use a 14-day course of oral prednisone 0.5 mg/kg each morning and taper only slightly during the interval. For example, start at 40 mg/d and taper by 10 mg every 3 days to 0 mg.

Antibiotics may be indicated when there is evidence of impetiginization. Topical mupirocin or an oral cephalosporin (e.g., cephalexin) or penicillinase-resistant penicillin (e.g., dicloxacillin) will often suffice.

Treatment with PUVA (psoralen plus UVA)/UVB or certain immune-modulating drugs (azathioprine, cyclosporine, methotrexate) has also been tried.

Pediatric Patient Considerations

Avoid high-potency steroids in children when the diagnosis is in doubt. Use lowest strength that will be effective.

High-Potency Topical Corticosteroids (Class 2)
Note: use on truncal and extremity skin for no more than 2 weeks.

- Fluocinonide cream, ointment—apply twice daily (15, 30, 60, 120 g)
- Clobetasol cream, ointment—apply twice daily (15, 60 g)

Midpotency Topical Corticosteroids (Classes 3 and 4)
- Triamcinolone cream, ointment—apply twice daily (15, 30, 60, 120, 240 g)
- Mometasone cream, ointment—apply twice daily (15, 45 g)

- Fluocinolone ointment, cream—apply twice daily (15, 30, 60 g)

Use mild-potency topical steroids on thinner skin and classes 6 and 7 steroids on the face and intertriginous areas (desonide cream, lotion or ointment twice daily).

Use steroid ointments with fewer preservatives if there seems to be flaring with multiple topical medications.

In severe cases involving large body areas, use a 14-day course of oral prednisone 0.5 mg/kg every morning and taper only slightly during the interval. For example, start at 40 mg/d and taper by 10 mg every 3 days to 0 mg.

There is no reason to use a very potent steroid combined with an antifungal agent.

Suggested Readings

Foy V, Weinkauf R, Whittle E, et al. Ethnic variation in the skin irritation response. *Contact Dermatitis*. 2001;45:346–349.

Rietschel RL, Fowler JF, eds. *Fisher's Contact Dermatitis*. 6th Ed. Hamilton, ON: BC Decker; 2008.

Robinson MK. Population differences in skin structure and physiology and the susceptibility to irritant and allergic contact dermatitis: Implications for skin safety testing and risk assessment. *Contact Dermatitis*. 1999;41:65–79.

Robinson MK. Population differences in acute skin irritation responses: Race, sex, age, sensitive skin and repeat subject comparisons. *Contact Dermatitis*. 2002;46:86–93.

Erythema Multiforme Minor

Mat Davey

■■ Diagnosis Synopsis

Erythema multiforme (EM) is an acute, self-limited inflammatory skin reaction characterized by the sudden onset of erythematous papules and plaques, commonly in an acral distribution. The lesions of EM are classically described as targetoid. In contrast to Stevens-Johnson syndrome (SJS) and toxic epidermal necrolysis (TEN), EM is most often precipitated by viral or other infectious pathogens, not medications. It is now recognized that EM does not progress to TEN. Two subtypes exist: EM major and EM minor. Key differences between the EM subtypes include mucosal involvement and systemic symptoms such as fever, arthralgias, and asthenia seen in the major subtype.

Most EM minor episodes are associated with a preceding herpes simplex virus (HSV-1 or HSV-2) outbreak occurring 1 to 3 weeks prior to development of EM lesions. In some cases, a preceding herpes outbreak is subclinical and not appreciated on history or exam; therefore, clinicians must maintain a high index of suspicion of HSV even in the absence of a known history of herpes infection. Other known precipitating pathogens include varicella, parapoxvirus, adenovirus, coxsackievirus, HIV, hepatitis, *Mycoplasma pneumoniae*, *Salmonella*, and *Histoplasma capsulatum*. Drugs are a rare cause of EM. While the etiology remains unclear, exposure to infection of genetically susceptible individuals with certain HLA subtypes may trigger aberrant cellular and humoral responses.

The progression of the cutaneous eruption of EM is usually complete within 72 hours. Lesions remain fixed for up to 2 weeks and resolve without sequela. Residual postinflammatory pigment changes may persist for months, especially in individuals with darker skin. Pruritus is a commonly associated feature. Patients are otherwise well with, at most, mild systemic symptoms consisting of low-grade fever, malaise, arthralgias, or myalgias.

EM can occur at any age but is most commonly seen in adolescents and young adults. A slight male predominance has been noted. The eruption is recurrent in at least 30% of patients. No ethnic or geographic predilection has been found.

◉ Look For

A symmetric eruption that may affect any cutaneous surface but favors the extremities, including the palms and soles. Lesions evolve over 24 to 48 hours. Early lesions consist of a well-defined, fixed, erythematous macule or papule that rapidly develops a dusky, grayish central discoloration (Fig. 4-417). Classical target lesions are <3 cm in diameter with three concentric components including a well-circumscribed erythematous border, a pale middle zone, and a dusky center disk or blister (Figs. 4-418 and 4-419). Atypical target lesions are poorly defined, circular, erythematous papules that have two distinct color zones. Individual lesions may reach several centimeters in diameter.

In darkly pigmented skin, lesions appear more violaceous than erythematous. Postinflammatory hyper/hypopigmentation may occur.

Mucosal involvement is not uncommon but is often limited to the oral cavity (Fig. 4-420). Oral lesions consist of erosions, indurated plaques, and targetoid lesions of the lips, tongue, and buccal mucosa.

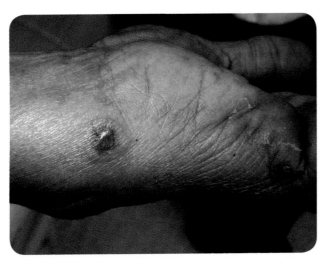

Figure 4-417 Targetlike vesicle on the palm in erythema multiforme minor.

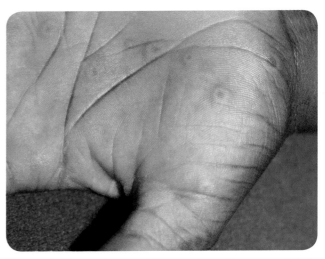

Figure 4-418 Erythema multiforme minor with several delicate target lesions on the palm.

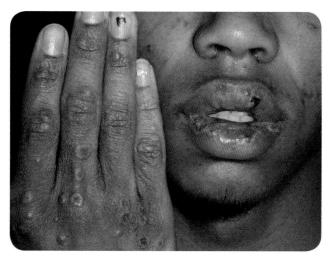

Figure 4-419 Erythema multiforme minor with target lesions on the dorsum of the hands and mucosal erosions.

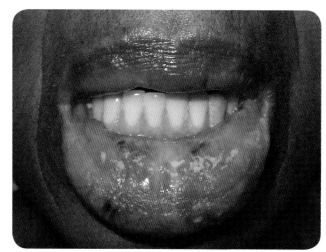

Figure 4-420 Diffuse mucosal erosions in erythema multiforme following labial herpes simplex.

Diagnostic Pearls

- Recurrent EM eruptions occur in over 30% of patients.
- In >70% of patients, a preceding episode of herpes outbreak is noted, with oral herpes being more common than genital herpes.
- Not all episodes of EM are preceded by a clinically evident herpes outbreak, and not all episodes of herpes outbreaks are followed by recurrent EM.

Differential Diagnosis and Pitfalls

Hypersensitivity Reactions

- Urticaria
- Kawasaki disease
- Fixed drug eruption
- Id reaction

Autoimmune Diseases

- Linear IgA bullous dermatosis
- Bullous pemphigoid
- Subacute cutaneous lupus erythematosus
- Urticarial vasculitis
- Henoch-Schönlein purpura

Annular Erythemas

- Erythema annulare centrifugum
- Erythema migrans (Lyme disease)

Infections and Infestations

- Viral exanthem
- Arthropod bites
- Disseminated bacterial or fungal infection
- Syphilis

Malignancies

- Lymphoma
- Leukemia
- Lymphomatoid papulosis

SJS/TEN

Histological features may not differentiate EM from SJS/TEN. Clinically, however, look for irregularly shaped, dusky red macular- or patchlike lesions on the trunk, face, and palms/soles. A positive Nikolsky sign can be found; mucosal involvement includes the eyes, lips, mouth, and genitalia. Look for hemorrhagic crust, bullae, and denudation in these areas. Systemic symptoms are commonly present but not invariable. Lesions are more pronounced on the trunk than on the extremities. Precipitating factors are usually medications.

Pediatric Patient Differential Diagnosis

EM minor is extremely rare in infants, and Kawasaki disease and urticaria should be strongly considered as alternative diagnoses. Infants with Kawasaki disease will appear ill and have a high fever. Urticarial lesions resolve and recur in different sites within 24 hours, whereas individual lesions of EM minor are static. Urticaria and Kawasaki disease may be associated with edema of the hands and feet, whereas EM minor is not.

Best Tests

- EM minor is largely a clinical diagnosis based on the history and the classic appearance and location of skin lesions. Skin biopsy for histological examination and direct immunofluorescence may help to rule out other bullous diseases.
- If grouped vesicles are present, culture them for HSV and/or perform HSV PCR.
- A thorough history should be obtained, searching for inciting factors (infections, drugs, and vaccinations) that the patient has been exposed to within 3 to 4 weeks of onset of the eruption. HSV infections usually occur 3 to 14 days prior to the onset of EM minor.

 Management Pearls

- Because EM minor is typically self-limited, it only requires symptomatic relief. Treat the underlying cause, which is usually recurring HSV infection. In recurrence, treating early in the course with systemic antiherpetic agents is a reasonable approach.
- Systemic corticosteroids are not recommended, as they may actually lead to continuing EM eruptions.

Therapy

Nonsteroidal anti-inflammatory drugs can be used for the relief of minor discomfort. Cool compresses may be soothing. Symptomatic relief can be provided with anti-inflammatory agents and oral antihistamines designed to suppress the inflammatory reaction and decrease pruritus.

Oral Antihistamines
- Hydroxyzine 25 mg p.o. three to four times daily, as needed
- Diphenhydramine hydrochloride 25 to 50 mg p.o. every 6 hours, as needed

Nonsedating Antihistamines
- Loratadine 10 mg p.o. daily
- Fexofenadine 60 mg p.o. twice daily
- Cetirizine hydrochloride 5 or 10 mg p.o. daily

For lesions on the trunk and extremities, midpotency (classes 3 and 4) topical steroids applied twice daily to individual lesions may control inflammation and itch. These agents should not be used on the face, genitals, or intertriginous areas; low- to moderate-potency (classes 5 to 7) topical steroids applied twice daily can usually control inflammation and itch in these areas.

Recurrent EM minor (greater than six attacks per year) may respond to long-term acyclovir (400 mg p.o. twice daily) or valacyclovir (500 mg p.o. daily). See HSV therapy sections for therapeutic options for primary or recurrent HSV infections.

In cases of refractory/recurrent EM minor failing to respond to HSV suppression, azathioprine (100 to 150 mg p.o. daily), dapsone (100 to 150 mg daily), and thalidomide (25 to 200 mg p.o. daily) have been reported to be useful.

Pediatric Patient Considerations

Systemic antihistamines (hydroxyzine 1 mg/kg at night and 0.5 mg/kg daily) and acetaminophen (15 mg/kg every 4 to 6 hours) usually control any pruritus or discomfort the child may have. Low- to moderate-potency (classes 5 to 7) topical steroids applied twice daily can usually control inflammation and itch in these patients.

Children experiencing recurrent episodes often have associated HSV infection and can be treated with suppressive doses of acyclovir (20 mg/kg/d for 6 to 12 months).

Suggested Readings

Ahdout J, Haley JC, Chiu MW. Erythema multiforme during anti-tumor necrosis factor treatment for plaque psoriasis. *J Am Acad Dermatol.* 2010;62:874–879.

Auquier-Dunant A, Mockenhaupt M, Naldi L, et al. Severe cutaneous adverse reactions. Correlations between clinical patterns and causes of erythema multiforme majus, Stevens-Johnson syndrome, and toxic epidermal necrolysis: Results of an international prospective study. *Arch Dermatol.* 2002;138(8):1019–1024.

Ayangco L, Rogers RS III. Oral manifestations of erythema multiforme. *Dermatol Clin.* 2003;21(1):195–205.

Roujeau JC. Erythema multiforme. In: Fitzpatrick TB, Wolff K, eds. *Fitzpatrick's Dermatology in General Medicine.* 7th Ed. New York, NY: McGraw-Hill; 2008:343–349.

Weston WL, Morelli JG. Herpes simplex virus-associated erythema multiforme in prepubertal children. *Arch Pediatr Adolesc Med.* 1997;151(10):1014–1016.

Erythema Toxicum Neonatorum

Alicia Ogram

▚ Diagnosis Synopsis

Erythema toxicum neonatorum (ETN) is a common, self-limited skin eruption of the newborn, usually beginning within 2 days of birth and resolving entirely within 6 to 14 days, without sequelae. Rarely, the eruption can present as late as 10 to 14 days of age or appear in preterm infants as they reach gestational maturity. ETN ordinarily affects term infants, and the incidence decreases with younger gestational age as well as birth weight.

Two variants have been described: erythematopapular and pustular. The eruption begins as erythema on the cheeks that rapidly spreads to the remainder of the face, trunk, and extremities. The palms, soles, and genitals are generally spared. A few hours after the erythema appears, evanescent macules arise within and adjacent to the erythema, soon coalescing to form a blotchy appearance which blanches on pressure and may resemble urticaria on the trunk. Persistent macules develop small central papules that change color from pink to yellow or white within 24 hours. Some papules develop in areas without erythematous macules. Many papules—mostly those on the trunk—transform to superficial pustules ranging from 2 to 4 mm in diameter and containing a pale yellow fluid.

ETN affects neonates of all races and ethnicities, but the incidence may vary in different regions of the world. The reported incidence ranges from 3.7% to 72%, with an average of one-third of term infants affected. In India, one study of 900 neonates found an incidence of 20.6%. A similar incidence of 23% was found in Italy. However, infants in Japan may have an incidence as high as 40.8% and Chinese neonates as high as 43.7%. In Iran, one study of 1,000 neonates found an incidence of 11.1%; however, these infants were evaluated at 48 hours of age or younger.

The etiology of ETN has not yet been elucidated. Some postulate allergy plays a role, given the predominance of eosinophilic infiltrate seen on histopathology. Environmental factors may also be involved, as one Chinese study demonstrated an increased incidence of ETN among male infants, infants born at term, first pregnancy births, births in the summer or autumn, infants fed with milk powder substitute or a mixed diet, and infants delivered vaginally. Recently, the idea that ETN may represent activation of the cutaneous immune system in response to penetration of commensal micro-organisms into the skin via hair follicles has gained favor. Many inflammatory mediators are involved, including IL-1 and IL-8; eotaxin; aquaporins 1 and 3; psoriasin; nitric oxide synthases 1, 2, and 3; and HMGB1.

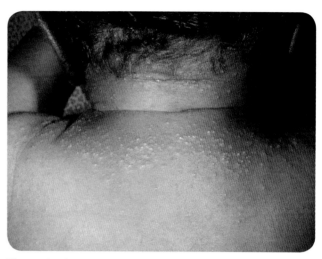

Figure 4-421 Erythema toxicum neonatorum: multiple tiny papules over large portions of the upper back.

◉ Look For

The characteristic lesion is a 1- to 2-mm pale pink to white to yellow papule or pustule with a large erythematous flare (Fig. 4-421). Early on, however, the rash may consist of blotchy, irregular erythematous macules. Any skin surface may be involved, but the palms and soles are usually spared.

●● Diagnostic Pearls

ETN is very rarely present at birth and rarely affects the palms and soles, distinguishing it from congenital candidiasis and transient neonatal pustular melanosis, in which this is characteristic. Lesions are usually evanescent, resolving within 1 to 2 weeks, and papules and pustules will often have surrounding erythema, which also contrasts with transient neonatal pustular melanosis.

?? Differential Diagnosis and Pitfalls

Vesiculopustular rashes in the neonate may be divided into infectious, transient, or persistent dermatoses.

Transient Noninfectious Pustular Dermatoses

- Transient neonatal pustular melanosis—Vesicles and pustules desquamate, leaving brown macules on the chin, neck, palms, and soles. Tzanck smear shows abundant neutrophils.

- Infantile acropustulosis—recurring crops of pustules on the hand and feet
- Pustular miliaria—generalized, grouped erythematous papules and pustules that increase in intertriginous areas; Tzanck smear shows predominance of lymphocytes.
- Neonatal acne—Closed comedones predominate. Gram stain shows bacteria and yeast.
- Pustular eruption in Down syndrome

Persistent Noninfectious Vesiculopustular Dermatoses

- Incontinentia pigmenti—rarely pustular; linear, irregular vesicular and bullous lesions over trunk and extremities
- Eosinophilic pustular folliculitis—crops of papules, vesicles, and pustules that crust, mostly on the scalp with some lesions on the trunk and extremities
- Langerhans cell histiocytosis—Generalized papules, vesicles, pustules, or nodules; biopsy shows Langerhans cells in the dermis with Birbeck granules on electron microscopy
- Pustular psoriasis
- Hyperimmunoglobulin E syndrome

Infectious Vesiculopustular Dermatoses

- Congenital cutaneous candidiasis—KOH shows pseudohyphae and spores.
- Superficial staphylococcal infection/impetigo bullosa—vesicles, pustules, and bullae on an erythematous base in the diaper area, neck, groin, and axilla. Gram stain shows Gram-positive cocci in clusters.
- *Listeria monocytogenes*—Widely disseminated granulomas can be present in early-onset (infected *in utero*) listeriosis. Late onset—grayish-white papulovesicular or pustular rash
- *Haemophilus influenzae*—Fulminant sepsis may present with petechial rash or tender pink macules, papules, and pustules.
- Group A streptococcal infection
- *Pseudomonas*—Most commonly found in children with immune deficiency, malnutrition, or severe burns. Classic lesion is ecthyma gangrenosum. Erythematous or purpuric macules progress to hemorrhagic blue-black bullae that rupture, leaving central necrosis.
- Cytomegalovirus—petechiae and purpura, generalized morbilliform or papulonodular eruption with blueberry muffin lesions
- Aspergillus
- Herpes simplex virus—grouped or single vesicles on erythematous bases in crops on skin and mucous membranes. Tzanck smear shows multinucleated giant cells.
- Neonatal varicella—crops of red macules, papules, vesicles, and pustules on erythematous bases that crust after 1 to 3 days. Tzanck smear shows multinucleated giant cells.

- *Malassezia (Pityrosporum)* folliculitis—follicular papules and sparse pustules on the scalp and face. KOH shows yeast cells budding monopolarly with a broad base.
- Scabies—rare; burrows on hands, feet, trunk, and genitalia. KOH shows *Sarcoptes scabiei* mites, eggs, or fecal particles.

✓ Best Tests

The diagnosis is usually clinically evident. If the clinical picture is unclear, a Tzanck smear with a Wright stain of pustular fluid will demonstrate numerous eosinophils. The cytologic specimen shows >50% eosinophils with a small number of neutrophils. Performing a Wright stain can also rule out viral infections caused by herpes simplex virus, varicella-zoster virus, and cytomegalovirus. A Gram stain without bacteria diminishes the possibility of bacterial infection, and likewise a KOH preparation without yeast diminishes the possibility of candidiasis.

Peripheral blood eosinophilia between 7% and 15% may exist. Histopathologic examination of erythematous macules shows superficial dermal edema with a mild diffuse and perivascular eosinophilic infiltrate. Biopsy of papules shows mild hyperkeratosis and more pronounced edema with eosinophilic infiltration. Pustules are subcorneal or intraepidermal and are usually associated with the pilosebaceous orifice. The superficial layer of the pilosebaceous unit is most intensely involved with sparing of the isthmus and inferior segment. Hair follicles and eccrine glands and ducts are strongly affected.

Management Pearls

Educate and reassure the parent that the eruption is benign and will resolve spontaneously and without sequelae.

Therapy

There is no recommended therapy other than parental reassurance, as ETN is a benign and transient eruption.

Suggested Readings

Akoglu G, Ersoy Evans S, Akca T, et al. An unusual presentation of erythema toxicum neonatorum: Delayed onset in a preterm infant. *Pediatric Dermatol.* 2006;23(3):301–302.

Boccardi D, Menni S, Ferraroni M, et al. Birthmarks and transient skin lesions in newborns and their relationship to maternal factors: A preliminary report from northern Italy. *Dermatology.* 2007;215:53–58.

Hidano A, Purwoko R, Jitsukawa K. Statistical survey of skin changes in Japanese neonates. *Pediatric Dermatol.* 1986;3(2):140–144.

Liu C, Feng J, Qu R, et al. Epidemiologic study of the predisposing factors in erythema toxicum neonatorum. *Dermatology.* 2005;210(4):269–272.

Marchini G, Hultenby K, Nelson A, et al. Increased expression of HMGB-1 in the skin lesions of erythema toxicum. *Pediatric Dermatol.* 2007;24(5):474–482.

Marchini G, Nelson A, Edner J, et al. Erythema toxicum neonatorum is an innate immune response to commensal microbes penetrated into the skin of the newborn infant. *Pediatric Res.* 2005;58(3):613–616.

Marchini G, Stabi B, Kankes K, et al. AQP1 and AQP3, psoriasin, and nitric oxide synthases 1–3 are inflammatory mediators in erythema toxicum neonatorum. *Pediatric Dermatol.* 2003;20(5):377–384.

Mengesha YM, Bennett ML. Pustular skin disorders, diagnosis and treatment. *Am J Clin Dermatol.* 2002;3(6):389–400.

Moosavi Z, Tahereh H. One-year survey of cutaneous lesions in 1000 consecutive Iranian newborns. *Pediatric Dermatol.* 2006;23(1):61–63.

Morgan AJ, Steen CJ, Schwartz RA, et al. Erythema toxicum neonatorum revisited. *Cutis.* 2009;83:13–16.

Nanda A, Kaur S, Bhakoo ON, et al. Survey of cutaneous lesions in Indian newborns. *Pediatric Dermatol.* 1989;6(1):39–42.

Van Praag MC, Van Rooij RW, Folkers E, et al. Diagnosis and treatment of pustular disorders in the neonate. *Pediatric Dermatol.* 1997;14(2):131–143.

Hand-Foot-and-Mouth Disease

Laurie Good

■■ Diagnosis Synopsis

Hand-foot-and-mouth disease (HFMD) is an acute, self-limited viral illness caused most commonly by coxsackievirus A16, although it can be caused by other coxsackieviruses and enteroviruses. It predominantly affects children, but adults can also develop the disease. The incubation period is short, ranging from 3 to 6 days. The illness begins with a mild fever, sore throat and mouth, cough, headache, malaise, and diarrhea and occasionally arthralgias. One or two days after the onset of fever, small oral vesicles develop. Later, vesicles appear on the hands, feet, and, occasionally, the buttocks.

The disease is highly contagious and often spreads via aerosolized droplets, nasal or oral secretions, or fecal material. Epidemic outbreaks usually occur from June to October. Though HFMD is typically self-limited, it can be complicated by encephalitis and other life-threatening complications. These include interstitial pneumonia, myocarditis, meningoencephalitis, and spontaneous abortion. Complications more commonly arise when the infectious agent is an enterovirus, especially enterovirus 71 (EV71), which has been identified as an increasingly common pathogen in HFMD epidemics throughout Asia in the last 20 years.

◉ Look For

Small erythematous macules appear on the oropharynx, later developing into 1- to 3-mm vesicles that ulcerate easily. Shallow ulcerations may involve the palate, tongue, gingiva, or buccal mucosa, and they are often painful. On average, approximately five to ten ulcers may be present.

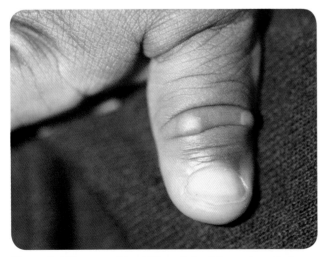

Figure 4-422 Two small hand blisters in hand-foot-and-mouth disease.

Lesions on the extremities begin as erythematous macules and then develop a central, yellow-gray, oval or football-shaped vesicle on an erythematous base (Fig. 4-422). Lesions are most prevalent on the palms and soles, but they can also be seen on the lateral and dorsal surfaces of fingers and toes as well as on the buttocks. Even tiny blisters on the palms and soles can be very painful.

●● Diagnostic Pearls

- Patients may have cervical or submandibular lymphadenopathy.
- Individual oval or elliptical cutaneous vesicles run parallel to skin lines (dermatoglyphics).

?? Differential Diagnosis and Pitfalls

- Varicella—The distribution of lesions as well as the morphology of individual lesions help to differentiate from cases of varicella.
- Erythema multiforme minor—presents with targetoid lesions as opposed to the oval or elliptical vesicles seen in HFMD. Patients frequently have coexisting herpes orolabialis.
- Dyshidrotic eczema—a more chronic dermatitis that presents as pruritic deep-seated vesicles involving the sides of the fingers

For oral lesions, consider:

- Herpes stomatitis
- Aphthous ulcers
- Streptococcal infection
- Candidal infection
- Herpangina—almost identical in systemic presentation with a flulike illness and mouth ulcers, but herpangina does not exhibit vesicles on the palms, soles, digits, and other skin sites. In herpangina, oral ulcers are confined to the posterior oral cavity mucosa.

For lesions on the hands, consider:

- Disseminated herpes simplex virus/zoster
- Papular acrodermatitis of childhood
- Meningococcemia—purpura and pustules
- Rocky Mountain spotted fever—purpura, not vesicular or eroded
- Subacute bacterial endocarditis—purpura
- Gonococcemia—pustular and purpuric

Best Tests

- HFMD is usually a clinical diagnosis; generally, no tests are required.
- If a CBC with differential is performed, white blood cell counts may be slightly elevated, and atypical lymphocytes may be present.
- The virus can be cultured from swabs of vesicles or mucosal surfaces and from stool specimens.
- Neutralizing antibodies may be detected during the acute phase of the illness, and complement-fixing antibodies can be isolated from convalescent sera.

 Management Pearls

This is a self-limited viral infection that needs to be treated only symptomatically, though certain causative agents, such as enteroviruses, have been linked to higher rates of complications and morbidity.

Therapy

Supportive therapy and reassurance are generally all that is required.

Oral pain may interfere with alimentation, and topical oral anesthetics (combination mouth rinses with diphenhydramine elixir, viscous lidocaine, and over-the-counter liquid antacids [all mixed 1:1:1]) are often needed. Encourage adequate hydration.

Antipyretics and oral analgesics (e.g., acetaminophen, ibuprofen) can be used to manage fever and arthralgias, if present.

Chinese literature presents evidence of the effectiveness of Qingre Xiehuo Tang (QXT), a traditional therapy, in the treatment of HFMD.

Suggested Readings

Xiang-hong H, Ming Z. Treatment of hand-foot-mouth disease by Qingre Xiehuo Tang: A clinical observation of 50 Cases. *N J Trad Chin Med.* 2004;20:354–355.

Xu J, Qian Y, Wang S, et al. EV71: An emerging infectious disease vaccine target in the Far East? *Vaccine* 2010;28(20):3516–3521.

Neonatal Herpes

Kamilah Dixon • Lynn McKinley-Grant

■■ Diagnosis Synopsis

Neonatal herpes simplex infections result most often from vertical transmission from the affected mother. While the transmission can occur in utero, intrapartum, or postnatally, intrapartum is the most common, representing 85% of neonatal herpes infections. The infection is spread when infants are exposed to the secretions of affected mothers in the birth canal. For this reason, it is imperative that early detection of HSV in pregnant women is performed to best prevent the spread of the infection. Both herpes simplex type 1 (HSV-1) and HSV-2 can cause neonatal herpes infections.

The symptoms are broad, including low birth weight, neurological complications, dissemination of disease to the liver and lungs, and HSV encephalitis. Many of the infants will present with the hallmark symptoms of vesicles that erupt, causing tender erosions that heal without scarring. These symptoms are often seen along with the more severe systemic complications. Rapid viral detection is necessary so that proper treatment can be started to help prevent detrimental neurological side effects. In the case of HSV encephalitis, the mortality rate is high, making prevention of neonatal herpes simplex of utmost concern.

There have been many hypotheses on how to best prevent infection in newborns, including early HSV serology testing in pregnant women, providing suppressive doses of antivirals to pregnant mothers near the time of delivery to prevent an outbreak, advocating for cesarean sections if the mother has herpes erosions near the birth canal, and preventing oral sex between individuals infected with oral herpes and pregnant women. While these methods may decrease the rates of neonatal herpes, they will not eliminate the spread of the virus completely.

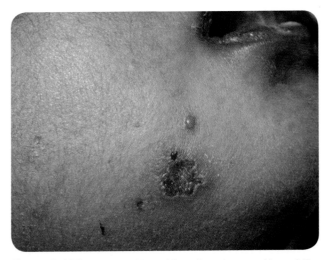

Figure 4-423 Neonate with vesicle and erosions on skin and lips due to herpes simplex virus.

Look For

Small, tender, grouped vesicles or erosions on an erythematous base that resolve without scarring (Fig. 4-423).

●● Diagnostic Pearls

Be aware of grouped vesicles or erosions that have a recurrent nature and resolve without scarring. When these symptoms present in a neonate who is experiencing more serious systemic signs of sepsis, HSV should be considered and empiric therapy should be initiated.

?? Differential Diagnosis and Pitfalls

- Varicella
- Listeriosis
- Gram-negative sepsis
- Group B streptococcal infection
- Staphylococcal infection

✓ Best Tests

In patients with lesions:

- Viral isolation in tissue culture is the gold standard. This must be done in patients with active lesions, preferably 2 to 7 days within the episode to ensure proper visualization.
- Tzanck smear
- Direct fluorescent antigen testing
- PCR-based clinical assays

In patients without lesions:

- Type-specific serology tests

▲▲ Management Pearls

If HSV is suspected, treatment should be initiated while you await test confirmation.

Therapy involves the following:

- Isolation
- IV antiviral therapy

Therapy

Disseminated/CNS Disease
Acyclovir 20 mg/kg IV every 8 hours for 21 days.

Disease Limited to Skin and Mucous Membranes
Acyclovir 20 mg/kg IV every 8 hours for 14 days.

Suggested Reading

Kimberlin DW. Herpes simplex infections of the newborn. *Semin Perinatol.* 2007;31(1):19–25.

Herpes Zoster (Shingles)

Naurin Ahmad

■■ Diagnosis Synopsis

Herpes zoster, commonly known as shingles, is a reactivation of a latent infection with the varicella-zoster virus (VZV), a member of the *Herpesviridae* family. After a primary infection (chickenpox), the virus lies dormant in dorsal root ganglia for life. Reactivation may be triggered by immunosuppression, certain medications, other infections, and even physical or emotional stress. The individual lifetime risk of developing herpes zoster is one in three.

The onset of cutaneous herpes zoster typically involves a 1- to 3-day prodrome of pain, tingling, pruritus, tenderness, or paresthesias in the affected sensory dermatome followed by a cutaneous eruption. In severe cases, the prodrome of thoracic dermatomal pain can simulate an acute myocardial infarction.

The eruption is typically that of erythematous, hemorrhagic, and clear papules and vesicles in the same dermatomal distribution, often coalescing. Herpes zoster is usually confined to a distinct dermatome but can also be found in multiple contiguous or noncontiguous dermatomes (zoster multiplex). There may be small islands of lesions at a distant location.

Among herpes zoster patients, 10% to 25% will have eye involvement, termed herpes zoster ophthalmicus. This variant involves the tissues innervated by the ophthalmic division of the trigeminal nerve. The presence of a localized vesicular rash at the nasal tip, known as Hutchinson sign, may aid in an early diagnosis. The sequelae of herpes zoster ophthalmicus can be devastating and include vision loss and chronic pain. Herpes zoster encephalitis usually appears in the first 2 weeks after the onset of lesions and has a 10% to 20% mortality rate.

The most common complication of herpes zoster is postherpetic neuralgia, defined as pain and neuropathic symptoms that persist beyond the resolution of the rash. This neuralgia is much more frequent in elderly patients with zoster. Risk factors include older age, presence of herpes zoster prodromal pain, and presence of severe pain in the initial clinical presentation of acute herpes zoster. The pain of postherpetic neuralgia can be intractable and debilitating, and one of the goals of treatment is to prevent its development.

Neuropathies may also occur and include peripheral motor neuropathies, neurogenic bladder, and diaphragmatic paralysis. These, however, are usually transient.

Lesions of zoster are also at risk for bacterial superinfection (particularly methicillin-resistant *Staphylococcus aureus*). In extreme cases, necrotizing fasciitis may occur.

Although there are some studies suggesting lower rates of herpes zoster in individuals of African descent and non-white Hispanics, this matter has not been definitively or systematically studied. The most practical issues concern the herpes zoster vaccine, which should be discussed with *all* patients, since the consequences of postherpetic neuralgia can be serious.

Geographic and ethnic factors have been reported in studies of the epidemiology of herpes zoster. Data from five multicenter clinical trials (total $N = 2,074$) revealed that non-white ethnic group and tropical region were each significantly associated with younger age at zoster onset. Upon further subgroup analysis, black and Asian patients from tropical regions had significantly younger mean ages of onset and greater rash duration at enrollment than those from temperate regions, even when controlled for sex and rash duration at enrollment. These results suggest that ethnicity and geographic region may be independent factors associated with age of onset in patients with herpes zoster.

Pediatric Patient Considerations

Herpes zoster has occurred in children receiving the varicella vaccine. However, varicella vaccine is recommended for all children without contraindications independent of ethnic or racial background.

Immunocompromised Patient Considerations

There is an increased incidence of zoster in the immunocompromised, such as AIDS and cancer patients, transplant recipients, and patients on long-term oral corticosteroids. There is also increased incidence and severity of herpes zoster and its complications in older patients due to a gradual decline in cell-mediated immunity.

In immunocompromised patients, herpes zoster may manifest with more atypical clinical presentations. These may include persistent crusted verrucous lesions in HIV-infected patients and postherpetic hyperhidrosis.

Disseminated zoster is more frequent in the immunocompromised population and occurs 5 to 10 days after the onset of dermatomal disease. It is defined as more than 20 lesions outside the initial dermatome of involvement. Associated symptoms can include pain, malaise, and headache.

The prevalence of herpes zoster has increased markedly in the last 30 years in South Africa and is possibly associated with HIV infection.

◉ Look For

Zoster is characterized clinically by the eruption of 2- to 5-mm grouped vesicles or small bullae on an erythematous base, usually (but not always) confined to a distinct

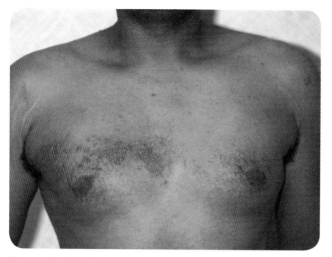

Figure 4-424 Dermatome-restricted blisters and papules are characteristic of herpes zoster.

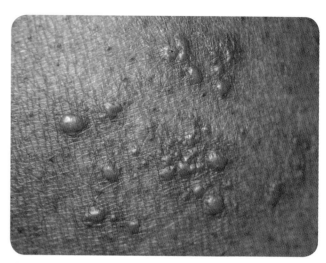

Figure 4-426 Numerous vesicles and hemorrhagic vesicles in facial herpes zoster.

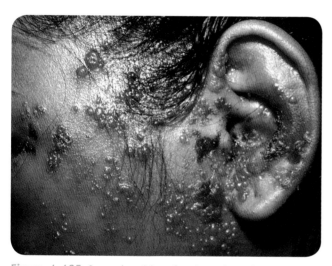

Figure 4-425 Grouped vesicles of various sizes with surrounding erythema in herpes zoster.

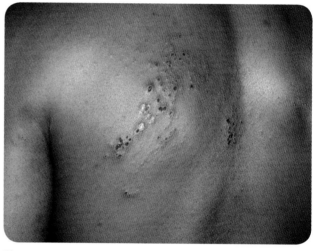

Figure 4-427 Dermatomal and disseminated lesions in a patient with HIV with herpes zoster.

dermatomal distribution without crossing the midline (Figs. 4-424 and 4-425).

Early lesions may be urticarial, grouped papules. Vesicles may be confluent, sparse, or discrete. Generally, vesicles become hemorrhagic, umbilicated, or pustular after several days (Fig. 4-426). The most frequently involved areas are the face in the trigeminal, especially ophthalmic, distribution as well as the trunk from T3 to L2. The lesions typically crust over and resolve after a 7- to 14-day course and are no longer infectious in the immunocompetent host.

Secondary scarring and dyspigmentation are common. Darkly pigmented patients may experience more apparent postinflammatory hyperpigmentation and keloidal scarring on the chest, back, upper arms, and face.

Regional adenopathy may be seen. Some patients may suffer acute segmental neuralgia, known as zoster sine herpete, without ever developing a skin eruption.

Immunocompromised Patient Considerations

If active lesions persist longer than 10 days despite therapy, consider an underlying immunodeficiency in the patient.

Dissemination can occur, particularly in immunocompromised patients, and be associated with multiple organ involvement (Fig. 4-427).

Additional CNS complications may include meningoencephalitis, myelitis, cranial nerve palsies, and, in some cases, may lead to cerebrovascular accidents from inflammation of cerebral vessels.

Diagnostic Pearls

- The Ramsay Hunt syndrome consists of vertigo, ipsilateral facial weakness, and deafness from involvement of the geniculate ganglion.
- Involvement of the nasociliary branch of the ophthalmic nerve increases the risk of ocular complications such as conjunctivitis, lid ulcerations, keratitis, glaucoma, optic neuritis, optic atrophy, and panophthalmitis.

 Differential Diagnosis and Pitfalls

- Herpes simplex virus (HSV) infection
- Cellulitis
- Allergic contact or irritant contact dermatitides
- Folliculitis
- Herpangina
- Insect bites
- Molluscum contagiosum
- Poxviruses (cowpox, monkeypox)
- Pyoderma gangrenosum
- Primary varicella infection
- During the prodromal phase, herpes zoster pain may mimic acute myocardial infarction or biliary colic.

 Best Tests

- There is no one standard method for diagnosing herpes zoster, although in most cases the disease is typically diagnosed clinically by appearance and distribution.
- The Tzanck smear is the most rapid and least expensive test. A smear is made of cells scraped from the base of the bullae, stained, and examined under the microscope for multinucleate giant cells.
- PCR can be useful for detecting viral DNA in difficult or complicated cases (encephalitis, zoster sine herpete).
- Direct immunofluorescence (DFA) may also be performed and is a more rapid (<24-hour) and sensitive test for HSV-1, HSV-2, and VZV. This test is performed by vigorously scraping the base of a vesicle with a sterile cotton-tipped swab or No. 15 blade and smearing the cells onto a glass slide from a DFA kit. The slide is then fixed (usually contained in a kit) and sent for immunofluorescence analysis. Individual slides must be sent for each virus suspected. Slides can be stored at room temperature for 24 hours after fixation, if needed.
- Electron microscopy is rarely used.
- Other special testing may be clinically indicated if lesions are resistant to therapy or patients deteriorate. These include HIV testing, lumbar puncture with CSF analysis, or MRI of the brain and/or spinal cord.

 Management Pearls

- Patients with active vesicular lesions can spread the infection to immunocompromised hosts and, if the patient is a health care provider, he/she should take a leave of absence from work.
- The following consultations may be needed: dermatology, neurology, infectious disease, and/or ophthalmology (herpes zoster ophthalmicus). In cases in which the ear is involved (herpes zoster oticus), an otolaryngology consult is warranted.
- The CDC Advisory Committee on Immunization Practices recommends a single dose of the live attenuated zoster vaccine, similar to varicella vaccine but 14 times more potent, for adults aged 60 or older, whether or not they have had a previous episode of herpes zoster. The vaccination decreases risk for both herpes zoster and postherpetic neuralgia.
- There is also some evidence that health care providers who are exposed to patients with herpes zoster may experience a boost in immunoprotection, and the risk of developing shingles may be decreased.

Immunocompromised Patient Considerations

The vaccine is contraindicated in the immunocompromised, those with an allergy to gelatin or neomycin, and those with active untreated tuberculosis.

Therapy

Antiviral therapy (acyclovir and prodrug forms), if administered in the first 72 hours after the onset of the first vesicle, can shorten the length and severity of the acute episode and may help to decrease the likelihood of developing postherpetic neuralgia. Antiviral therapy is the mainstay of treatment and is most effective in reducing sequelae and duration of disease if started within 72 hours, but benefit has been shown even when therapy was delayed. Three main oral antivirals used are acyclovir 800 mg p.o. every 4 hours for 7 to 10 days (frequently given five times daily), famciclovir 500 mg p.o. every 8 hours for 7 days, and valacyclovir 1,000 mg p.o. every 8 hours for 7 days.

Wet-to-dry dressings with sterile saline solution, aluminum acetate, or Burow soaks can help to alleviate cutaneous symptoms. This should be applied to the affected skin for 30 to 60 minutes four to six times daily.

Antihistamines and topical anti-itch lotions may also be used as an antipruritic agent. Domeboro soaks may help to dry out weeping or oozing blisters.

A single published study supports the use of amitriptyline (25 mg daily) as an adjunct to an antiviral agent in acute herpes zoster to decrease the incidence of and pain associated with subsequent postherpetic neuralgia. Physicians should also take into account the risk factors for developing postherpetic neuralgia in certain patient populations (elderly, severe pain in the acute episode of herpes zoster, and presence and severity of prodromal pain).

Patients routinely require pain control. Nonsteroidal anti-inflammatory agents and opioid narcotics may be added for pain relief. Topical pain control can be achieved with EMLA cream, lidocaine patches, capsaicin, and nerve blocks. Other medications used for neuropathic pain include gabapentin and tricyclic antidepressants. Corticosteroids do not appear to prevent postherpetic neuralgia but can be used in severe cases to reduce inflammation.

Scarring, atrophy, and dyspigmentation are often long-term consequences of zosteriform eruptions and can be more prominent in darkly pigmented patients. Case reports in Asian patients demonstrated improvement in atrophic, depressed plaques of the forehead from a prior herpes zoster infection with injection of pneumatic hyaluronic acid (one-shot 0.2-mL volume of HA and an 80% pressure power with a 10- × 10-mm square-shaped tip).

Immunocompromised Patient Considerations

Hospital admission should be considered for any of the following situations: severe symptoms, immunosuppression, and more than two dermatomes involved. This group of patients may benefit from intravenous acyclovir as the initial therapy for herpes zoster. Patients should then switch over to an oral agent (valacyclovir or famciclovir) after initial clinical improvement is noted and lesions have crusted over.

Suggested Readings

Hartshorne ST. Dermatological disorders in Johannesburg, South Africa. *Clin Exp Dermatol*. 2003;28(6):661–665.

Kang JH, Ho JD, Chen YH, et al. Increased risk of stroke after a herpes zoster attack: A population-based follow-up study. *Stroke*. 2009;40(11):3443–3448.

Kim BJ, Yoo KH, Kim MN. Successful treatment of depressed scars of the forehead secondary to herpes zoster using subdermal minimal surgery technology. *Dermatol Surg*. 2009;35(9):1439–1440.

Nagasako EM, Johnson RW, Griffin DR, et al. Geographic and racial aspects of herpes zoster. *J Med Virol*. 2003;70(Suppl 1):S20–S23.

Schmader K, George LK, Burchett BM, et al. Racial differences in the occurrence of herpes zoster. *J Infect Dis*. 1995;171(3):701–704.

Whitley RJ. A 70-year-old woman with shingles: Review of herpes zoster. *JAMA*. 2009;302(1):73–80.

Bullous Impetigo

Meaghan Canton Feder

▪▪ Diagnosis Synopsis

Bullous impetigo is a superficial infection of the skin that is usually caused by phage group II *Staphylococcus aureus*. It is primarily seen in newborns, but can affect all ages. In adults it presents as a painful red rash with fragile large bullae that rupture, leaving "honey-colored" crusted lesions. Constitutional symptoms are rare and mild if they do occur. Outbreaks tend to occur during the summer months and in warmer, humid climates. *S. aureus* can secondarily infect the lesions of varicella and atopic dermatitis, causing a bullous presentation.

Methicillin-resistant *S. aureus* (MRSA) first emerged as an important nosocomial pathogen in the 1960s. In more recent years, outbreaks of community-acquired MRSA have been described increasingly among healthy individuals lacking the traditional immunocompromised risk factors for such infections.

Pediatric Patient Considerations

Bullous impetigo usually affects newborn infants within the first 2 weeks of life. It is often very contagious. Infants present with bullae, usually on the hands or face, and develop fever and diarrhea. If the infection is not treated, they can develop pneumonia or meningitis; the condition can even result in death.

Immunocompromised Patient Considerations

MRSA can be seen more frequently in immunocompromised patients. Bullous impetigo can be an early sign of HIV infection.

◉ Look For

The lesions in bullous impetigo are large, flaccid, serous or yellow fluid-filled bullae that usually present in adults on the trunk or extremities (Fig. 4-428). They rarely affect the scalp. The superficial bullae rapidly progress and are easily denuded, leaving moist red erosions that evolve rapidly to honey-colored crusts. The lesions are well demarcated with no surrounding erythema. There are usually no constitutional symptoms in adults. Atopic dermatitis is common in African Americans, and *S. aureus* can be a secondary infection, causing bullous impetigo.

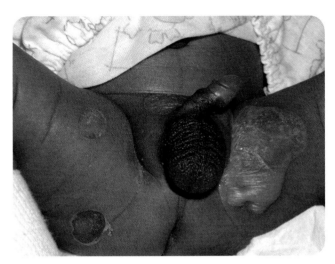

Figure 4-428 Bullous impetigo with large intact and eroded bullae.

Pediatric Patient Considerations

Newborn babies usually present with bullae similar to those of adults; bullae are typically located on the hands or face but can appear anywhere on the body. Usually, but not initially, newborns have a fever with no other constitutional symptoms.

●● Diagnostic Pearls

Bullous impetigo usually occurs in warmer, humid climates. It can be very contagious and can spread through direct contact.

Pediatric Patient Considerations

In the pediatric population, bullous impetigo is very contagious and can spread through contact. It is often seen in children playing contact sports, such as wrestling. Also consider a concurrent secondary dermatosis, such as scabies, poison ivy, an insect bite, atopic dermatitis, or trauma that leads to impetigo. Primary varicella can present as bullous varicella due to coinfection with *S. aureus*.

?? Differential Diagnosis and Pitfalls

- Bullous dermatitis—If the rash is persistent and recurrent, consider a primary bullous disease such as pemphigus vulgaris, bullous pemphigoid, epidermolysis bullosa acquisita, linear IgA dermatosis, or dermatitis herpetiformis.

- Contact dermatitis—usually small vesicles in distinct location. If poison ivy, vesicles will be in linear formation and pruritic.
- Herpes simplex virus—Perform viral culture.
- Burns—Take detailed history and ask about trauma.
- Stevens-Johnson syndrome
- Bullous tinea—Perform KOH to rule out tinea.
- Drug eruption
- Varicella—usually small, discrete, umbilicated vesicles that can cover all body surface areas including the mouth
- Bullous lupus erythematosus—Ask about history of lupus.

✓ Best Tests

- The provider can perform a Gram stain of blister fluid. The stain will show neutrophils with Gram-positive cocci in chains or clusters.
- The provider can send a bacterial culture and antibiotic sensitivity to the laboratory. However, if there is a strong suspicion of bacterial infection, then do not wait for results to treat infection.

Pediatric Patient Considerations

The provider can perform a Gram stain of blister fluid or can send a bacterial culture and antibiotic sensitivity to the laboratory.

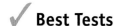

Management Pearls

- Bullous impetigo can be very contagious, and the use of standard precautions can decrease the spread of infection. The infected individuals should use separate towels and soap. They should perform gentle wound cleaning with good hygiene to prevent the spread of infection. If large areas of skin are denuded, consider intravenous fluid replacement. If in the hospital, healthcare workers should use standard and contact precautions, including isolation of patient, wearing gloves and a gown, limiting patient transport, and avoidance of sharing patient-care equipment.
- Early treatment is also important to avoid scarring from loss of skin and to decrease postinflammatory hyperpigmentation on darker skin types.

Pediatric Patient Considerations

The pediatric patient should avoid direct contact with other children and avoid all contact sports. The patient should also be taught to wash hands and to avoid sharing towels and soap.

Therapy

Bullous impetigo should be treated early with systemic antibiotics.

- Erythromycin 250 mg p.o. four times daily for 1 week
- Dicloxacillin 250 to 500 mg p.o. four times daily for 1 week
- Cephalexin 250 to 500 mg p.o. four times daily for 1 week
- Clindamycin 300 mg p.o. three times daily for 10 days

MRSA is resistant to stand ard cephalosporins and penicillins. For bullous impetigo caused by MRSA, consult current CDC guidelines due to rapidly changing treatment recommendations.

Pediatric Patient Considerations

Bullous impetigo should be treated early with systemic antibiotics in the pediatric population.

- Erythromycin 30 to 50 mg/kg/d p.o. divided into four times daily for 1 week
- Dicloxacillin 25 to 50 mg/kg/d p.o. divided into four times daily for 1 week
- Cephalexin 25 to 50 mg/kg/d p.o. divided into four times daily for 1 week
- Clindamycin 10 to 30 mg/kg/d p.o. divided into three times daily for 10 days

MRSA is resistant to standard cephalosporins and penicillins. For bullous impetigo caused by MRSA, consult current CDC guidelines, as treatment recommendations are rapidly changing.

Suggested Readings

James WD, Berger TG, Elston DM, eds. Infections caused by Gram-positive organisms, impetigo contagiosa, bullous impetigo, and ecthyma. In: *Andrews' Diseases of the Skin: Clinical Dermatology*. 10th Ed. Philadelphia, PA: Saunders Elsevier; 2006:255–259.

Nakaminami H, Noguchi N, Ikeda M, et al. Molecular epidemiology and antimicrobial susceptibilities of 273 exfoliative toxin-encoding-gene-positive *Staphylococcus aureus* isolates from patients with impetigo in Japan. *J Med Microbiol.* 2008;57(10):1251–1258.

Pawun V, Jiraphongsa C, Puttamasute S, et al. An outbreak of hospital-acquired *Staphylococcus aureus* skin infection among newborns, Nan Province, Thailand. *Euro Surv Eur Commun Dis Bull.* 2009;14(43).

Rayner C, Munckhof WJ. Antibiotics currently used in the treatment of infections caused by *Staphylococcus aureus. Intern Med J.* 2005;36(2):142–143.

Steer AC, Tikoduadua LV, Manalac EM, et al. Validation of an integrated management of childhood illness algorithm for managing common skin conditions in Fiji. *Bull Work Health Org.* 2009;87(3):173–179.

Larva Migrans

Stephanie Diamantis

◼◼ Diagnosis Synopsis

Cutaneous larva migrans (also known as creeping eruption, creeping verminous dermatitis, sandworm eruption, plumber's itch, and duck hunter's itch) is a parasitic infestation of the epidermis caused by larvae of hookworms that infect domestic dogs and cats or humans. The disease is most commonly found in tropical climates, with high incidence observed in southeastern United States, Central and South America, Africa, and the Caribbean. The most common organisms are *Ancylostoma braziliense*, *Ancylostoma caninum*, and *Uncinaria stenocephala*. Larva migrans is acquired by walking barefoot on soil or sand contaminated with dog or cat feces that contains the larvae. After contact with the skin, larvae penetrate the skin and migrate through the epidermis in a serpiginous, or "snakelike," fashion. The infection is almost always confined to the outermost layers of the skin and very rarely penetrates to subcutaneous tissues or spreads throughout the body, as humans are incidental hosts.

Cutaneous findings are characterized by intensely pruritic, serpiginous tracts localized primarily to the ankles and feet; however, other areas of the body that have contacted infected soil may be involved (e.g., buttocks, abdomen). Itching begins within hours to days of exposure, and migration usually occurs after 4 days. Lesions are often edematous, erythematous papules and may have associated vesicles and bullae. The majority of patients present with more than one lesion, and lesions migrate at a rate of 1 to 2 cm/d. As humans are "dead-end" hosts, the infection is generally self-limited and resolves within weeks to months. Treatment is limited to symptomatic relief of intense pruritus. Bacterial superinfection can occur as a result of scratching. Systemic symptoms are rare but may include coughing or wheezing.

◉ Look For

Pruritic, raised, red, serpiginous, curvilinear trails with or without papules and/or vesicles (Figs. 4-429–4-431). Migration of the larvae in the epidermis occurs at a rate of approximately 2 cm/d.

Eruption is most commonly located over the ankles and feet but can be found on the buttocks, genitals, hands, or any area with direct contact with sand or soil.

◉◉ Diagnostic Pearls

- History of skin exposure to the ground or sand in warm climates. Ask about history of travel.

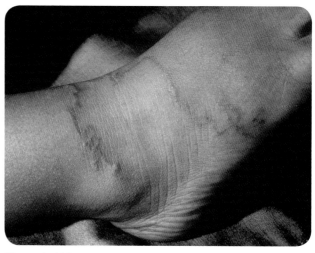

Figure 4-430 Multiple larval tracts with a serpiginous configuration on the foot.

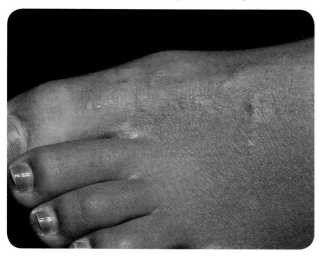

Figure 4-429 Small red papules and one small vesicle in cutaneous larva migrans.

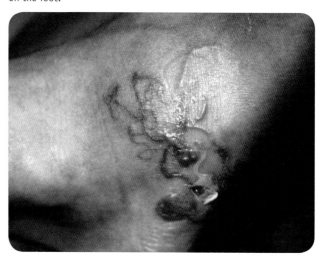

Figure 4-431 Complex interweaving of larva tracks with vesicles and frank erosions.

- Lesions may erupt upon the change of seasons with an increase in temperature (weeks to months after exposure).
- Systemic involvement is rare.

?? Differential Diagnosis and Pitfalls

- Cercarial forms of nonhuman schistosomes
- Seabather's eruption—involves areas of the body covered by the bathing suit
- Larval forms of marine coelenterates
- Portuguese man-of-war or jellyfish stings
- Strongyloides infestation—migrates much more quickly (5 to 10 cm/h)
- Erythema annulare centrifugum
- Erythema chronicum migrans
- Figurate erythemas
- Contact dermatitis
- Tinea pedis—hyphae evident on KOH prep
- Myiasis
- Loiasis
- Impetigo
- Dracunculiasis
- Gnathostomiasis
- Scabies—look for burrows
- Swimmer's itch
- Dermatophytosis

✓ Best Tests

The diagnosis of cutaneous larva migrans is made clinically.

Biopsy is not recommended, as the serpiginous tract lags behind the movement of the worm, typically leading to negative or nonspecific histopathology. Rarely, peripheral eosinophilia may be present.

▲▲ Management Pearls

- Preventative measures include wearing shoes and sitting on a towel or chair at the beach.

- Attempts at surgical extraction or treatment with liquid nitrogen should be avoided because the skin findings are a delayed reaction to the parasite (i.e., the worm is not directly under the lesion in most cases).
- This infection is self-limited and will eventually resolve without therapy after several weeks; however, due to the intense pruritus and risk of superinfection, treatment is recommended.

Therapy

Preferred treatments include:

- Ivermectin 200 µg/kg by mouth daily for 1 to 2 days
- Albendazole 400 to 800 mg by mouth daily for 3 to 5 days

Oral thiabendazole is also an option for treatment but is not as well-tolerated as ivermectin or albendazole and is poorly effective with one-time dosing. Frequent side effects include nausea, vomiting, diarrhea, and headache.

Topical 10% to 15% thiabendazole solution or ointment is available and is well tolerated. Dosing schedule is as follows: apply three times per day for at least 15 days, including the area about 2 cm beyond the leading edge of the serpiginous trail. Effectiveness is limited in widespread lesions or hookworm folliculitis.

Suggested Readings

Caumes E. Treatment of cutaneous larva migrans. *Clin Infect Dis.* 2000;30:811–814.

Heukelbach J, Feldmeier H. Epidemiological and clinical characteristics of hookworm-related cutaneous larva migrans. *Lancet Infect Dis.* 2008;8:302–309.

O'Brien BM. A practical approach to common skin problems in returning travelers. *Travel Med Infect Dis.* 2009;7(3):125–146.

Patel S, Sethi A. Imported tropical diseases. *Dermatol Ther.* 2009;22: 538–549.

Wilson ME, Caumes E. Helminthic infections. In: Wolff K, Goldsmith LA, Katz SI, Gilchrest BA, Paller AS, Leffell DJ, eds. *Fitzpatric k's Dermatology in General Medicine.* 7th Ed. New York, NY: McGraw Hill; 2008: 2011–2029.

Lymphangioma Circumscriptum (Microcystic Lymphatic Malformation)

Chris G. Adigun

■■ Diagnosis Synopsis

Lymphatic malformations (LMs) consist of vesicles or cysts filled with lymphatic fluid. Macrocystic LMs, formerly known as cystic hygroma, are larger than 1 cm in diameter. Microcystic LM, formerly known as lymphangioma circumscriptum, lymphangioma simplex, verrucous hemangioma, and angiokeratoma circumscriptum, is a benign congenital disorder that consists of dilated superficial lymphatic channels or large cysts filled with lymphatic fluid. Microcystic LMs occur as a result of an error in the morphogenesis of the lymphatic vessels, leading to a disorder of lymph drainage. However, the exact etiology of this error is unknown. Subcutaneous lymphatic cisterns communicate through dilated channels with the skin's surface to form localized clusters of translucent vesicles that contain clear or serosanguineous lymphatic fluid. Unlike venous malformations, microcystic LMs do not swell with the Valsalva maneuver but rather swell periodically, often in association with viral illnesses. Microcystic LMs form in utero and are, thus, present at birth or become more apparent in early childhood. Most are diagnosed before the age of 2. At times, these lesions are not detected until complications arise, such as infection or bleeding. Microcystic LMs can occur as combined lymphatic and vascular malformations. These combined lesions are more commonly seen in the head region and can interfere with normal development of the jaw.

The presentation of microcystic LMs can vary greatly, usually depending on the site and depth. Distribution of microcystic LMs is most commonly on the face, although they may occur on the proximal extremities, groin, axilla, or oral or genital areas. Lesions tend to grow proportionally and, thus, enlarge with age, which may delay the diagnosis. These lesions may intermittently leak lymphatic fluid, and they can bleed and become purple or nodular.

Microcystic LMs have a propensity to appear on the face, especially in the mandibular area, and may cause facial asymmetry. Sepsis is a serious complication that may occur in lesions close to the alimentary tract, such as the face and pelvis. Other locations that can cause extracutaneous complications include intraorbital LM, which can cause exophthalmia and ocular dystopia, or LM on the tongue, which can impair speech and produce halitosis.

Intervention is typically not necessary unless lesions are symptomatic. The most common symptoms include pain, inflammatory flares, minor bleeding, and recurrent episodes of cellulitis. Historically, surgical treatment was the treatment of choice for microcystic LM, although recurrence was frequent and surgical morbidity was considerable, as the entire lesion needed to be excised. Newer therapies, including the use of sclerosing agents, have shown promising long-term results.

⦿ Look For

Multiple grouped or contiguous 2- to 4-mm pink, red, translucent, or black (hemorrhagic) thick-walled vesicles, the appearance of which has been likened to that of "frog spawn" (Figs. 4-432–4-435). These lesions appear fluid-filled but are firm to palpation and typically do not rupture. Oral mucosal lesions may have thick walls and contain a milky-appearing fluid. Lesions may also appear verrucous. Uncommonly, lesions may present with a well-defined bruiselike area that occurs due to bleeding into subcutaneous cysts that are not apparent unless filled with blood.

The lesions are most commonly encountered on the face but may occur on the proximal extremities, trunk, axilla, and in the oral cavity. Anogenital lesions, including the vulva and scrotum, are also frequently reported.

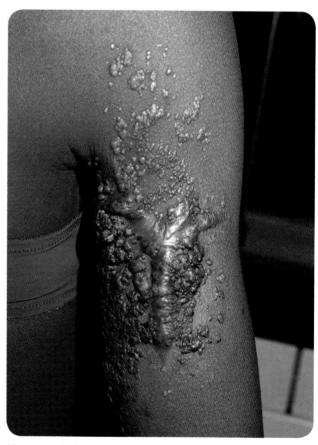

Figure 4-432 Lymphangioma circumscriptum with clear lymph-containing vesicles and darker blood-containing vesicles.

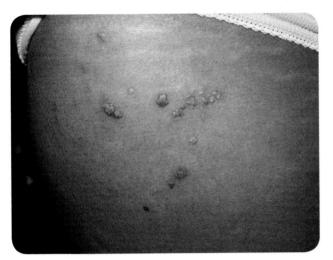

Figure 4-433 Lymphangioma circumscriptum with clear vesicles.

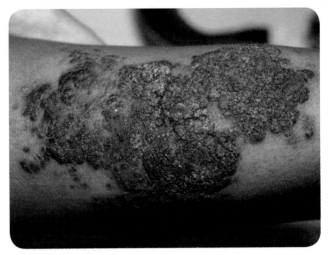

Figure 4-435 Lymphangioma circumscriptum with predominantly blood-filled vesicles.

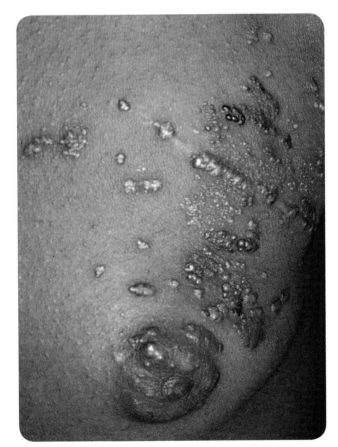

Figure 4-434 Lymphangioma circumscriptum with predominantly clear vesicles.

 Diagnostic Pearls

- Although the lesions appear similar to vesicles, they are often straw-colored or blood-tinged. They also do not break as easily as true vesicles. Lesions are generally long-standing, with intermittent draining of serosanguineous lymphatic fluid.
- The lesions of lymphangioma circumscriptum tend to expand and increase in number with age, which may be a diagnostic challenge if the patient reports that it is a new lesion rather than one that is present from birth.
- Lesions may be verrucoid and appear to be deeply pigmented in patients with dark skin, whereas the color would appear more hemorrhagic in light skin. There is a report of a 2-year-old Sri Lankan boy—with presumably darkly pigmented skin—who was diagnosed and treated for a viral wart in Australia. In addition, there are two other reports of patients of Indian heritage and darkly pigmented skin with microcystic LMs that were misdiagnosed as molluscum contagiosum and genital warts.

?? Differential Diagnosis and Pitfalls

- Venous ectasias
- Metastatic carcinoma
- Melanoma
- Angiosarcoma
- Hemangioma
- Verruca vulgaris
- Condyloma acuminata
- Molluscum contagiosum
- Allergic contact dermatitis
- Herpes simplex virus (HSV)
- Incontinentia pigmenti
- Acquired lymphectasia due to radiotherapy, Crohn disease, postsurgical fibrosis, or infections such as scrofuloderma or erysipelas

In an adult with darkly pigmented skin, also consider the following:

- Epidermal nevus
- Sarcoidosis

Pediatric Patient Differential Diagnosis

- Fibro- or rhabdomyosarcoma— if rapidly growing
- Infantile hemangioma—would be well-demarcated, less vesicular/translucent
- Venous malformation—would have a bluer color and more deep component
- Angiokeratomas
- Epidermal nevus
- Teratoma
- Verruca vulgaris
- Molluscum contagiosum
- Incontinentia pigmenti
- HSV

✓ Best Tests

- Skin biopsy will demonstrate characteristic histopathology of dilated, flat, endothelium-lined channels that are typically thin; the diagnosis can be made on clinical appearance alone.
- Ultrasonography may aid in determining the depth and extent of the lesions prior to surgical intervention. MRI and lymphangiography have been used to locate lymphatic cisterns in preparation for excision. MRI is the gold standard for this purpose, and lesions demonstrate hyperintensity in T2-weighted images.

▲▲▲ Management Pearls

- If the lesion is asymptomatic, adopting a "watch and wait" policy is reasonable.
- Surgical intervention is typically undertaken for cosmetic reasons, although other indications include pain, recurrent bleeding, and infections.
- Although microcystic LM is considered a benign entity, there are extremely rare case reports of malignant tumor appearance within this malformation. Risk of malignant change is greatest in malformations previously treated with irradiation.
- For surgical intervention, wide excision is needed, as recurrence following surgery is frequent.

- If a patient undergoes sclerotherapy for a lesion and has recurrent swelling, studies show that if these patients undergo a second procedure, their rate of another recurrence is significantly lower.

Therapy

If treatment is desired for aesthetic reasons or symptomatic lesions (painful, bleeding, recurrent infections), historically, wide local excision was the treatment of choice. At this time, all other therapies are considered noncurative but palliative for symptoms and cosmetic appearance. Therapies that have proven successful include electrocautery, cryotherapy, sclerotherapy, and laser vaporization (carbon dioxide laser). Pulsed dye laser has been reported as effective in treating smaller superficial cutaneous blebs. A good cosmetic outcome was also reported with intense pulsed light therapy. However, recurrence rates are high with all therapeutic modalities.

Multiple sclerosant drugs have been employed, including ethanol, sodium tetradecyl sulfate, OK-432, bleomycin, and doxycycline. In the United States, ethanol is a commonly used sclerosant. However, this treatment has limitations when used in children, as the volume of ethanol that can be injected safely is often too small to be effective. Current literature evaluating the use of doxycycline shows that it is safe for all ages, and studies have shown it to be more effective than other sclerosants in eliminating cysts of microcystic LMs. A recent retrospective review of percutaneous treatment with doxycycline for microcystic malformations, both primary and after surgical intervention, shows excellent outcomes, with all patients who underwent the procedure having complete resolution of the microcysts. The success of this treatment was further confirmed by sonography or MRI.

Complicating skin and soft tissue infections should be treated with appropriate antibiotics.

In patients with darkly pigmented skin, proper counseling should be performed prior to any form of laser or sclerotherapy, as scarring and dyspigmentation occur at high rates in this treatment population.

Suggested Readings

Burrows PE, Mitri RK, Alomari A, et al. Percutaneous sclerotherapy of lymphatic malformations with doxycycline. *Lymphat Res Biol.* 2008;6 (3–4):209–216.

Davies D, Rogers M, Lam A, et al. Localized microcystic lymphatic malformations—ultrasound diagnosis. *Pediatr Dermatol.* 1999;16(6): 423–439.

Gupta S, Radotra BD, Javaheri SM, et al. Lymphangioma circumscriptum of the penis mimicking venereal lesions. *J Eur Acad Dermatol Venereol.* 2003;17(5):598–600.

Halder RM, Nootheti PK. Ethnic skin disorders overview. *J Am Acad Dermatol.* 2003;48(6 Suppl):S143–S148.

Jackson BA. Lasers in ethnic skin: A review. *J Am Acad Dermatol.* 2003;48(6 Suppl):S134–S138.

Nayler SJ, Rubin BP, Calonje E, et al. Composite hemangioendothelioma: A complex, low-grade vascular lesion mimicking angiosarcoma. *Am J Surg Pathol.* 2000;24(3):352–361.

Shiels WE II, Kang DR, Murakami JW, et al. Percutaneous treatment of lymphatic malformations. *Otolaryngol Head Neck Surg.* 2009;141(2):219–224.

Tulasi NR, John A, Chauhan I, et al. Lymphangioma circumscriptum. *Int J Gynecol Cancer.* 2004;14(3):564–566.

Verma SB. Lymphangiectasias of the skin: Victims of confusing nomenclature. *Clin Exp Dermatol.* 2009;34(5):566–569. Epub 2009 May 18.

Miliaria Crystallina

Saurabh Singh

▪▪ Diagnosis Synopsis

Miliaria is a common disorder caused by the occlusion of eccrine sweat ducts. There are different clinical patterns of miliaria depending on the level of occlusion.

Miliaria crystallina results from blockage of the eccrine sweat ducts in the stratum corneum, corresponding to the formation of asymptomatic, pinpoint, fragile vesicles. Superficial occlusion is thought to result from increased hydration compounded with humidity and sweating. When the occlusion of the sweat duct is deeper in the epidermis, miliaria rubra (prickly heat), miliaria pustulosa, or miliaria profunda may result.

Miliaria crystallina is most common in neonates, but is seen in adults in the setting of hospitalized and/or bedridden patients with high fever and excessive sweating. It also follows sunbathing, warming in a hot tub, occlusion of the skin from dressings, and restrictive clothing. The use of occlusive products prior to exercise may induce this condition as well. It is also more common in tropical climates and is frequently seen in patients who have recently moved to a tropical climate from a more temperate climate.

The primary triggers for the development of miliaria are high heat, humidity, and febrile illnesses. These precipitants can lead to excessive sweating causing overhydration of the stratum corneum. The blockage of the eccrine glands results in leakage of sweat in either the dermis or epidermis.

Bacteria normally present on the skin, such as *Staphylococcus aureus* or *S. epidermis*, are also believed to be involved in the pathogenesis of miliaria. Periodic acid-Schiff–positive diastase-resistant material has been found in the intraductal plug.

Pediatric Patient Considerations

Miliaria crystallina commonly affects neonates <2 weeks of age. Neonates, usually around the sixth or seventh postnatal day, are thought to have a predisposition to miliaria because of immature eccrine ducts that easily rupture when sweating occurs; however, the occurrence of this condition prior to the fourth day of life is extremely rare. There have been three cases of congenital miliaria crystallina reported in black newborns. In these cases, it has been hypothesized that the disease results from the occlusion of sweat glands *in utero*.

◉ Look For

Miliaria crystallina presents with tiny, clear, superficial, noninflammatory vesicles that are 1 to 2 mm in diameter (occasionally larger) (Figs. 4-436–4-438). They appear

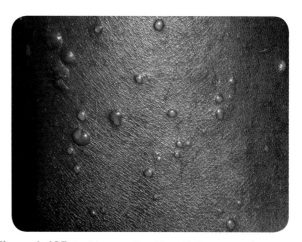

Figure 4-437 Rapid onset of vesicles of miliaria crystallina (biopsy proven).

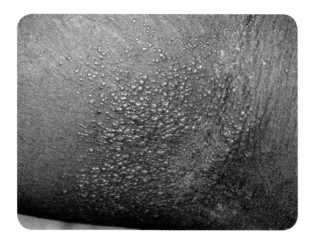

Figure 4-436 Multiple thin-roofed noninflammatory vesicles of miliaria crystallina.

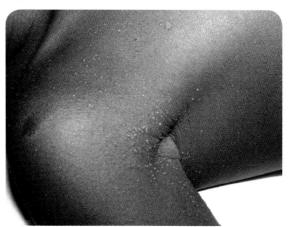

Figure 4-438 Miliaria crystallina in a child with sickle cell anemia and fever.

within days to weeks of exposure to warm, humid weather. The vesicles are fragile and do not persist, resolving within hours to days. They may become confluent and most commonly involve areas occluded by clothing or bedding. After the vesicles rupture, they may leave behind areas of fine desquamation.

Diagnostic Pearls

- Vesicles are very fragile and rupture easily. Lesions are most prominent in areas occluded by bedding or clothing (e.g., the back in bedridden patients).
- Patients will often have a history of a recent high fever or a visit/move to a tropical climate.

Differential Diagnosis and Pitfalls

Miliaria crystallina can be caused by various entities, including hot and humid conditions such as the tropics, incubators in neonatal nurseries, and febrile illnesses.

Vesicular drug eruption has also been associated with crystalline miliaria. Bethanechol, a drug that induces sweating, can cause miliaria. A combination of days to weeks of fever leading to profuse sweating and the use of cholinergic drugs, such as neostigmine, that stimulate glandular secretion can induce miliaria. Patients in the ICU are often on beta blockers in addition to alpha 1- and alpha 2-adrenergic catecholamines. The effect of the intrinsic sympathomimetic activity from a beta blocker may result in increased pressure within the eccrine ducts, enhancing sweat flow and contributing to the development of miliaria crystallina. Opiates can also have a similar effect by stimulating the parasympathetic nervous system. Other drugs such as clonidine and isotretinoin have been linked to cases of miliaria. More recently, doxorubicin was reported as a cause of miliaria crystallina after the fifth day of chemotherapeutic administration. These drugs may create an environment where sweat glands become blocked, making the patient susceptible to developing miliaria crystallina. There are several entities that a clinician should consider when diagnosing miliaria.

- Lesions may resemble toxic epidermal necrolysis with the presence of desquamation; however, miliaria crystallina does not have the intense erythema, mucosal involvement, or systemic illness associated with toxic epidermal necrolysis.
- Varicella presents with vesicles on an erythematous base (e.g., "dewdrops on a rose petal") and with lesions in different stages.
- Folliculitis manifests as follicular-based pustules.
- Herpes simplex or herpes zoster presents with painful crops of vesicles that often occur near a mucosal surface or in a dermatomal distribution, respectively.

Pediatric Patient Differential Diagnosis and Pitfalls

- Vesicular drug eruptions—larger tense vesicles
- Eosinophilic pustular folliculitis
- Acute generalized exanthematous pustulosis—pustules are opaque, not clear as in miliaria

Best Tests

- A skin biopsy will confirm the diagnosis but is usually not necessarily based on the clinical history and physical examination.
- If there is concern for infection, a culture is appropriate.

Management Pearls

Treat any underlying causes of fever, and avoid occlusive clothing or products. Keep the patient in a cool environment; provide air conditioning, if possible.

Pediatric Patient Considerations

Overdressing of young children is a common cause of this condition; make sure to ask the parents and recommend fewer clothes if this etiology seems possible.

Therapy

- Miliaria crystallina is usually asymptomatic and self-limited; treatment in most cases is not required.
- Cool baths or showers may enhance patient comfort. Encourage patients to wear loose-fitting clothing and expose the involved skin to the air, if possible. Antipyretics can help control fever and prevent subsequent miliaria formation. Patients should avoid heavy emollients, as they may exacerbate the problem.

Suggested Readings

Anbu AT, Williams S. Miliaria crystallina complicating staphylococcal scalded skin syndrome. *Arch Dis Child*. 2004;89(1):94.

Godkar D, Razaq M, Fernandez G. Rare skin disorder complicating doxorubicin therapy: Miliaria crystallina. *Am J Ther*. 2005;12(3):275–276.

Haas N, Martens F, Henz BM. Miliaria crystallina in an intensive care setting. *Clin Exp Dermatol*. 2004;29(1):32–34.

Haas N, Henz BM, Weigel H. Congenital miliaria crystallina. *J Am Acad Dermatol*. 2002;47(5):S270–S272.

Sato K, Kang WH, Saga K, et al. Biology of sweat glands and their disorders. II. Disorders of sweat gland function. *J Am Acad Dermatol*. 1989;20:713–726.

Transient Neonatal Pustular Melanosis

Alicia Ogram

■■ Diagnosis Synopsis

Transient neonatal pustular melanosis (TNPM) is an idiopathic pustular disease of term newborns. Lesions begin *in utero* as pustules that then rupture, leaving behind collarettes of scale and hyperpigmented macules. Depending on the eruption's stage of evolution, infants are born with a combination of pustules, scale, and hyperpigmented macules. Sometimes, the vesiculopustular stage is not noticed, as fragile pustules may be easily wiped away. The pustules and scale resolve within 2 weeks of birth, leaving behind hyperpigmented macules that persist for several months. New lesions do not form after delivery.

The disorder is present at birth in 4% to 5% of black infants and in 0.1% to 0.3% of white infants. Boys and girls are affected equally. The etiology is unknown, though a few authors have noted an increased incidence of placental squamous metaplasia in mothers giving birth to children with the disorder.

(●) Look For

Look for vesiculopustules without surrounding erythema presenting at birth (Figs. 4-439 and 4-440). They measure 2 to 6 mm and rupture easily, leaving behind pigmented macules and collarettes of scale or brown crust (Fig. 4-441). Typically, pustules, collarettes of scale, and hyperpigmented macules are all present simultaneously at birth. The hyperpigmentation is usually not observed in white infants. The macules may spontaneously fade within 3 to 4 weeks or persist for several months. Commonly affected areas include the chin, neck, upper chest, lower back, buttocks, abdomen,

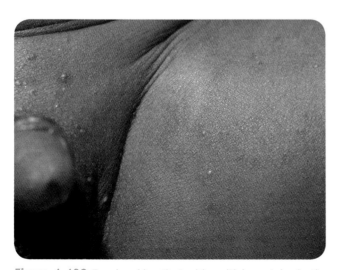

Figure 4-439 Two-day-old patient with multiple pustules in the groin in transient neonatal pustular dermatosis.

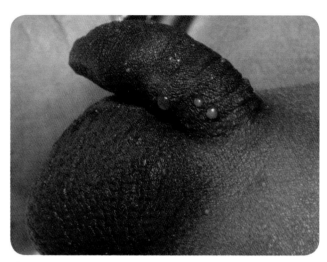

Figure 4-440 Transient neonatal pustular dermatosis with clear vesicles and pustules on the penis.

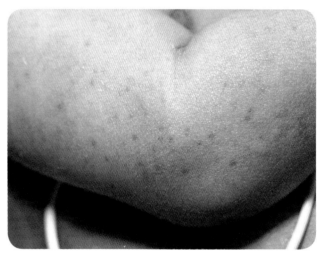

Figure 4-441 The pustules of transient neonatal pustular dermatosis heal with hyperpigmentation.

and thighs, but all areas may be affected. Palms and soles are often involved. There are no systemic symptoms.

●● Diagnostic Pearls

The pustules of TNPM are very fragile and often rupture upon removal of the vernix caseosa. Pustules may rupture *in utero* as well. Because new lesions do not form after delivery, pustules may not be present on examination, leading one to consider the diagnosis of multiple cutaneous lentigines. The hyperpigmented macules of TNPM, however, are less well defined than lentigines and are often surrounded by collarettes of scale in the first days of life. Furthermore, even when part of a syndrome (LEOPARD syndrome, Carney syndrome, or

Peutz-Jeghers syndrome), lentigines tend to be few at birth and develop progressively thereafter, whereas the hyperpigmented macules of TNPM are numerous at birth and fade over time.

TNPM may also be confused with erythema toxicum neonatorum, which, unlike TNPM, is almost never present at birth and has significant underlying erythema.

Differential Diagnosis and Pitfalls

If Mainly Consisting of Scale

- Bullous impetigo
- Staphylococcal scalded skin syndrome
- Ichthyosis bullosa of Siemens
- Postmaturity desquamation

If Mainly Consisting of Pigmented Macules

- Multiple lentigines
- LEOPARD syndrome
- Carney complex
- Peutz-Jeghers syndrome
- Multiple melanocytic nevi

If There Are Many Pustules

- Infectious vesiculopustular dermatoses
- Congenital cutaneous candidiasis
- Superficial staphylococcal infection
- *Listeria monocytogenes*
- *Haemophilus influenzae*
- Group A streptococcal infection
- *Pseudomonas*
- *Cytomegalovirus*
- *Aspergillus*
- Herpes simplex virus
- Neonatal varicella
- Scabies

Transient Noninfectious Vesiculopustular Dermatoses

- Neonatal pustular melanosis
- Miliaria crystallina and rubra
- Neonatal acne
- Acropustulosis of infancy
- Pustular eruption in Down syndrome

Persistent Noninfectious Vesiculopustular Dermatoses

- Incontinentia pigmenti
- Eosinophilic pustular folliculitis
- Langerhans cell histiocytosis
- Hyperimmunoglobulin E syndrome
- Pustular psoriasis

Best Tests

A Tzanck smear with a Wright stain of pustular fluid demonstrates polymorphic neutrophils and occasional eosinophils. A skin biopsy is not necessary to make the diagnosis, but if performed will show intracorneal and subcorneal pustules with collections of polymorphic neutrophils and occasional eosinophils under a thickened stratum corneum. The dermis remains uninvolved until late stages when postinflammatory changes such as increased melanin within basal keratinocytes and melanophages can be seen.

▲▲ Management Pearls

Parents should be reassured that this is a benign, nonscarring, self-limited disease that is not associated with any internal problems.

Therapy

No specific therapy is recommended because TNPM resolves spontaneously without sequelae. Parents should be reassured that the hyperpigmented macules will disappear within several weeks to months.

Suggested Readings

Mengesha YM, Bennett ML. Pustular skin disorders, diagnosis and treatment. *Am J Clin Dermatol.* 2002;3(6):389–400.

Van Praag MC, Van Rooij RW, Folkers E, et al. Diagnosis and treatment of pustular disorders in the neonate. *Pediatric Dermatol.* 1997;14(2): 131–143.

Staphylococcal Scalded Skin Syndrome

Chris G. Adigun

◼◼ Diagnosis Synopsis

Staphylococcal scalded skin syndrome (SSSS), or Ritter disease, is an acute, potentially life-threatening disease caused by epidermolytic toxins A and B, released by phage group II strains of *Staphylococcus aureus*. It is a toxin-mediated infection characterized by initial skin tenderness, followed by the development of flaccid bullae and subsequent skin detachment. Most commonly, toxins produced by focal infection of the nasopharynx, conjunctivae, perineum, or umbilicus disseminate hematogenously, leading to widespread desquamation. A prodrome of fever, sore throat, malaise, and irritability often occurs prior to the onset of bullae and skin sloughing.

SSSS is mainly a disease of infants and children aged younger than 6 years, likely due to their decreased renal ability to excrete the toxin. There is also a reported higher incidence seen in boys. With appropriate antibiotics, SSSS can resolve over 1 to 2 weeks. However, many adults who suffer from SSSS have underlying medical problems such as renal insufficiency, immunodeficiency, diabetes mellitus, or alcoholism. Mortality rates are estimated at 60% or even higher in the adult population.

In the United States, phage group II staphylococci are the most common toxin-producing strains. These phage group II strains are either methicillin sensitive or methicillin resistant and produce exotoxins—epidermolytic toxins A and B (ETA and ETB)—that cause cleavage within the epidermis with subsequent superficial epidermal sloughing. ETA and ETB are serine proteases that cleave the extracellular domain of desmoglein 1, a cell-adhesion molecule that binds keratinocytes together in the upper part of the epidermis. ETA-producing strains are more commonly associated with bullous impetigo, whereas ETB-producing strains are associated with SSSS. Note that bullous impetigo and toxic shock syndrome (TSS) are also toxin-mediated diseases that are considered within the same spectrum of SSSS. The key difference is that bullous impetigo is a localized infection, with epidermolytic toxin—usually ETA—acting within only focal areas of infection. Bacterial culture of bullae in bullous impetigo will reveal *S. aureus*, whereas affected skin in SSSS is sterile. In the case of TSS, the toxin produced by the infection acts as a superantigen rather than an epidermolytic toxin, and is typically TSS toxin 1 rather than ETA and/or ETB. This leads to severe illness, with shock, sepsis, and multiorgan failure.

The natural history of SSSS is characterized by the following:

- Prodromal symptoms and/or purulent rhinorrhea, conjunctivitis, otitis media, or skin infection
- Facial erythema that generalizes to the body in <48 hours, characterized by exquisite skin tenderness
- Bullae development and positive Nikolsky sign
- Epidermal sloughing within 48 hours after bullae develop
- Desquamation that continues for up to 5 days
- Re-epithelialization, without scarring, completed over the following 2 weeks

Newborns are believed to have particularly increased susceptibility to SSSS, not only because of their decreased renal ability to excrete the epidermolytic toxin but also because they have a lack of neutralizing antibodies. When SSSS does occur in the newborn, the majority of cases present between 3 and 7 days of age. There has been only one reported case of congenital SSSS. Symptoms occur acutely, with sudden onset of fever, irritability, skin tenderness, and characteristic cutaneous eruption. Symptoms of SSSS can be seen following an initial presentation consistent with bullous impetigo. Full recovery occurs in most cases. Sepsis, temperature, and fluid and electrolyte abnormalities are possible, and hospitalization for IV antibiotics and fluid/electrolyte monitoring is essential. Multisystem involvement may occur with sepsis.

Immunocompromised Patient Considerations

Immunocompromised patients are at significant risk for development of SSSS and even TSS.

◉ Look For

SSSS typically begins with a sudden onset of fever, irritability, cutaneous tenderness, and diffuse erythema that is accentuated at the flexures and perioral area. This is described as a scarlatiniform eruption and may be subtle. However, the skin tenderness is marked and may be so severe that infants will refuse to be held. This is followed within days by the development of superficial paperlike wrinkling that progresses to large, fragile bullae and desquamation that is also accentuated at the flexures and perioral area (Figs. 4-442–4-445). The underlying skin is moist and erythematous. Patients classically develop radial fissuring around the eyes, mouth, and nose. In more severe cases, the entire cutaneous surface may be involved with bullae and erosions. Mild cases may display only mild erythema and superficial desquamation. Mucosal surfaces are never affected.

Diagnosis in patients with darkly pigmented skin may be delayed, unfortunately, as the initial erythematous eruption is difficult to detect. These patients may present only with skin tenderness, such as a baby refusing to be held. In this circumstance, regardless of the apparent lack of skin findings, a focus of infection should be searched for, and close monitoring should be implemented.

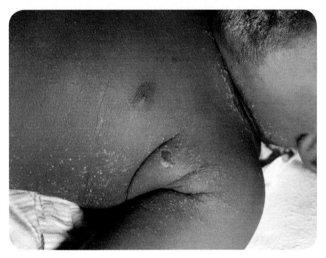

Figure 4-442 SSSS with desquamation and pustules.

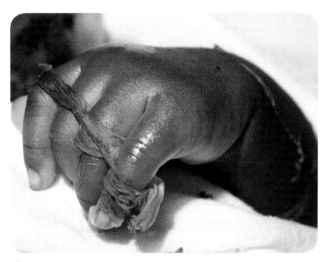

Figure 4-443 Eleven-month-old patient with glovelike desquamation of the hands from SSSS.

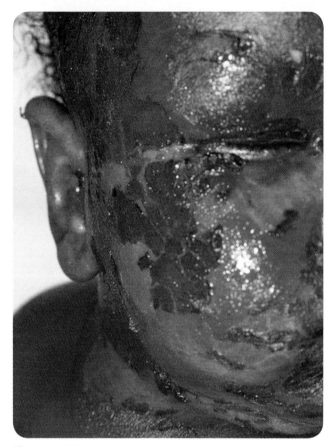

Figure 4-444 Extensive facial desquamation in SSSS.

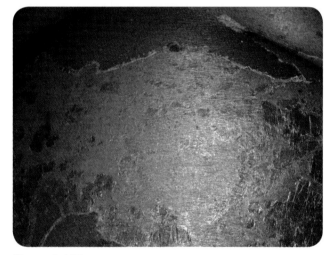

Figure 4-445 Late desquamation after SSSS.

 Diagnostic Pearls

- SSSS is mainly a clinical diagnosis; thus, thorough physical examination is critical for the correct diagnosis. The typical early patient is an irritable child/adult with skin tenderness and erythema around the mouth and localized to the neck, axillae, and perineal creases.
- Evaluate the eyes, nose, mouth, umbilicus, middle ear, and intertriginous areas for a pyogenic focus of infection, although the source of infection is rarely found.
- Bullae and Nikolsky sign (extension of bullae with gentle pressure) may be present over erythematous and nonerythematous skin.
- The bullae of SSSS are very fragile and rupture easily with gentle pressure, unlike many other bullous diseases in which bullae are tense and do not rupture with gentle pressure.

- Keep in mind that the fluid from the widespread bullae is sterile.
- Fever may be present, but infants and children do not appear toxic or severely ill unless they have developed other complications such as sepsis or pneumonia.
- White blood cell count may be elevated or normal.
- In contrast to TEN, SSSS never has mucosal erosions.

- If necessary, diagnosis may be confirmed with ELISA for the toxin or frozen section skin biopsy to show the intra-epidermal acantholysis.
- Very mild forms of the disease exist, with desquamation and circumoral pallor as the major findings.

?? Differential Diagnosis and Pitfalls

- Bullous impetigo—localized with honey-colored crusted plaques and with bacteria present in bullae
- TSS—high fever and severe systemic symptoms including vomiting and diarrhea; hypotension quickly ensues; diffuse scarlatiniform exanthem that starts on the trunk (in contrast to head/neck in SSSS)
- Kawasaki disease—fever lasting more than 5 days with oral mucosal changes, conjunctival injection, and cervical lymphadenopathy
- Toxic epidermal necrolysis (TEN)/Stevens-Johnson syndrome—drug induced, high fever, skin tenderness, mucosal involvement, and skin detachment about 1 to 3 weeks after the inciting medication is started
- Scarlet fever—1 mm erythematous papules, always elevated WBC with left shift, eosinophilia in up to 20% of patients
- Necrotizing fasciitis—rapidly progressing necrosis of fascia and subcutaneous fat
- Graft versus host disease—history of transplant or transfusion in an immunodeficient patient
- Drug eruption–associated desquamation—history of drug rash, desquamation occurs as erythema resolves, Nikolsky sign negative, and limited to areas of prior erythema
- Nutritional deficiency—subacute to chronic onset with failure to thrive and systemic symptoms
- Sunburn
- Keratolysis exfoliativa—acrally limited
- Boric acid poisoning
- Methylmalonic acidemia
- Ichthyosis bullosa of Siemens—present at birth and persists despite appropriate antibiotics
- Epidermolytic hyperkeratosis—present at birth and persists despite appropriate antibiotics
- Epidermolysis bullosa—onset at birth; does not improve with antibiotics
- Congenital syphilis

Immunocompromised Patient Differential Diagnosis

Immunocompromised patients may present with systemic symptoms such as hemodynamic instability and are at risk for complications including sepsis, fluid/electrolyte abnormalities, and death.

✓ Best Tests

- The erythrocyte sedimentation rate is elevated; WBC may be normal or elevated.
- Gram stain and culture should be obtained of presumed sites of infection, including nasal and throat swabs, conjunctivae, blood, plus any suspected areas, in order to determine the source of the infection. Fluid from bullae should be sterile.
- Tzanck smear will show acantholytic cells in SSSS (absent in TEN).
- Frozen section of skin biopsy and histopathologic examination provides a rapid diagnosis. SSSS shows superficial epidermal cleavage at the level of the granular layer, whereas TEN will reveal full-thickness necrosis down to the dermal-epidermal junction.
- The toxins responsible for SSSS can be identified by ELISA, latex agglutination assays, or PCR.

▲▲▲ Management Pearls

- Use parenteral penicillinase-resistant antistaphylococcal antibiotics, supportive skin care, IV fluids, and admission to the ICU or burn unit depending on severity.
- The underlying focus of staphylococcal infection is not always obvious, and treatment is often initiated based on the characteristic clinical picture. Cover eroded areas with Aquaphor ointment or petroleum jelly.
- The skin is very tender like with sunburn. Minimize handling and apply ointments only as tolerated.
- The blister is superficial and does not cause scarring. Full recovery occurs in 1 to 2 weeks.
- Parents need to be advised that because the blistering is superficial, the hyperpigmentation that they may see is usually temporary.
- Approximately 20% to 40% of the population is an asymptomatic carrier of *S. aureus* (nares, axillae, perineum). These individuals may be responsible for outbreaks (e.g., in the neonatal intensive care unit), and, in such cases, efforts should be made to identify and treat carriers.
- Although the superficial bullae and widespread desquamation heal without scarring, patients with SSSS who have darkly pigmented skin may experience postinflammatory hyperpigmentation. This should resolve with time, with an average time of 50 days. However, if persistent, appropriate interventions for dark skin should be employed. For hyperpigmentation, bleaching agents such as hydroquinone 4%, tretinoin 0.5%, triamcinolone 0.1%, superficial salicylic acid peels, glycolic acid peels, and kojic acid (which recently became available in the United States) may be appropriately employed, and all have shown efficacy for the treatment of postinflammatory hyperpigmentation in darker skin types.

Precautions: Standard and Contact. (Isolate patient, wear gloves and a gown, limit patient transport, and avoid sharing patient-care equipment.)

Therapy

Use only nonadherent dressings such as petroleum-impregnated gauze on areas of denuded epidermis.

Identify susceptibility of organism when possible. If susceptibility is unknown, use a penicillinase-resistant penicillin such as nafcillin or methicillin. Use penicillin G if the organism is susceptible. Use macrolides or aminoglycosides in patients with penicillin allergy. Mode of administration (oral vs. parenteral) is dictated by degree of severity.

- Nafcillin or oxacillin (150 mg/kg/d IV in four divided doses) for 5 to 7 days
- A macrolide such as azithromycin (500 mg IV daily for 2 days, then 250 to 500 mg p.o. daily to complete a course of 7 to 10 days) is an alternative.
- Vancomycin IV—2 to 3 g/d (20 to 45 mg/kg/d) in divided doses every 6 to 12 hours; maximum 3 g/d; note: dose requires adjustment in renal impairment

Change to oral penicillins after 1 to 2 days to avoid possible phlebitis—amoxicillin or dicloxacillin 500 mg p.o. four times daily.

Pediatric Patient Considerations

Mild cases can be treated with oral antibiotics (i.e., dicloxacillin, cephalexin, or clindamycin) as outpatients but need to be followed closely.

In preterm neonates, the use of intravenous immunoglobulin (IVIG) may be warranted, as the presence of anti-epidermolytic toxin antibodies in commercial IVIG preparations has been documented. This has been employed in a case report, with presumed success.

Suggested Readings

Halder RM, Nootheti PK. Ethnic skin disorders overview. *J Am Acad Dermatol.* 2003;48(6 Suppl):S143–S148.

Kapoor V, Travadi J, Braye S. Staphylococcal scalded skin syndrome in an extremely premature neonate: A case report with a brief review of literature. *J Paediatr Child Health.* 2008;44(6):374–376.

Murray RJ. Recognition and management of Staphylococcus aureus toxin-mediated disease. *Intern Med J.* 2005;35(Suppl 2):S106–S119.

Nishifuji K, Sugai M, Amagai M. Staphylococcal exfoliative toxins: "Molecular scissors" of bacteria that attack the cutaneous defense barrier in mammals. *J Dermatol Sci.* 2008;49(1):21–31. [Epub 2007 Jun 19.]

Odugbemi TO, Ajasin MA, Ogunbi O. Staphylococcal scalded skin syndrome in Nigerian children: A report of three cases. *J Trop Med Hyg.* 1976;79(12):260–263.

Patel GK. Treatment of staphylococcal scalded skin syndrome. *Expert Rev Anti Infect Ther.* 2004;2(4):575–587.

Stanley JR, Amagai M. Pemphigus, bullous impetigo, and the staphylococcal scalded-skin syndrome. *N Engl J Med.* 2006;355(17):1800–1810.

Stevens-Johnson Syndrome and Toxic Epidermal Necrolysis

Suzanne Berkman

■■ Diagnosis Synopsis

Stevens-Johnson syndrome (SJS) and toxic epidermal necrolysis (TEN) are rare severe reactions that represent one end of a spectrum of clinically and pathogenically related blistering skin diseases that are often drug induced. SJS is characterized by <10% of body surface area (BSA) involvement and carries a 1% to 5% mortality risk. TEN involves >30% BSA and carries a 25% to 35% mortality risk. SJS-TEN overlap occurs when 10% to 30% BSA is involved. They are closely related although their precise pathomechanism is still unknown.

Medications are implicated in over 95% of patients with TEN. The most common drugs include nonsteroidal anti-inflammatory drugs, antibiotics, anticonvulsants, and allopurinol. Additional causes, albeit rare, include immunizations and infections. SJS may be triggered by drugs, as in TEN, or infection. A strong association between allopurinol-induced SJS and TEN and the HLA-B*5801 allele has been observed in Han Chinese, Thai, and Japanese populations with high frequency of this allele. There is a strong association in the Han Chinese population between the HLA-B*1502 allele and SJS and TEN induced by carbamazepine, a drug commonly prescribed for the treatment of seizures. This allele is commonly seen in many other Asian populations; however, it is unclear whether it is a marker for severe outcomes in these groups. SJS has been reported in two children in Ghana following antimalarial treatment. An outbreak of SJS/TEN associated with mebendazole and metronidazole used for helminthiasis prophylaxis among Filipino laborers in Taiwan has been reported.

Infectious associations include mycoplasma pneumonia, herpes simplex virus (HSV), influenza, orf, coxsackievirus, echovirus, Epstein-Barr virus, yersinia, tuberculosis, histoplasmosis, and coccidioidomycosis. X-ray therapy of certain tumors is also a documented association.

SJS and TEN, when drug induced, are associated with the host's inability to detoxify drug metabolites. This results in a cell-mediated immune response that activates cytotoxic T cells, subsequently inducing keratinocyte apoptosis via cell surface death receptor signaling (membrane-bound or soluble Fas-Fas ligand [FasL] interaction).

SJS/TEN can affect all ages and races/ethnicities and has a slight female predominance (1.5:1). Risk factors that confer a worse prognosis include extent of BSA involved at the time of diagnosis, older age, malignancy, AIDS, number of medications, and elevated serum urea, glucose, and creatinine levels.

Typically, within 3 weeks of receiving an inciting medication, patients develop systemic toxicity characterized by fever, headache, mucositis, and conjunctivitis. Rapid development of a generalized, dusky, erythematous eruption with subsequent detachment of large areas of skin ensues. Ocular, oral, and genital mucosae are affected in more than 90% of cases. Involvement of the respiratory and gastrointestinal (GI) tracks with resultant pneumonia and GI bleeding may occur.

Rapid identification and withdrawal of the offending drug and transfer to a burn unit with aggressive supportive care are the most critical steps in management. Death is usually due to sepsis, adult respiratory distress syndrome, GI bleeding, or pulmonary embolism. Re-epithelialization begins a few days after the epidermis is sloughed. Most of the epidermis is re-epithelialized after 2 to 3 weeks with no scarring over most areas. However, mucous membrane erosions may persist for months.

◉ Look For

- Less than 10% BSA involvement in SJS; >30% BSA involvement in TEN
- Isolated, irregularly shaped, dusky erythematous macules on the trunk, face, and palms/soles; these are largely coalescing in TEN (Figs. 4-446–4-449).
- Erythroderma, which is manifested in dark skin types by deep and dark colors. This may be a subtle finding in patients with darker skin tones.
- Atypical target lesions may be seen.
- Flaccid bullae and sheetlike sloughing of the epidermis (Figs. 4-450 and 4-451)
- Positive Nikolsky sign—Tangential mechanical pressure of an erythematous macule leads to epidermal-dermal detachment.

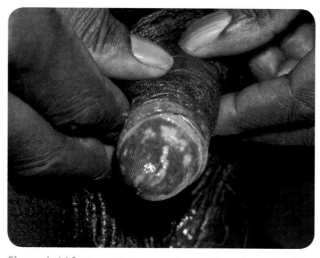

Figure 4-446 Stevens-Johnson syndrome with erosions and vesicles of glans.

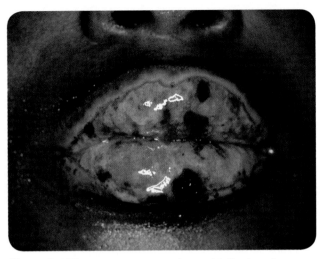

Figure 4-447 Stevens-Johnson syndrome with lip ulcerations.

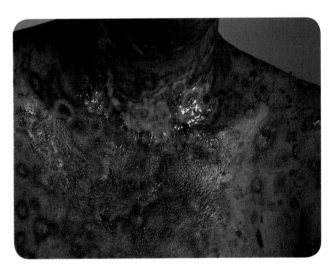

Figure 4-448 Stevens-Johnson syndrome with erosions, ulcers, and targetlike hyperpigmented macules.

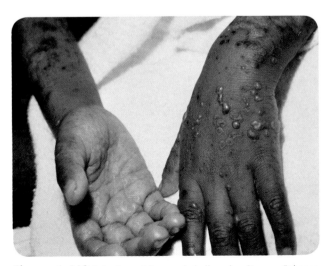

Figure 4-449 Intact vesicles and bullae in Stevens-Johnson syndrome.

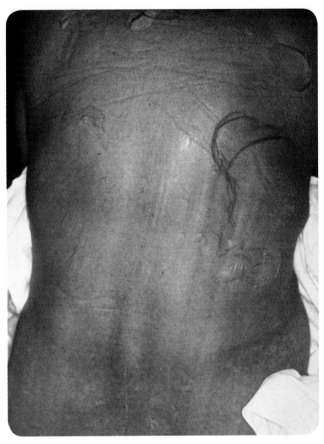

Figure 4-450 Peeling of skin with minimum trauma is characteristic of toxic epidermal necrolysis.

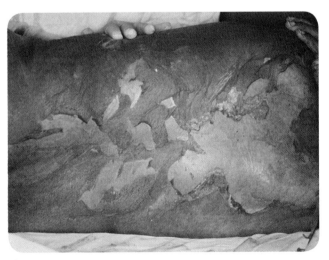

Figure 4-451 Progression of skin lesions of patient in Fig. 4-450 with a deep erosion of toxic epidermal necrolysis.

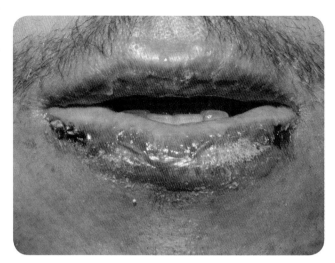

Figure 4-452 Upper and lower lip ulcerations from toxic epidermal necrolysis in an Asian man with AIDS.

- Mucosal involvement of the eyes, lips, mouth, and genitalia—Look for hemorrhagic crust, bullae, and denudation. In one third of cases, mucous membrane changes precede cutaneous changes by 1 to 3 days (Fig. 4-452).
- Pseudomembranous conjunctival erosions are common. Urethral or vaginal bleeding may occur.
- Systemic symptoms are commonly present in SJS; they are invariably present in TEN.

Diagnostic Pearls

The clinician should be aware of nonvisual signs of mucosal involvement including painful swallowing, painful micturition, and diarrhea. The blisters are characteristically flaccid, break easily, and can be extended laterally by slight tangential pressure (Asboe-Hansen sign).

?? Differential Diagnosis and Pitfalls

- Erythema multiforme (EM)—EM has characteristic target lesions (three concentric colors that are round and well demarcated) that occur on the extremities more often than on the trunk. Precipitating factors are usually infectious (HSV, mycoplasma) and not medications. Note that EM is *not* considered within the same disease spectrum as SJS/TEN and confers no risk of progressing to TEN. Nikolsky sign is negative.
- Staphylococcal scalded skin syndrome (SSSS)—usually occurs in newborns, infants, and young children. Mucous membranes and palms/soles are spared. The exfoliated skin is significantly more superficial (subcorneal vs. epidermal-dermal split). Nikolsky sign can be positive.
- Acute generalized exanthematic pustulosis (AGEP)—Look for neutrophilia, eosinophilia, and almost confluent erythema with overlying nonfollicular pustules. Nikolsky sign can be positive. Histology will clearly differentiate AGEP from SJS/TEN.
- Linear IgA disease—Look for tense blisters. Direct immunofluorescence (DIF) will demonstrate linear IgA deposition. DIF is negative in SJS/TEN.
- Generalized fixed drug eruption—Look for erythematous plaques that develop on the lips, face, distal extremities, and genitalia 1 to 2 weeks after drug ingestion. Oral mucosa can be involved. Histology will differentiate fixed drug eruption from SJS/TEN.
- Toxic shock syndrome (TSS) and toxic–shocklike syndrome—Look for sudden onset of exanthematous eruption. Histology will help differentiate TSS and SJS/TEN.
- Drug reaction with eosinophilia and systemic symptoms (DRESS)—Look for facial edema (hallmark of DRESS), eosinophilia, hepatitis, and other viscera.
- Bullous pemphigoid—Widespread tense bullae, usually in patients >60 years old
- Pemphigus vulgaris
- Paraneoplastic pemphigus—significant involvement of the vermilion border
- Dermatitis herpetiformis—extremely pruritic
- Sweet syndrome
- Acute graft versus host disease—Look for history of bone marrow transplant.

✓ Best Tests

- Skin biopsy will aid in confirming the diagnosis. Early-stage biopsy demonstrates apoptotic keratinocytes throughout the epidermis. Late-stage biopsy demonstrates subepidermal blisters and full-thickness epidermal necrosis.
- Patients with SJS/TEN require ongoing monitoring for infection, end organ damage, and electrolyte disturbances. Frequent determinations of CBC, comprehensive serum electrolytes, BUN and creatinine, transaminases, and urine output should be performed. Swabs from potentially infected areas and blood and urine cultures are necessary. Baseline chest films and GI studies are needed to follow possible respiratory and GI tract involvement.

▲▲ Management Pearls

Patients with SJS/TEN require intensive care or burn unit level care. The primary goals are to provide fluid/nutritional support and pain control and monitor for infection. The use of systemic corticosteroids is controversial. Many authorities believe that they offer no clinical benefit and may increase the rate of complications. Necessary consultations include dermatology, ophthalmology, burn or wound care specialist, and nutrition. There is no role for prophylactic antibiotics, but monitor for and promptly treat any identified infections.

The SCORTEN severity-of-illness score allows for prediction of disease severity and prognosis. It analyzes seven known risk factors including:

- Age > 40
- Heart rate > 120 bpm
- Malignancy
- Involved BSA > 10%
- BUN > 10 mEq/L
- Serum bicarbonate < 20 mEq/L
- Blood glucose > 252 mg/dL

Mortality estimates are based on the number of the above criteria that are met:

- 0 to 1 factor ≥ 3.2%
- 2 factors ≥ 12.1%
- 3 factors ≥ 35.3%
- 4 factors ≥ 58.3%
- 5 or more factors ≥ 90%

Therapy

Early diagnosis of SJS/TEN and rapid identification and discontinuation of the inciting drug is of paramount importance. The faster the inciting drug is discontinued, the more favorable the prognosis. Supportive therapy in a burn unit is the mainstay of treatment. No universally accepted specific therapies exist. Consultation with a dermatologist or other experienced specialist is recommended.

Supportive care:

- Wound care—Consider nanocrystalline gauze materials containing silver ions (nonadherent) or petrolatum-based gauze pads.
- Fluid and electrolyte management—Correct for transepidermal water loss.
- Nutritional supplementation
- Temperature management
- Superinfections—Patients with SJS/TEN are at high risk for sepsis and infection. Patients should be pan-cultured (skin, blood, urine, and any arterial lines and catheters) routinely throughout hospital stay. Note that systemic antibiotics are not used prophylactically.
- Ocular care—Vigorous lubrication and lysis of any adhesions that develop. Immediately request an ophthalmologic consult to decrease risk of irreversible ocular damage.
- Pain relief with opioid analgesics. There may also be considerable pruritus as the skin re-epithelializes. This can be controlled with antihistamines.

Specific therapies:

- Corticosteroids—Data regarding the use of steroids are mixed, and their use remains controversial.
- Intravenous immunoglobulin (IVIG)—It has been shown that IVIG can block Fas-mediated keratinocyte apoptosis via inhibition of binding between Fas and FasL. The majority of the literature reports improved mortality when IVIG is used in the setting of TEN. However, there have been at least four reports showing no benefit or even an increase in mortality when IVIG was used in the treatment of TEN. In the studies suggesting a beneficial effect, IVIG was used at a total dose of at least 2 g/kg over 3 to 4 days. Thromboembolic events, acute renal failure, anaphylaxis, and aseptic meningitis are potential rare side effects of therapy. If possible, check IgA levels prior to initiating therapy, as anaphylaxis can ensue in patients with IgA deficiency.
- Plasmapheresis—Mixed findings; consider adjunct with IVIG.

Suggested Readings

Bachot N, Revuz J, Roujeau JC. Intravenous immunoglobulin treatment for Stevens-Johnson syndrome and toxic epidermal necrolysis: A prospective noncomparative study showing no benefit on mortality or progression. *Arch Dermatol*. 2003;139:33–36.

Bastuji-Garin S, Fouchard N, Bertocchi M, et al. SCORTEN: A severity of illness score for toxic epidermal necrolysis. *J Invest Dermatol*. 2000;115:149–153.

Ghislain PD, Roujeau JC. Treatment of severe drug reactions: Stevens-Johnson syndrome, toxic epidermal necrolysis and hypersensitivity syndrome. *Dermatol Online J*. Available at: http://dermatology.cdlib.org. Accessed November 17, 2008.

Murphy JT, Purdue GF, Hunt JL. Toxic epidermal necrolysis. *J Burn Care Rehabil*. 1997;18:417–420.

Paul C, Wolkenstein P, Adle H, et al. Apoptosis as a mechanism of keratinocyte death in toxic epidermal necrolysis. *Br J Dermatol*. 1996;134:710–714.

Pereira FA, Mudgil AV, Rosmarin D. Toxic epidermal necrolysis. *J Am Acad Dermatol*. 2007;56:181–200.

Prins C, Kerdel FA, Padilla RS. Treatment of toxic epidermal necrolysis with high dose intravenous immunoglobulin: Multicenter retrospective analysis of 48 consecutive cases. *Arch Dermatol*. 2003;139:39–43.

Revuz J. New advances in severe adverse drug reactions. *Dermatol Clin*. 2001;19:697–709.

Viard I, Wehrli P, Bullani R. Inhibition of toxic epidermal necrolysis by blockade of CD95 with human intravenous immunoglobulin. *Science*. 1998;282:490–493.

Graft Versus Host Disease

Ivy Lee

▪▪ Diagnosis Synopsis

Graft versus host disease (GVHD) refers to organ dysfunction resulting from the introduction of foreign immunocompetent lymphocytes from the graft (peripheral blood stem cells, cord blood, bone marrow or solid organ transplants or blood transfusions) into an immunologically compromised host.

Risk factors for GVHD include increasing age, adjuvant donor lymphocyte infusion, HLA mismatch, gender mismatch, nonmyeloablative conditioning, and peripheral blood stem cell transplant. There have been conflicting studies on whether the incidence and severity of GVHD differ among ethnic groups. Two retrospective studies demonstrated increased incidence and severity of GVHD among African Americans and nonwhites, while two comparative studies showed that there were no statistically significant differences in the risk for chronic GVHD or overall survival among different ethnic groups. There is a 50% risk of GVHD even with a perfect (6/6) HLA match. GVHD is a major source of morbidity and mortality among transplant recipients.

GVHD most frequently involves the skin, liver, and/or intestinal mucosa. Cutaneous GVHD has both an acute and a chronic form. Acute disease typically occurs within 1 to 3 weeks of transplantation and often presents as a morbilliform eruption that may progress to erythroderma or, rarely, a toxic epidermal necrolysis–like picture. Chronic cutaneous GVHD presents more than 3 months after transplantation and has protean manifestations.

⦿ Look For

Acute GVHD

Acute GVHD of the skin most commonly presents as perifollicular morbilliform erythematous macules that may evolve into papules and coalesce over time. Oropharyngeal or ocular mucositis, diarrhea, and hepatitis may accompany the morbilliform eruption.

The severity of acute GVHD is determined by the total body surface area affected and is graded as follows:
Stage 1—<25% of body surface involved
Stage 2—25% to 50% of the skin surface involved
Stage 3—generalized erythroderma
Stage 4—generalized erythroderma with bullae formation (positive Nikolsky sign) and desquamation

Chronic GVHD

Chronic GVHD may present with predominantly epidermal, dermal, or subcutaneous changes.

Epidermal variants include clinical mimickers of lichen planus, lupus erythematosus, ichthyosis, papulosquamous diseases, keratosis pilaris, poikiloderma, or acral erythema (Figs. 4-453–4-457). Dermal involvement may mimic lichen sclerosus, and subcutaneous variants often present with sclerosis with prominent rippling and fasciitis with contractures and/or decreased range of motion. Lesions may be diffuse or limited in distribution with a predilection for flexural and frictional areas. Patients with chronic

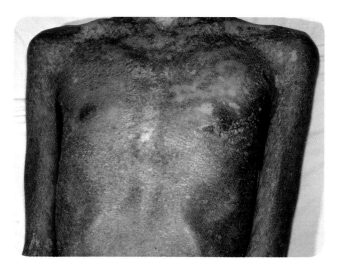

Figure 4-453 Chronic graft versus host disease with sclerosis, hypopigmentation, and hyperpigmentation.

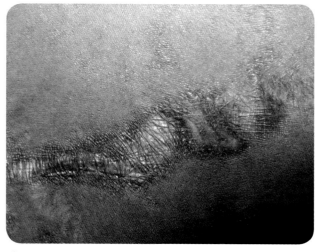

Figure 4-454 Hypertrophic and atrophic scars in graft versus host disease.

421

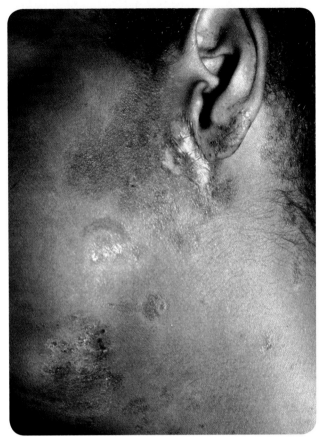

Figure 4-455 Atrophy and hyperpigmentation on cheek and ear in graft versus host disease (same patient as Fig. 4-454).

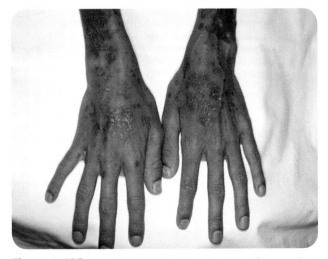

Figure 4-456 Symmetrical lichenoid papules in graft versus host disease (same patient as Fig. 4-453).

GVHD may also have alopecia and nail loss and nail plate distortions.

Associated findings include oral ulcers, xerostomia, xerophthalmia, and fatigue.

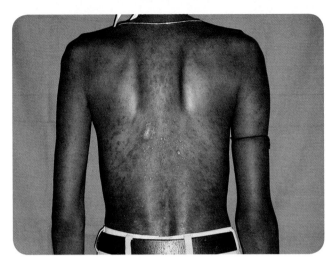

Figure 4-457 Scattered hyperpigmented and hypopigmented lesions in graft versus host disease.

 Diagnostic Pearls

The clinical and histological presentation of GVHD is protean and nonspecific.

Diagnosis is based on index of suspicion in conjunction with the clinical presentation.

 Differential Diagnosis and Pitfalls

In the immunocompromised, differentiating between GVHD and an acute drug eruption can be difficult.

Differential diagnoses for acute GVHD include the following:

- Viral exanthem
- Contact dermatitis
- Drug eruption
- Engraftment syndrome
- Lupus erythematosus
- Pemphigus
- Bullous pemphigoid
- Exfoliative dermatitis
- Stevens-Johnson syndrome
- Toxic epidermal necrolysis
- Staphylococcal scalded skin syndrome

Differential diagnoses for chronic GVHD include the following:

- Lichen planus
- Lichenoid drug eruption
- Morphea
- Lichen sclerosus
- Scleroderma
- Burn

Best Tests

- The clinical impression should be confirmed by skin biopsy.
- Elevated hepatic transaminases and bilirubin are expected in acute GVHD and sometimes occur with or without hyperbilirubinemia in chronic GVHD. In late chronic GVHD, autoantibodies such as antinuclear antibodies, anti–smooth muscle antibodies, and rheumatoid factor may appear, along with circulating immune complexes. Many patients will need to be followed with serial examinations of their hepatic and hematopoietic functions.

 Management Pearls

- Refer patient to a hematologist or dermatologist who has had experience with GVHD; large centers are usually the best.
- Extracorporeal photopheresis (ECP) or phototherapy (psoralens and UVA [PUVA] or UVA-1) is used for both the treatment and prevention of the disease. Approximately 50% of patients will respond to therapy. Daily ultraviolet protection and antiviral and antifungal prophylaxis are also important.
- Care of the patient with GVHD is multidisciplinary, often involving clinicians in such specialties as hematology/oncology, dermatology, transplant medicine, gastroenterology, ophthalmology, gynecology, and rehabilitation. Patients require close monitoring of their immunosuppressive regimens, primary disease status, and for complications such as infections and secondary malignancies.

Therapy

Prophylaxis
One of the most common regimens to prevent the development of acute GVHD consists of a combination of methotrexate (standard protocols for GVHD prophylaxis are available) and cyclosporine (5 to 10 mg/kg p.o. daily). Other combinations using sirolimus, mycophenolate mofetil, and systemic corticosteroids have also been used.

Treatment of Acute GVHD
Once acute GVHD has developed, systemic corticosteroids are considered first-line treatment. Prednisone 1 to 2 mg/kg p.o. daily or methylprednisolone 2 mg/kg IV daily in divided doses should be added to an optimized dose of cyclosporine until the GVHD is under control. If there is no response to corticosteroids, consider mycophenolate mofetil (1 to 2 g p.o. daily), tacrolimus (0.03 to 0.1 mg/kg p.o. daily), or antithymocyte globulin (15 mg/kg IV daily for 5 days). Certain biologics (alemtuzumab, infliximab, etanercept), PUVA, or ECP may also be tried as adjuvant therapy. Treating this disorder is best left to those with experience with this disorder.

Supportive measures include ceasing oral intake and placing the patient on total parenteral nutrition, antiviral and antibiotic prophylaxis, and analgesia. In patients with only mild acute GVHD limited to the skin, topical corticosteroids and antipruritics may be used for symptom relief.

Treatment of Chronic GVHD
A standard treatment for chronic GVHD consists of systemic corticosteroids (prednisone 1 to 2 mg/kg p.o. daily) plus a calcineurin inhibitor such as cyclosporine (5 to 10 mg/kg p.o. daily) or tacrolimus (0.03 mg/kg daily). In patients not responsive to corticosteroids, thalidomide (100 to 300 mg p.o. nightly) or tacrolimus (0.03 to 0.1 mg/kg p.o. daily) alone or in combination with mycophenolate mofetil (1 to 2 g p.o. daily) can be tried. The lichenoid variants of chronic GVHD may respond well to PUVA or UVA-1, whereas the sclerodermatous and subcutaneous variants may respond better to extracorporeal photochemotherapy or oral retinoids (acitretin 10 to 75 mg p.o. daily). Hydroxychloroquine, cyclophosphamide, and anti–TNF-alpha biologic agents have also been used. Supportive care consists of careful attention to nutrition, dental hygiene, skin integrity, and physical rehabilitation, if needed.

Suggested Readings

Baker KS, Loberiza FR, Yu H, et al. Outcome of ethnic minorities with acute or chronic leukemia treated with hematopoietic stem-cell transplantation in the United States. *J Clin Oncol.* 2005;23(28):7032–7042.

Easaw SJ, Lake DE, Beer M, et al. Graft-versus-host-disease. Possible higher risk for African American patients. *Cancer.* 1996;78(7):1492–1497.

Filipovich AH, Weisdorf D, Pavletic S, et al. National Institutes of Health Consensus development project on criteria for clinical trials in chronic graft-versus-host disease: I. Diagnosis and staging working group report. *Biol Blood Marrow Transplant.* 2005;11(12):945–956.

Karanth M, Begum G, Cook M, et al. Increased acute GvHD and higher transplant-related mortality in non-caucasians undergoing standard sibling allogenic stem cell transplantation. *Bone Marrow Transplant.* 2006;37(4):419–423.

Oh H, Loberiza FR, Zhang MJ, et al. Comparison of graft-versus-host-disease and survival after HLA-identical sibling bone marrow transplantation in ethnic populations. *Blood.* 2005;105(4):1408–1416.

Varicella

Randa Khoury

Varicella may be seen in the unimmunized and the immunosuppressed and is discussed in detail here. Two other diseases with similar clinical presentations are smallpox and vaccinia. Smallpox is a result of laboratory exposure or bioterrorism, and vaccinia is seen in those vaccinated for smallpox, usually military personnel, or those closely associated with the vaccinated individual, such as family members. For discussion on smallpox and vaccinia, see VisualDx online. (If you are a first-time online user, go to www.essentialdermatology.com/pigmented; if you already have set your password, go directly to www.visualdx.com/visualdx.)

Diagnosis Synopsis

Varicella, also known as chickenpox, is a self-limited viral infection caused by varicella-zoster virus (VZV), a member of the *Herpesviridae* family. Prior to the clinical implementation of the varicella vaccine, more than 99% of adults aged 40 and older had evidence of previous infection. Transmission occurs via airborne respiratory droplets or direct contact with vesicular fluid. The incubation period ranges from 10 to 20 days.

A prodrome of malaise, myalgias, and mild fever is typically followed by an acute eruption of pruritic, erythematous macules and papules that start on the face, oral mucosa, and scalp and spread to the trunk and extremities. The lesions rapidly evolve into 1- to 3-mm vesicles with clear serous fluid on an erythematous background. The hallmark of chickenpox is the presence of lesions in various stages of development. Older lesions will evolve to form pustules and serous crusts that heal within 10 days time.

In healthy individuals, the clinical course is most commonly benign and self-limited. Varicella is highly contagious, and the infected individual has the potential to infect others until all cutaneous lesions have completely crusted over. The most common complication is secondary bacterial infection with subsequent scarring. In immunocompromised individuals, varicella can cause significant morbidity and mortality, and patients often present with more hemorrhagic and purpuric lesions. Complications in immunocompetent and immunocompromised individuals include the following:

- Central nervous system—encephalitis, Reye syndrome, acute cerebellar ataxia
- Pulmonary—varicella pneumonia and acute respiratory distress syndrome
- Hepatic—viral hepatitis
- Cutaneous—herpes zoster and postherpetic neuralgia
- Additional rare complications include myocarditis, pancreatitis, glomerulonephritis, uveitis, optic neuritis, and vasculitis.

Congenital varicella infection can cause a wide range of fetal abnormalities, with the highest risk of abnormalities seen in the first trimester. Congenital abnormalities include the following: ocular abnormalities, cortical atrophy, low birth weight, cicatricial skin lesions, hypoplastic limbs, and psychomotor retardation.

Due to widespread use of the varicella vaccine since 1995 for children, incidence of varicella infection has decreased in the United States, and cases that do occur tend to be milder than in those who have not been vaccinated.

Look For

Note: In dark-skinned patients, it may be more difficult to appreciate erythema, which can appear deep red or red-purple. Trauma to pruritic vesicles may result in hypertrophic or keloid scarring.

In children, typical varicella begins with a 1- to 3-day prodrome of fever and malaise followed by a rapidly progressive vesiculopustular eruption. The eruption is characterized by crops of erythematous macules that develop central papules and progress into 2- to 3-mm diameter vesicles, pustules, and crusts within 12 to 48 hours (Figs. 4-458–4-461). Crops of lesions continue to develop over 3 to 4 days before becoming completely crusted over in 6 to 7 days. The pathognomonic picture is that of a centrally focused eruption with lesions in all stages of evolution simultaneously. Lesions may concentrate within areas of inflammation, such as a sunburn or dermatitis. Mucous membranes may also be involved with 2- to 3-mm shallow ulcerations. Patients typically develop 250 to 500 lesions.

In adults with varicella, look for:

- Erythematous macular eruption that evolves to papules and then vesicles with a surrounding halo of erythema,

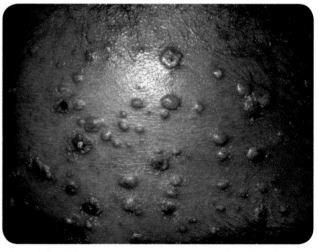

Figure 4-458 Varicella with vesicles, umbilicated vesicles, and hemorrhagic vesicles.

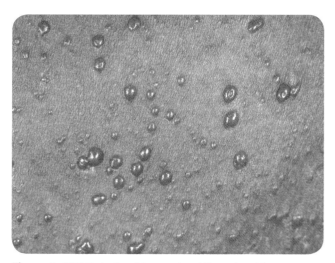

Figure 4-459 Varicella with several umbilicated vesicles.

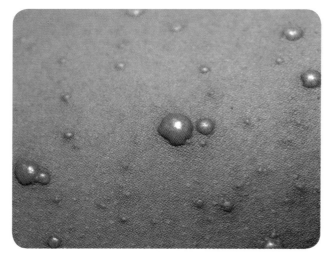

Figure 4-460 Vesicles of different sizes and some pustules in varicella.

known as "dewdrops on a rose petal." Tens to hundreds of lesions can be present on one individual.

- Mucous membranes, palms, and soles can be involved, but the disease burden is greater on the face, scalp, and trunk.
- Vesicles are usually discrete, unlike the clustered vesicles seen in herpes simplex or in herpes zoster.
- Simultaneous appearance of lesions in different stages of evolution is the hallmark of varicella infection.
- Vesicles become cloudy, appearing pustular, and then crust over, with healing completed within 1 to 3 weeks.

Diagnostic Pearls

The varicella vesicle is classically described as "a dewdrop on a rose petal." The vesicle is thin-walled and easily broken.

Differential Diagnosis and Pitfalls

- Herpes simplex virus (HSV)—Grouped vesicles on an erythematous base. Request direct fluorescence antigen (DFA) testing (DFA HSV, in contrast to DFA VZV) and viral culture. Look for more localized lesions in HSV at site of primary infection.
- Hand-foot-and-mouth disease (coxsackievirus)—vesicular eruption of palms and soles
- Echovirus
- Impetigo—honey-colored crusts with larger plaques and erosions
- Rickettsialpox—check serologies; transmitted by the house mite
- Pityriasis lichenoides et varioliformis acuta (PLEVA)—asymptomatic crops of erythematous papules that spontaneously resolve within weeks and recur at a later time
- Drug eruption—Often present with urticarial, exanthematous, or vesicular/bullous lesions. Eosinophilia

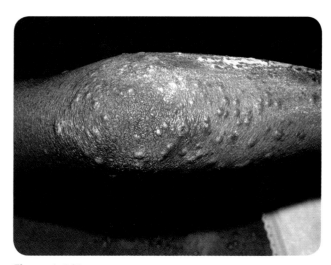

Figure 4-461 Varicella in a patient with atopic dermatitis.

on CBC and histology are often seen (but not an invariable finding). Look for nonsteroidal anti-inflammatory drugs, sulfonamides, and penicillin in medication history.

- Gianotti-Crosti syndrome (in children)—Lesions are monomorphic edematous papules (in contrast to various stages of lesions seen with varicella).
- Contact dermatitis—does not have prodromal symptoms and will be localized to site of contact (in contrast to disseminated distribution seen in VZV)
- Vasculitis—Check for RF, ANA, anti-ds DNA, ANCA, cryoglobulins, C3 and C4 levels, and clinical course that does not resolve over several weeks.
- Eczema herpeticum—hemorrhagic crusted papules and vesicles overlying eczematous skin, usually on the face; history of atopic dermatitis or Darier disease
- Miliaria—no viral symptoms; lesions do not rapidly progress to pustules and crusts

- Insect bite reactions—larger papules and vesicles; lesions do not rapidly progress to pustules and crusts; favor exposed sites
- Molluscum contagiosum—no viral symptoms; lesions do not rapidly progress to pustules and crusts
- Variola (smallpox)—all lesions at the same stage, favors extremities

✓ Best Tests

- If smallpox is suspected, this is a potential public health emergency and immediate infectious disease consultation is required. These diagnoses can often be made clinically, but a number of investigations are available to confirm the clinical impression.
- For varicella, DFA testing of skin lesion scrapings is more sensitive and specific than a Tzanck preparation, although the Tzanck will give more immediate results. Tzanck smears may be positive in 100% of cases, but false positives can be a problem. DFA is a rapid (<24-hour) and sensitive test for HSV-1, HSV-2, and VZV. This test is performed by vigorously scraping the base of a vesicle with a sterile cotton-tipped swab or No. 15 blade and smearing the cells onto a glass slide from a DFA kit. The slide is then fixed (usually contained in a kit) and sent for immunofluorescence analysis. Individual slides must be sent for each virus suspected. Slides can be stored at room temperature for 24 hours after fixation if needed.
- Viral culture of vesicular fluid
- Serologic studies are often used to confirm past infection and to assess current susceptibility. Among these are a latex agglutination assay, an enzyme-linked immunosorbent assay (ELISA), an indirect fluorescent antibody test, a radioimmunoassay, a neutralization test, and a fluorescent antibody to membrane antigen (FAMA) test.
- Consider obtaining a chest X-ray with respiratory signs and symptoms and, likewise, perform a lumbar puncture on patients with neurologic signs and/or symptoms. PCR can be used to detect viral DNA in the cerebrospinal fluid.

▲▲ Management Pearls

- The pruritus from varicella can lead to atrophic scars if excoriated. If pruritus is intense, systemic antihistamines (e.g., hydroxyzine or diphenhydramine) are more effective than the traditional calamine lotion.
- *Note:* The CDC Advisory Committee on Immunization Practices recommends that all health care workers ensure that they are immune to varicella as nosocomial transmission of varicella is a well-recognized problem. If susceptible persons must enter the room of a patient known or suspected to have varicella, they should wear respiratory

protection (N95 respirator). Persons immune to varicella need not wear respiratory protection.
- Nonimmune pregnant women who have had contact with a person with varicella should receive varicella-zoster immune globulin (VZIG) for postexposure prophylaxis.
- Consult with an infectious disease specialist in complicated cases. Certain patients may require hospitalization.

Precautions: Standard and Airborne. (Isolate patient in a negative pressure room, wear respiratory protection [N95 mask], and limit patient transport.)

Therapy

Varicella

Symptomatic treatment consists of antipyretics (acetaminophen), cool compresses and baths, calamine lotion, and systemic antihistamines:

- Diphenhydramine hydrochloride (Benadryl) (25, 50 mg tablets or capsules): 25 to 50 mg nightly or every 6 hours as needed
- Hydroxyzine (Atarax) (10, 25 mg tablets): 12.5 to 25 mg every 6 hours as needed
- Cetirizine hydrochloride (Zyrtec) (5, 10 mg tablets): 5 to 10 mg/d
- Loratadine (Claritin) (10 mg tablets and RediTabs): 10 mg tablet or RediTab once daily

Acyclovir and related compounds can lessen the severity of acute infection and decrease the incidence of complications. Consideration should be given to administration of these agents in adults and especially those with risk factors such as chronic lung disease or immunosuppression.

- Acyclovir 800 mg p.o. five times daily for 7 days
- Famciclovir 500 mg p.o. three times daily for 7 days
- Valacyclovir 1,000 mg p.o. three times daily for 7 days
- Foscarnet 40 mg/kg IV every 8 hours for 10 days given as an infusion over 1 hour for patients who have developed resistance to acyclovir

A live, attenuated varicella vaccine imparts protective antibody formation in 96% of patients immunized (0.5 mL SC twice in adults; second dose is given 4 to 8 weeks after the first).

Treat any secondarily infected lesions with the appropriate topical or systemic antibiotics.

For children, symptomatic treatment for varicella includes oral antihistamines (hydroxyzine 2 mg/kg/d divided three times a day), calamine lotion, trimming of fingernails to discourage scratching, and acetaminophen (15 mg/kg four times daily) for fever and pain.

Antiviral therapy is reserved for those with severe varicella or at risk for severe varicella. Adolescents, children receiving intermittent or aerosolized corticosteroids, those on long-term salicylate therapy, and patients with chronic skin or lung disease may be given a closely monitored course of oral acyclovir (20 mg/kg four times daily for 5 days). All severely affected and immunosuppressed patients should be given intravenous acyclovir until no new lesions appear for more than 48 hours. Foscarnet may be given to resistant cases.

Passive immunization with VZIG is recommended as postexposure prophylaxis (within 96 hours of exposure) for immunocompromised children.

Varicella vaccine may be given to normal children within 5 days of exposure to prevent or ameliorate varicella. A recent study suggests that children of African descent are less likely than white or Asian children to develop herpes zoster, or shingles, after receiving the varicella vaccine. This is consistent with previous studies showing lower rates of herpes zoster in black versus white adults. There is a suspected genetic cause behind these findings, although no specific gene has been identified.

Suggested Readings

Chartrand SA. Varicella vaccine. *Pediatr Clin North Am.* 2000;47(2): 373–394.

Harbecke R, Oxman MN, Arnold BA, et al. A real-time PCR assay to identify and discriminate among wild-type and vaccine strains of varicella-zoster virus and herpes simplex virus in clinical specimens, and comparison with the clinical diagnoses. *J Med Virol.* 2009;81(7):1310–1322.

McCrary ML, Severson J, Tyring SK. Varicella zoster virus. *J Am Acad Dermatol.* 1999;41(1):1–14; quiz 15–16.

Nahass GT, Goldstein BA, Zhu WY, et al. Comparison of Tzanck smear, viral culture, and DNA diagnostic methods in detection of herpes simplex and varicella-zoster infection. *JAMA.* 1992;268(18):2541–2544.

Nguyen HQ, Jumaan AO, Seward JF. Decline in mortality due to varicella after implementation of varicella vaccination in the United States. *N Engl J Med.* 2005;352(5):450–458.

Schwartz RA, Jordan MC, Rubenstein DJ. Bullous chickenpox. *J Am Acad Dermatol.* 1983;9(2):209–212.

Snoeck R, Andrei G, De Clercq E. Current pharmacological approaches to the therapy of varicella zoster virus infections: A guide to treatment. *Drugs.* 1999;57(2):187–206.

Tseng HF, Smith N, Marcy SM, et al. Risk factors of herpes zoster among children immunized with varicella vaccine: results from a nested case-control study. *Pediatr Infect Dis J.* 2010;29(3):205–208.

Vázquez M, Shapiro ED. Varicella vaccine and infection with varicella-zoster virus. *N Engl J Med.* 2 005;352(5):439–440.

Vinzio S, Lioure B, Goichot B. Varicella in immunocompromised patients. *Lancet.* 2006;368(9554):2208.

Porphyria Cutanea Tarda

Arden Fredeking

Diagnosis Synopsis

Porphyria cutanea tarda (PCT) is the most common porphyria and is caused by an acquired (type I) or inherited autosomal dominant (type II) deficiency of uroporphyrinogen decarboxylase, the fifth of eight enzymes in the heme biosynthetic pathway. In most cases of PCT, even inherited cases, liver toxicity (e.g., from alcoholism, exogenous estrogens from contraceptives or hormone replacement, hepatitis C virus infection, iron overload, liver tumors) causes or exacerbates the effects of the enzymatic deficiency. Photoexcitable uroporphyrins accumulate in the skin and cause damage, with clinical manifestations of skin fragility, blistering, hypertrichosis, scarring, and sclerodermoid features. Patients may also notice a reddish urine discoloration. Though historically associated with male alcoholics, awareness of PCT in women with liver disease or women who take exogenous estrogen has increased. The disease usually begins in middle age, sooner in alcoholics. There is no apparent predisposition in any ethnicity. Sun exposure—specifically ultraviolet light (wavelength 400 to 410 nm)—plays a major role in lesion development, as photoexcited porphyrins generate the reactive oxygen species that damage the skin.

Because sun exposure is a major factor in lesion development, the incidence of PCT is higher in the springtime and summer months. Higher incidence of PCT is reported in patients with HIV. The Bantus of South Africa have a high incidence of PCT; however, it is unusual in African Americans.

PCT can appear as vesicular lesions, bullae, milia, and atrophic scars, usually on the hands and other sun-exposed areas, with erythematous hyperpigmentation at the site of previous blisters.

Look For

Tense vesicles, bullae and resultant scars, and milia (small superficial cysts) on the dorsum of the hands and sun-exposed surfaces (Figs. 4-462–4-466). Hypertrichosis of the lateral cheeks and temples is another important finding in PCT. Look for periorbital violaceous suffusion as well as scars and mottled pigmentation in areas of prior lesions. Advanced disease has sclerodermoid features. The morphology of PCT in darker skin types is similar to that in lighter skin types.

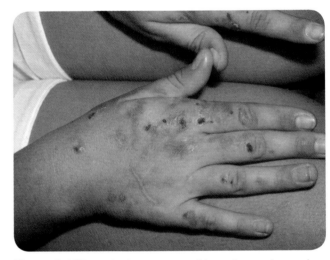

Figure 4-463 Porphyria cutaneous with erosions and scars in a common location for this disease.

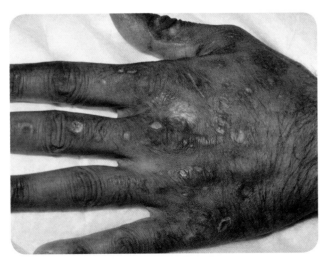

Figure 4-462 Porphyria cutanea tarda with erosions, scars, and a few milia.

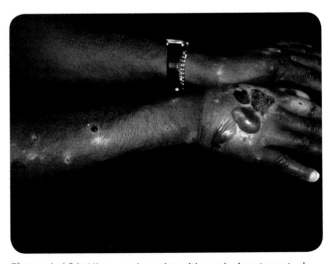

Figure 4-464 Blisters and scarring with porphyria cutanea tarda.

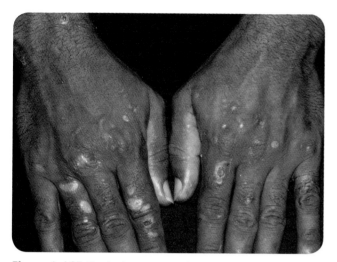

Figure 4-465 Porphyria cutanea tarda with erosions, hypopigmentation, and milia of different sizes.

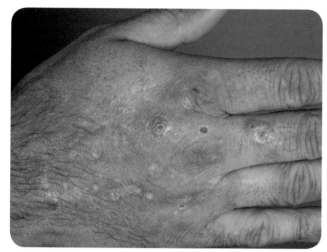

Figure 4-466 Porphyria cutanea tarda with milia, erosions, and ulcers.

Diagnostic Pearls

- To establish a tentative diagnosis of PCT, immediately examine the patient's urine with a Wood lamp after acidifying it with 10% HCl or acetic acid. Look for an orange-red fluorescence. This test is not particularly sensitive, however, and many tests are falsely negative.
- In the absence of intact bullae, heavily crusted erosions are very suggestive of PCT.

?? Differential Diagnosis and Pitfalls

- Rarely, patients may have increased dermal fibrosis, resulting in skin that resembles the skin of patients with scleroderma, but they do not have associated gastrointestinal (GI) or renal abnormalities.

- Pseudoporphyria secondary to certain drugs (nonsteroidal anti-inflammatory drugs, vitamin A derivatives, immunosuppressants, and chemotherapeutic agents)—Patients have normal porphyrin levels.
- Variegate porphyria (VP)—May present with skin findings identical to PCT, but patients are also at risk for acute porphyric (neuro) crises not seen in PCT. VP is more common in whites of South African descent and may be differentiated from PCT by the pattern of porphyrins in urine, plasma, and fecal specimens (ratio of urine uroporphyrin to coproporphyrin is approximately 1:1 in VP but up to 8:1 in PCT).
- Hepatoerythropoietic porphyria—childhood onset with rare autosomal recessive uroporphyrin decarboxylase deficiency
- Erythroprotoporphyria—It is the second most common porphyria seen in clinical practice, falling just behind PCT. There is no gender predominance, and it is found in all races and ethnic groups. Most affected patients present in early childhood with sun sensitivity and, at times, an urticarial-type reaction. Infants and children classically develop intense burning pain from sun-exposed skin following brief exposure in the spring and summer. This is differentiated from PCT by finding increased levels of protoporphyrin without increased levels of coproporphyrin in the RBCs, stool, or both. Urinary porphyrins will be normal because protoporphyrin is not excreted into the urine.
- Hereditary coproporphyria
- Hydroa vacciniforme
- Bullous lupus erythematosus
- Photodrug eruption
- Epidermolysis bullosa
- Epidermolysis bullosa acquisita
- Acute dermatomyositis
- Polymorphous light eruption
- Morphea
- Contact dermatitis
- Bullous pemphigoid
- Bullous fixed drug eruption
- Bullous arthropod bites

✓ Best Tests

Serum porphyrins should be analyzed. Uroporphyrins and coproporphyrins can also be measured from a quantitative 24-hour urine collection or fecal specimens.

Skin biopsy may be suggestive but is not diagnostic.

Other tests to consider include the following:

- 24-hour urine porphyrin collection reveals levels of porphyrins that range from a few hundred (300 µg) to several thousand micrograms.
- The ratio of uroporphyrins to coproporphyrins in PCT is typically 3:1 to 5:1, which distinguishes it from VP.

429

- Hematologic and iron studies, including serum ferritin and liver function tests
- In the case of anuric patients on hemodialysis, one can use the Wood lamp while the patient is on dialysis to look for pink or coral fluorescence while body fluids are in the dialysis tubing.
- Hepatitis serology (high association of HCV with PCT)
- HIV testing
- Hemochromatosis gene analysis
- Liver imaging or biopsy to identify underlying causative liver pathology
- Fasting blood glucose and antinuclear antibodies (sometimes elevated in PCT)
- Alpha-fetoprotein may be useful as a screen for hepatocellular carcinoma
- Use urine porphyrin levels to monitor response to therapy

▲▲ Management Pearls

- Stress the importance of sun avoidance.
- Work with the patient to reduce or eliminate alcohol use. Optimize the management of any hepatitis, if present. Encourage a decrease in consumption of iron-containing foods. Eliminate the use of estrogen, if possible. Ensure adequate vitamin C intake.
- Depending on the extent of disease and underlying factors, consultations with specialists in hematology, gastroenterology (hepatology), and dermatology may be needed.

Therapy

- Emphasize sun avoidance and the use of broad-spectrum sunscreens such as zinc oxide or titanium dioxide. Sunscreens must cover the lower-wavelength visible spectrum (i.e., ultraviolet light between 400 and 410 nm) to be helpful in PCT.
- First-line specific treatment consists of phlebotomy and antimalarial drugs.

Serial Phlebotomy

Approximately 500 mL of blood should be removed weekly or biweekly (as the patient tolerates) until the hemoglobin reaches a value of 10 to 11 g/dL or until serum iron has reached 60 µg/dL. Many patients demonstrate serum or liver iron overload.

Antimalarials

- Chloroquine (low dose)—125 mg twice weekly or hydroxychloroquine 200 mg twice weekly; usually more than a year of therapy is required. The patients must have their visual fields monitored by ophthalmology every 6 months.
- Other therapies to consider include chelation with desferrioxamine and subcutaneous erythropoietin (50–100 units/kg three times weekly) for those who are anemic, in order to facilitate intermittent phlebotomy.

Suggested Readings

Bardia A, Swanson EA, Thomas KG. 66-year-old woman with painless vesicular lesions. *Mayo Clin Proc.* 2009;84(7):639–642.

Mosterd K, Henquet C, Frant J. Porphyria cutanea tarda as rare cutaneous manifestation of hepatic metastases treated with interferon. *Int J Dermatol.* 2007;46(Suppl 3):19–21.

Thapar M, Bonkovsky H. The diagnosis and management of erythropoietic protoporphyria. *Gastroenterol Hepatol.* 2008;8:4.

Neonatal Candidiasis

Chris G. Adigun

▪▪ Diagnosis Synopsis

Congenital cutaneous candidiasis is an *in utero*–acquired infection with *Candida* species. Neonates present within the first 24 hours of life with either isolated cutaneous or simultaneous cutaneous and systemic disease. This should be differentiated from *neonatal candidiasis*, which is an infection that occurs after birth and is usually seen after the first week of life. In term infants, the infection is almost uniformly limited to the skin and resolves uneventfully with topical antifungals alone. However, preterm infants, especially those younger than 26 weeks' gestation or with extremely low birth weight (<1,000 g), are at high risk for systemic disease and death despite appropriate therapy. Furthermore, these infants are at risk of neurodevelopmental impairment due to systemic infection of *Candida*. Prompt recognition and initiation of treatment is critical in these circumstances to prevent potentially devastating outcomes.

◉ Look For

Characteristically, neonatal candidiasis begins as a morbilliform eruption that may be completely macular or consist of some combination of 2 to 4 mm erythematous macules, papulovesicles, and pustules on an erythematous base (Figs. 4-467–4-470). The borders are often well demarcated. Over days, the eruption becomes more papular, vesicular, and, occasionally, bullous. Lesions coexist in different stages of evolution and cover the face, trunk, buttocks, and extremities, favoring the skin folds. The palms, soles, and nails are often affected, whereas the diaper area and oral mucosa are usually spared. In term infants, the rash generally resolves with desquamation within 2 weeks, persisting longest on the palms and soles. Care must be taken to make the proper diagnosis in infants with darker skin types, as neonatal candidiasis may be confused with transient neonatal pustular melanosis.

In premature infants, it tends to be more severe, being more widespread and progressing more rapidly to vesicles and bullae. Patients sometimes present with diffuse, erythematous, burnlike areas that rapidly become eroded.

Systemically infected neonates may show signs of sepsis, including lethargy, poor perfusion, hypotonia, temperature instability, development of or worsening respiratory distress, an elevated white blood count with a left shift, thrombocytopenia, persistent hyperglycemia, or glycosuria. The clinical signs of sepsis may be very subtle, and one should maintain a high index of suspicion in high-risk infants (i.e., infants who are preterm or with very low birth weight; have had prolonged treatment with broad-spectrum antibiotics, prolonged endotracheal intubation, or central intravascular catheters; or have widespread cutaneous involvement or major congenital malformations).

●● Diagnostic Pearls

- The finding of pustules on the skin of a preterm infant, neonate, or full-term infant with signs of sepsis may be suggestive of systemic infection with *Candida* species. A septic infant with pustules should prompt a diagnostic workup for candidemia.
- Unlike erythema toxicum neonatorum, the palms and soles are often involved.

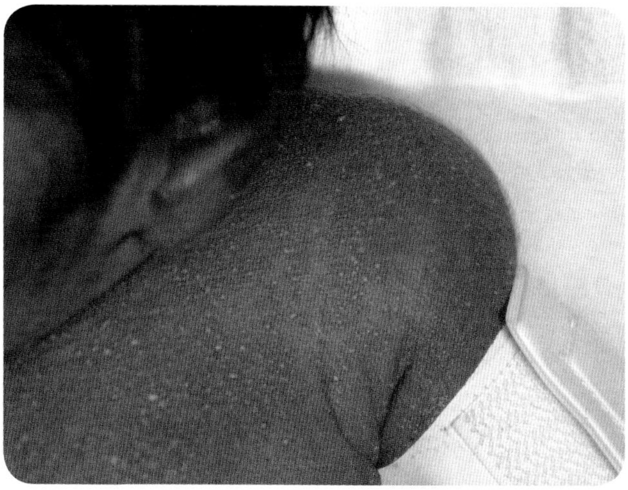

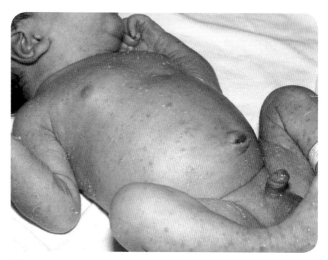

Figure 4-467 Neonatal candidiasis with shoulder pustules that were culture and biopsy positive.

Figure 4-468 Multiple trunk papules and pustules in neonatal candidiasis.

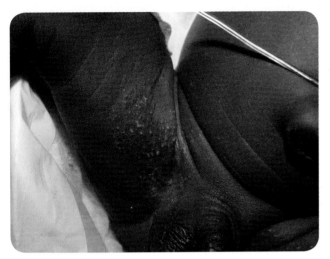

Figure 4-469 Multiple pustules in neonatal candidiasis.

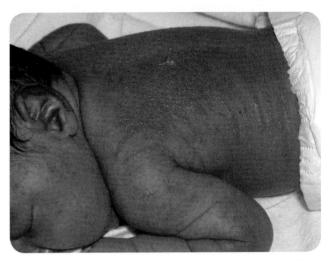

Figure 4-470 Multiple papules and pustules in neonatal candidiasis.

?? Differential Diagnosis and Pitfalls

Vesiculopustular rashes in the neonate may be divided into infectious, transient, or persistent dermatoses. The first goal in all vesiculopustular eruptions in the neonate is to rule out infectious etiologies.

Infectious Vesiculopustular Dermatoses

- Superficial staphylococcal infection
- *Listeria monocytogenes*
- *Haemophilus influenzae*
- Group A streptococcal infection
- *Pseudomonas*
- Cytomegalovirus
- *Aspergillus*
- Herpes simplex virus
- Neonatal varicella
- Scabies

Transient Noninfectious Vesiculopustular Dermatoses

- Erythema toxicum neonatorum
- Transient neonatal pustular melanosis
- Miliaria crystallina and rubra
- Neonatal acne
- Acropustulosis of infancy
- Pustular eruption in Down syndrome

Persistent Noninfectious Vesiculopustular Dermatoses

- Incontinentia pigmenti
- Eosinophilic pustular folliculitis
- Langerhans cell histiocytosis
- Hyperimmunoglobulin E syndrome
- Pustular psoriasis

✓ Best Tests

Even when the diagnosis is clinically obvious, confirmation by potassium hydroxide (KOH) is rapidly and easily performed. Other studies may include smears (Wright stain, Gram stain, direct fluorescent antibodies, and Tzanck), and cultures (bacterial, viral, and fungal) of vesicular contents should be performed for all infants with vesiculopustular eruptions to both narrow the differential diagnosis and rule out infection. In neonatal candidiasis, the KOH prep would reveal yeast and pseudohyphae, the fungal culture would grow *Candida* species, and the Wright stain would reveal inflammatory cells; all other tests would be negative. Biopsies are rarely indicated.

In infants—most frequently preterm infants—with signs of sepsis, in addition to bacterial blood cultures, blood should be sent for fungal cultures as well to investigate for *Candida* species.

▲▲ Management Pearls

All preterm infants with neonatal candidiasis, even when otherwise asymptomatic, should have a complete workup for systemic disease, including cultures from the blood, urine, and cerebrospinal fluid. Because term infants almost uniformly recover uneventfully, only those with systemic signs require more thorough evaluation.

Therapy

Topical imidazole antifungal creams, such as ketoconazole, are sufficient for term infants without systemic signs. Prompt systemic therapy should be initiated immediately in all infants with respiratory distress and/or demonstrating laboratory signs of sepsis, such as elevated leukocyte count with an increase in immature forms, or persistent hyperglycemia and glycosuria. Current systemic antifungal therapies include amphotericin B, flucytosine, and fluconazole. Amphotericin B is considered the mainstay of antifungal therapy for candidemia in the neonatal intensive care unit.

Current research has investigated the benefit of fluconazole prophylaxis in high-risk infants (i.e., preterm, <1,000 g), due to the high risk of mortality and neurodevelopmental impairment even with prompt or empiric treatment. Recent meta-analyses have illustrated that the incidence of *Candida* infections was lowered, as was all-cause mortality, with the initiation of fluconazole prophylaxis.

Given that the gut reservoir is the site from which dissemination of *Candida* species starts in preterm infants, recent interest has focused on the use of probiotics for the treatment of candidiasis and other diseases in neonatal patients. Basic science research has shown that probiotics have been effective in preventing *Candida* gut colonization and systemic dissemination in mice models, and a recent pilot trial in human preterm neonates has demonstrated that *Lactobacillus casei* subsp. *rhamnosus* GG (LGG) administered in the first month of life significantly reduces enteric *Candida* colonization. There is a need for further investigation into this arena, but it is promising for the possible role of LGG in the prevention of fungal disease in preterm neonates.

Although many studies have investigated their efficacy in candidal diaper dermatitis, many antifungal agents are not FDA approved in infancy. This does not mean that they are not recommended or used in infancy; they simply do not carry FDA approval. FDA-approved systemic antifungals in infancy include nystatin suspension for oral administration, IV miconazole, and fluconazole.

Suggested Readings

Kaufman DA. Fluconazole prophylaxis: can we eliminate invasive Candida infections in the neonatal ICU? *Curr Opin Pediatr.* 2008;20(3):332–340.

Kaufman DA, Cuff AL, Wamstad JB, et al. Fluconazole prophylaxis in extremely low birth weight infants and neurodevelopmental outcomes and quality of life at 8 to 10 years of age. *J Pediatr.* 2010 Dec 17. [Epub ahead of print].

Manzoni P. Use of Lactobacillus casei subspecies Rhamnosus GG and gastrointestinal colonization by Candida species in preterm neonates. *J Pediatr Gastroenterol Nutr.* 2007;45(Suppl 3):S190–S194.

Manzoni P, Monstert M, Agriesti G, et al. Neonatal fungal infections: the state of the art. *J Chemother.* 2007;19(Suppl 2):42–45.

Wang SM, Hsu CH, Chang JH. Congenital candidiasis. *Pediatr Neonatol.* 2008;49(3):94–96.

Zaoutis T, Walsh TJ. Antifungal therapy for neonatal candidiasis. *Curr Opin Infect Dis.* 2007;20(6):592–597.

Scleroderma and CREST Syndrome

Sabrina Newman

■■ Diagnosis Synopsis

Scleroderma

Scleroderma, or systemic sclerosis, is an autoimmune connective tissue disease with sclerotic changes of the skin and some internal organs. The etiology is unknown, but the disease is characterized by autoantibody production, abnormal fibrosis, and vascular dysfunction. The disease is observed in all ages, but the age of onset is usually between 30 and 50 years.

Scleroderma can affect the connective tissue of any organ, including the skin, gastrointestinal tract, lungs, kidneys, joints, muscles, heart, and blood vessels. Pulmonary disease is the leading cause of mortality, and gastrointestinal involvement is the leading cause of morbidity. Additional common clinical features include esophageal fibrosis and dysmotility, arthralgias, and Raynaud phenomenon. Less common manifestations include hypertensive renal crisis, pulmonary hypertension, interstitial lung disease, and cardiomyopathy.

There are two major subsets of scleroderma: limited scleroderma and diffuse scleroderma. Note that limited and diffuse refer to the degree of cutaneous involvement and that both subsets demonstrate internal organ involvement. Internal organ involvement occurs decades after initial diagnosis in the limited form and within 5 years in the diffuse form, carrying a worse prognosis. Additional risk factors that confer a worse prognosis include internal organ involvement at presentation, male gender, sclerotic changes of the trunk, elevated ESR, recent African ancestry, and older age at presentation.

The major diagnostic criterion for scleroderma is symmetric sclerosis of the skin proximal to the metacarpophalangeal or metatarsophalangeal joints. Minor criteria include bibasilar pulmonary fibrosis, sclerodactyly, substance loss of the finger pad, and digital pitting scars. Scleroderma is mainly a clinical diagnosis with one major criterion or two minor criteria satisfying the American College of Rheumatology classification. Autoantibodies assist in the diagnosis. More than 90% of patients with limited or diffuse scleroderma will demonstrate elevated antinuclear antibody (ANA) titers with a discrete speckled or nucleolar pattern. Additional autoantibodies include anti-Scl-70 antibody, which confers an increased risk for pulmonary involvement; anticentromere antibodies, which are more often seen with limited disease; and anti-RNP antibodies, which are more often seen with diffuse disease.

Scleroderma is about 1.5 times more frequent in individuals of African descent than whites, with a female-to-male ratio of 4:1. Disease presentation and course differ in black patients, with earlier onset, a more severe course, and increased mortality. According to a US study, the incidence of diffuse cutaneous scleroderma in black patients is about 20 cases per million per year, with peak age of onset at 35 to 44 years, compared to incidence in whites of 8 cases per million per year, with peak age of onset at 45 to 55. This may be due to black patients being more likely to have diffuse—rather than limited—cutaneous systemic scleroderma. In addition, lung function is often worse in black patients. There is a greater prevalence of anti-topoisomerase I antibodies, anti-RNP, and anti-Ro antibodies in black patients, although the frequency of anticentromere antibodies is less compared to whites. Some studies have suggested that black patients have shorter disease duration, possibly because limited scleroderma, which is less frequent in black patients, has a more prolonged course.

Variants of limited scleroderma:

- CREST syndrome (calcinosis, Raynaud phenomenon, esophageal dysmotility, syndactyly, and telangiectases) refers to a subset of patients with limited scleroderma. See below.
- Systemic sclerosis sine scleroderma is limited scleroderma with internal organ involvement and positive serologies but no cutaneous disease.
- Morphea is a cutaneous disorder with histology similar to that of scleroderma but without systemic manifestations.
- Linear forms of scleroderma (linear scleroderma) affect an extremity or even the face (Perry-Romberg syndrome) and often have associated soft tissue and even bone changes. Methotrexate is used to treat this disorder in children and adolescents.

CREST Syndrome

CREST syndrome is a connective tissue disease and a more benign, localized variant of scleroderma. The acronym includes the most common features: **C**alcinosis cutis, **R**aynaud phenomena, **E**sophageal dysfunction, **S**clerodactyly, and **T**elangiectasia. Patients have dysphagia, chronic heartburn, dyspnea, joint contractures, and diminished exercise capacity. Patients with CREST syndrome have a lower frequency of cardiac and renal involvement and a more prolonged survival than patients with scleroderma.

Other manifestations associated with CREST include pulmonary hypertension, autoimmune hepatitis, biliary cirrhosis, and sicca syndrome. Some patients may have what is termed "overlap disease," in which CREST occurs in conjunction with another autoimmune condition. CREST is more common in women, especially during middle age and the childbearing years. Certain ethnic groups are also predisposed, including Choctaw Native Americans and persons of Japanese descent.

⦿ Look For

Scleroderma

Cutaneous changes include:

- Induration and taut, shiny skin. This is usually seen first in the fingers and hands and can lead to joint contractures (Fig. 4-471).
- Pigmentary changes including diffuse hyperpigmentation as well as depigmentation with sparing of perifollicular skin, giving a salt-and-pepper appearance. This is especially common on the back and legs (Fig. 4-472).
- Telangiectases that are most commonly seen on the lips, palms, and proximal nail folds. (Of note, the telangiectases are flat, in contrast to the raised telangiectases observed in hereditary hemorrhagic telangiectasia.) Matted telangiectases can be found on palms and lips. Prominent proximal nail fold capillaries are present in nearly all patients; they frequently have sausage-shaped vessels with magnification. They can be visualized with an ophthalmoscope and show both loss of capillary and dilated capillaries.
- Calcinosis cutis of the fingers or other pressure points is a deposition of calcium in the tissues, presenting clinically as hard nodules that may exude a white chalky substance if ruptured.
- Raynaud phenomenon resulting in cutaneous ulcers of the digits. Acutely, this can appear as transient red, blue, or white changes in the skin of the fingers or toes. This may be the earliest clinical sign of vascular involvement of scleroderma.
- The face may develop a characteristic "beaklike" appearance to the nose and a reduced oral aperture. As the disease progresses, there is a paucity of wrinkling as the skin thickens and the patient's face develops a masklike stiffness.
- Sclerodactyly and joint contractures with loss of skin creases and in some cases digital necrosis (Fig. 4-473).

- Limited cutaneous scleroderma usually involves the distal extremities and may involve the face and neck. The diffuse form of scleroderma has additional sclerotic changes of the trunk and proximal extremities.

CREST Syndrome

- Diffuse, hard, smooth plaques localized to the hands and the lower face.
- Calcinosis cutis is often seen with hard, white skin nodules found on the hands and elbows.
- Facial hyperpigmentation and lack of wrinkles are characteristic of this disorder.
- Telangiectases of the face, fingers, palms, and mucous membranes are prominent in CREST (Fig. 4-474).
- Dilated nail fold capillaries are common.
- Sclerodactyly with ulcerations and/or scarring of the fingertips is seen frequently.

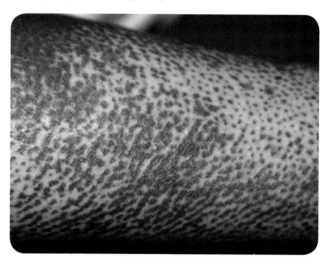

Figure 4-472 Salt-and-pepper hypopigmentation of scleroderma, with retained perifollicular pigment.

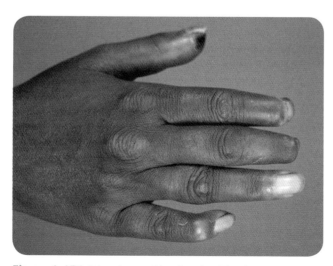

Figure 4-471 Scleroderma with sclerosis of hands, amputation of distal second digit, and infarction of distal thumb.

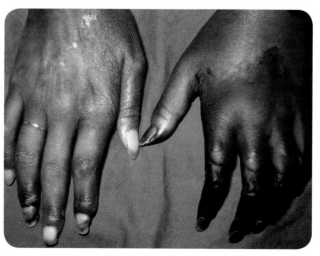

Figure 4-473 Digital necrosis in scleroderma.

435

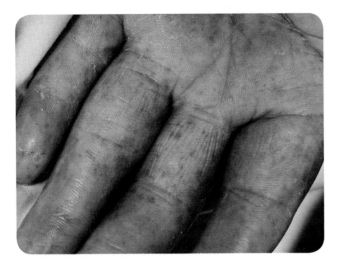

Figure 4-474 Multiple telangiectatic mats on the palm, some of which are hyperpigmented, in CREST syndrome.

Diagnostic Pearls

Scleroderma

- Because many of the features of scleroderma are nonspecific, care must be taken to consider other clinical diseases that overlap with scleroderma. These include overlap with rheumatoid arthritis, systemic lupus erythematosus (SLE), dermatomyositis, polymyositis, and, rarely, vasculitis (Fig. 4-475). Consideration of additional serologies is important if symptoms of these other conditions are present.
- The combination of sclerosis with hyperpigmentation and hypopigmentation in a salt-and-pepper pattern is diagnostic. The skin finding of scleroderma can be mimicked by porphyria cutanea tarda and syndromes from external exposures such as toxic oil syndrome and contaminated tryptophan.

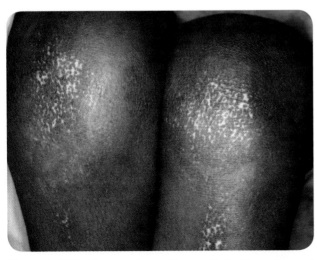

Figure 4-475 Sclerodermatomyositis in patient with carcinoma of the colon.

CREST Syndrome

Not all clinical signs of the syndrome need be present, although the vascular and esophageal manifestations occur most commonly. Raynaud phenomenon is often the first symptom to develop. Clinical calcinosis is less common, but digital calcification can be seen on X-ray of hands.

?? Differential Diagnosis and Pitfalls for Scleroderma and CREST

- CREST syndrome
- Generalized morphea—asymmetric induration, no Raynaud phenomenon, no systemic involvement
- Scleredema—ANA negative, no Raynaud phenomenon, no systemic involvement
- Scleromyxedema—ANA and anticentromere negative, no Raynaud phenomenon, no sclerodactyly
- Porphyria cutanea tarda and syndromes from external exposures such as toxic oil syndrome and contaminated tryptophan can mimic the skin finding of scleroderma.
- Generalized myxedema
- Chronic graft versus host disease—ANA negative, vascular abnormalities such as Raynaud phenomenon absent
- Eosinophilic fasciitis—ANA negative, no Raynaud phenomenon, no facial involvement
- Nephrogenic fibrosing dermopathy—recent history of radiologic imaging with gadolinium-based intravenous contrast in patients with renal insufficiency or renal transplant; ANA negative, no sclerodactyly, no Raynaud phenomenon
- Stiff skin syndrome—characteristic sparing of the hands and feet, develops during early childhood, systemic involvement rare
- Phenylketonuria—rarely has localized plaques of sclerosis
- Polyvinyl chloride exposure—ANA negative, cutaneous changes reverse with cessation of exposure
- Carcinoid syndrome—diarrhea and flushing common
- Cutaneous T-cell lymphoma
- Telangiectases on face and lips resemble hereditary hemorrhagic telangiectasia.
- Calcinosis cutis can occur in dermatomyositis (especially the juvenile form), and it may have prominent red and purple atrophic lesions that can be confused with scleroderma.

✓ Best Tests

Scleroderma

- A skin biopsy is not required for diagnosis but may help.
- ANAs are present in the majority of patients. Anticentromere antibodies (more common in limited disease)

and anti-Scl-70 antibodies (anti-topoisomerase I, only seen in diffuse disease) may be seen. Anti-Scl-70 is associated with pulmonary fibrosis but will be positive in only approximately 25% of patients. Other autoantibody tests may be useful, including anti-U3RNP, anti-fibrillin, and anti-PM-Scl. These antibodies are often associated with overlap syndromes.

- A greater prevalence of anti-topoisomerase I antibodies, anti-RNP, and anti-Ro antibodies are seen in African Americans; the frequency of anticentromere antibody is less in African Americans compared to whites.

Additional screening to consider includes:

- Renal—urinalysis, BUN, creatinine clearance
- Pulmonary—pulmonary function tests and high-resolution CT
- Cardiac—right heart catheterization, echocardiogram
- Gastrointestinal—esophagogastroduodenoscopy, manometry, small bowel follow-through, barium swallow

CREST Syndrome

- Perform a thorough history and physical examination.
- Skin biopsy (usually unnecessary) demonstrates increased dermal collagen.
- The Scl-70 (anti-topoisomerase) antinuclear antibody is present in 30% of cases.
- Speckled anticentromere antibodies in nucleus are a frequent finding.
- Patients will also exhibit abnormal esophageal motility tests.
- Further testing may be needed to rule out more extensive systemic involvement, such as tests of renal, lung, and/or cardiac function.

▲▲▲ Management Pearls

Scleroderma

- The approach to the patient with scleroderma should be multidisciplinary. A rheumatologist should be involved. Depending on the manifestations and course of the disease, other specialties may need to be consulted (dermatology, nephrology, pulmonology, gastroenterology, or hand surgery).
- An experienced physician should be monitoring and treating internal organ involvement because effective therapies exist, particularly for early pulmonary and renal disease. Hypertension in renal disease can now be controlled in most cases with ACE inhibitors. Internal organ changes include:
  - Pulmonary hypertension and interstitial pulmonary fibrosis
  - Hypertensive renal crisis

- Cardiomyopathy
- Esophageal dysmotility
- Sicca syndrome
- Myositis
- Neither scleroderma nor CREST has been associated with internal malignancies, so cases of overlaps with dermatomyositis need careful internal evaluations.
- Supportive measures are important. Patients should be kept warm to minimize Raynaud phenomenon. Any ulcers should be kept clean and dry.
- Encourage patients with dysphagia or reflux to eat smaller, more frequent meals. Advise smoking cessation, if applicable.
- Patients often require extensive occupational and physical therapy to maintain their range of motion and prevent contractures.
- Long-term follow-up is required to ensure proper assessment of the extent of internal disease.

CREST Syndrome

Patient Education Points

- As most patients have Raynaud phenomenon, be sure that they protect their hands and feet from cold, both indoors and out. Encourage patients to stay active and abstain from smoking.
- Patients with esophageal symptoms should eat small meals of soft foods and avoid foods that exacerbate reflux such as caffeine, alcohol, chocolate, and spicy foods.
- Liberal use of moisturizers and emollients can help soothe dry skin.
- Consultation with an occupational therapist and a plastic or orthopedic surgeon may be needed to address severe cases of sclerodactyly.

Therapy

Scleroderma
The systemic complications of scleroderma should be managed in conjunction with a rheumatologist. Note that scleroderma is a challenging disease to treat, particularly the cutaneous manifestations. Therapies have demonstrated efficacy in treating the lungs and kidneys.

Drugs that are used include the following:

- Corticosteroids, immunomodulators, immunosuppressants and antimetabolites, photophoresis, and statins to treat digital ulcerations
- Endothelin receptor antagonists have been used more recently.
- Other agents used include phosphodiesterase type 5 inhibitors and penicillamine.

(Continued)

Important treatment adjuncts include:

Raynaud phenomenon—nifedipine XL (30 mg p.o. daily) or a different calcium channel blocker, losartan (50 mg p.o. daily), intravenous alprostadil (prostaglandin E_1), or sildenafil by those trained in that modality

Emollients and antihistamines for pruritus:

- Diphenhydramine hydrochloride (25, 50 mg tablets or capsules): 25 to 50 mg nightly or every 6 hours as needed
- Hydroxyzine (10, 25 mg tablets): 12.5 to 25 mg every 6 hours or as needed
- Cetirizine hydrochloride (5, 10 mg tablets): 5 to 10 mg/d
- Loratadine (10 mg tablets) once daily

Gastroesophageal reflux—antacids (calcium carbonate), H2 blockers (ranitidine, famotidine), and proton pump inhibitors (omeprazole, pantoprazole)

Patients should be aggressively monitored for hypertension and placed on an ACE inhibitor as soon as it is detected to prevent a renal crisis.

CREST Syndrome

- As there is no cure for CREST syndrome, treatment is aimed at ameliorating symptoms.
- Laser (pulsed dye or potassium titanyl phosphate) for cutaneous improvement of telangiectases. *Caution:* this could potentially exacerbate the disease.
- Calcinosis cutis may be excised. Treatment success has also been achieved using extracorporeal shock wave lithotripsy (ESWL) and the carbon dioxide laser.

Consider an H2 blocker (famotidine, ranitidine) or a proton pump inhibitor (omeprazole, pantoprazole) for reflux symptoms.

- Calcium channel blockers for Raynaud phenomenon—nifedipine 10 to 20 mg/d alone or in combination with pentoxifylline (400 mg three times daily). The serotonin reuptake inhibitor venlafaxine (75 mg/d) also has been used.
- Sclerodactyly may respond to UVA phototherapy.
- Aerosolized iloprost may benefit select patients with CREST syndrome–related pulmonary hypertension.
- Relaxin and extracorporeal photophoresis may have a role in severe cases.

Suggested Readings

Jacobe HT, Cayce R, Nguyen J. UVA1 phototherapy is effective in darker skin: A review of 101 patients of Fitzpatrick skin types I–V. *Br J Dermatol.* 2008;159:691–696.

Krieg T, Takehara K. Skin disease: A cardinal feature of systemic sclerosis. *Rheumatology.* 2009;48:iii14–iii18.

Kuwana M, Kaburaki J, Arnett FC, et al. Influence of ethnic background on clinical and serologic features in patients with systemic sclerosis and anti-DNA topoisomerase I antibody. *Arthritis Rheum.* 1999;42:465–474.

Matucci-Cerinic M, Steen V, Nash P, et al. The complexity of managing systemic sclerosis: Screening and diagnosis. *Rheumatology.* 2009;48: iii8–iii13.

Mayes MD. Scleroderma epidemiology. *Rheum Dis Clin N Am.* 2003;29: 239–254.

Nietert PJ, Mitchell HC, Bolser MB, et al. Racial variation in clinical and immunological manifestations of systemic sclerosis. *J Rheumatol.* 2006; 33:263–268.

Nietert PJ, Silver RM, Mitchell HC, et al. Demographic and clinical factors associated with in-hospital death among patients with systemic sclerosis. *J Rheumatol.* 2005;32:1888–1892.

Radiation Dermatitis

Lowell A. Goldsmith

▪▪ Diagnosis Synopsis

Radiation-induced dermatitis is typically caused by radiotherapy for underlying malignancies. It may also result from exposure to radiation during long and multiple interventional procedures such as coronary angiography, embolization procedures, and indwelling catheter placements. Radiation-induced skin injury occurs instantaneously following radiation exposure and is due to impairment of functional stem cells, endothelial cell changes, inflammation, and epidermal cell apoptosis and necrosis. Pigmentation is of no protection against ionizing radiation.

Radiosensitizing agents act concomitantly to worsen skin damage. Pathophysiologic mechanisms leading to radiation-induced dermatitis can be classified as acute or chronic.

Acute Radiation Dermatitis

This occurs within 90 days of exposure. The patient may have changes ranging from faint erythema and dry desquamation to skin necrosis and ulceration, depending on the severity of the reaction. The National Cancer Institute has developed a four-stage criterion for the classification of acute radiation dermatitis.

Chronic Radiation Dermatitis

This is an extension of the acute process and can lead to long-lasting and often permanent impairment of the skin's ability to heal, which can be due to compromised cellular dysfunction with atrophy and fibrosis.

Onset may occur from 15 days to 10 years after the beginning of the procedure. There is no increased predilection for radiation injuries between men and women. The predominance in men of radiation dermatitis merely reflects the higher incidence of coronary artery disease and subsequent increased use of fluoroscopic procedures for therapeutic purposes. There are no racial or ethnic differences in susceptibility to radiodermatitis.

Radiation Recall

This is a well-documented phenomenon that occurs at sites of previous radiation therapy, after an antineoplastic agent (e.g., methotrexate, etoposide) is given. The reaction may occur weeks to years after radiation. As in acute radiation dermatitis, it is graded according to the severity of the cutaneous reaction and ranges from erythema to necrosis, ulceration, and hemorrhage. It tends to occur when cytotoxic agents are used following the completion of radiotherapy. Radiation recall has also been seen after the use of drugs such as nonsteroidal antiestrogens, interferon alfa 2b, and antituberculosis drugs.

Risk Factors for Radiation Dermatitis in the General Population

- Poor nutritional status
- Problems with skin integrity
- Overlapping skin folds
- Prolonged or multiple procedures requiring radiation exposure
- Increased exposure, especially in obese patients (Larger patients require higher doses of radiation and are, therefore, more susceptible to developing skin changes.)
- Total radiation doses of >55 Gy, or large individual doses per fraction (>3 to 4 Gy/dose)
- Concurrent cetuximab therapy in patients receiving radiation for head and neck malignancies

Certain diseases and syndromes increase the risk of radiation dermatitis:

- Connective tissue diseases (systemic lupus erythematosus, scleroderma, or mixed connective tissue diseases)—Peripheral blood lymphocytes from patients with rheumatoid arthritis, systemic lupus erythematosus, and polymyositis are more radiosensitive and exhibit greater DNA damage after irradiation. Thus, the presence of connective tissue disease is a contraindication to radiation therapy.
- Diseases with reduced cellular DNA capability, such as hereditary nevoid basal cell carcinoma
- Diseases involving chromosomal breakage syndromes, like Fanconi anemia and Bloom syndrome
- Homozygosity for the ataxia telangiectasia gene
- Infectious diseases—Patients with HIV show a reduced tolerance of the skin and mucous membranes to treatment. They develop not only cutaneous changes at lower doses but also more significant systemic problems.
- Diabetes mellitus
- Radiosensitizing drugs (e.g., paclitaxel or docetaxel) given before or up to 7 days after radiation therapy increase cellular damage.

Secondary cutaneous malignancy may also result from radiation therapy. The most common type occurring is basal cell carcinoma.

Immunocompromised Patient Considerations

An increased rate of cutaneous reactions, including bullous eruptions, has been reported in patients with HIV receiving radiotherapy.

◉ Look For

Acute Radiation Dermatitis

The cutaneous changes seen here depend on the timing of the appearance of symptoms. Signs will be localized to the site of radiation, but be sure to examine both portals of entry and exit sites.

Early Changes (Days to Weeks)

- Erythema—may be hard to appreciate in highly pigmented skin
- Dermal necrosis
- Edema and blister formation
- Desquamation
- Acute ulceration
- Alopecia (Fig. 4-476)
- Epilation—initially the loss of growing hairs that have a distinct microscopic appearance

Late Changes (Months to Years)

- Hypopigmentation
- Hyperpigmentation
- Telangiectasia
- Skin induration
- Alopecia—can be a scarring alopecia
- Epidermal atrophy, fragility
- Recurrent erosions
- Severe ulceration
- Scarring

Very Late Changes

- Necrosis
- Chronic ulceration
- Squamous cell carcinoma

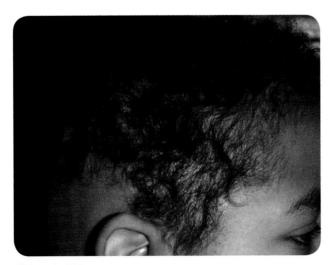

Figure 4-476 Radiation-induced alopecia.

440

Chronic Radiation Dermatitis

Symptoms may not appear for months to years after exposure. Some changes are temporary, such as the edematous peau d'orange (pock marking) appearance of breast skin following radiation. Other changes, such as postinflammatory hypopigmentation or hyperpigmentation, may persist or take longer to resolve.

Signs of Chronic Radiation Dermatitis

- Xerosis
- Hyperkeratosis
- Desquamation
- Telangiectasia
- Permanent loss of nail and skin appendages, including alopecia and/or decreased or absent sweating/loss of sweat glands
- Fibrosis leading to tissue retraction, limitation of movement, and pain

●● Diagnostic Pearls

Radiation dermatitis typically shows a geometric pattern on the skin that follows the field of exposure. Circle and square shapes are common patterns. Changes may appear at portals of both entry and exit.

?? Differential Diagnosis and Pitfalls

Acute

- Dermatitis
- Allergic contact dermatitis
- Cellulitis/erysipelas
- Carcinoma erysipeloides
- Primary/autoimmune blistering disease

Chronic

- Poikilodermatous mycosis fungoides
- Morphea
- Lichen sclerosus et atrophicus
- Graft versus host disease (chronic, sclerodermatous)
- Carcinoma en cuirasse
- Scleredema
- Scleromyxedema
- Nephrogenic systemic fibrosis

A prodromal nonspecific dermatitic eruption at the irradiation portal should not be interpreted as radiation dermatitis.

Management Pearls

Radiation necrosis caused by high-dose radiotherapy is difficult to manage due to impaired healing and superinfection that occurs in these tissues.

Prevention

Skin damage may be prevented or minimized by the following actions:

- Continuous surveillance of X-ray dose
- Keeping irradiated areas as small as possible

Therapy

Treatment will vary according to the severity of skin injury and whether it is acute or chronic radiation dermatitis.

Acute Radiation Dermatitis

Early changes of erythema and dry desquamation should be treated symptomatically to prevent progression to moist desquamation. The site should be washed with either water alone or water combined with a low-pH soap. Washing limits bacterial presence, thereby reducing chances of superantigen-induced inflammation. Petroleum-based emollients used to treat skin dryness are usually better tolerated than a cream form.

Later changes of erosions and ulcers involve the use of dressings, which serve the purpose of absorbing secretions, protecting against contamination, and pain control.

- Hydrocolloid dressing can be used for wounds that are minimally exudative.
- Alginate or foam dressings are for wounds that are highly exudative.
- Radioemulsions (thought to be radioprotective), such as trolamine, act by stimulating macrophages to remove necrotic tissue, promote fibroblast formation, and reduce vascular alteration and promote epithelial cell proliferation. Although controlled studies show no clinical radioprotective effect, patients express satisfaction with these ointments.
- Ionic silver pads or topical antibiotics may be used for infected wounds.

Avoid neomycin, a frequent cause of allergic contact dermatitis. Patients should limit the use of topical irritants such as perfumes and deodorants. They should wear clothes that fit well but do not stick to the skin.

Systemic treatment with pentoxifylline 400 to 800 mg p.o. three times daily and/or pyridoxine 50 to 150 mg twice daily may be helpful.

Chronic Radiation Dermatitis

Debridement of the ulcer can be achieved in a number of ways:

- Mechanical debridement involves removing eschars with the patient under local anesthesia.
- Enzymatic debridement or autolytic dressings may also be used (DuoDERM or Tegasorb).
- Oral antibiotics may be necessary for infected wounds.
- Chronic fibrosis may be minimized by physical therapy and deep massage.
- Intramuscular injections of liposomal copper/zinc superoxide dismutase twice a week for 2 weeks have shown some regression of fibrosis.
- Hyperbaric oxygen therapy leads to re-epithelialization of small areas in addition to reducing pain, edema, erythema, and lymphedema.
- Pulsed dye laser treatment may be used for radiation-induced telangiectasia.
- Deep ulceration may require surgical debridement with skin grafting.

Suggested Readings

Aistars J, Vehlow K. Radiation dermatitis. *Oncology (Williston Park)*. 2007;21(8 Suppl):41–43.

Frazier TH, Richardson JB, Fabré VC, et al. Fluoroscopy-induced chronic radiation skin injury: a disease perhaps often overlooked. *Arch Dermatol*. 2007;143(5):637–640.

Giro C, Berger B, Bölke E, et al. High rate of severe radiation dermatitis during radiation therapy with concurrent cetuximab in head and neck cancer: results of a survey in EORTC institutes. *Radiother Oncol*. 2009;90(2):166–171.

Hivnor CM, Seykora JT, Junkins-Hopkins J, et al. Subacute radiation dermatitis. *Am J Dermatopathol*. 2004;26(3):210–212.

Hymes SR, Strom EA, Fife C. Radiation dermatitis: clinical presentation, pathophysiology, and treatment 2006. *J Am Acad Dermatol*. 2006;54(1):28–46.

Jain S, Agarwal J, Laskar S, et al. Radiation recall dermatitis with gatifloxacin: a review of literature. *J Med Imaging Radiat Oncol*. 2008;52(2):191–193.

Smith ML. Environmental and sports-related skin diseases. In: Bolognia J, Jorizzo JL, Rapini RP, eds. *Dermatology*. 2nd Ed. St. Louis, MO: Mosby/Elsevier; 2008:1356–1357.

Smith KJ, Skelton HG, Tuur S, et al. Increased cutaneous toxicity to ionizing radiation in HIV-positive patients. Military Medical Consortium for the Advancement of Retroviral Research (MMCARR). *Int J Dermatol*. 1997;36(10):779–782.

Striae and Steroid Atrophy

Sridhar Dronavalli

■■ Diagnosis Synopsis

Striae

Striae distensae, or stretch marks, are due to thinning or atrophic defects in the dermis, typically in areas of repeated or prolonged skin stretching. The etiology likely involves the interplay of mechanical stress, hormones, and genetics. Striae are commonly located on the abdomen, thighs, and buttocks, or in areas where the skin stretches excessively.

Periods of rapid growth, such as puberty, pregnancy, weight lifting, rapid weight gain, and adolescent growth spurts, are common triggers. Striae also commonly occur in the setting of obesity. As 60% to 70% of the US population is labeled as overweight or obese, the prevalence of striae from obesity is estimated at 40%. Since obesity is more common in African Americans, Hispanics, and Native Americans, striae are frequently encountered in darker skin types. Striae occurring on the abdomen and breasts are common in pregnancy. The skin findings themselves are only of cosmetic concern, but they may indicate an underlying disease state (such as Cushing syndrome). Striae tend to flatten and become less conspicuous over time.

Steroid Atrophy

Steroid atrophy refers to thinning of the skin from exposure to corticosteroids. Generalized thinning can occur as the result of long-term oral or inhaled steroid use. Localized thinning occurs following the direct application of topical steroids to the skin. Steroid atrophy can be seen as early as 1 week after starting superpotent topical steroids under occlusion and as soon as 2 weeks with less potent agents. Atrophied skin may also be found over areas where intralesional steroids have been injected. Striae can also occur in thinned skin.

◉ Look For

Striae

Striae are flat or depressed, wrinklelike thinning of the skin in a longitudinal configuration, parallel to lines of skin relaxation (Figs. 4-477–4-481). They are often multiple and symmetric. The lesions are initially pink to violaceous and raised (striae rubra), then later become less colored, and finally appear as a skin-colored, depressed scar (striae alba). When due to endogenous or exogenous corticosteroid excess, striae can be larger and widespread. In adolescent boys, they tend

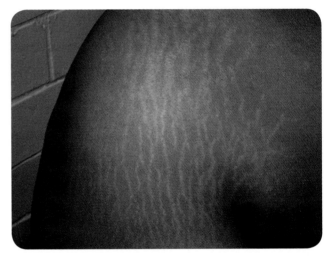

Figure 4-478 Hypopigmented stage of striae around the shoulder.

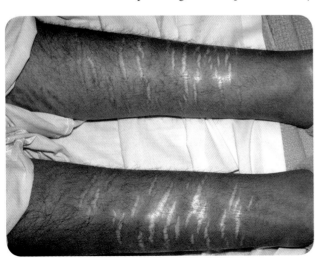

Figure 4-477 Depigmented stage of topical corticosteroid-induced striae.

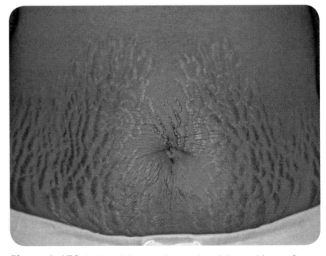

Figure 4-479 Striae with smooth atrophy, giving a shiny surface.

442

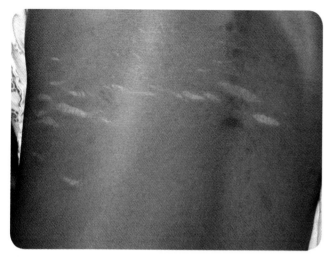

Figure 4-480 Pigmented stage of striae.

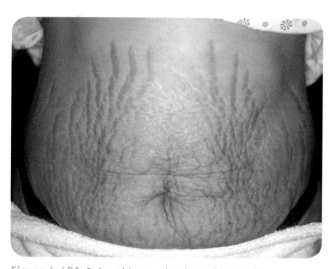

Figure 4-481 Striae with secondary hyperpigmentation.

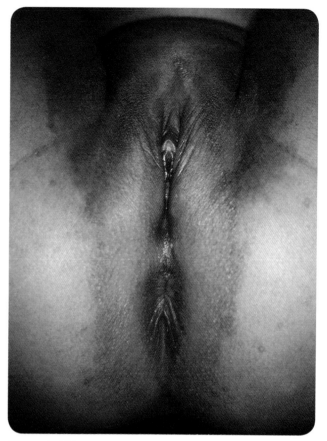

Figure 4-482 Perineal atrophy due to use of an ultra–high-potency topical steroid.

to occur on the thighs, shoulders, and lumbosacral region. In adolescent girls, they tend to occur on the proximal thighs, breasts, and buttocks.

Striae may be more prominent with a more violaceous color in darker skin.

Pediatric Patient Considerations

Children often present with striae during growth spurts.

Steroid Atrophy

Prolonged application of topical steroids results in areas of thin, loose, fragile skin (Fig. 4-482). Additionally, the skin appears shiny and transparent, with superficial blood vessels readily apparent. The most common sites are the face, axilla, groin, medial thigh, and perirectal areas.

Patients who use systemic steroids for a prolonged time may present with crepe paper–like, easily traumatized and bruised skin. These findings are more pronounced in areas of chronic sun exposure, like the face and forearms.

Patients who use anabolic steroids may present with striae along hypertrophied areas, in a similar manner to children during rapid growth phases.

Diagnostic Pearls

- Striae due to Cushing syndrome are typically widespread and larger and have a more violaceous color. In addition, patients will have several other signs and symptoms, including central obesity, a fat pad on the back of the neck ("buffalo hump"), a round face ("moon face"), skin thinning, acne, superficial skin infections, and hyperhidrosis. Patients will also have endocrine abnormalities and hypertension.
- The striae of obesity tend to be narrower and less atrophic than those related to Cushing syndrome.
- Striae in unusual locations, such as the face or axillae, are likely due to topical application of steroids.

Striae appear in specific directions depending on the area:

- Hips—transverse
- Buttocks—oblique
- Lumbosacral region—transverse
- Breasts—radiated from the nipple
- Shoulders—oblique

?? Differential Diagnosis and Pitfalls

For striae:
- Anetoderma
- Lichen sclerosus et atrophicus
- Linear focal elastosis
- Lipoatrophy
- Use of superpotent topical steroids

Additional considerations for steroid atrophy:

- Radiation-induced changes
- Chronic sun damage

✓ Best Tests

- Both striae and steroid atrophy are clinical diagnoses based on history and physical exam.
- Skin biopsy is very rarely needed but will differentiate striae from anetoderma, lichen sclerosus et atrophicus, lipoatrophy, and linear focal elastosis.
- If there is concern for Cushing syndrome, consider obtaining a serum ACTH level, a 24-hour urine free cortisol level, and a plasma cortisol level.

▲▲ Management Pearls

- Extensive laboratory testing is rarely indicated.
- There is essentially no therapy that will remove these lesions.
- Reassurance and observation are often all that are necessary in patients who are not overly concerned about the cosmetic appearance of their striae.
- Sun protection will reduce the added atrophy-inducing effects of ultraviolet light.

Pediatric Patient Considerations

Patients should be informed that striae improve over months to years.

Therapy

Tretinoin cream has been shown to decrease the length and width of striae and improve their overall appearance. Pulsed dye laser therapy may decrease the erythema associated with striae. Caution should be exercised in treating dark-skinned patients with laser therapy, given the risk of significant pigmentary alteration. Alternative treatments include excimer laser, intense pulsed light treatments, microdermabrasion, copper bromide laser, and chemical peels containing glycolic acid.

For steroid atrophy, no treatment is indicated, but the steroid cream or oral steroids should be stopped if possible. Topical retinoids may be helpful in reversing some of the superficial changes.

Suggested Readings

Alster T. "Laser treatment of hypertrophic scars, keloids, and striae." *Dermatol Clin.* 1997;15:3:419–429.

Arem A, Kischer C. Analysis of striae. *Plast Reconstr Surg.* 1980;65:1: 22–229.

Hengge U, Ruzicka T, Schwartz R, et al. Adverse effects of topical glucocorticoids. *J Am Acad Dermatol.* 2006;54:1:1–15.

James WD, Berger TG, Elston DM, eds. *Andrews' Diseases of the Skin: Clinical Dermatology.* 10th Ed. Philadelphia, PA: Saunders Elsevier; 2006.

Maari C, Powell J. Atrophies of connective tissue. In: Bolognia JL, Jorizzo JL, Rapini RR, eds. *Dermatology.* 2nd Ed. St. Louis, MO: Mosby/Elsevier; 2008:1539–1548.

Singh G, Kumar LP. Striae distensae. *Indian J Dermatol Venereol Leprol.* 2005;71(5):370–372.

Yosipovitch G, DeVore A, Dawn A. Obesity and the skin: skin physiology and skin manifestations of obesity. *J Am Acad Dermatol.* 2007;56(6): 901–916.

Necrobiosis Lipoidica and Diabetic Dermopathy

Lowell A. Goldsmith

Both of these conditions are associated with diabetes mellitus and have undiscovered pathophysiologies.

■ Diagnosis Synopsis

Necrobiosis Lipoidica

Necrobiosis lipoidica (NL) is a disorder with dermal inflammation and thinning. The percentage of patients with diabetes at the time of presentation ranges from 11% to 65%. Many more patients will have impaired glucose tolerance, develop diabetes at a later date, or have a positive family history of diabetes. However, this disorder may occur in patients who are not diabetic.

NL typically presents with asymptomatic shiny, red-brown patches on the shins. Occasionally, ulcerations and pain will occur after trauma (Figs. 4-483 and 4-484). Lesions slowly enlarge over the course of months to years. NL may occur at any age, and there is no racial predilection. Females are affected three times as often as males.

Treatment for NL is palliative; the disease process is chronic and progressive.

Diabetic Dermopathy

Diabetic dermopathy, commonly known as shin spots, is found in 50% of diabetics and is the most common cutaneous finding in patients with diabetes mellitus. Trauma is also thought to be a causative factor. The incidence of diabetic dermopathy ranges from 5% to 9% in patients with diabetes mellitus. There is no clear variation of incidence between diabetic dermopathy in patients with non-insulin-dependent diabetes mellitus and those with insulin-dependent diabetes mellitus.

There is a correlation between the presence of skin lesions and the number of microangiopathic complications (retinal, neuropathic, and/or nephrogenic) present. As the number of complications present increases from 1 to 3, so does the number of lesions. The incidence of diabetic dermopathy in patients with all three complications is much higher than in patients with just one complication.

Lesions do not itch or cause pain. Control of blood sugar levels does not affect the outcome of the lesions.

Diabetic dermopathy is diagnosed less frequently in darker-skinned individuals, perhaps because the macules are more difficult to discern.

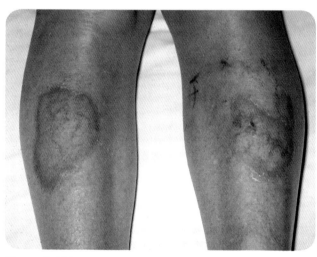

Figure 4-483 Atrophic annular lesions in NL.

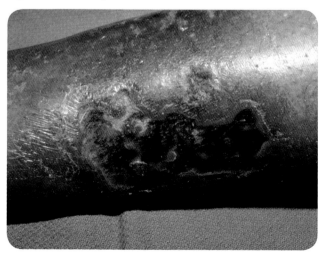

Figure 4-484 Ulceration and eschar in NL.

◉ Look For

Necrobiosis Lipoidica

The presenting lesions of NL are often red-brown papules or nodules that enlarge over time. NL may also present as similarly colored patches or plaques.

Over time, lesions coalesce into plaques and become yellow-brown, waxy, and atrophic centrally. Prominent telangiectases are characteristic.

Ulcers can occur at the sites of trauma and may be painful.

NL most commonly affects the pretibial area, but other common locations are the ankles, calves, thighs, and feet. Lesions are usually bilateral. They have also been reported on the face, scalp, trunk, and arms.

Diabetic Dermopathy

Diabetic dermopathy presents as few or many macules, patches, and papular lesions that are dark brown to reddish-brown in color at the anterior lower legs (Fig. 4-485).

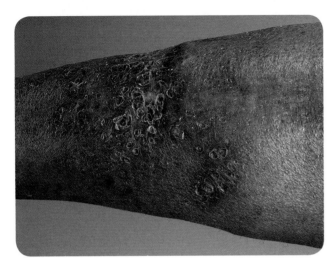

Figure 4-485 Irregular scarring and hyperpigmentation of diabetic dermopathy.

They are usually oval, round, or linear in shape and smooth and well demarcated, though some papules can have scale or hemorrhagic crusts. They vary in size from 0.5 cm in diameter to large patches covering most of the shin. Older lesions are covered with a thin scale and appear atrophic and hyperpigmented.

 ## Diagnostic Pearls

Necrobiosis Lipoidica

NL tends to develop at an earlier age in patients with preexisting diabetes. Koebnerization (lesions developing at trauma sites) may take place in NL. Upper extremity lesions tend to be more papulonodular in appearance.

Diabetic Dermopathy

The presence of well-demarcated, hyperpigmented, atrophic scars on the shins of a diabetic patient strongly point to a diagnosis of diabetic dermopathy.

?? Differential Diagnosis and Pitfalls

Necrobiosis Lipoidica

- Cellulitis or erysipelas
- Abscess
- Botryomycosis
- Majocchi granuloma
- Pretibial myxedema
- Granuloma annulare
- Contact dermatitis

- Sarcoidosis
- Xanthomas
- Diabetic dermopathy
- Stasis dermatitis
- Rheumatoid nodules
- Necrobiotic xanthogranuloma
- Pyoderma gangrenosum
- Sweet syndrome
- Calciphylaxis
- Vasculitis
- Panniculitis, including erythema nodosum
- Morphea
- Lichen sclerosus
- Leprosy
- Deep fungal infections

Diabetic dermopathy

- Stasis dermatitis
- NL—This entity also occurs on the shins but has a more yellow color and a firm, waxy consistency as discussed above.
- Granuloma annulare
- Lichen planus
- Postinflammatory hyperpigmentation
- Psoriasis
- Neurotic excoriations
- Capillaritis (Schamberg disease)
- Lichen amyloidosis
- Vasculitis

✓ Best Tests

Necrobiosis Lipoidica

Biopsy is characteristic.

Diabetic dermopathy

Diabetic dermopathy is a clinical diagnosis based on the appearance and location of the typically macular (occasionally papular) lesions.

 ## Management Pearls

Necrobiosis Lipoidica

- In diabetics, the severity (or frequency) of the disease does not correlate with the degree of glycemic control. Nevertheless, glucose control in diabetics should be optimized and smoking stopped. Diabetics with NL have higher rates of retinopathy and neuropathy.

- Some advocate a glucose tolerance test for patients presenting with NL.
- Squamous cell cancers have been rarely reported in lesions of NL, related to trauma and chronic ulceration.

Diabetic Dermopathy

Because lesions are asymptomatic, management of diabetes is the main concern.

Therapy

Necrobiosis Lipoidica

Numerous therapies have been tried, but a substantial body of evidence to recommend some definitively over others is lacking.

Intralesional triamcinolone and 0.1% betamethasone under occlusion have demonstrated some success, as have the antiplatelet agents aspirin and dipyridamole. Systemic corticosteroids tapered over 5 weeks were effective in a small case series, though hyperglycemia was a reported side effect. There are single case reports and small series reporting the efficacy of pentoxifylline, topical tacrolimus, infliximab, psoralen plus UVA (PUVA), tretinoin, ticlopidine, mycophenolate mofetil, nicotinamide, clofazimine, and perilesional heparin injections.

Pulsed dye laser has been used to successfully treat prominent telangiectases.

In diabetics, ulcer prevention with leg rest, support stockings, and glucose control is important. If ulcers should develop, the same basic principles of meticulous wound care as for all diabetics apply.

Cyclosporine 2.5 mg/kg/d has healed ulcerated NL in a few cases, as has GM-CSF.

Surgical excision with split-thickness skin grafting should be kept as a last resort for recalcitrant ulcers.

A theoretical basis for the use of inhibitors of the gli-1 oncogene (including tacrolimus and sirolimus), which is upregulated in NL, has been described and may guide future therapeutic investigations.

Diabetic Dermopathy

Blood sugar control is of paramount importance.

Suggested Readings

Ahmed I, Goldstein B. Diabetes mellitus. *Clin Dermatol.* 2006;24(4): 237–246.

Körber A, Dissemond J. Necrobiosis lipoidica diabeticorum. *CMAJ.* 2007;177(12):1498.

Köstler E, Porst H, Wollina U. Cutaneous manifestations of metabolic diseases: Uncommon presentations. *Clin Dermatol.* 2005;23(5):457–464.

Marinella MA. Necrobiosis lipoidica diabeticorum. *Lancet.* 2002;360 (9340):1143.

McDonald L, Zanolli MD, Boyd AS. Perforating elastosis in necrobiosis lipoidica diabeticorum. *Cutis.* 1996;57(5):336–338.

Moreno-Arias GA, Camps-Fresneda A. Necrobiosis lipoidica diabeticorum treated with the pulsed dye laser. *J Cosmet Laser Ther.* 2001;3(3): 143–146.

Morgan AJ, Schwartz RA. Diabetic dermopathy: A subtle sign with grave implications. *J Am Acad Dermatol.* 2008;58(3):447–451.

Romano G, Moretti G, Di Benedetto A, et al. Skin lesions in diabetes mellitus: Prevalence and clinical correlations. *Diabetes Res Clin Pract.* 1998;39(2):101–106.

Yorav S, Feinstein A, Ziv R, et al. Diffuse necrobiosis lipoidica diabeticorum. *Cutis.* 1992;50(1):68–69.

Neonatal Lupus Erythematosus

Stephanie Diamantis

■■ Diagnosis Synopsis

Neonatal lupus erythematosus is an autoimmune disorder of the newborn caused by maternal autoantibodies. Anti-SSA/Ro, anti-SSB/La, and anti-U1RNP antibodies can be found in both the fetal and maternal circulation. The main concern in patients with neonatal lupus is congenital heart block, which is irreversible in almost all cases. Elevated liver enzymes, thrombocytopenia, anemia, and neutropenia may also be seen. These will resolve as the maternal antibodies are cleared, usually between the ages of 6 and 8 months.

◉ Look For

At birth or shortly thereafter, erythematous, scaly plaques appear in a periorbital or forehead distribution, though they may appear anywhere (Figs. 4-486 and 4-487). These lesions are present at birth in two-thirds of patients; the remainder of the time they appear by the age of 5 months. Lesions generally heal within a year and may be associated with telangiectasia and atrophy.

●● Diagnostic Pearls

Look for periorbital plaques that seem to worsen with the infant's first sun exposure.

?? Differential Diagnosis and Pitfalls

- Seborrheic dermatitis
- Tinea faciei
- Bloom syndrome

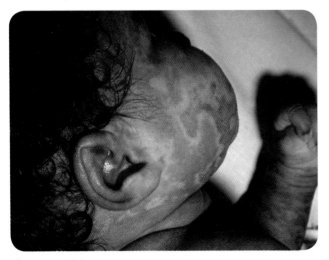

Figure 4-486 Neonatal lupus erythematosus with erythema and hypopigmentation.

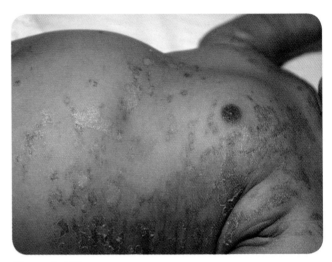

Figure 4-487 Erythema and scaling in neonatal lupus erythematosus (same patient as Fig. 4-486).

- Rothmund-Thomson syndrome
- Congenital rubella
- Congenital syphilis

✓ Best Tests

- Maternal and patient serum should be checked for ANA, anti-SSA/Ro, anti-SSB/La, and anti-U1RNP antibodies.
- A CBC with differential and liver function tests should be checked. An ECG and echocardiogram should be obtained to rule out cardiac involvement.
- Skin biopsy will demonstrate histologic features of lupus.

▲▲ Management Pearls

As soon as neonatal lupus is suspected, pediatric cardiology should be consulted to evaluate for cardiac involvement.

Therapy

Avoid sun exposure and use sunscreen if infant will be exposed. Midpotency topical corticosteroids may be helpful for the skin rash. No other treatment is required, as the skin lesions will resolve by the age of 6 to 8 months.

Suggested Readings

James WD, Berger TG, Elston DM, eds. Cutaneous vascular diseases. In: *Andrews' Diseases of the Skin: Clinical Dermatology*. 10th Ed. Philadelphia, PA: Elsevier; 2006:816–817.

Lee LA. Lupus erythematosus. In: Bolognia JL, Jorizzo JL, Rapini RP, eds. *Dermatology*. 2nd Ed. St. Louis, MO: Mosby/Elsevier; 2008:601–613.

Erythrasma and Intertrigo

Mat Davey

◼◼ Diagnosis Synopsis

Erythrasma

Erythrasma is a common chronic superficial bacterial infection of the skin caused by *Corynebacterium minutissimum*. It is characterized by distinct superficial hyperpigmented or erythematous patches localized to intertriginous areas, especially of the axillae, genitocrural crease, and interdigital web space of the toes. Lesions are often asymptomatic, although pruritus may be present, especially when it affects the genitocrural region. A "disciform" variant (large disklike lesions) usually occurs outside of the intertriginous areas and is associated with type 2 diabetes mellitus. Obesity, diabetes mellitus, immunosuppression, a history of atopy, and hyperhidrosis are risk factors. All age groups may be affected, but incidence increases with age. The highest incidence is seen in regions of high humidity, especially in the tropics.

Intertrigo

Intertrigo is a chronic inflammatory condition of approximating or opposing skin surfaces (intertriginous skin) presenting in a distribution similar to that of erythrasma, but it is also common in the inframammary areas of women. Clinically, affected skin is erythematous with associated weeping, maceration, crusting, or erosions. The affected areas may itch or burn. It is most frequently seen in obese and/or diabetic patients and is induced or exacerbated by any conditions causing increased warmth, wetness, and friction. Incontinence is a predisposing factor in intertrigo of the perineum and genitocrural folds, and there is significant overlap with diaper dermatitis. Hot and/or humid weather exacerbates the condition. Intertrigo is often complicated by superficial skin infection with yeast or bacteria. There is no predilection in either sex or any ethnicity. It is typically seen at the extremes of age.

◉ Look For

Erythrasma

In erythrasma, look for well-demarcated, reddish-brown, almost flat plaques with fine scale predominately located in the axillae, inframammary folds, and in the genitocrural creases. In patients with darker skin, the involved areas usually have an overlying fine, grayish scale (Figs. 4-488–4-490). A common site of involvement is the interdigital web spaces of the feet (especially between the fourth and fifth toes), which display macerated, white plaques often associated with surrounding yellowish hyperkeratosis.

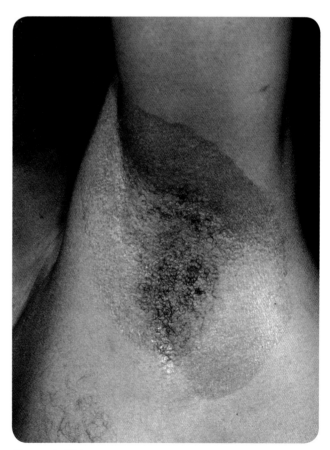

Figure 4-489 Sharply bordered plaque of erythrasma in the axilla of a middle-aged woman.

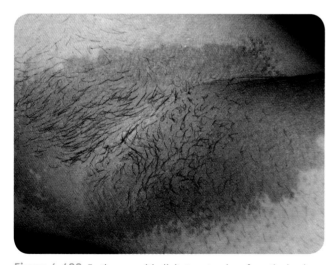

Figure 4-488 Erythrasma with digitate extensions from the borders.

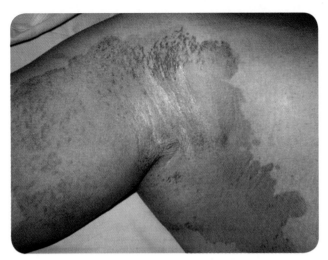

Figure 4-490 Sharply bordered plaque of erythrasma in the axilla.

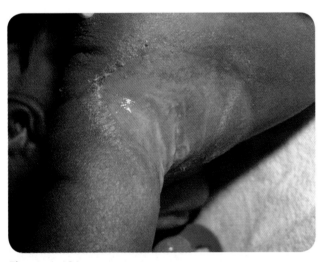

Figure 4-491 Intertrigo in an infant: a large superficial erosion with a shiny, sharply defined border.

Intertrigo

In intertrigo, look for erythema or erosions of opposing skin surfaces, such as the axillae, groin, perineum, inframammary creases, and abdominal folds (Fig. 4-491). Lesions may progress to maceration and crusting. Fissuring may occur following erosion. Pustules or vesicles usually indicate secondary infection (*Candida*, *Staphylococcus*, or other). There may be coexistent satellite pustular lesions in the case of intertrigo with candidal involvement.

Pediatric Patient Considerations

In infants who are obese, erythrasma and intertrigo may occur in neck creases, in the popliteal or antecubital fossae, as well as in the thigh and groin folds, and less commonly under pendulous breasts or abdominal folds.

 Diagnostic Pearls

Erythrasma and Intertrigo

- In erythrasma, plaques are usually sharply marginated, non-inflammatory plaques with minimal, if any, redness or erythema. Intertrigo is typically more inflammatory in nature, with erythema and serous discharge/crust often present.
- Erythrasma and intertrigo are not mutually exclusive; they commonly occur together.

 Differential Diagnosis and Pitfalls

Erythrasma and Intertrigo

- Inverse psoriasis
- Seborrheic dermatitis
- Candidiasis
- Fungal infections (tinea corporis/pedis)
- Tinea versicolor
- Acanthosis nigricans
- Allergic or contact dermatitis (including diaper dermatitis)
- Confluent and reticulated papillomatosis
- Langerhans cell histiocytosis
- Inverse lichen planus
- Hailey-Hailey disease

 Best Tests

Erythrasma and Intertrigo

- If a Wood lamp (UVA lamp) is available, the diagnosis of erythrasma is confirmed by coral red (pink-red) fluorescence due to the presence of coproporphyrin III produced by the organism. Bathing may result in removing the superficially deposited fluorescing coproporphyrins and can result in a false-negative Wood light exam.
- KOH preparations of skin scrapings should be performed to evaluate for concomitant yeast/fungal infection. In the case of erythrasma, scrapings will often show chains of bacilli. Stain with methylene blue to facilitate identification of these bacilli.
- If the diagnosis is not straightforward or recalcitrant to the below therapies, biopsy may be necessary to evaluate for other causes such as inverse psoriasis.

 Management Pearls

Erythrasma and Intertrigo

- With erythrasma, washing with an antibacterial soap may both treat active infections and prevent recurrences.

- In cases of intertrigo, conservative/preventative measures are aimed at eliminating friction, moisture, and warmth. Patients should keep skin folds exposed to the air when feasible, or tuck cotton or linen towels/cloths between them. Instruct patients to avoid tight clothing and hot/humid environments.
- Compresses with 1:40 Burow solution or dilute vinegar followed by fanning may help keep skin dry and soothe irritation. Castellani paint, another drying agent, may also be tried.

Therapy

Erythrasma

In cases of erythrasma, treatment may include any of the following:

- Topical imidazole creams—miconazole, clotrimazole, or econazole applied to affected areas twice daily for 2 weeks
- Topical antibiotics—topical erythromycin solution 2%, topical clindamycin solution 2%, or topical fusidic acid cream 2% applied twice daily for 2 weeks
- Benzoic acid 6%, salicylic acid 3% (Whitfield's ointment)—apply twice daily for 4 weeks; may be irritating
- Oral antibiotics are only necessary for severe or widespread infections—erythromycin 250 mg p.o. every 6 hours for 5 to 7 days

Intertrigo

Intertrigo is best treated with conservative/preventative measures. Concomitant infection should be treated, if present. In addition, a barrier cream applied as a thick coat to the affected areas may be utilized. Examples include:

- Zinc oxide
- Petrolatum

If a strong inflammatory component of intertrigo is present, consider addition of the following:

- A low-potency corticosteroid (1% hydrocortisone, desonide)—Apply twice daily until inflammation resolves. Note: Care must be taken with use of topical steroids in occluded areas because of increased risk of cutaneous side effects (i.e., striae) and increased systemic absorption.

An adsorbent powder may be used to reduce moisture but should be rinsed off daily to avoid irritation.

Suggested Readings

Craft NC, Lee PK, Zipoli MT, et al. Superficial cutaneous infections and pyodermas. In: Fitzpatrick TB, Wolff K, eds. *Fitzpatrick's Dermatology in General Medicine.* 7th Ed. New York, NY: McGraw-Hill; 2008:1708–1709.

Holdiness MR. Management of cutaneous erythrasma. *Drugs.* 2002;62(8): 1131–1141.

James WD, Berger TG, Elston DM, eds. *Andrews' Diseases of the Skin: Clinical Dermatology.* 10th Ed. Philadelphia, PA: Saunders Elsevier; 2006:267–268.

Yosipovitch G, DeVore A, Dawn A. Obesity and the skin: Skin physiology and skin manifestations of obesity. *J Am Acad Dermatol.* 2007;56(6):901–916.

Ischemic Ulcer (Arterial Ulcer)

Lynn McKinley-Grant

▪▪ Diagnosis Synopsis

Ischemic (or arterial) ulcers are a type of vascular ulcer caused by inadequate blood supply to the skin, usually the result of progressive atherosclerosis (peripheral vascular disease) or rarely arterial embolization. They predominantly involve the lower legs.

Ischemic ulcers are often chronic and quite painful relative to other types of ulcers. Their occurrence may be precipitated by seemingly trivial trauma or localized pressure. The incidence of ischemic ulcers increases with advancing age. Patients with ischemic ulcers due to peripheral vascular disease will often give a history of claudication. Risk factors for the development of these ulcers include diabetes mellitus, smoking, hyperlipidemia, obesity, rheumatoid arthritis, coronary artery disease, hypertension, male gender, and sedentary lifestyle. The goals of therapy include pain relief, wound healing, avoidance of amputation via revascularization, and risk factor modification.

Critical limb ischemia (CLI) is defined by the presence of >2 weeks of limb pain at rest from ischemia, tissue loss due to ischemia, or ischemic ulceration. Clinicians must be aware of the need for rapid revascularization, modifications in medical therapy, and wound care to minimize loss of limbs and loss of life in these patients.

◉ Look For

Look for an ulceration with a pale base and well-demarcated, "punched-out"–appearing borders, most often involving the tips of the toes, the dorsal aspect of the foot, bony prominences, or the heel (Fig. 4-492). The ulcer bed may

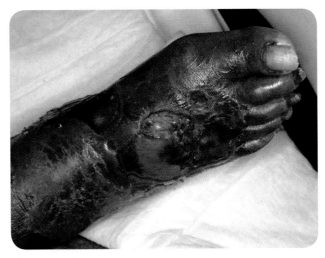

Figure 4-492 Multiple arterial ulcers with thick adherent crusts, some of which are hemorrhagic.

contain a small amount of grayish-white granulation tissue that bleeds only minimally upon manipulation. There may be dry eschar or gangrene and exudate is minimal. Tendons and other deep structures may be exposed.

Associated skin findings may include persistent cyanosis or pallor, loss of hair, atrophy, or skin fissures. The extremities are often cool to the touch, distal pulses are diminished, and capillary refill is delayed (more than 3 to 4 seconds). Toe nails may be thickened and irregular. Elevation pallor and dependency rubor are signs of limb ischemia.

●● Diagnostic Pearls

- The patient may report pain when supine, which is relieved by dependency of the extremity (e.g., dangling the affected limb off the edge of the bed).
- Elevation of the extremities (45 degrees for 1 minute) will result in pallor, while lowering the limbs to a dependent position for 10 to 15 seconds leads to rubor.
- A general rule that has stood the test of time: Ischemic ulcers tend to occur on the lateral malleoli, whereas venous ulcerations have a predilection for the medial malleoli.

?? Differential Diagnosis and Pitfalls

The differential diagnosis includes other disease processes in which ulceration is a prominent feature:

- Venous ulcers/venous insufficiency (approximately 70% to 80% of lower extremity ulcers)
- Neurogenic (diabetic) ulcers
- Emboli such as cholesterol or foreign materials
- Sickle cell anemia (hemoglobin S) and other abnormal hemoglobins must be considered in highly pigmented patients.
- Buerger disease should be considered in younger patients
- Pressure (decubitus) ulcers
- Infections (e.g., ecthyma, Old World leishmaniasis and New World leishmaniasis, cutaneous anthrax, cutaneous diphtheria)
- Vasculitis (thromboangiitis obliterans, vasculitides associated with connective tissue diseases such as scleroderma or systemic lupus erythematosus, especially with paraproteins, cryoglobulins, and cryofibrinogens, etc.)
- Hypercoagulable states and other hematologic diseases
- Erythema nodosum
- Necrobiosis lipoidica
- Frostbite
- Burn
- Trauma
- Pyoderma gangrenosum

- Neoplasms (basal cell carcinoma, squamous cell carcinoma, cutaneous T-cell lymphoma)
- Bites (e.g., brown recluse spider)
- Factitial ulcer
- Radiodermatitis

Best Tests

Ankle-brachial index (ABI)—The ABI is a noninvasive tool used to diagnose peripheral arterial disease and will aid in differentiating arterial from venous insufficiency. Specifically, the ABI measures the systolic blood pressures (BPs) in the ankle and the arm using a Doppler probe and a BP cuff.

How to Obtain the Brachial Systolic Blood Pressure

The patient should be at rest in the supine position for 5 minutes. Place the lower end of the BP cuff about 1 inch above the antecubital fossa. Locate the brachial artery and apply the probe gel over the artery. Place the tip of the probe into the gel until consistent and characteristic arterial sounds are heard. Inflate the BP cuff to 20 mm Hg above the blood pressure at which arterial sounds disappear. Slowly deflate the BP cuff until arterial sounds are obtained on the Doppler. Repeat on the other arm. The higher of the two brachial systolic pressures will be used to calculate the ABI. In individuals with normal vascular anatomy, less than a 10-mm Hg difference between the two arms is observed.

How to Obtain the Ankle Systolic Blood Pressure

Place the lower end of the BP cuff about 2 inches above the medial malleolus. Locate the posterior tibial pulse and perform the same procedure as described above. Now identify the dorsalis pedis artery and perform the same procedure. Repeat on the other leg. The highest of the systolic pressures will be used to calculate the ABI.

ABI Calculation

There should now be three values for each side: a brachial, posterior tibialis, and dorsalis pedis artery systolic blood pressure for the right side and left side. Take the highest brachial artery value. This will be the denominator. For the lower extremity values, take the highest value, whether it is the posterior tibialis or the dorsalis pedis, of the right side, and divide it by the brachial value. Repeat for the left side.

Interpretation

- Normal ABI: 1.0 to as high as 1.3
- Noncompressible calcified vessel: values > 1.3
- Positive peripheral arterial disease: value < 0.9

An ABI <0.9 has 100% specificity and 95% sensitivity for detecting angiogram-positive peripheral arterial disease. There is ≥ 50% stenosis in one or more major arteries.

An ABI of 0.40 to 0.90 indicates obstruction associated with claudication.

An ABI <0.4 represents severe ischemia.

Other Tests to Consider Include:

- Duplex ultrasound
- Formal contrast angiography
- CT or MR angiography
- Consider obtaining a skin biopsy in particularly recalcitrant ulcers to rule out malignancy
- Glycosylated hemoglobin (HbA1c) determination (for occult diabetes)

▲▲▲ Management Pearls

- A biopsy of any leg ulcer should be undertaken with caution. Like the ulcer itself, the biopsy site will often experience difficulty with wound healing. Because carcinoma is in the differential, however, ulcers that do not heal after 4 to 6 months of optimal therapy should have a biopsy taken from the ulcer edge.
- Patients with ischemic ulcers typically require referral to a vascular surgeon and occasionally a plastic surgeon. Podiatry referrals are also indicated for foot ulcers.
- Patients may experience some relief of pain from raising the head of the bed 4 to 6 inches while resting.
- Avoid vasoconstrictive drugs such as nonselective beta-blockers.
- Compression should *not* be employed in the treatment of ischemic ulcers.

Therapy

General Principles
- Optimize the management of or eliminate exacerbating factors (diabetes, smoking, hypertension, hyperlipidemia, etc.), and encourage exercise as tolerated.
- Take measures to reduce risk of death from coronary artery disease and further morbidity from peripheral vascular disease:
  - Antiplatelet therapy with aspirin or clopidogrel
  - Selective beta-blockers
  - Lipid-lowering therapy—goal LDL cholesterol < 100 mg/dL and in very high-risk patients < 70 mg/dL
- Meticulous foot care
- Weight-offloading devices as directed by a podiatrist
- Antibiotics (topical or systemic) when clinically indicated for secondarily infected ulcers

(Continued)

453

- Any ulcer with extensive slough or necrotic tissue should be débrided, whether by surgical or enzymatic means:
  - Sharp surgical removal of nonviable tissues and surrounding callus
  - Remove thick eschar only when separating at wound edge
  - Topical collagenase preparations may be useful
- Adequate pain control

Specific Treatments

- Wound dressings—As ischemic ulcers tend to have slough but low levels of exudate, hydrogel dressings, such as Nu-Gel, IntraSite, and Curasol, that rehydrate wounds and promote autolytic debridement are most appropriate.
- Surgical revascularization, including endovascular procedures (angioplasty, stenting, catheter-based plaque excision) or open lower extremity bypass, is the mainstay of therapy in patients who are acceptable surgical candidates. Nonhealing ulcerations and gangrene as well as rest pain and worsening claudication are indications for surgery.
- Skin graft and flap coverage of chronic ulcers often fail but are sometimes improved following surgical revascularization.
- Vacuum-assisted wound closure is useful for large wounds but is contraindicated in patients with friable, thin skin or neoplastic ulcers.
- Amputation is indicated in selected patients.

- The following modalities currently have limited evidence to support their use: oral zinc, hyperbaric oxygen, electrotherapy and electromagnetic therapy, biosurgery (myiasis) with sterile maggots, intermittent pneumatic compression in poor surgical candidates refusing amputation, and noncontact, low-frequency ultrasound.

Note: Current evidence does not support the use of drugs such as pentoxifylline or iloprost.

Suggested Readings

Belch JJ, Topol EJ, Agnelli G, et al., Prevention of atherothrombotic disease network. Critical issues in peripheral arterial disease detection and management: A call to action. *Arch Intern Med.* 2003;163(8):884–892.

Hiatt WR. Medical treatment of peripheral arterial disease and claudication. *N Engl J Med.* 2001;344(21):1608–1621.

Hopf HW, Ueno C, Aslam R, et al. Guidelines for the prevention of lower extremity arterial ulcers. *Wound Repair Regen.* 2008;16(2):175–188.

Nelson EA, Bradley MD. Dressings and topical agents for arterial leg ulcers. *Cochrane Database Syst Rev.* 2007;(1):CD001836.

Phillips T. Ulcers. In: Bolognia J, Jorizzo JL, Rapini RP, eds. *Dermatology.* 2nd Ed. St. Louis, MO: Mosby/Elsevier; 2008:1597–1610.

Sieggreen MY, Kline RA. Arterial insufficiency and ulceration: Diagnosis and treatment options. *Adv Skin Wound Care.* 2004;17(5 Pt 1):242–251; quiz 252–253.

Slovut DP, Sullivan TM. Critical limb ischemia: Medical and surgical management. *Vasc Med.* 2008;13(3):281–291.

Takahashi PY, Kiemele LJ, Jones JP. Wound care for elderly patients: Advances and clinical applications for practicing physicians. *Mayo Clin Proc.* 2004;79(2):260–267.

Pressure Ulcer (Decubitus Ulcer)

Suzanne Berkman

▪▪ Diagnosis Synopsis

Pressure ulcers, previously termed decubitus ulcers, are also commonly referred to as pressure sores and bed sores. Pressure ulcers are localized areas of tissue necrosis that usually develop over a bony prominence as a result of prolonged pressure.

Pressure ulcers affect from 1.5 to 3 million people in the United States at an annual cost of approximately 5 billion dollars. They occur more commonly in the elderly, patients who have had surgery for hip fracture, and patients with spinal cord injury. Hospitalized African Americans have an age-dependent higher prevalence of pressure ulcers compared with whites. Risk factors include diabetes mellitus, peripheral vascular disease, cerebrovascular disease, sepsis, and hypotension. Hispanics have also been shown to have a higher prevalence of pressure ulcers than non-Hispanic whites in nursing homes. Barriers to medical treatment and poor social support may contribute to differences in prevalence rates for pressure ulcers among ethnic minorities.

Factors promoting pressure ulcer formation include the following:

- Pressure—This is the primary contributive factor leading to formation of ulcers. The length of time over which high pressures are sustained is also important.
- Friction—This results in damage to superficial layers of skin, and intraepidermal blisters leading to superficial skin erosions. Friction can occur when a patient is pulled across a bedsheet or when a patient wears a badly fitting prosthetic device.
- Shearing forces—These are generated by the motion of bone and subcutaneous tissue relative to the skin, which is prevented from moving because of friction (as seen when the head of the bed is raised to more than 30 degrees or when a seated patient slides down a chair).
- Moisture—Moist surfaces predispose to ulcer formation in two ways: they increase the effects of pressure, friction, and shear; and they cause maceration of the skin, thereby increasing the incidence of ulcer formation fivefold. These conditions are from perspiration, urinary or fecal incontinence, or leakage from a wound site.

Pressure ulcers are classified according to the extent of tissue damage:

- Stage I—Nonblanching erythema of intact skin.
- Stage II—Partial-thickness skin loss, with loss of the epidermis and some of the dermis. No slough or necrotic tissue present.
- Stage III—Full-thickness loss of skin and damage to or necrosis of subcutaneous tissues. Damage extends down to but not through the underlying fascia.
- Stage IV—Full-thickness loss of skin with extensive destruction, tissue necrosis, and damage to bone, muscle, or other supporting structures.

Recently, two more stages of pressure ulcer formation have been added (per the National Pressure Ulcer Advisory Panel; http://www.npuap.org/pr2.htm):

- Deep tissue injury—Localized area of discolored skin that is purple or maroon-red in color. It is nonblanching with an intact dermis, and the skin feels boggy.
- Unstageable pressure ulcers—Full-thickness tissue loss in which the base of the ulcer is covered by slough or an eschar, and therefore the true depth of the damage cannot be estimated until these are removed. (**Note:** stable eschar—no erythema present, dry, and adherent—on the heels should *not* be removed, as it serves as a natural cover.)

Risk factors leading to pressure ulcer formation are as follows:

- Limited mobility
- Malnutrition
- Anemia
- Advanced age
- Fecal or urinary incontinence
- Smoking
- Dry skin
- Altered skin perfusion—decreased in cases of shock or increased if patient has edema due to fluid overload
- Acute illness leading to temporary immobility
- Chronic systemic illness
- Terminal illness
- Degenerative neurologic disease
- Increased weight
- Sudden decrease in weight
- Altered mental status
- Prolonged pressure

Simultaneous treatment with the following medications can also predispose to ulcer formation:

- Corticosteroids
- Sedatives
- Analgesics
- Antihypertensives

When a patient presents with a pressure ulcer, the following steps should initially be followed:

1. Assess the stage of the ulcer, and record it according to the ICD-9 codes.
2. Record the ulcer location according to the ICD-9 codes.
3. Carry out an assessment using the Braden or Norton scale, tools for predicting pressure ulcer risk. This determines the prevention measures taken and the type of pressure-reducing support surfaces used.
4. Monitor the progress daily.

When assessing a pressure ulcer, take note of the following factors:

- Location of the ulcer
- Size of the ulcer, including the length, width, and depth
- Stage of the ulcer
- Appearance of the ulcer bed, if visible—Observe the tissue color and whether it appears moist. The wound bed color for healthy granulating tissue is pink-red and cobblestone-like. A red and smooth wound bed is indicative of clean but nongranulating tissue. Unhealthy granulation tissue is dark red and bleeds on contact.
- Wound edges—Look carefully at the edge of the ulcer for evidence of induration, maceration, rolling edges, and redness.
- Skin around the edges of the ulcer—The periwound skin should be assessed for color, texture, temperature, and integrity of the surrounding skin.
- Drainage—If exudate is present, note the color and amount.
- Presence of necrotic tissue or eschar
- Presence of complicating features, such as undermining, tunneling, and tracts
- Any odor emanating from the ulcer
- Presence or absence of pain

Look For

Although classically pressure ulcers are located on the sacrum or heels, be sure to assess other pressure points, such as the occiput, back of the ears, and elbows.

Clinical appearance will vary according to the stage of the ulcer:

- Stage I—Nonblanching erythema. Epidermis appears normal. Site of the impending ulcer appears as an area of persistent redness in lighter-skinned people, whereas in darker-skinned individuals, the skin may appear as an area of persistent red-blue or purple tones.
- Stage II—Epidermis is lost. Lesion appears as an abrasion, denuded blister, or superficial erosion.
- Stage III—Full-thickness loss of skin extending into the subcutaneous tissue (Fig. 4-493). May extend into the fascia but does not involve it. May be visible as a crater, and a little slough or necrotic tissue may be visible.
- Stage IV—Full-thickness loss of skin with extensive necrosis extending into muscle, bone, joint capsule, or tendon (Figs. 4-494 and 4-495).
- Deep tissue injury—Skin may appear as a localized area of purple or maroon discoloration or as a blood-filled blister due to damage of underlying soft tissue.
- Unstageable pressure ulcer—Full-thickness tissue loss, but the base of the ulcer is covered by slough (yellow, green, brown) or by eschar (black, brown, tan).

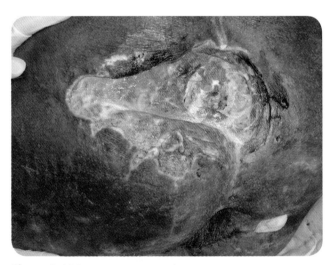

Figure 4-494 Stage IV pressure ulcer.

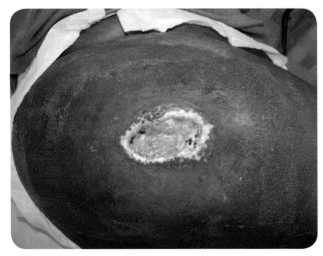

Figure 4-493 Ulcer due to pressure: stage III.

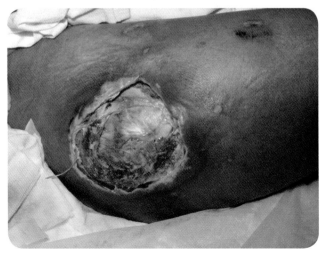

Figure 4-495 Stage IV pressure ulcer.

Erythema can be subtle in darker skin and may appear as a slightly different color, or the skin may be slightly darker than normal. Discoloration, warmth, induration, or hardness of skin may be the only signs of a stage I ulcer in people with darker skin tones.

Nonblanchable erythema may not be visible in darkly pigmented skin. Rather, the damaged area of skin may appear darker than the surrounding skin and may be indurated, edematous, and shiny. Color changes may range from violaceous to blue rather than erythematous. When compressed, the color of pressure-damaged dark skin does not blanch. Thus, the definition of stage I pressure ulcers as "nonblanchable erythema" may contribute to the underdiagnosis of low-grade pressure ulcers in ethnic minorities, which may then progress untreated to higher-grade ulcers. This likely contributes to the higher rates of high-grade ulcers observed in African Americans and Hispanics. Technology to assess the blanch response in skin of color is currently under investigation.

 ## Diagnostic Pearls

Diagnosis of a pressure ulcer is based on its location and the history of the patient. Presence of an ulcer at specific pressure points, such as the sacrum, heel, or occipital scalp, in conjunction with a history of hip fracture or being confined to bed because of either prolonged systemic illness or spinal cord injury should alert one to the diagnosis of pressure ulcer.

?? Differential Diagnosis and Pitfalls

- Pyoderma gangrenosum
- Squamous cell carcinoma
- Vasculitis
- Ecthyma gangrenosum
- Neurogenic (or diabetic) ulcer
- Stasis ulcer
- Ischemic ulcer
- Factitial ulcer
- Herpetic ulcer
- Basal cell carcinoma

 ## Best Tests

The diagnosis is based on a clinical assessment of the patient. However, the patient should undergo a full physical examination to identify any underlying factors that may be exacerbating wound development.

The following diagnostic studies should be carried out:

- CBC
- ESR

- HbA1c
- Nutritional assessment including
  - Albumin
  - Prealbumin
  - Transferrin levels
  - Serum protein
- Metabolic assessment including
  - Zinc levels
  - Copper levels
- Urinalysis
- Wound cultures should be taken if there are signs of possible infection. The value of taking a wound culture, however, is debatable. If infection is suspected, treat with a broad-spectrum antibiotic.
- Biopsy of the ulcer may be performed to rule out malignancy or an alternative diagnosis in the case of a long-standing ulcer.
- Imaging studies may be employed to detect underlying complications such as osteomyelitis. This is particularly relevant in cases with deep pressure ulcer sores in which bone is exposed.
- Viral culture for herpes simplex virus (HSV) or direct fluorescence antigen (DFA) testing should be performed when erosive HSV infection is suspected.

▲▲ Management Pearls

- Prevention is the best form of management:
  - Turn patients at least every 2 hours; rotate them to a 30-degree oblique position.
  - Avoid elevation of the head of the bed to >30 degrees.
  - Patients who are chair bound should be properly positioned.
  - Alleviate pressure over bony prominences, and protect skin from maceration secondary to incontinence or sweating.
  - Patients at risk should be placed on a special pressure-reduction surface, not on an ordinary mattress.
  - Maintain personal hygiene of patient.
  - Ensure adequate nutrition and hydration of patient.
  - Manage urinary and fecal incontinence by using a skin barrier cream to avoid contamination of intact skin. Also, collecting pouches may be used or catheterization may be considered in incontinent patients.
  - Avoid dragging the patient across the bed, and instead use lifting devices such as bed linen or a trapeze.
  - Massaging reddened areas over bony prominences should not be carried out, and this must be emphasized to the patient.
- Continuous assessment of the pressure ulcer is imperative; assessment should be performed at least once a day. More frequent reassessment may be required if the patient does not show steady improvement.

- The size of the ulcer may increase as it improves, especially if there was a lot of necrotic tissue at the base. This increase, however, should occur in the context of the ulcer looking healthier and cleaner.
- If the ulcer worsens, multidisciplinary management is necessary, involving allied health professionals such as specialized wound care nurses, physical and occupational therapists, social workers, and dieticians. In addition, physicians in such specialties as geriatrics, general or plastic surgery, and rehabilitation may also be consulted.

Avoid the use of topical antibiotics that include neomycin. Allergic contact dermatitis is a frequent complication in the treatment of skin ulcers and erosions.

Therapy

Prevention Plan
Prevention is the single most important factor. Assess patients at risk for developing pressure ulcers using the Braden Scale (an assessment tool to identify hospitalized patients at risk for ulcer development). The protocols for management of the patient will vary according to their Braden Scale categorization.

The Norton Scale
Physical condition—Rated from 1 to 4, where 1 is very bad and 4 is good.

Mental condition—Rated from 1 to 4, where 1 is in stupor and 4 is alert.

Activity—Rated from 1 to 4, where 1 is bed bound and 4 is ambulant.

Mobility—Rated from 1 to 4, where 1 is immobile and 4 is fully mobile.

Incontinent—Rated from 1 to 4, where 1 is doubly incontinent and 4 is not incontinent.

The Braden Scale
Sensory perception—Rated from 1 to 4, where 1 is perception is completely limited and 4 is no impairment.

Moisture—Rated from 1 to 4, where 1 is constantly moist and 4 is rarely moist.

Activity—Rated from 1 to 4, where 1 is bedfast and 4 is walks frequently.

Mobility—Rated from 1 to 4, where 1 is completely immobile and 4 is no limitation.

Nutrition—Rated from 1 to 4, where 1 is very poor nutrition and 4 is excellent nutrition.

Friction and shear—Rated from 1 to 3, where 1 is the presence of a problem and 3 is no apparent problem.

The scale determines the protocols for management. A score of 18 or lower indicates a patient at risk.

Management Protocols
Not at risk (19 to 23)

At Risk (score <15 to 18)

Frequent turning

Maximal remobilization

Protect heels

Manage moisture, nutrition, and friction and shear.

Pressure-reduction support surfaces if bed or chair bound, and should include foam or gel mattress

Moderate Risk (13 to 14)

Turning schedule

Use foam wedges for 30-degree lateral positioning.

Pressure-reduction support surface can include either the foam or gel mattress or the alternating or low-air-loss system.

Maximal pressure reduction

Protect heels—Elevate, use splint.

Manage moisture, nutrition, friction, and shear.

High Risk (10 to 12)

Increase frequency of turning.

Supplement with small shifts.

Pressure-reduction support surface should include alternating or low-air-loss systems.

Use foam wedges for 30-degree lateral positioning.

Maximal remobilization

Protect heels—Elevate, use splint.

Manage moisture, nutrition, friction, and shear.

Very High Risk (9 or below)

All of the above plus the following: use pressure-relieving surface if patient has intractable pain or severe pain exacerbated by turning, or if there are additional risk factors.

The use of the air-fluidized bed, the Clinitron, is highly recommended.

For discussion on managing ulcers, see VisualDx online. (If you are a first-time online user, go to www.essentialdermatology.com/pigmented; if you already have your password set up, go directly to www.visualdx.com/visualdx.)

Suggested Readings

Flanagan M. How can you accurately assess pressure damage on patients with darkly pigmented skins? *J Wound Care*. 1996;5:454.

Fogerty M, Guy J, Barbul A, et al. African Americans show increased risk for pressure ulcers: A retrospective analysis of acute care hospitals in America. *Wound Repair Regen*. 2009. [Epub ahead of print]

George B, Malkenson G. Pressure ulcers, a clinical review. *Rehab Manag*. 2008;21:16–19.

Gerardo MP, Teno JM, Mor V. Not so black and white: nursing home concentration of Hispanics associated with prevalence of pressure ulcers. *J Am Med Dir Assoc*. 2009;10:127–132.

Kanji LF, Wilking SVB, Phillips TJ. Pressure ulcers. *J Am Acad Dermatol*. 1998;38:517–538.

Lapane KL, Jesdale W, Zierler S. Racial differences in pressure ulcer prevalence in nursing homes. *J Am Geriatr Soc*. 2005;53:1077–1078.

Matas A, Sowa MG, Taylor V, et al. Eliminating the issue of skin color in assessment of the blanch response. *Adv Skin Wound Care*. 2001;14:180–188.

Norton D. Calculating the risk: Reflections on the Norton Scale. *Decubitus*. 2:24, 1989.

Saladin LK, Krause JS. Pressure ulcer prevalence and barriers to treatment after spinal cord injury: Comparisons of four groups based on race-ethnicity. *Neuro Rehabilitation*. 2009;24:57–66.

Factitial Dermatitis and Factitial Ulcers

Nasir Aziz

▪▪ Diagnosis Synopsis

Factitial Dermatitis

Factitial dermatitis, or dermatitis artefacta, is a factitious disorder that results when the patient consciously induces self-inflicted cutaneous injury to fulfill an unconscious psychological need.

To diagnose a factitious disorder, the *Diagnostic and Statistical Manual of Mental Disorders* requires that the following three criteria be met: (a) intentional production or feigning of physical or psychological signs or symptoms, (b) motivation for the behavior is to assume the sick role, and (c) absence of external incentives for the behavior (e.g., economic gain, avoiding legal responsibility, and improving physical well-being).

Physicians must rely on clinical presentation, careful observation, and detailed history from the patient and family. It is common for these patients to refuse psychiatric referrals, which may leave the burden on dermatologists alone. The patient provides a "hollow history" and is often unwilling to provide details about the eruption. The patient may appear indifferent towards his or her condition, a phenomenon known as "la belle indifference."

There usually are no prodromal symptoms as the lesions appear fully formed and in the same stage. Lesions can take on bizarre shapes, depending on the method of injury. They may have sharp angles, geometric borders, and surface necrosis that fail to conform to any known dermatological disorder. Lesions occur in areas easily accessible to the hands of the patient, and may be solitary or bilateral and symmetrically distributed. In fact, indirect diagnostic confirmation may be obtained by witnessing healing of lesions after isolation with occlusive dressings.

Factitial Ulcer

Factitial ulcers (a manifestation of dermatitis artefacta) occur secondary to a patient digging, excoriating, or generally manipulating his or her own skin.

Patients will not admit to creating the lesions, which are usually more elaborate than simple excoriations. Factitial ulcers should be differentiated from malingering, in which lesions are created deliberately for secondary gain, such as collecting disability or obtaining prescriptions.

The diagnosis of self-abuse tends to occur more frequently in women and in those working in health care. Such patients may inject foreign substances into their skin, leading to ulceration. The psychological profile of the patient with self-induced skin disease is the patient with a dependent and manipulative personality or borderline personality disorder.

The patients' typical lack of concern for how disfiguring the lesions appear is out of proportion to the reality of their presentation. The patient history never seems to add up to explain the unusual cutaneous findings. There is also a lack of findings to support the diagnosis of an alternative ulcerative process.

The lesions are often produced by digging, picking, biting, cutting, injecting, and puncturing. More serious wounds can be complicated by gangrene, abscess formation, or other life-threatening infections. Treatment is often challenging and requires a multidisciplinary approach.

◉ Look For

Factitial Dermatitis

Look for unusual and bizarre inflammatory plaques and erosions. Scaly and crusted plaques will typically have geometric, linear, angular, or curving shapes (Figs. 4-496–4-499).

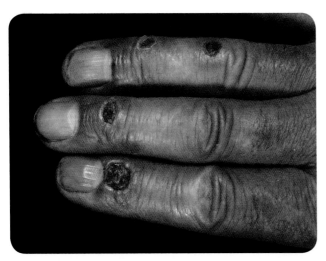

Figure 4-496 Very regular borders and no history of primary lesions suggest factitial etiology.

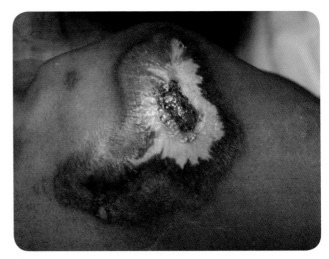

Figure 4-497 Factitial ulcer with irregular outline.

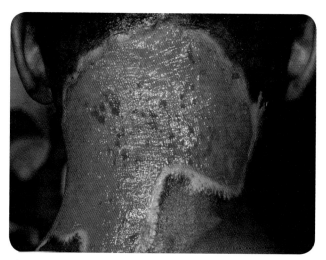

Figure 4-498 Large superficial ulceration with geometric borders is suggestive of self-induced etiology.

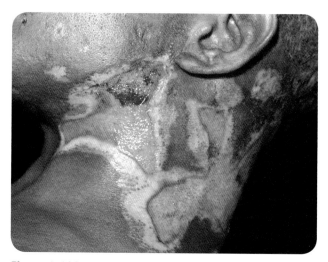

Figure 4-499 Multiple irregular ulcerations, some with linear borders characteristic of self-induced skin disease; earlier lesions on the periphery show prominent hypopigmentation.

Plaques are almost always within reach of the dominant hand. The patient will not tell you how he or she produces the lesions. The patient essentially creates a synthetic disease.

Factitial Ulcer

Look for bizarre distributions and geometric-shaped ulcers. The surrounding skin is usually normal. There may be scarring or postinflammatory hyperpigmentation at sites of older lesions, especially in darker-skinned patients. As with factitial dermatitis, lesions are usually in anatomical sites that are readily accessible to the dominant hand.

 Diagnostic Pearls

Factitial Dermatitis

There is an absence of external incentives (e.g., financial gain, obtaining narcotics) for inducing the lesions.

Factitial Ulcer

Carefully examine the patient for neuropathy. For example, in trigeminal neuralgia, where the ganglion has been destroyed by disease or therapy (such as injection with alcohol), the lack of sensation can predispose the tissue to destruction. These usually have a characteristic distribution, often around the nasal ala, whereas factitious ulcers have a wider distribution. Also, a careful neurological examination will reveal sensory abnormalities in the distribution of the trigeminal nerve.

?? Differential Diagnosis and Pitfalls

Factitial Dermatitis

- Münchhausen syndrome, a form of factitial dermatitis where the patient compulsively causes medical and/or surgical injuries to obtain money, drugs, and hospitalization
- Contact dermatitis
- Vasculitis
- Impetigo
- Arthropod reaction
- Delusions of parasitosis
- Lesch-Nyhan disease (self-mutilation by biting the lips, fingertips and shoulders) associated with an inherited abnormality of uric acid metabolism
- Burns
- Bullous diseases

Factitial Ulcer

- There are a number of skin disorders that worsen due to trauma (pathergy). Consider diagnoses such as Behçet disease and pyoderma gangrenosum.
- Repetitive skin trauma in a patient with a neuropathy
- Factitious disorder or Münchhausen syndrome by proxy is the intentional production or feigning of physical or psychological signs or symptoms by the patient's caregiver.
- Malingering
- Acne excoriée
- Vasculitis
- Lesch-Nyhan disease (self-mutilation by biting the lips, fingertips, and shoulders)
- Abuse
- Neurotic excoriations
- Scabies

Pediatric Patient Considerations

Self-injurious behaviors in children with autism, mental retardation, and Tourette syndrome can also create lesions mimicking factitious ulcers.

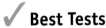 **Best Tests**

Swab crusted plaques for bacterial culture. A skin biopsy will confirm a clinical diagnosis. If the lesions heal when covered by an occlusive dressing and reappear when exposed, suspect the diagnosis.

 Management Pearls

See these patients often for their skin disease. Do not confront them, as they will feel threatened and not follow up. Gradually gain their trust by treating their skin manifestations and by offering empathy and reassurance. Once a stable physician–patient relationship has been established, recommend consultation with a mental health professional.

Therapy

Cover lesions with occlusive dressings (i.e., Unna boot). Involve the patient in the wound care regimen as much as possible. Optimize the management of any secondary complications, such as infection.

Patients with factitial dermatitis benefit from psychiatric therapy and follow-up. However, most patients are resistant to being seen by a mental health professional. Broach the topic of psychiatric consultation once a trusting relationship has been established. Psychodynamic, behavioral, cognitive, or insight-oriented psychotherapies may be helpful.

Psychotropic medications, when used by those familiar with using those medications, include selective serotonin reuptake inhibitors (SSRIs) and pimozide or olanzapine (2.5 to 5 mg daily) and may be useful in certain cases.

Therapy should be targeted at the underlying psychiatric issues. SSRIs have shown favorable responses in decreasing obsessive-compulsive disorder manifestations.

Suggested Readings

Koblenzer CS. Dermatitis artefacta. Clinical features and approaches to treatment. *Am J Clin Dermatol.* 2000;1:47–55.

Medina AC, Sogbe R, Gómez-Rey AM, et al. Factitial oral lesions in an autistic paediatric patient. *Int J Paediatr Dent.* 2003;13(2):130–137.

Setyadi HG, Cohen PR, Schulze KE, et al. Trigeminal trophic syndrome. *South Med J.* 2007;100(1):43–48.

Walia NS. Dermatitis artefacta: Three case reports. *Ind J Derm Ven Leprol.* 2006;51:39–41.

Pyoderma Gangrenosum

Laurie Good

◼◼ Diagnosis Synopsis

Pyoderma gangrenosum (PG) is an inflammatory, noninfectious, ulcerative neutrophilic dermatosis of uncertain etiology commonly misdiagnosed as an aggressive skin infection. Classically, pustules form and evolve to ulcers with a necrotic, undermined margin. PG can affect any age and has a number of differing clinical presentations, though four clinical variants are recognized: pustular, ulcerative, bullous, and vegetative. Fever, toxicity, and pain are common. Extracutaneous manifestations may take the form of sterile neutrophilic abscesses, such as in the lungs, heart, GI tract, liver, eyes, CNS, and lymphatic tissue.

Though the exact cause is unknown, PG is associated with a number of systemic illnesses in about half the cases, most commonly ulcerative colitis or Crohn disease; it can also be associated with arthritis, myeloma, leukemia, monoclonal gammopathy, Wegener granulomatosis, collagen vascular disease, Behçet disease, and other disorders. There is no racial or gender predilection for PG itself, though the diseases with which PG has shown an association can vary in prevalence by ethnicity and race. For example, ulcerative colitis has a relatively high prevalence in white patients. However, to date, ulcerative colitis has only been reported in association with PG in a handful of cases in Africans (two Nigerian patients and two black South African patients). Ulcerative colitis and Crohn colitis are also less common in the Asian population; thus one might expect ulcerative colitis–associated PG to occur less commonly in these ethnic groups.

The disease occurs most often in middle-aged adults. PG tends to be self-limited, and although first-line therapies are widely accepted, alternative therapeutic recommendations are largely based on anecdotal evidence. Surgical intervention is a common exacerbating factor because skin trauma can lead to worsening disease through the poorly understood "pathergy" phenomenon. PG can have either an acute or chronic course and result in extensive scarring, which can be keloidal or have dyspigmentation, especially in patients with darker skin types.

Pediatric Patient Considerations

Though lower in frequency (3% to 4% of all cases), PG can occur in infants and children. In this population, perianal and genital regions are commonly affected. In one case series of 14 patients in Senegal, an unusually high frequency of PG was observed in children (30%), but this has not been observed elsewhere.

◉ Look For

The skin lesions of PG typically begin as extremely painful, solitary nodules or deep-seated pustules that rupture and form a shaggy ulcer (Figs. 4-500–4-503). Often, there are pustules that do not progress to ulcerative lesions. The border of the ulcer has a deep violaceous or dusky color and is usually undermined. The ulcer extends peripherally with a bright erythematous or violaceous halo. Oral aphthae, ulcerative lesions of the oral mucosa, and ulcerative lesions of the vulva and eyes are possible. Necrosis is a common feature. As the ulcer progresses, a purulent coating commonly forms over the center of the ulcer. The ulcer may become secondarily infected and have a foul odor.

Variants of PG include pustular and bullous variants that can resemble Sweet syndrome. Vegetative forms have been described. Infrequently, PG can present in the form

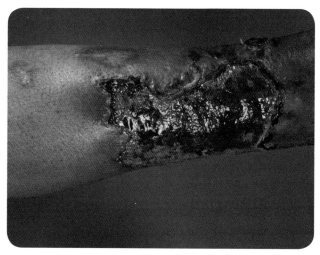

Figure 4-500 Pyoderma gangrenosum with irregular undermined border.

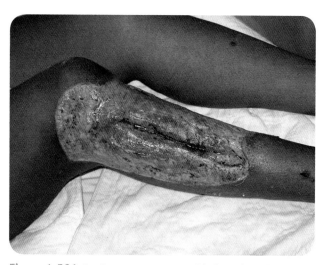

Figure 4-501 Pyoderma gangrenosum with deep ulceration.

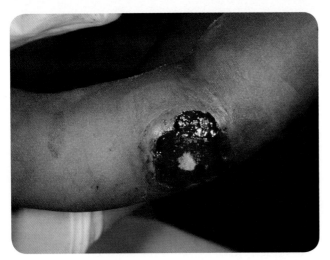

Figure 4-502 Two-year-old patient with classic pyoderma gangrenosum with wide purple border with extensive undermining.

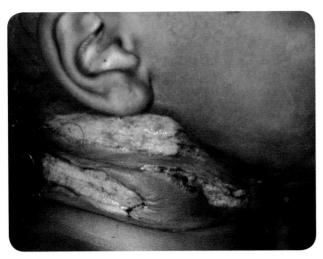

Figure 4-503 Same patient as Figure 4-502 with multiple neck ulcerations of pyoderma gangrenosum.

of suppurative panniculitis. With all variants, there may be eventual spontaneous healing with thin, atrophic scars.

The lesions of PG most commonly occur on the extremities, but can occur on the buttocks, face, arms, hands, scalp, genitals, or elsewhere. Patients with darker skin types may heal with hypopigmented or hyperpigmented scars.

Pediatric Patient Considerations

Presentations are no different in children than they are in adults, except that the distribution tends to be in the perianal and genital regions rather than lower extremities.

Diagnostic Pearls

The characteristic ulcer edge is undermined, and the base can be deep and is usually purulent. PG shares with Behçet disease and Sweet syndrome the occurrence of pathergy or the invocation of lesions by trauma to the skin such as a needle stick biopsy procedure, or even insect bites. PG ulcerations are often mistaken for infectious processes, but debridement will make the lesions larger. This history, or the history of an ulcerative wound following even minor trauma, should raise suspicions for PG.

?? Differential Diagnosis and Pitfalls

- Pustules/nodules
- Cellulitis
- Folliculitis
- Furuncle
- Insect or spider bite
- Sporotrichosis
- Mycobacterium marinum infection
- Impetigo
- Panniculitis
- Sweet syndrome (acute febrile neutrophilic dermatosis)
- Bromoderma

Ulcers

Infectious causes of ulcers can mimic PG. PG is in the family of neutrophilic skin disorders, which includes Sweet syndrome, subcorneal pustular dermatosis, and Behçet disease. As many infectious processes can cause a similar picture (e.g., progressive bacterial synergistic gangrene, North American blastomycosis, other deep fungal infections, amebiasis, sporotrichosis, atypical mycobacteria, etc.), PG is a diagnosis of exclusion.

- Aphthous stomatitis
- Acute febrile neutrophilic dermatosis
- Calciphylaxis—rapidly progressive, can be associated with eschars
- Chancroid—usually present around genital skin
- Churg-Strauss syndrome
- Cutaneous anthrax—develops to an eschar and is a medical emergency
- Cutaneous diphtheria
- Herpes simplex virus (HSV)—usually grouped, punched-out erosions
- Ecthyma
- Ecthyma gangrenosum
- Leukocytoclastic vasculitis
- Factitial ulcer—sharp geometric borders
- Factitial panniculitis

- Squamous cell carcinoma—associated with keratotic plaques
- Lymphoma
- Venous or arterial ulcerations
- Wegener granulomatosis
- Traumatic ulceration
- Necrobiosis lipoidica—usually associated with atrophic plaques
- Tertiary syphilis

If a patient has traveled to tropical countries within the last 6 months, diagnoses such as leishmaniasis, tropical ulcer, and Buruli ulcer must be considered.

Because PG may be a relapsing and remitting condition with treatment, atrophic, hyperpigmented, and hypopigmented scarring may occur. These scars may resemble scars from leukocytoclastic vasculitis or atrophie blanche.

Immunocompromised Patient Considerations

The differential diagnosis for an immunocompromised patient also includes:

- Chronic HSV
- Ulcerative Kaposi sarcoma

✓ Best Tests

Because PG is a diagnosis of exclusion, testing should be undertaken to rule out similar or associated disorders. Routine investigations to evaluate for systemic disease may include the following:

- CBC ± peripheral blood smear
- Serum electrolytes
- Liver function tests
- Urinalysis
- ANCA, ANA, antiphospholipid antibody, and rheumatoid factor
- Serum and/or urine protein electrophoresis

Skin biopsy with culture for bacteria and fungi should be performed to rule out infectious etiologies. Cultures should be taken for analysis of viruses and atypical mycobacteria as well as bacteria and fungi. It is important to note that secondary infections in PG ulcers may lead to positive bacterial cultures, despite the fact that this infection is not the primary cause of the ulcers. Histopathology typically reveals a dense neutrophilic skin infiltrate, necrosis, and hemorrhage. Leukocytoclastic vasculitis may be observed in some biopsy specimens.

▲▲ Management Pearls

- Because pathergy is often causative of new or enlarging ulcers in PG, do not débride a PG wound; this will only result in increasing its size.
- Surgical therapy and elective surgeries should be avoided, if possible. If surgical therapy is required, it should be performed only in conjunction with immunosuppressive therapy. Autologous skin grafts should be avoided due to the risk of inducing PG at the donor sites.
- The inflammatory bowel disease that may be associated with PG can be subtle and requires a full evaluation, even in the absence of signs and symptoms. Referral to a gastroenterologist is indicated for possible endoscopy and management. The lesions of PG respond to treatment of underlying rheumatoid arthritis or ulcerative colitis. Improvement of the underlying inflammatory disease may clear the PG or make treatment easier.
- Other consultants may be needed: ophthalmologist, rheumatologist, oncologist, general, or plastic surgeon. Evaluate on a case-by-case basis.

Therapy

Effective treatment of any underlying medical condition will often ameliorate the lesions of PG. Referral to dermatology for management is often indicated for multiple lesions or widespread disease.

Systemic corticosteroids are the mainstay of therapy, as corticosteroids can arrest the rapid enlargement of the ulcers of PG.

For more detailed information about therapy, see VisualDx online. (If you are a first-time online user, go to www.essentialdermatology.com/pigmented; if you already have your password set up, go directly to www.visualdx.com/visualdx.)

Suggested Readings

Alese OB, Irabor DO. Pyoderma gangrenosum and ulcerative colitis in the tropics. *Rev Soc Bras Med Trop.* 2008;41(6):664–667.

Diallo M, Kane A, Sy N, et al. Pyoderma gangrenosum in Dakar: About 14 cases. *Dakar Medical.* 2005;50(2):52.

Goh K, Xiao SD. Inflammatory bowel disease: A survey of the epidemiology in Asia. *J Dig Dis.* 2009;10(1):1–6.

Li LF. Treatment of pyoderma gangrenosum with oral Tripterygium wilfordii multiglycoside. *J Dermatol.* 2000;27(7):478–481.

Ruocco E, Sanguiliano S, Gravino AV, et al. Pyoderma gangrenosum: An updated review. *J Eur J Dermatol Venereol.* 2009;23(9):1008–1017.

Smith EH, Essop AR, Segal I, et al. Pyoderma gangrenosum and ulcerative colitis in black South Africans. Case reports. *S Afr Med J.* 1984;66(9):341–343.

Soft Tissue Tumors

Laurie Good • Pooja Sodha • Lynn McKinley-Grant • Chris G. Adigun

Connective tissue nevi and lipomas, including their variants, are discussed in this section. For discussions on fibrous hamartomas and smooth muscle hamartomas, see VisualDx online. (If you are a first-time online user, go to www.essentialdermatology.com/pigmented; if you already have your password set up, go directly to www.visualdx.com/visualdx.)

■■ Diagnosis Synopsis

Connective Tissue Nevi

Connective tissue nevi are lesions in which the normal dermal composition is altered. In connective tissue nevi, collagen, elastin, or glycosaminoglycans can predominate in excess. They may be present at birth or arise during childhood or adulthood, and can be found anywhere on the body. Connective tissue nevi can be found in normal individuals, or they can be associated with an underlying syndrome or disorder.

Connective tissue nevi have been described in association with tuberous sclerosis (shagreen patches) and in a familial cutaneous collagenoma syndrome. Rarely present at birth, shagreen patches of tuberous sclerosis tend to develop during childhood and are most commonly located on the lower back. The incidence of tuberous sclerosis is accepted to be about 1:25,000 in the white population, but little is known about its epidemiology in other racial or ethnic groups. A study that accessed the single national health insurance database in Taiwan demonstrated a prevalence of only 1:95,136 in this Chinese population, suggesting that shagreen patches may be less common in the Chinese population.

In European and North American literature, about 40% of tuberous sclerosis patients have a shagreen patch, while studies in Indian populations found higher prevalences, for example, 66.7% and 80%.

When found on the plantar surface, connective tissue nevi may be part of the Proteus syndrome. They have also been associated with multiple endocrine neoplasia (MEN I). Buschke-Ollendorf elastomas are another form of connective tissue hamartoma associated with benign bony lesions. Nevus mucinosis is a form of connective tissue nevi seen with Hunter syndrome, a severe lysosomal storage disease.

Lipomas

Lipomas are benign tumors of slow-growing mature fat cells commonly found in subcutaneous tissues. They are the most common soft tissue tumor, accounting for nearly 50% of all soft tumors with an incidence of approximately 1%. Based on microscopic findings, they may be classified as lipomas, angiolipomas, spindle cell lipomas, pleomorphic lipomas, adenolipomas (containing eccrine sweat glands), or lipomas with

hibernoma (brown fat, occurring more commonly in arms and neck). Rarely, lipomas may be found within or between muscle planes. The term pseudolipoma is used to denote the prolapse of unencapsulated fat through a fascial tear.

Clinically, lipomas present as soft, rubbery, freely mobile subcutaneous masses demarcated by a thin fibrous capsule without overlying skin change. They are most often solitary but can be multiple. They can occur anywhere on the body where fat is found, with the highest predilection for the trunk, back, extremities, and abdominal wall, but rarely on the head and neck. They can be small (most are <5 cm) to quite large (>10 cm) and occasionally are multilobular, weighing as much as 1 kg. Lipomas are usually asymptomatic; however, large tumors may compress nerves, limit normal tissue movement, or cause lymphedema with discomfort and pain. Tumors with a vascular component (angiolipomas) also tend to be painful; pain may be precipitated by cold. They grow slowly to a stable size and do not spontaneously regress.

Solitary idiopathic lipomas are more common in women, whereas multiple lipomas are more often seen in men. These lesions commonly present between the third and seventh decade, rarely before puberty. They may grow with weight gain, but do not shrink with weight loss. Since the fat in lipomas is not available for metabolism, excessive weight loss may make the lesion more prominent. Deeper lesions may become more visible on muscle contraction. Some lipomas are familial and have autosomal dominant inheritance. Malignant transformation is rare.

Lipomas increase with diabetes, obesity, and hypercholesterolemia.

Multiple lipomas are associated with several rare syndromes:

- Diffuse lipomatosis—characterized by the infiltration of nonencapsulated fat into multiple tissues including muscle, skin, fascia, and bone. This entity can be seen in association with tuberous sclerosis
- Familial multiple lipomatosis—characterized by multiple encapsulated lipomas in several family members
- Proteus syndrome—characterized by multiple hamartomas (including lipomas) and disproportionate overgrowth of multiple tissues
- Hemihyperplasia/multiple lipomatosis syndrome—characterized by multiple lipomas, asymmetric tissue overgrowth, capillary malformations, and accentuation of plantar skin creases
- Benign symmetric lipomatosis (Madelung disease)—characterized by symmetric fat deposits around and above the shoulders; associated with alcoholism
- Adiposis dolorosa (Dercum disease)—characterized by multiple painful lipomas in postmenopausal women; associated with weakness and depression

- Gardner syndrome—characterized by multiple lipomas, colon polyposis, odontomas, epidermoid cysts, osteomas, leiomyomas, desmoid fibromatosis, and hypertrophy of the retinal pigment epithelium
- Bannayan-Riley-Ruvalcaba syndrome—characterized by multiple lipomas, macrocephaly, intestinal polyposis, lentigines of the penis, and hemangiomas

Angiolipomas are an important variant of lipomas. They comprise approximately 5% to 17% of all lipomas and occur more commonly in people with multiple lipomas. They are benign localized growths of adipose and vascular tissue, averaging about 5 cm in size. Familial transmission of this lesion has been reported. Whether incidence is greater in men or women is still unclear. Clinically, angiolipomas are designated as noninfiltrating and infiltrating, the former being more common. These lesions are more likely to cause pain, postulated to be neuropathic in origin.

Angiolipomas present after puberty, typically in the second or third decades. Common sites include the trunk and extremities. Occurrences have been associated with protease inhibitor use and new-onset diabetes mellitus. They may be found in the kidneys in association with tuberous sclerosis and account for <1% of spinal tumors, in which case they may be associated with spina bifida. Later in life, they may present with CNS findings of acute back pain with abnormal neurologic findings (weakness, hyperreflexia, spasticity).

Pediatric Patient Considerations

In children and infants, lipoblastomas can be found typically in the subcutaneous tissue of the distal lower extremities.

Nevus lipomatosus superficialis (NLS) is a rare benign hamartoma composed of ectopic mature fat tissue in the dermis and is discussed in detail on VisualDX online.

Look For

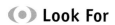

Connective Tissue Nevi

Slightly elevated nodules or flat-topped plaques are usually yellowish in color, indicating high elastic tissue content. Their size ranges from several millimeters to several centimeters. They may be clumped or grouped together, and they may be solitary or disseminated (Figs. 4-504 and 4-505). Lesions may be centered around hair follicles, forming a "cobblestone" appearance.

Lipomas

Discrete, solitary or multiple, mobile, soft encapsulated nodules with no overlying color change or punctum (Fig. 4-506). Sometimes feels like a group of small worms.

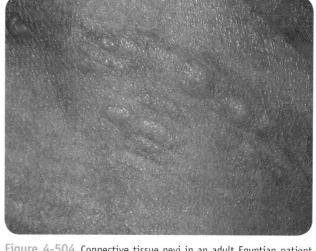

Figure 4-504 Connective tissue nevi in an adult Egyptian patient without associated genetic diseases.

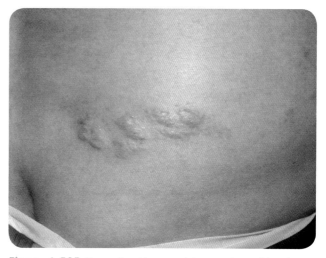

Figure 4-505 Connective tissue nevi in a patient with tuberous sclerosis.

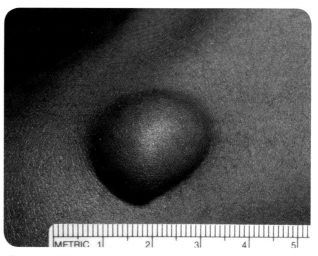

Figure 4-506 Large soft lipoma in a 16-year-old male patient.

467

Sizes vary, but may range from 1 to 10 cm. The tumors are fluctuant to touch and often lobulated. They tend to be subcutaneous but rarely intramuscular or intermuscular. Osseous involvement is rare. They occur most commonly on the back, shoulders, and upper extremities.

Sonographic finding is of hyperechogenic mass, but distinguishing the capsule may be difficult. Heterogeneic components can be discerned within the fat lobule.

CT/MRI are optimal modalities for identifying lipomas because of the fat content. On CT, lipomas appear as well-defined homogenous densities.

Pediatric Patient Considerations

Look for solitary or multiple soft, round to ovoid, lobulated tumors with the typical slippery edge. The tumors are painless and freely movable. Overlying skin can be pinched up.

It is important to differentiate from NLS (clusters of soft skin-colored to yellowish papuloplaques or nodules on the thighs, gluteal region, and lumbosacral region).

Look for spinal dysraphism in the case of congenital centrally located lumbosacral lipomas.

Diagnostic Pearls

Connective Tissue Nevi

Clinically and histologically, the differences between connective tissue nevi and surrounding skin can be subtle, but in patients with darker pigmentation, there is typically a greater degree of contrast that provides higher visibility of such lesions.

Lipomas

- Lipomas are usually not tender; angiolipomas are tender and may have a faint overlying erythema.
- Malignant lesions tend to be tethered to the overlying skin and are, therefore, less mobile.
- Lipomas may grow during times of weight gain, but do not decrease in size during weight loss.

?? Differential Diagnosis and Pitfalls

Connective Tissue Nevi

- Fibromatoses
- Fibrous hamartoma of infancy
- Infantile myofibromatosis
- Dermatofibromas
- Smooth muscle hamartomas

Lipomas

- Epidermoid cyst—There is no overlying skin change, nor are there ostia or dilated pores as would be seen in an epidermoid cyst. Cysts are usually firmer and more superficial.
- Metastatic malignancy—usually much firmer to the touch
- Liposarcoma—considered to arise *de novo*, not as a consequence of benign lipoma; differentiated from lipoma by histologic presence of lipoblasts, mitoses, pleomorphism, and high cellularity. They commonly occur in lower extremities and retroperitoneum and can become quite large. Lipomas occurring at less common sites, such as intramuscular, may be confused with this.
- Subcutaneous fat necrosis
- Angiomyolipomas—on histology, would have smooth muscle cell proliferation along with adipose and vascular tissue
- Abscess—One would expect to see accompanying erythema and induration.
- Leiomyoma—well-defined smooth muscle proliferation; usually more superficial, smaller, and multiple
- Dermatofibroma
- Glomus tumor
- Teratoma
- Blue rubber bleb nevus syndrome
- Nodular fasciitis
- Rheumatoid nodule
- Erythema nodosum
- Sarcoidosis neurofibroma—soft skin-colored papule or papulonodule that can be moved in lateral (side to side) direction but not along the direction of the nerve. The pathognomonic "buttonhole" sign is positive.
- Epidermal cyst—cystic swelling with dilated pores or punctum. Overlying skin cannot be pinched up.

✓ Best Tests

Connective Tissue Nevi

Skin biopsy—An area of poorly demarcated increased dermal collagen, without an apparent increase in fibroblasts, may be seen. There may be increased, decreased, or normal elastic fibers.

Lipomas

- This diagnosis can often be made on clinical grounds (nearly 85% of the time). If the diagnosis is in doubt or there is concern for malignancy, perform a biopsy.
- A CT scan can help distinguish lipoma from liposarcoma.

Pediatric Patient Considerations

In children, biopsy the lesion. Ultrasound may be used to distinguish from vascular and cystic lesions.

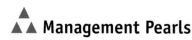

▲▲ Management Pearls

Connective Tissue Nevi

- Full exam is necessary in patients with connective tissue nevi to rule out any associated conditions, especially in cases with multiple lesions, shagreen patches, and Hunter syndrome.
- Referral to orthopedics in case of bony involvement (Buschke-Ollendorf syndrome)
- Referral to neurology if Hunter syndrome or tuberous sclerosis is suspected
- Ophthalmology referral for tuberous sclerosis patients, as potential for retinal hamartomas exists

Lipomas

Often, a lipoma can be fully excised through a small skin opening utilizing a "squeeze" technique. A 6-mm punch or stab incision can be made over the lipoma and then, through a combination of manual expression and curettage, the entire lipoma can be removed through the small opening. Recurrence is rare. Lipomas can be left alone. Malignant transformation of cutaneous lipomas is extremely rare.

Therapy

Connective Tissue Nevi

No specific therapy is necessary for the actual nevi, unless the lesions are of significant cosmetic concern. Clinicians should be aware of the increased risk of keloidal scarring and hypopigmentation when using surgical or laser interventions in patients with darker skin types.

Lipomas

Lipomas do not have to be treated, but if they are progressively enlarging, excise them when they are small. Use the squeeze technique as above or make a small elliptical incision overlying the lipoma. Make sure to excise the tumor and its fibrous capsule fully to prevent recurrence.

Liposuction has also been used for treatment of larger lesions. The advantage of liposuction is smaller incisions with less subsequent scarring. Recurrence is higher, particularly if residual tumor components are not completely removed.

Intralesional corticosteroids are sometimes employed to shrink smaller lipomas by inducing fat atrophy.

Depigmentation of the overlying skin may occur, which may be of significance in darker skin.

Surgical management remains treatment of choice. Complications include seroma, hemorrhage, infection, ecchymosis, scarring, and focal deformity. After excision, recurrence rate is approximately 5%.

Pediatric Patient Considerations

A lipoma can often be fully excised through a small skin opening. A 6-mm punch biopsy can be used over the lipoma and then, through a combination of manual expression and curettage, the entire lipoma can be removed through the small opening.

Liposuction has been used for treatment of larger lesions.

Suggested Readings

Aust MC, Spies M, Kall S, et al. Lipomas after blunt soft tissue trauma: Are they real? analysis of 31 cases. *Br J Dermatol.* 2007;157:92–99.

Brenn T. Neoplasms of subcutaneous fat. In: Fitzpatrick TB, Wolff K, eds. *Fitzpatrick's Dermatology in General Medicine.* 7th Ed. New York, NY: McGraw-Hill; 2008:1190–1194.

Dalal KM, Antonescu CR, Singer S. Diagnosis and management of lipomatous tumors. *J Surg Oncol.* 2008;97(4):298–313.

Ghosh S, Bandyopadhyay D, Chatterjee G, et al. Mucocutaneous changes in tuberous sclerosis complex: A clinical profile of 27 Indian patients. *Ind J Dermatol.* 2009;54(3):255.

Guaraldi G, Orlando G, Squillace N, et al. Prevalence of and risk factors for pubic lipoma development in HIV-infected persons. *J Acquir Immune Defic Syndr.* 2007;45(1):72–76.

Halder RM, Nootheti PK. Ethnic skin disorders overview. *J Am Acad Dermatol.* 2003;48(6 Suppl):S143–S148. Review.

Hong CH, Darling TN, Lee CH. Prevalence of tuberous sclerosis complex in Taiwan: A national population-based study. *Neuroepidemiology.* 2009;33(4):335–341.

Kransdorf, Mark J. Benign soft-tissue tumors in a large referral population: Distribution of specific diagnoses by age, sex, and location. *Am J Roentgenol.* 1995;164:395–402.

Pinski KS, Roenigk HH. Liposuction of lipomas. *Dermatol Clin.* 1990;8(3):483–492.

Rahman GA, Abdulkadir AY, Yusif IF. Lipomatous lesions around the shoulder: Recent experience in a Nigerian Hospital. *Int J Shoulder Surg.* 2009;3.1:13–15.

Silistreli OK, Durmuş EU, Ulusal BG, et al. What should be the treatment modality in giant cutaneous lipomas? Review of the literature and report of 4 cases. *Br J Plast Surg.* 2005;58(3):394–398.

Suga H, Eto H, Inoue K, et al. Cellular and molecular features of lipoma tissue: Comparison with normal adipose tissue. *Br J Dermatol.* 2009;161:819–825.

Cysts

Pooja Sodha • Lynn McKinley-Grant

Diagnosis Synopsis

An epidermoid (epidermal inclusion cyst, keratinous cyst, or sebaceous cyst) is a benign tumor of ectodermal origin that may become symptomatic in the later decades of life. The lesion grows due to the continuous desquamation of epithelial cells into the cavity.

An epidermoid cyst can arise anywhere on the body, but most are reported on the face, scalp, neck, trunk, upper back, genitals, or in the mouth. They have a semisolid mixture of macerated keratin and lipids surrounded by a stratified squamous epithelial wall. The contents may be expressed as soft "cheesy" material. They may appear at any age, although they are commonly diagnosed prior to the fourth decade. An epidermoid cyst is usually asymptomatic and is more common in men, with a higher incidence among individuals of African descent than those of Northern European descent. Infection of the cyst can develop spontaneously or after rupture and may be painful. Rarely, malignancies such as basal cell carcinoma, squamous cell carcinoma (SCC), and mycosis fungoides have developed within these cysts.

In African American and Asian Indian populations, epidermal cysts are more commonly pigmented. In one study of 125 cysts in pigmented skin, 63% of cysts were pigmented, closely resembling the overlying skin color. Injury or rupture of the cysts can precipitate an inflammatory reaction, resulting in darkening of the lesion. In the same study, cysts that occurred in areas along skin closure, where epidermal sequestration occurred prior to melanocyte migration in the embryo, were devoid of pigment. Nonpigmented epidermal cysts occur most commonly on the face along the frontal, maxillary, and mandibular prominences; along the most distal parts of the body (to which migration is a longer process);

and in scrotal regions. This can be important to differentiate from other less benign pigmented lesions.

Epidermodysplasia verruciformis, a rare cutaneous infection from HPV-6 and HPV-8, presents with epidermal inclusion cysts in darkly pigmented skin; this is different from the presentation in white patients, in whom plaques and papules may progress to SCC.

Dermoid cysts arise from two embryonic germ layers, thereby commonly involving the adjacent adnexae, such as nails, and, like epidermal cysts, have an epithelial lining.

Pediatric Patient Considerations

Epidermoid cysts are a feature of several hereditary syndromes, such as Gardner syndrome, pachyonychia congenita, and the basal cell nevus syndrome, all of which commonly present with multiple cysts. Because it is rare to see an "ordinary" epidermoid cyst in a prepubertal patient, in such cases other diagnoses should be carefully considered.

Look For

A dome-shaped, well-circumscribed, firm but smooth skin-colored nodule that is freely movable on palpation and sometimes has a small, dilated punctum. Occasionally, a thick, cheesy material with a foul odor can be expressed. The cyst can be well defined or irregular due to prior rupture, scarring, and regrowth. The lesion is not pulsatile or reducible.

They can be located almost anywhere but are common on the face, neck, scalp, or trunk (Figs. 4-507–4-510).

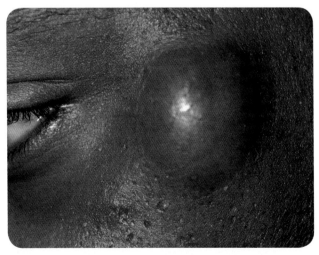

Figure 4-507 Tense epidermal cyst on the temple.

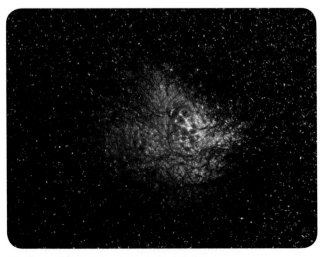

Figure 4-508 Pilar cyst in a typical location.

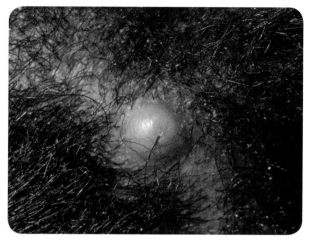

Figure 4-509 Smooth-surface pilar cysts on the scalp; frequently, there is some associated alopecia.

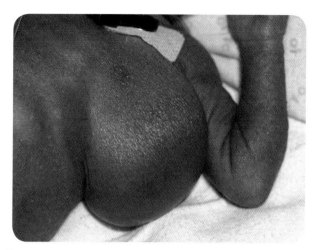

Figure 4-511 Large cystic hygroma in a typical location in a neonate.

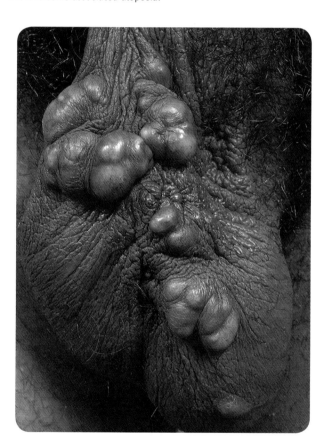

Figure 4-510 Multiple sebaceous cysts on the scrotum.

Pediatric Patient Considerations

The cyst is generally one-half to several centimeters in diameter. If manipulated or inflamed, the cyst can appear infected, with erythema and tenderness. Cystic hygromas are large cystlike structures usually on the posterior neck (Fig. 4-511).

Diagnostic Pearls

- Careful examination will frequently show a porelike opening (also known as a central punctum). The lesion usually has a consistency a little firmer than the adult eyeball.
- Sudden pain or swelling may be related to bleeding, infection, or the rupture of the cyst contents into the surrounding tissue. The content of the cyst, when exposed to air, has a foul-smelling odor.
- The presence of multiple epidermoid cysts and a family history of the same should lead to the consideration of a heritable condition such as Gardner syndrome, which is associated with GI polyps and malignancy.
- In pigmented skin, the cyst may parallel the color of the overlying skin.

Pediatric Patient Considerations

Sudden pain or swelling may be related to the rupture of the cyst contents into the surrounding tissue, leading to a vigorous foreign body inflammatory response and not true infection.

Differential Diagnosis and Pitfalls

- Dermoid cyst
- Eruptive vellus hair cyst
- Lipoma
- Pilar cysts
- Pilomatrixoma

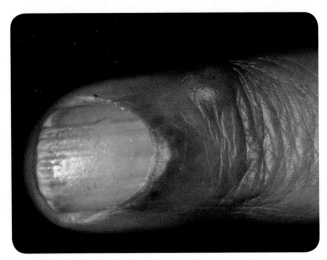

Figure 4-512 Small myxoid cyst in a typical location.

- Steatocystoma
- Trichilemmal cyst
- Myxoid cyst—a benign ganglion of the distal interphalangeal joint (Fig. 4-512). Solitary, rounded, flesh-colored or translucent papule or nodule that may feel relatively firm or be somewhat fluctuant. Fluid inside the cysts is viscous, clear to yellowish, and may be expressed. It results from degeneration of connective tissue associated with osteoarthritic joints. Prevalent in women and the elderly, and occurs more frequently on the fingers than on the toes.
- Rheumatoid nodule
- Calcinosis cutis
- Cutaneous metastatic malignancy
- Favre-Racouchot syndrome
- Gardner syndrome—The presence of multiple epidermoid cysts in an individual and a positive family history of the same should lead to the consideration of Gardner syndrome, a heritable disorder associated with GI malignancy.
- Superficial lymph nodes—can be palpated within the subcutaneous fat and are found along the course of lymphatics
- Dermoid cysts—result from anomalies in embryonic closure zones, comprising ectodermal and mesodermal components. Present at birth. Surgical removal or biopsy of a cyst over the midline should not be attempted without proper imaging to rule out intraspinal, intracranial, or intraorbital connection. 7% occur on the head, most commonly in the periorbital region and along the nasal bridge, rarely on the scalp.
- Pilar cysts (trichilemmal cysts)—may be clinically indistinguishable from epidermoid cysts, but often have no punctum, can be associated with ulceration, and are easily enucleated. More common in women and typically found on the scalp. Histological differentiation with infiltration of inflammatory cells and fibroblasts and foci of calcification (25%). When it proliferates, can be confused with SCC. Autosomal dominant transmission has been reported.

- Pilomatrixoma—usually presents as a solitary skin-colored to faint blue nodule, frequently found on the head or upper trunk in children. Arises from follicle matrix cells. Can be differentiated from epidermal and dermoid cysts by irregular nodules and earlier age of presentation. Firmness is a reflection of calcification within this benign tumor. Surface may become ulcerated. Sometimes associated with myotonic dystrophy.
- Lipomas—soft, mobile subcutaneous nodules of adipose tissue with normal overlying epidermis
- Steatocystomas—occur as asymptomatic single or multiple cysts on the chest, axillae, and/or groin that may drain an oily substance if punctured. Multiple steatocystomas are seen in some patients with pachyonychia congenita.
- Bronchogenic cysts—most frequently found in the suprasternal notch, and they represent sequestered respiratory epithelium during embryological development.
- Thyroglossal duct cysts (TGDCs)—embryological remnants that fail to regress after fetal descent of the thyroid gland from foramen cecum. This is the most common cervical malformation in children. TGDCs present in childhood, with a median age of 5.6 years, as midline, painless, soft masses near the hyoid bone. There is no sex predominance. At least half of childhood cases present when the TGDC is complicated by infection, in which case the cysts may be painful. Cysts may rarely cause life-threatening airway obstruction. Thyroid hormone levels should be checked if these cysts are so diagnosed, as these patients may be hypothyroid.
- Branchial cleft cysts—present in the second or third decade as a nodule in the preauricular area, mandibular region, or along the anterior border of the sternocleidomastoid muscle. Resulting from incomplete closure of the branchial clefts in the 4 to 8 weeks of embryonic development.
- Milia—small keratin-filled papular lesions, 1 to 2 mm, that may be present in the neonate; arise spontaneously or secondary to trauma

✓ Best Tests

- The diagnosis can usually be made clinically. With pressure or a small incision, a yellow, cheesy material can be expressed from the cyst. Skin biopsy can confirm the diagnosis by demonstrating characteristic histopathology but is usually not necessary. However, skin biopsy in dark skin is preferable to rule out alternative cause for pigmentation.
- Ultrasound is another modality suitable for certain anatomical regions. Sonographic characteristics include a well-circumscribed mass surrounded by a hyperechoic ring and alternating areas of hyperechogenicity and hypoechogenicity due to central and peripheral

calcifications within the lesion. Ultrasound is the modality of choice when delineating cystic features.
- CT/MRI is a useful technique to rule out intracranial involvement but is usually not necessary.
- In case of infection, obtain cultures and sensitivities, if possible, from any cysts.

Pediatric Patient Considerations

In children, if the punctum is present over a typical lesion, no test is necessary. Skin biopsy may be performed if diagnosis is unclear. Cystic lesions present over the midline may require imaging to rule out central nervous system connection prior to surgical intervention.

▲▲▲ Management Pearls

- Cyst rupture with associated inflammation is often misdiagnosed as an "infection" of the cyst. Cultures are usually negative, and treatment with antibiotics is not required.
- Incision and drainage can provide immediate reduction in the cyst, but without removing the epidermal lining, the cyst will refill with layers of soft keratin. There are three surgical interventions: wide excision, punch biopsy excision, and minimal excision. If the cyst wall is not completely removed, the cyst will likely recur. In the case of an inflamed cyst, it is generally preferable to delay the procedure until the inflammation has subsided.
- If there is any concern for associated malignancy (e.g., rapid growth, ulceration), remove the cyst entirely, and send the specimen for pathologic analysis.

Pediatric Patient Considerations

If the child is young, defer therapy of an asymptomatic, stable, nonfacial cyst until older.

Therapy

Asymptomatic lesions require no treatment.

Symptomatic cysts can be excised in an elliptical fashion, or a punch biopsy can be used to create a small skin opening followed by curettage to remove the entire cyst wall. Incision and drainage are used for only temporary relief. With wide excision, the entire cyst (along with the wall) can be excised surgically. For small cysts (<1 cm), a minimal excision technique with a 3-mm incision line has shown to be effective with minimal scarring (particularly useful with cysts of the face). Patients should be advised of the possibility of keloidal scarring, especially for lesions on the face and upper trunk.

In cases of recurrence, two iodine crystals can be placed within the center of the cyst via the punctum. Over the course of a few weeks, the cyst darkens and hardens, permitting easy removal of the entire cyst. Though inexpensive and effective, this technique involves brief cosmetic changes and clinical follow-up.

An infected cyst should be treated with systemic antibiotics prior to surgical intervention. The choice of antibiotic should be tailored to the suspected organism.

For methicillin-sensitive *Staphylococcus aureus* infection, a first-generation cephalosporin:

- Cephalexin 500 mg p.o. four times daily for 10 to 14 days

For methicillin-resistant *S. aureus* (MRSA):

- Refer to current CDC guidelines, as treatment recommendations are rapidly changing.

Inflamed cysts that are not infected may respond to intralesional triamcinolone, but incision and drainage is preferred to remove the "foreign body" (keratinous debris) causing the inflammatory reaction.

Pediatric Patient Considerations

Surgical dissection around the wall of a noninflammatory cyst is the best way to permanently remove lesions.

Some have used a punch biopsy to create a small skin opening and then curetted the cyst wall. This technique is sometimes effective and can reduce the incision size.

If the cyst is inflamed, resist the urge to incise and express (this usually results in only temporary relief). Intralesional triamcinolone (3 to 5 mg/mL) and oral tetracycline (only in children older than 8) can be effective in decreasing inflammation of a symptomatic/ruptured lesion.

Appropriate dosages of systemic antibiotics for children may be necessary, as outlined in Chapter 5.

Suggested Readings

Armon N, Shamay S, Maly A, et al. Occurrence and characteristics of head cysts in children. *Open Access J Plast Surg.* 2010;10:305–312. Open Science Co. LLC, 22 May 2010. Web. 15 June 2010. <http://www.eplasty.com/index.php?option=com_content&view=article&id=449&catid=15&Itemid=116>.

Chang SJ, Sims J, Murtagh FR, et al. Proliferating trichilemmal cysts of the scalp on CT. *Am J Neuroradiol.* 2006;27:712–714.

Mehrabi D, Leonhardt JM, Brodell RT. Removal of keratinous and pilar cysts with the punch incision techniques: Analysis of surgical outcomes. *Dermatol Surg.* 2002;28.8:673–677.

Pryor SG, Lewis JE, Weaver AM, et al. Pediatric dermoid cysts of the head and neck. *Otolyaryngol Head Neck Surg.* 2005;132:938–942.

Ramagosa R, De Villiers E-M, Fitzpatrick JE, et al. Human papillomavirus infection and ultraviolet light exposure as epidermoid inclusion cyst risk factors in a patient with epidermodysplasia verruciformis? *J Am Acad Dermatol.* 2008;58(5 Suppl 1):S68.e1-6.

Shet T, Desai S. Pigmented epidermal cysts. *Am J Dermatopathol.* 2001;23.5:477–481.

Yang H-J, Yang K-C. A new method of facial epidermoid cyst removal with minimal incision. *J Eur Acad Dermatol Venereol.* 2009;23:887–890.

Zuber TJ. Minimal excision technique for epidermoid (sebaceous) cysts. *Am Fam Phys.* 2002;65.7:1409–1412.

Ecthyma

Meaghan Canton Feder

▪▪ Diagnosis Synopsis

Ecthyma is considered a deeper form of impetigo. It is an ulcerative bacterial skin infection caused by group A beta-hemolytic streptococci and is often secondarily associated with staphylococci. Unlike impetigo, which only affects the stratum corneum, ecthyma extends into the dermis and results in a scar.

Clinically, the lesions of ecthyma appear as vesicles or pustules that ulcerate and crust over. Ecthyma is usually seen in pediatric and geriatric populations and presents most often on the lower extremities. Risk factors for ecthyma are immunosuppression, diabetes, poor hygiene, overcrowding, malnutrition, and humidity. It can also present at the site of preexisting trauma, such as a bug bite or a neglected superficial skin wound. It has also been seen in military trainees in tropical climates on lower legs.

Immunocompromised Patient Considerations

Ecthyma is usually seen in immunocompromised patients, such as those with diabetes or HIV infection. It is also seen in environments with crowded living conditions and poor hygiene.

◉ Look For

The lesions of ecthyma commonly begin as small fluid-filled vesicles or vesicopustules that are usually found on the dorsal feet, shins, legs, or buttocks. As the vesicles enlarge, they rupture, and thick gray-yellow crusts cover the lesions (Fig. 4-513). If the crusts are removed, superficial ulcers are revealed with depressed, raw bases and raised edges. The ulcers heal within a few weeks leaving scars. Localized lymphadenopathy is commonly present in these patients.

Immunocompromised Patient Considerations

Immunocompromised patients are more at risk for these ulcers to develop into gangrene.

▪▪ Diagnostic Pearls

- Look for a few lesions localized to one area on the lower legs that have persisted for weeks to months with adherent crusts and punched-out ulcers.

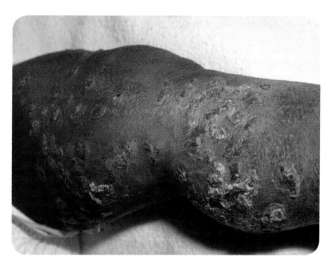

Figure 4-513 Deep and superficial crusted lesions of streptococcal ecthyma.

- There should be no other obvious signs of cellulitis.
- Regional lymphadenopathy is commonly present.

?? Differential Diagnosis and Pitfalls

- The disorder is similar to streptococcal impetigo but is differentiated by deeper components.
- Ecthyma should be differentiated from ecthyma gangrenosum, which is caused by *Pseudomonas* sepsis, is potentially life-threatening, and evolves over hours to days.
- Methicillin-resistant *Staphylococcus aureus* (MRSA) infections
- Pyoderma gangrenosum
- *Mycobacterium marinum* infection
- Leishmaniasis
- Insect bites/insect bite reactions—could be initial cause of trauma
- Sporotrichosis
- Lymphomatoid papulosis
- Papulonecrotic tuberculids
- Tungiasis

✓ Best Tests

- Gram stain and bacterial culture and antibiotic sensitivity of lesions will reveal Gram-positive cocci representing group A streptococci with or without *Staphylococcus aureus*.
- Skin biopsy is rarely needed but, if performed, will show dermal necrosis and inflammation with a granulomatous perivascular infiltrate.

Management Pearls

- The wound should be cleaned with soap and water. Saline soaks should be used to remove crusts. Mupirocin or bacitracin ointment should be applied to the ulcer twice a day. The patient should be educated on ulcer healing as an atrophic scar.
- Proper hygiene is the most important measure in the prevention of ecthyma.
- Nonsuppurative complications of streptococcal skin infections include glomerulonephritis and scarlet fever.

Therapy

Ecthyma should be treated with systemic antibiotics depending on the bacterial culture sensitivity. Usually, treatment consists of dicloxacillin or a first-generation cephalosporin.

- Dicloxacillin—250 mg four times daily for 10 days
- Erythromycin—333 mg three times daily for 10 days
- Azithromycin—two tabs for 1 day then one tablet per day for 4 days
- Cephalexin—250 mg four times daily for 10 days

Care for local wounds with gentle cleansing and the application of mupirocin or bacitracin ointment twice daily as combined therapy.

Suggested Readings

James WD, Berger TG, Elston DM, eds. Infections caused by Gram-positive organisms, impetigo contagiosa, bullous impetigo, and ecthyma. In: *Andrews' Diseases of the Skin: Clinical Dermatology.* 10th Ed. Philadelphia, PA: Saunders Elsevier; 2006:255–259.

Rayner C, Munckhof WJ. Antibiotics currently used in the treatment of infections caused by *Staphylococcus aureus. Intern Med J.* 2005;36(2):142–143.

Wasserzug O, Valinsky L, Klement E, et al. A cluster of ecthyma outbreaks caused by a single clone of invasive and highly infective *Streptococcus pyogenes. Clin Infect Dis.* 2009;48(9):1220–1222.

Erythema Nodosum

Mat Davey

Diagnosis Synopsis

Panniculitis refers to an inflammatory disorder primarily localized in the subcutaneous fat. Erythema nodosum (EN) represents the most common type of inflammatory panniculitis. It typically presents as symmetric, tender, subcutaneous nodules in the pretibial region of the lower legs. The majority of cases are idiopathic, although precipitating factors including endogenous or exogenous stimuli may be identified. Streptococcal infections are by far the most common etiologic factor in children, while sarcoidosis, inflammatory bowel disease, and drugs (particularly oral contraceptives) are more commonly implicated in adults. Other triggers include lymphoproliferative malignancies, connective tissue diseases, and pregnancy. Bacterial, viral, fungal, and protozoal infections may cause EN, with tuberculosis remaining an important cause in areas of endemic disease.

Löfgren syndrome, a condition associated with sarcoidosis, consists of a febrile illness with EN and bilateral enlargement of the hilar glands. It occurs more commonly in women, especially during pregnancy.

Upper respiratory tract infection or flulike symptoms may precede or accompany the development of the eruption. Arthralgias are reported by a majority of patients, regardless of the etiology of EN. The eruption persists for 3 to 6 weeks and spontaneously regresses without ulceration, scarring, or atrophy. Recurrences may occur, especially with repetition of the precipitating factors. EN can occur at any age, but most cases occur between the ages of 20 and 45. Women outnumber men 3 to 6:1. No specific ethnic predilection exists except for the underlying diseases (e.g., sarcoidosis being more common in African Americans).

Pediatric Patient Considerations

In children, the most common cause of EN is streptococcal infection. A number of cases remain idiopathic or are associated with similar conditions as seen in adults. Childhood cases of EN mirror those in adults, although faster resolution (often within 14 to 18 days) is noted. Before puberty, EN occurs in boys and girls in equal proportions, though it rarely occurs before age 2 years; however, after puberty, the female-to-male ratio is similar to adults, with females outnumbering males.

In younger children especially, physical factors such as cold exposure or trauma may lead to panniculitis. Subcutaneous fat necrosis of the newborn has been associated with difficult labor and childbirth, perinatal hypothermia/hypoxia, maternal diabetes, preeclampsia,

and seizures, all of which may lead to disintegration and destruction of the subcutaneous fat. Lesions are not typically present at birth but develop over the first few weeks of life. It may occur in both premature and term infants. Infants are afebrile and without systemic symptoms. Lesions resolve spontaneously within 2 to 3 months. Hypercalcemia may appear weeks to months after the appearance and resolution of the skin lesion.

Cold panniculitis is the crystallization of subcutaneous fat with subsequent inflammation in response to cold injury. The typical scenario is an infant or young child who has had prolonged cold exposure to the cheeks or limbs from low ambient temperatures, local therapeutic application of cold (e.g., during cardiac surgery), or other cold exposure (e.g., from a popsicle). Children of African descent are especially prone to developing cold panniculitis. Lesions resolve without sequelae over several days to weeks.

Look For

In EN, look for erythematous, tender subcutaneous nodules and plaques, usually 2 to 5 cm in diameter. They are initially bright red and slightly elevated. In people with darker skin, the lesions are often more dusky red or violaceous (Figs. 4-514–4-516). They usually have a smooth and "deep-seated" appearance. A pretibial symmetric distribution is the most common, but lesions may appear on the thighs, buttocks, or extensor arms, and occasionally on the face and neck. Over a period of 1 to 3 weeks, the lesions become flatter

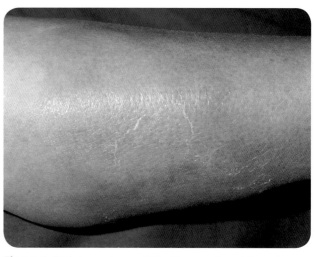

Figure 4-514 Large plaque of EN with a very fine white scale.

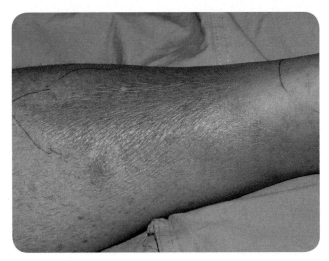

Figure 4-515 Sixty-two-year-old woman with bilateral lower extremity nodules of EN.

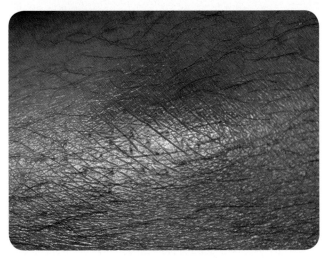

Figure 4-517 Bruiselike lesion of EN.

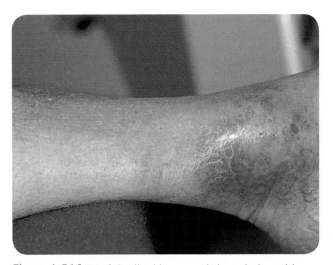

Figure 4-516 EN of the distal legs can mimic stasis dermatitis.

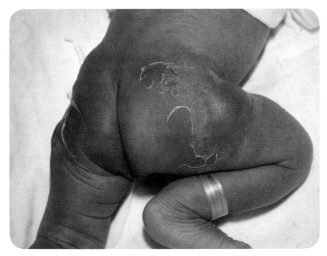

Figure 4-518 Large nodule of subcutaneous fat necrosis.

and evolve to a purple/livid or red-brown color, which may mimic a bruise (contusiforme) (Fig. 4-517). Lesions never ulcerate (unlike nodular vasculitis). Postinflammatory hyper/hypopigmentation is common among those with darker skin types. Even in uncomplicated cases of EN, adenopathy, including hilar adenopathy on chest X-ray, may occur.

Pediatric Patient Considerations

In EN, lesions appear similar to those seen in adults.

In subcutaneous fat necrosis of the newborn, look for tender, firm, rubbery, red nodules that typically appear on the back, buttocks, cheeks, and extremities (Fig. 4-518). Nodules can be greater than a centimeter,

and in rare instances, broad areas of fat necrosis can occur. As lesions progress, they may develop a brownish color. Large nodules can develop fluctuance.

In cold panniculitis, look for painful, firm, red-to-violaceous, ill-defined, 1- to 3-cm, indurated nodules that form 1 to 3 days after cold exposure (Figs. 4-519 and 4-520). The cheeks are the most common site of involvement. The buttocks and other fatty areas, especially the scrotum of obese prepubertal boys, may be affected.

●● Diagnostic Pearls

Sarcoidosis is frequently associated in familial cases of EN.

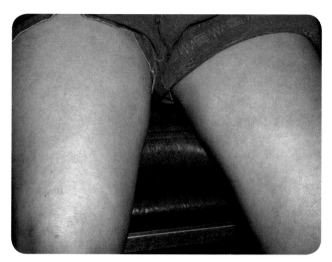

Figure 4-519 Cold panniculitis from snow sledding.

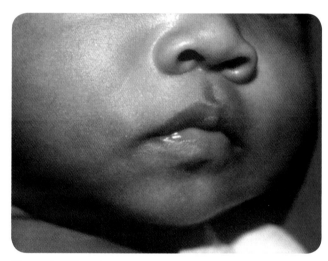

Figure 4-520 Cold panniculitis due to external cold exposure.

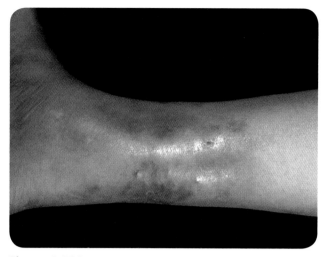

Figure 4-521 Erythema induratum with extensive subcutaneous involvement on the lower extremities and development of tuberculous cervical lymph nodes.

- Sarcoidosis
- Infections—cellulitis, erysipelas, tinea (Majocchi granuloma), deep fungal
- Insect bites
- Erythema multiforme
- Urticaria
- Cutaneous polyarteritis
- Erythema induratum (nodular vasculitis) (Fig. 4-521)
- Subcutaneous granuloma annulare
- Rheumatoid nodules
- Eosinophilic cellulitis
- Sweet syndrome
- Pretibial myxedema
- Necrobiosis lipoidica
- Pseudolymphoma and some forms of lymphoma
- Lipodermatosclerosis

Pediatric Patient Considerations

- In children with EN, inquire about antecedent upper respiratory infection or sore throat.
- In subcutaneous fat necrosis of the newborn, lesions often occur over bony prominences.
- In cold panniculitis, the development of lesions occurs 12 to 72 hours after cold exposure. Exposure of the face to subfreezing temperatures results in symmetric involvement of the cheeks, whereas local exposure to ice (e.g., a popsicle) will result in unilateral cheek involvement.

Pediatric Patient Differential Diagnosis

- Henoch-Schönlein purpura—generally not tender
- Child abuse
- Subcutaneous granuloma annulare
- Nodular vasculitis
- Metastatic neuroblastomas

?? Differential Diagnosis and Pitfalls

- Trauma
- Superficial migratory thrombophlebitis

✓ Best Tests

- Most cases of EN can be diagnosed clinically. When in doubt, a punch skin biopsy (deep enough to include the subcutaneous fat) will confirm the diagnosis.

- In patients with recurrent EN, a secondary cause should be suspected. A basic procedure including careful medical history taking, a physical examination for peripheral synovitis, two consecutive ASO determinations, a tuberculin skin test, and chest radiography may be sufficient to diagnose secondary EN.

Pediatric Patient Considerations

- As in adults, most cases of panniculitis are diagnosed clinically, but when in doubt, a punch skin biopsy (deep enough to include the subcutaneous fat) will confirm a diagnosis. In infants with subcutaneous fat necrosis, fine needle aspiration and magnetic resonance imaging have been reported to aid in the diagnosis.
- If EN is suspected, throat culture, ASO titer, or EBV titer may help identify the underlying etiology.

▲▲ Management Pearls

- In patients with EN, spontaneous resolution occurs in most cases. Bed rest and limb elevation are important alleviating measures. Anti-inflammatory medications are often useful therapies for pain. Vigorous exercise or other physical activities should be avoided, as they may lengthen recovery time.
- Care must be taken to identify and treat any underlying causes of the condition in order to prevent relapse.

Pediatric Patient Considerations

- EN, subcutaneous fat necrosis of the newborn, and cold panniculitis are all self-limiting conditions in which spontaneous resolution occurs. No specific therapies are required. As in adults, limiting physical activities may hasten resolution.
- In the case of subcutaneous fat necrosis of the newborn, periodic serial serum calcium levels should be followed for the first 3 to 4 months of life, as hypercalcemia may appear weeks to months after the appearance and resolution of the skin lesions.

Therapy

- Nonsteroidal anti-inflammatory agents may be helpful in controlling pain and discomfort associated with EN: aspirin 325 to 650 mg p.o. every 4 to 6 hours, ibuprofen 400 to 800 mg p.o. every 6 to 8 hours, naproxen 275 mg p.o. every 6 to 8 hours, or indomethacin ER 25 to 50 mg p.o. three times daily.
- Colchicine (0.6 mg twice daily) has been successful in the treatment of acute lesions. Applying potent topical corticosteroids (classes 1 and 2) with plastic cling wrap occlusion at night may help to reduce inflammation. Intralesional corticosteroids have also been of some benefit in recalcitrant lesions. Systemic corticosteroids have been used on rare occasion but are contraindicated unless infectious etiologies are ruled out.
- In refractory situations, potassium iodide (400 to 900 mg/d) has been successful (but is contraindicated in pregnancy) as has hydroxychloroquine (200 mg twice daily). Isolated case reports have touted the success of the following treatments: dapsone, erythromycin, infliximab, and mycophenolate mofetil.

Suggested Readings

García-Porrúa C, González-Gay MA, Vázquez-Caruncho M, et al. Erythema nodosum: Etiologic and predictive factors in a defined population. *Arthritis Rheum.* 2000;43(3):584–592.

Gonzalez-Gay MA, Garcia-Porrua C, Pujol RM, et al. Erythema nodosum: A clinical approach. *Clin Exp Rheumatol.* 2001;19(4):365–368. PubMed ID: 11491490.

James WD, Berger TG, Elston DM, eds. *Andrews' Diseases of the Skin: Clinical Dermatology.* 10th Ed. Philadelphia, PA: Saunders Elsevier; 2006: 487–492.

Mahe E, Girszyn N, Hadj-Rabia S, et al. Subcutaneous fat necrosis of the newborn: A systematic evaluation of risk factors, clinical manifestations, complications and outcome of 16 children. *Br J Dermatol.* 2007;156(4):709–715. PubMed ID: 17493069.

Mana J, Marcoval J. Erythema nodosum. *Clin Dermatol.* 2007;25(3): 288–294. PubMed ID: 17560306.

Requena L, Yus ES, Kutzner H. Panniculitis. In: Fitzpatrick TB, Wolff K, eds. *Fitzpatrick's Dermatology in General Medicine.* 7th Ed. New York, NY: McGraw-Hill; 2008:569–585.

Gout

Stephanie Diamantis

Diagnosis Synopsis

Gout is the systemic deposition of monosodium urate crystals in tissues due to hyperuricemia. Elevated uric acid levels can be caused by overproduction of uric acid from purine catabolism or insufficient excretion by the kidneys. The deposition of urate crystals in tissues leads to inflammation and subsequent tissue damage. Men aged 40 to 50 are most commonly affected and may have a family history of gout. Other risk factors include renal insufficiency, hypertension, obesity, increased alcohol consumption, medications (e.g., diuretics), lymphomas, leukemias, tumor lysis syndrome, and hemolysis. African Americans are reported as being at higher risk for gout, but the association is weakened when the increased incidence of hypertension in this population is taken into account.

The most common sites involved are the skin and joints. Gout can present in an acute and chronic form: acute gouty arthritis or chronic tophaceous gout, respectively. The acute form presents as a painful, swollen, warm, tender, and erythematous joint. Most common joints include the great toe, ankle, wrist, and knee. The majority of attacks involve one joint. Chronic tophaceous gout presents most commonly on the joints or helix of the ear. Smooth or multilobulated nodules can ulcerate, leading to extrusion of a chalklike substance.

Complications include joint destruction and nephropathy.

Look For

Acute gout often presents with a single joint that is hot, red, tender, and occasionally edematous. The most commonly affected joints are the great toe, ankle, wrist, and knee.

Chronic tophaceous gout can occur years after the initial gouty attack. The nodules of gout vary in size and are yellow or cream in color (Fig. 4-522). It is common to have nodules that break down, heal, and then develop again. These deposits are mostly found overlying joints, tendons, or cartilage: for example, the rims of the ears (helix and antihelix), the distal toe and finger joints, the Achilles tendon, or the olecranon or prepatellar bursae.

Diagnostic Pearls

There is a male preponderance of the disease. Tophi in women are rare but do occur. The most common site of a first attack of acute gout is the great toe (podagra).

?? Differential Diagnosis and Pitfalls

Acute Gouty Arthritis

- Pseudogout (chondrocalcinosis)
- Septic arthritis
- Psoriatic arthritis
- Reactive arthritis
- Osteoarthritis
- Cellulitis
- Chondrodermatitis nodularis helicis (can often get a history of pressure in the area affected)
- Acute paronychia
- Osteomyelitis
- Rheumatoid nodule

Chronic Tophaceous Gout

- Rheumatoid nodules
- Calcinosis cutis
- Tendinous xanthomas
- Chondrodermatitis nodularis helicis
- Squamous cell carcinoma

✓ Best Tests

Gout

- Biopsy or aspirate with polarizing microscopy—Finding the characteristic needle-shaped negatively birefringent crystals of monosodium urate in the joint fluid confirms the diagnosis.
- Biopsy for histopathologic analysis—Gouty deposits have a characteristic amorphous appearance in the subcutaneous tissue.
- Plain radiographs of the affected joint(s)
- Elevated serum uric acid level—Note that this test is not particularly sensitive or specific for diagnosis of gout.

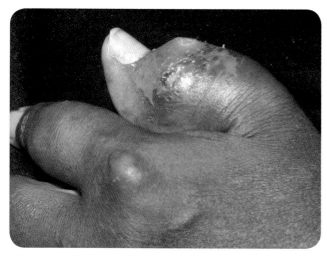

Figure 4-522 Gouty tophi and arthritis.

- White blood cell count (in joint fluid and blood) and erythrocyte sedimentation rate are usually elevated during acute attacks.

▲▲ Management Pearls

- Patients with gout should avoid foods high in purines, such as anchovies, organ meats, asparagus, oatmeal, cocoa, mushrooms, and spinach. Alcohol consumption should be limited to two drinks per day.
- As there are many causes of mild elevations in the serum uric acid, biopsy of presumptive lesions is necessary to avoid missing an infiltrative disease or a malignancy.

Therapy

Acute
- Rest and elevate affected joint, if possible.
- Nonsteroidal anti-inflammatory drugs (NSAIDs)—Ibuprofen (preferred) 800 mg p.o. three times daily for 5 days, indomethacin 50 mg p.o. four times daily for 5 days, or another NSAID at maximum dose. Doses must be lowered in cases of renal insufficiency, and NSAIDs are contraindicated in patients with known peptic ulcer disease.
- Colchicine—0.6 to 1.2 mg p.o. initial dose, then 0.6 mg p.o. every 1 to 2 hours until attack improves or gastrointestinal symptoms develop. Maximum total dose equals 4 to 6 mg.
- Steroids—Reserve for patients in whom NSAIDs or colchicine may be contraindicated or ineffective. Triamcinolone acetonide 60 mg IM or prednisone 20 to 40 mg p.o./IM daily.
- Intra-articular steroids, such as triamcinolone hexacetonide, may be used to treat a single inflamed joint.

Chronic
The main indication for long-term prophylactic treatment is recurrent attacks (i.e., three or more per year). Goal serum urate ≤6 mg/dL.

- Colchicine—0.6 to 1.2 mg p.o. daily for 1 to 2 weeks prior to initiating hypouricemic therapy; continue for several months after hypouricemic therapy has begun. Some patients will require long-term colchicine in addition to hypouricemics.
- Allopurinol—For overproducers of uric acid, 300 to 900 mg p.o. daily.
- Probenecid—For persons with decreased excretion of uric acid, 0.5 to 1 g p.o. twice daily.
- A 24-hour urine collection is often useful in determining which hypouricemic agent is indicated.

Rarely, surgical intervention is required secondary to joint destruction.

Suggested Readings

Haverstock CL, Jorizzo JL. Rheumatoid arthritis, rheumatic fever and gout. In: Wolff K, Goldsmith LA, Katz SI, et al., eds. *Fitzpatrick's Dermatology in General Medicine*. 7th Ed. New York, NY: McGraw Hill; 2008:1575–1577.

Hochberg MC, Thomas J, Thomas DJ, et al. Racial differences in the incidence of gout. The role of hypertension. *Arthritis Rheum*. 1995;38(5):628–632.

Kim KY, Ralph Schumacher H, Hunsche E, et al. A literature review of the epidemiology and treatment of acute gout. *Clin Ther*. 2003;25(6):1593–1617.

Sutaria S, Katbamna R, Underwood M. Effectiveness of intervention for the treatment of acute and prevention of recurrent gout—a systematic review. *Rheumatology*. 2006;10:1093.

Tourat DM, Sau P. Cutaneous deposition diseases, part II. *J Am Acad Dermatol*. 1998;39(4):527–544.

Hidradenitis Suppurativa

Laurie Good

■■ Diagnosis Synopsis

Hidradenitis suppurativa (HS), or acne inversa, is a destructive, chronic, relapsing, painful, inflammatory disorder of the terminal follicular epithelium in apocrine gland-bearing regions of the body. Previously, this disease was thought to be due to bacterial infection, but it has now become clear that it is a noninfectious acneiform disease. It is believed that follicular occlusion leads to trapping of follicular contents, rupture, and inflammation of the dermis, with bacterial superinfection in some cases. HS is most common in young women, and associations between HS and cigarette smoking, as well as obesity, have been found. A familial form of the disease has been supported by studies, including a molecular genetic study of four generations affected by HS in a large Chinese family, through which a novel HS locus on chromosome 1p21.1–1q25.3 was identified. With a prevalence of up to 1% in some population-based studies, HS is a commonly encountered disease.

The nodules of HS are seen most commonly on the buttocks, breasts, and in the groin and axillae. Onset occurs after puberty, and mechanical (shaving) or chemical (deodorant) irritation can exacerbate the condition. In patients with chronic HS, squamous cell carcinoma, anemia, and interstitial keratitis may develop.

Interestingly, HS shares a common etiology (severe inflammation, occlusion of the follicle, and scarring) and clinical features with dissecting cellulitis of the scalp and acne conglobata; often more than one of these conditions occur in the same patient. Dissecting cellulitis predominantly affects African American men in their second to third decades, is characterized by scalp pustules, nodules, and abscesses with coalescing, draining sinuses, and results in scarring alopecia. Acne conglobata is a cystic, nodular, abscess-forming acne on the chest, back, shoulders, arms, buttocks, and face that often renders keloidal scars and does so more readily in patients with darker skin types. Collectively, HS, dissecting cellulitis, and acne conglobata are referred to as the follicular occlusion triad. A pilonidal cyst is another condition of follicular occlusion found in some patients with HS, leading some physicians to recognize a follicular occlusion tetrad.

While rare, several syndromes have also been associated with HS, a few of which are more severe or occur with a higher prevalence in African American or Afro-Caribbean patients. SAPHO (synovitis, acne, pustulosis, hyperostosis, osteitis) syndrome is most severe in African American patients with HS. Analogous to SAPHO syndrome is a seronegative arthritis occurring in conjunction with the follicular occlusion triad. Additionally, spondyloarthropathy in association with HS and acne conglobata (plus or minus dissecting cellulitis) most commonly affects African American or Afro-Caribbean men in their 30s and 40s. Skin manifestations can occur just prior to arthritis, or precede it by more than 20 years. Crohn disease has also been demonstrated to have an association with HS, as has a complex known as PAPA (pyogenic arthritis, pyoderma gangrenosum, and acne).

Pediatric Patient Considerations

Most patients affected by HS do not experience symptoms until after puberty.

◉ Look For

Firm, tender, red to dark brown nodules, cysts, and sometimes large sinuses under the surface of the skin (Figs. 4-523–4-526). These sinuses can drain pus, which is often malodorous, resulting in social isolation and/or depression. Lesions are seen mostly on the groin, axillae, buttocks, and inframammary area. Axillae involvement is more common in women, and anogenital involvement is more common in men. Rarely, lymphatic fibrosis can result, causing

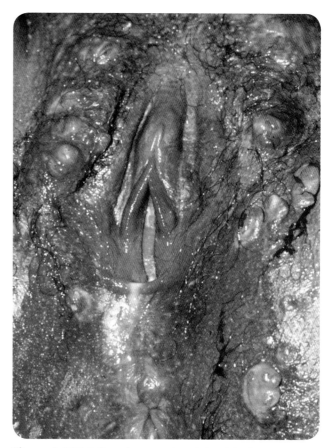

Figure 4-523 Inflamed cysts and eroded nodules in HS involving the vulva.

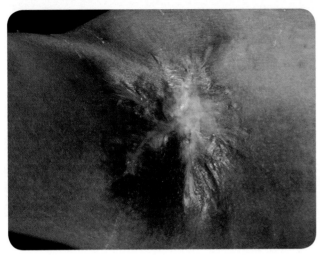

Figure 4-524 Fibrotic hypopigmented and hyperpigmented lesion of HS of the axilla.

scrotal or penile lymphedema. Premenstrual flares are not uncommon. The disease is rarely seen on the chest, scalp, or lower extremities. Perianal sinuses can involve the rectum and anus. Vaginal and urethral fistulas can develop.

Pediatric Patient Considerations

The double comedone has been noted on flexural surfaces of children, and some believe it is a precursor lesion in those who will progress to HS after puberty.

Diagnostic Pearls

- Double comedones on a single lesion (similar to the acne conglobata complex) are very suggestive of this diagnosis.
- Only half of bacterial cultures will demonstrate pathogens.
- Involvement of the axillae is more common in women, and involvement of the anogenital region is more common in men. It is most common in young women, and premenstrual flares are not uncommon.

?? Differential Diagnosis and Pitfalls

- Epidermoid cysts
- Bartholin cyst infection
- Crohn disease (cutaneous perianal disease)
- Granuloma inguinale
- Ulcerative colitis
- Tuberculosis
- Tularemia
- Scrofuloderma
- Actinomycosis
- Lymphogranuloma venereum

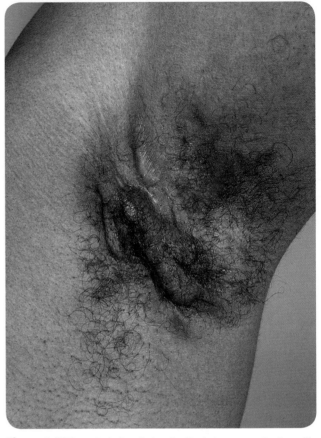

Figure 4-525 Typical chronic longitudinal sinus tracts in the axilla in HS.

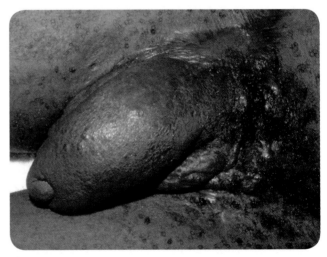

Figure 4-526 Sinuses, cysts, and penile edema in HS of the groin.

- Furuncles
- Carbuncles
- Dermoid cyst

HS can be distinguished from other entities on its differential diagnosis through the age of onset (shortly after puberty), the characteristic lesion distribution, lack of systemic symptoms, relapsing nature, unresponsiveness to antibiotics, and failure to isolate a single bacterial species (often HS cultures yield numerous species) on culture and stain.

Pediatric Patient Considerations

Special consideration should be given to patients under 11 who develop HS, as this is very rare and could indicate congenital adrenal hyperplasia or precocious puberty. Cases of HS in childhood do occur, however, in the absence of endocrine abnormalities or obesity.

✓ Best Tests

- The diagnosis is usually made on clinical grounds without a need for biopsy.
- Gram stain, culture, and sensitivity can be performed on any pus/exudate, as superinfection may occur. Additionally, histologic studies can rule out other entities on the differential diagnosis of HS, as results will be nonspecific in HS.
- When in doubt, skin biopsy may aid in making the diagnosis.

▲▲ Management Pearls

- Advise patients that treatment can be difficult, but, with limited disease, conservative measures can be effective.
- Surgical excision is often the ideal treatment for extensive, recurrent disease. Very wide unroofing and debridement of individual sinus tracts, allowing for healing by secondary intention, is best. Incision and drainage may offer temporary relief from individual lesions but are generally avoided because cysts will simply re-form. When severe, refer to a dermatologist or surgeon who has special training in treating this disease.
- Patients should be counseled on the risk of hypertrophic and keloidal scar formation after surgical intervention for HS. Keloids are more likely to develop in patients with darker skin types. If this should occur, intrakeloidal corticosteroid injections can be used, but efficacy is debatable and patient-specific.
- Instruct patients to avoid tight-fitting clothing and excessive friction to the involved areas. Encourage weight loss in the obese and smoking cessation in cigarette smokers.
- Squamous cell carcinoma may develop in scars after many years, and occurs almost exclusively on the buttocks of HS-affected men. Because of the deep-seated nature of the cancer's origin, diagnosis may be delayed, carrying a poor prognosis.
- Because of the severity of the disease and the foul odor of the drainage, social isolation and/or depression is commonly seen. Attention should be given to pain management and social factors.

Therapy

First-line treatments are antibiotics and surgery:

- Consider oral tetracycline (500 mg twice daily) or minocycline (100 mg twice daily) or doxycycline (100 mg twice daily) for months.
- Topical clindamycin 2% solution applied twice daily to affected areas may help with early lesions or between flares.
- Surgical techniques include the excision of affected tissues and exteriorization of sinus tracts. Simple incision and drainage of large cysts may be performed with the recognition that the rate of recurrence is extremely high. Additionally, it should be considered that keloids are more likely to develop in patients with more deeply pigmented skin types. If this should occur, intrakeloidal corticosteroid injections can be used, but efficacy is debatable and patient-specific.

- Second-line therapies include intralesional triamcinolone to active cysts and nodules (triamcinolone 3 to 10 mg/mL), as well as hormonal therapy (in women only) with either cyproterone acetate alone or in combination with ethinylestradiol, though efficacy has not been consistently demonstrated. The antiandrogenic effect is likely behind any observed efficacy, and as such, oral contraceptives may be beneficial in women as well. Finasteride (5 mg/d for 3 months) may be useful in patients of both sexes.
- Isotretinoin 1 mg/kg daily has been beneficial in some patients as has acitretin 25 mg twice daily. Systemic anti-inflammatory agents such as corticosteroids and cyclosporine are occasionally used to palliate symptoms. Dapsone at daily doses from 25 to 150 mg has been proven effective in a small series of patients. Biologic agents such as the anti-TNF drugs infliximab and etanercept have shown great promise in recent small studies.
- Other techniques with some reported success include carbon dioxide laser ablation and liposuction.

- Suggested empiric antibiotics for the treatment of superinfections include oral clindamycin (300 mg twice daily) or dicloxacillin (500 mg three times daily). Metronidazole is commonly used to treat anaerobic superinfections, but there is little evidence base to support this.
- Attention to psychosocial ramifications of this disease is crucial. Depression is not uncommon, and patient suffering likely exceeds that of most common chronic skin diseases.

Pediatric Patient Considerations

Botulinum A toxin has reportedly been used with success in a prepubescent girl with severe HS. Other cases have had success with surgical management.

Suggested Readings

Alikhan A, Lynch PJ, Eisen DB. Hidradenitis suppurativa: A comprehensive review. *J Am Acad Dermatol.* 2009;60:539–561.

Bhalla R, Sequeira W. Arthritis associated with hidradenitis suppurativa. *Ann Rheum Dis.* 1994;53:64–66.

Feito-Rodriguez M, Sendagorta-Cudos E, Herranz-Pinto P, et al. Prepubertal hidradenitis suppurativa successfully treated with botulinum toxin A. *Dermatol Surg.* 2009;35:1300–1302.

Gao M, Wang PG, Cui Y, et al. Inversa acne (hidradenitis suppurativa): A case report and identification of the locus at chromosome 1p21.1–1q25.3. *J Invest Dermatol.* 2006;126(6):1302–1306.

Leybishkis B, Fasseas P, Ryan KF, et al. Hidradenitis suppurativa and acne conglobata associated with spondyloarthropathy. *Am J Med Sci.* 2001;321(3):195–197.

Mengesha YM, Holcombe TC, Hansen RC. Prepubertal hidradenitis suppurativa: Two case reports and review of the literature. *Pediatr Dermatol.* 1999;16(4):292–296.

Revuz J. Hidradenitis suppurativa. *J Eur Academic Dermatol Venereol.* 2009;23(9):985–998.

Scheinfeld NS. A case of dissecting cellulitis and a review of the literature. *Dermatol Online J.* 2003;9(1):8.

Steinhoff JP, Cilursu A, Falasca GF, et al. A study of musculoskeletal manifestations in 12 patients with SAPHO syndrome. *J Clin Rheumatol.* 2002;8(1):13–22.

Thein M, Hogarth MB, Acland K. Seronegative arthritis associated with the follicular occlusion triad. *Clin Exp Dermatol.* 2004;29:545–562.

Cutaneous T-Cell Lymphomas

Rodolfo E. Chirinos

Lymphocytic infiltrates are common in many skin diseases. Some of the diseases may be preneoplastic or frankly neoplastic. In this chapter, the discussion is concentrated on mycosis fungoides (MF) and its potential precursors, including large plaque parapsoriasis. For discussions on related conditions such as lymphomatoid papulosis, pseudolymphoma and pityriasis lichenoides chronica, see VisualDx online. (If you are a first-time online user, go to www.essentialdermatology.com/pigmented; if you already have your password set up, go directly to www.visualdx.com/visualdx.)

Diagnosis Synopsis

Cutaneous T-Cell Lymphomas

Primary cutaneous lymphomas are the second most common form of extranodal non-Hodgkin lymphoma and can be divided into T-cell and B-cell lymphomas that involve the skin and various extracutaneous sites. Cutaneous T-cell lymphomas (CTCLs) account for at least 80% of these lymphomas, with MF being the most common variant.

Mycosis Fungoides

Mycosis fungoides along with its clinical variants comprises the majority of all CTCL cases and will be discussed in this review.

MF is the most common type of CTCL and accounts for nearly half of all cases. MF is approximately twice as common in men as in women, and gender differences in incidence increase with age. African Americans have twice the incidence of whites, though this difference decreases with age. MF is mostly seen in older adults (median age at presentation is 50 to 55 years), although any age group may be affected. Onset of disease may occur at an earlier age (before age 40) in African American and Hispanic women. Children and adolescents are hardly ever affected. Although the clinical course of MF is usually indolent, with slow progression over years to decades, African American patients, especially women with early-onset disease, have a worse prognosis than other groups

The diagnosis of MF in its patch or early plaque phase may be difficult to make because pathologic findings may be subtle. Multiple biopsies may be required to confirm the clinical suspicion, and in most cases, the definitive diagnosis must be established by clinicopathologic correlation. Although the etiology remains unclear, the most commonly postulated hypothesis is that CTCL represents a model of chronic antigen stimulation. Extracutaneous involvement correlates with generalized lesions and lymphadenopathy and erythroderma.

A hypopigmented variant of MF is seen primarily in people of African descent but has been reported in those of Asian, Indian, and Latin American descent also.

Sézary Syndrome

Sézary syndrome (SS) is the leukemic and advanced stage of CTCL, characterized by infiltrative or exfoliative erythroderma, generalized lymphadenopathy, and neoplastic Sézary cells (i.e., lymphocytes with hyperconvoluted cerebriform nuclei) in the skin and/or peripheral blood. Associated features include severe pruritus, lichenification, palmoplantar hyperkeratosis, ectropion, nail dystrophy, and hepatosplenomegaly. Flow cytometric immunophenotyping analyses of peripheral blood demonstrating a CD4:CD8 ratio of ≥10, an absolute count of ≥1,000 Sézary cells/μL, and evidence of T-cell clonality are diagnostic criteria.

Large Plaque Parapsoriasis

Large plaque parapsoriasis (parapsoriasis en plaque) is a cutaneous T-cell lymphoproliferative disorder and often a preliminary stage of CTCL. It is a chronic inflammatory eruption seen most often in middle-aged and elderly patients. It may be slightly more common in men. Parapsoriasis is so named for its appearance: the scaly patches and plaques may resemble psoriasis. Although the disease is quite indolent, it may progress to CTCL after a number of years, and therefore treatment is warranted.

There continues to be debate over the definition of parapsoriasis. A small plaque variant also exists, and some clinicians consider pityriasis lichenoides chronica and pityriasis lichenoides et varioliformis acuta (PLEVA) to be a part of the same disease spectrum. Small plaque parapsoriasis, rarely if ever, progresses to MF or CTCL. To add to the confusion, sometimes both large and small plaque variants of parapsoriasis are referred to as parapsoriasis en plaque.

Look For

Cutaneous T-Cell Lymphomas

In darker skin tones, look for brownish-red plaques with sharply marginated borders and minimal to moderate scale (Figs. 4-527–4-532). CTCL can present as a limited disease with patches or thin plaques or can be severe with cutaneous nodules and ulcerating tumors. The latter is usually more accelerated and has a poor prognosis. Many African Americans have a long history of generalized eczematoid or psoriasiform dermatitis before being diagnosed with CTCL. An uncommon hypopigmented variant of CTCL that occurs almost exclusively in African American or Asian patients

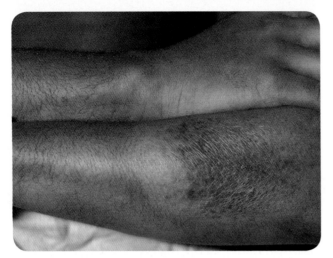

Figure 4-527 MF with poorly delimited hyperpigmented plaques on arms.

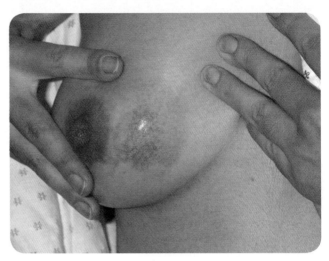

Figure 4-528 Mottled erythematous plaque of MF.

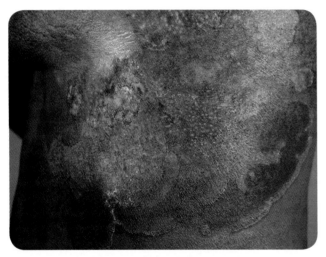

Figure 4-529 Scaling and eroded plaques of MF.

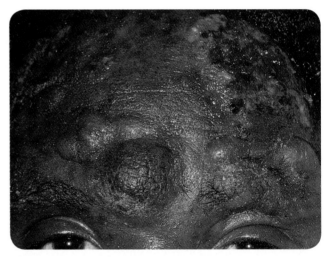

Figure 4-530 MF with hyperpigmented nodules and ulcerations.

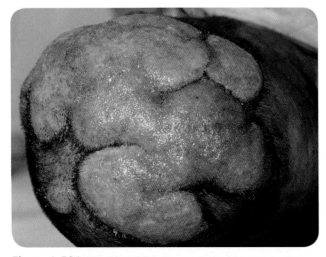

Figure 4-531 MF with multiple large scalp nodules.

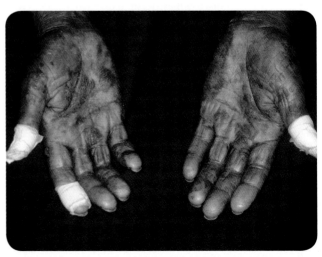

Figure 4-532 MF with hyperpigmented palmar plaques.

and has an earlier age of onset including children presents with ill-defined hypopigmented macules and patches with variable scale.

Mycosis Fungoides

- Persistent and/or progressive erythematous patches and plaques with fine scale and variation in shape and size (usually from 5 to 20 cm) that anatomically favor the buttocks and sun-protected areas of the trunk and limbs (i.e., flanks, breasts, inner arms/thighs, and periaxillary areas)
- Associated features include pruritus, poikiloderma (i.e., mottled pigmentation, telangiectases, and epidermal atrophy resembling cigarette paper wrinkling), and ulceration.
- Lesions of tumor stage disease are typically violaceous, exophytic, mushroom-shaped tumors that predominantly affect the face and body folds. Lesions often undergo ulceration or necrosis and secondary infection. Interestingly, pruritus may decrease in intensity.

Sézary Syndrome

- Erythroderma and generalized lymphadenopathy
- Associated features include extreme pruritus, lichenification, palmoplantar hyperkeratosis, ectropion, and nail dystrophy.
- Often, alternating bands of pigment and erythema and uninvolved skin around flexural areas known as the "deck chair sign" or "folded luggage" sign
- Infiltrative plaques occurring on the face may result in exaggeration of normal skin folds known as a lionlike face or leonine facies.

Large Plaque Parapsoriasis

Large (5 to 10 cm) brown-red oval, round, or irregularly shaped plaques with minimal scale (Fig. 4-533). Plaques may have a cigarette paper-like wrinkling that corresponds

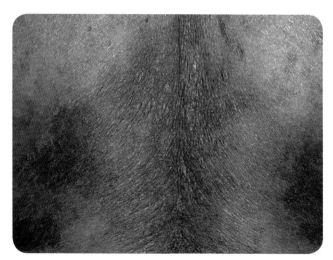

Figure 4-533 Large plaques of parapsoriasis may be an early stage of, or may evolve into, MF.

to epidermal atrophy. Lesions are most frequently seen on the buttocks, lower extremities, and trunk.

 Diagnostic Pearls

Cutaneous T-Cell Lymphomas

Lesions may be less prominent on sun-exposed areas (e.g., extensor arms) than on sun-protected areas (e.g., flexor forearm, beneath the breasts). Early disease may appear as chronic red, scaling patches on the buttocks. Such lesions may have nondiagnostic histopathology and respond to sunlight, artificial UV irradiation, or topical corticosteroids.

Diagnosis

- The most important thing is to differentiate CTCL from benign conditions. This requires a strategy that incorporates clinical, histological, and immunophenotyping findings.
- Ideal biopsy: 4- to 8-mm punch biopsy in previously untreated skin that is representative of the cutaneous lesions. Alternatively, an excisional biopsy can be performed.
- Because the conversion from premalignant to malignant phase often runs an indolent course, repeated biopsies may be necessary.
- Immunophenotyping utilizes fluorescently tagged antibodies that recognize cell surface markers. For example, CD4 or CD8 surface expression in neoplastic T cells assists in making the diagnosis.
- Molecular studies for T-cell receptor (TCR) gene rearrangements: This should be used in conjunction with the overlying clinical, histological, and immunophenotyping landscape. Note that clonal T cells can be found in benign inflammatory conditions such as lichen sclerosus et atrophicus, lichen planus, and PLEVA, and hence identification of a TCR clone supports but never exclusively confirms a diagnosis of CTCL.
- Assessment of peripheral blood for Sézary cells (in cases where skin is not diagnostic, especially T4) including Sézary cell prep, flow, cytometry and PCR for TCR gene rearrangement.

Classification

- Once a clinical-histological diagnosis is made, the type of T-cell lymphoma should be determined, because varying CTCLs carry different prognoses and treatment strategies.
- Refer to WHO-EORTC Classification.

Staging

- Complete skin examination for assessment of percent body surface area and type of skin lesion (patch/plaque, tumor, erythroderma).
- Palpation of peripheral lymph node regions as well as for organomegaly or masses

489

- CBC with differential and Sézary screen (i.e., Sézary cell prep), complete metabolic panel, serum LDH, and peripheral blood analyses for immunophenotyping and TCR gene rearrangement studies
- Imaging studies include a chest X-ray for IA or limited IB stage of disease (refer to VisualDx online for staging guidelines). CT of the neck/chest/abdomen/pelvis with contrast or integrated whole body PET/CT should be considered for advanced IB or higher stage of disease, large cell transformation or folliculotropic MF, lymphadenopathy, or abnormal lab studies.
- Biopsy of suspicious lymph nodes or suspected extracutaneous sites
- A bone marrow biopsy is not required for staging but is used to document visceral disease in those suspected to have marrow involvement and patients with unexplained hematologic abnormalities.

Large Plaque Parapsoriasis

Clinically, the presence of dilated blood vessels and atrophy suggests CTCL. The lesions of large plaque parapsoriasis frequently have a "bathing suit" distribution. Lesions with atrophy are seen in dermatomyositis, making it important to look for muscle weakness.

?? Differential Diagnosis and Pitfalls

Cutaneous T-Cell Lymphomas

- Psoriasis—Look for erythematous silver-scaled plaques, nail oil-drop changes, and nail pitting. A family history of psoriasis is often noted. CTCL and psoriasis are histologically different, and a biopsy will aid in the diagnosis.
- Atopic dermatitis—Patients are often aware of their atopic history, which commonly starts in childhood. Look for lichenified plaques on the flexural surfaces and neck.
- Superficial fungal infections (e.g., tinea corporis)—Look for erythematous annular plaques that have a raised leading scale at the border. Central clearing is more common in tinea corporis. Perform a fungal KOH of scales from skin scraping.
- Drug eruption—Drug eruptions often present with urticarial, exanthematous, or vesicular/bullous lesions. Systemic symptoms include fever, lymphadenopathy, and facial edema. Eosinophilia on CBC and histology are often seen but not a consistent finding. Look for nonsteroidal anti-inflammatory drugs (NSAIDs), sulfonamides, and penicillin in medication history.
- Seborrheic dermatitis—Look for a chronic history of erythema and/or greasy scales on the glabella, melolabial folds, and/or retroauricular areas.
- Chronic contact dermatitis—Look for pink, red, or violaceous plaques with or without vesicles.

- Pityriasis lichenoides chronica (Fig. 4-534)—may have scaling and hypopigmented plaques. Biopsy will be necessary.
- Cutaneous lymphoma and pseudolymphoma (Fig. 4-535)—Papules and plaques may resemble nodules of MF. Pseudolymphomas are often drug induced, and a thorough drug history should be obtained. Refer to VisualDx online for a list of the drugs that can cause pseudolymphoma.
- Pityriasis rubra pilaris (PRP)—Look for orange-red, waxy-like palmoplantar hyperkeratosis. Islands of sparing (i.e., normal skin within larger plaques) are characteristically seen in PRP. CTCL and PRP are histologically different, and a biopsy will aid in the diagnosis.
- PLEVA—Look for papules and nodules in various stages of healing. Central necrosis can be noted in some papules, like lymphomatoid papulosis.
- Lymphomatoid papulosis—papulonecrotic lesions that are usually discrete and have minimal scale

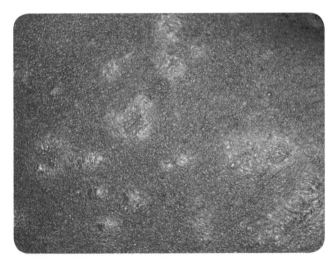

Figure 4-534 Scaling and hypopigmented lesions of pityriasis lichenoides chronica.

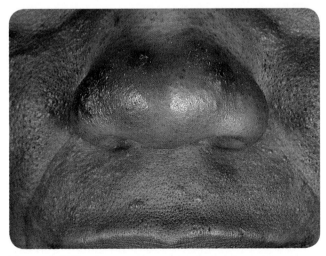

Figure 4-535 Infiltrated papules and plaques of pseudolymphoma.

- Vasculitis—purpuric or hemorrhagic papules and plaques. Check for RF, ANA, anti-DS-DNA, ANCA, cryoglobulins, complement (C3, C4) levels.
- Varicella—prodrome of mild fever, malaise, and myalgias followed by an eruption of pruritic erythematous macules and papules. Lesions rapidly evolve into pin-sized vesicles with clear serous vesicles surrounded by narrow red halos. Lesions are seen in all stages of development. Varicella does not recur.
- Secondary syphilis—generalized scaling papules and plaques. Lesions can involve the palms and soles. Obtain an RPR and determine if history of chancre exists.
- Dermatitis herpetiformis—Look for pruritic papules and plaques over the extensor surfaces and/or retroauricular areas. Direct immunofluorescence will show granular IgA deposition within the dermal papillae.
- Disseminated HSV—often begins with a prodrome of intense pain and more often than not is associated with pruritus or hyperesthesia. Look for a painful eruption of vesicles on an erythematous base in immunocompromised patients. Obtain a viral culture and direct fluorescent antibody, ideally from the underside of an intact vesicle or from a ruptured vesicle.
- Pityriasis rosea—Inquire into recollection of a herald patch. Look for scaly papules and/or plaques on the trunk. Crusts and vesicles/bullae are not a common finding.
- Lichen planus—Look for very pruritic, flat-topped violaceous papules with fine scale. Disease is associated with hepatitis C infection.
- Erythroderma of other causes
- Cutaneous B-cell lymphomas
- Paget disease
- Pagetoid melanoma
- Lepromatous leprosy
- Sarcoidosis
- Leishmaniasis
- Chronic actinic reticuloid
- Dermatomyositis
- Lichen simplex chronicus
- Prurigo nodularis
- Erythema chronicum migrans
- Nummular eczema

Hypopigmented Variant of Mycosis Fungoides

- Vitiligo
- Pityriasis alba
- Tinea versicolor
- Sarcoidosis
- Postinflammatory hypopigmentation
- Progressive macular hypomelanosis
- Leprosy

Pitfalls

Previous treatment with phototherapy, topical corticosteroids, and immunosuppressants can profoundly change the histology of the lesion; however, early CTCL, like many of the diseases in the differential diagnosis, will partially clear or completely clear with topical corticosteroids or phototherapy.

 ## Best Tests

Cutaneous T-Cell Lymphomas

- Skin biopsy for basic histology, immunophenotyping, and TCR gene rearrangement analysis.
- CBC with differential and Sézary screen (i.e., Sézary cell prep), complete metabolic panel, serum LDH, and peripheral blood analyses for immunophenotyping and TCR gene rearrangement studies.
- Consider obtaining HTLV-1/2 serology, as this virus can cause lesions that appear similar to MF.
- Patients with clinically abnormal lymph nodes (≥1.5 cm or firm, irregular, clustered or fixed) should have them biopsied and examined by the same methods as the skin specimen(s).

Large Plaque Parapsoriasis

- Skin biopsy will not show the classic changes of CTCL, but immunophenotyping analysis and T-cell gene rearrangement analysis may demonstrate a T-cell clone.
- Consider obtaining a CBC with differential. An increased lymphocyte count or the presence of Sézary cells suggests MF/CTCL.

 ## Management Pearls

The detailed management and therapy of all these conditions are discussed online and are usually done in conjunction with a dermatologist or hematologist/oncologist.

Therapy

See online discussion.

Suggested Readings

Akaraphanth R, Douglass MC, Lim HW. Hypopigmented mycosis fungoides: treatment and a 6 ½-year follow-up of 9 patients. *J Am Acad Dermatol.* 2000;42:33–39.

Drews R, Samel A, Kadin ME. Lymphomatoid papulosis and anaplastic large cell lymphomas of the skin. *Sem Cutan Med Surg.* 2000;19(2):109–117.

Droc C, Cualing HD, Kadin ME. Need for an improved molecular/genetic classification of CD30+ lymphomas involving the skin. *Cancer Control.* 2007;14(2):124–132.

Hinds GA, Heald P. Cutaneous T-cell lymphoma in skin of color. *J Am Acad Dermatol.* 2009;60(3):359–375.

Horwitz SM, et al. Review of the treatment of mycosis fungoides and Sézary syndrome: A stage-based approach. *J Natl Compr Canc Netw.* 2008;6(4):436–442.

Kazakov DV, et al. Clinicopathological spectrum of mycosis fungoides. *J Eur Acad Dermatol Venereol.* 2004;18(4):397–415.

Keehn CA, et al. The diagnosis, staging, and treatment options for mycosis fungoides. *Cancer Control.* 2007;14(2):102–111.

Kempf W. CD30+ lymphoproliferative disorders: Histopathology, differential diagnosis, new variants, and simulators. *J Cutan Pathol.* 2006;33(Suppl 1): 58–70.

Kim EJ, et al. Mycosis fungoides and Sézary syndrome: An update. *Curr Oncol Rep.* 2006;8(5):376–386.

LeBoit PE. Lymphomatoid papulosis and cutaneous CD30+ lymphoma. *Am J Dermatopathol.* 1996;18(3):221–235.

Olsen E, et al. Revisions to the staging and classification of mycosis fungoides and Sézary syndrome: A proposal of the international society for cutaneous lymphomas (ISCL) and the cutaneous lymphoma task force of the European organization of research and treatment of cancer (EORTC). *Blood.* 2007;110(6):1713–1722.

Pimpinelli N, et al. Defining early mycosis fungoides. *J Am Acad Dermatol.* 2005;53:1053–1063.

Siegel RS, et al. Primary cutaneous T-cell lymphoma: Review and current concepts. *J Clin Oncol.* 2000;18(10):2152–2168.

Morphea

Tess Nasabzadeh

▚ Diagnosis Synopsis

Morphea, also known as localized scleroderma, is a connective tissue disease characterized by skin thickening with increased collagen deposition. The disease is usually self-limited with spontaneous improvement in skin lesions after 3 to 5 years. Symptoms range from pruritus and skin tightness to functional impairment from contractures and psychological distress from cosmetic deformity.

Morphea is classified into five main subtypes: plaque morphea, generalized morphea, bullous morphea, linear scleroderma, and deep morphea. Linear scleroderma is the most common subtype in children, while plaque morphea is the most common subtype in adults.

The etiology of morphea is not fully understood. It is thought to be an autoimmune process, and recent studies suggest a role for chimerism. Transforming growth factor β, interleukin-4, and connective tissue growth factor are thought to be responsible for the excess fibroblast proliferation and matrix production. Inciting factors include mechanical trauma, vaccinations, insect bites, prior infection with *Borrelia* spp., irradiation, and local hypoxemia from chronic venous insufficiency. There have been a few reports of an association between morphea and chronic hepatitis C. This purported association may be especially relevant for the health care practitioner caring for those of ethnic skin, because hepatitis C disproportionately affects minority populations in the United States.

Morphea is a rare disease with a prevalence of about 3 cases per 100,000 people. Women are affected two to three times more frequently than men. While whites account for the majority of patients in some studies, it is unclear whether this represents a true ethnic difference or whether homogenous sample populations and the potential of dark skin to mask the initial inflammation of morphea contribute to these statistics. A retrospective study in Dallas, TX, where 20.9% of the population is African American, revealed that only 4.5% of those patients diagnosed with morphea were African American. Similar results were found in a study that reviewed the charts of 136 patients from a children's hospital dermatology department. Specifically, 82% of the morphea patients were white, 12% were Hispanic, 3% were African American, and 3% were Asian. The overall patient population of the dermatology department in this study was composed of 60% whites, 15% Hispanics, 12.5% African Americans, and 12.5% Asians.

While morphea has traditionally been approached as a disease confined to the skin, it is now known that a significant percentage of patients have extracutaneous disease or concomitant autoimmune disease. The fact that 20% of morphea patients have extracutaneous involvement supports the idea that morphea and systemic sclerosis reside on opposite sides of the spectrum of a single disease state. Dysphagia, articular involvement, and Raynaud phenomenon occur most commonly in the generalized subtype, whereas neurologic and ocular complications occur most commonly in the linear subtype. Concomitant autoimmune diseases in morphea patients include psoriasis, vitiligo, inflammatory bowel disease, diabetes, and thyroiditis. Numerous autoantibodies are found in morphea patients. While the prognostic significance is not always clear, antihistone antibodies may correlate with disease activity, and rheumatoid factor in the setting of adult generalized morphea may correlate with disease severity.

Pediatric Patient Considerations

When linear scleroderma occurs on the frontoparietal scalp or paramedian forehead it is referred to as *en coup de sabre*. Children with *en coup de sabre* may develop Parry-Romberg syndrome, also known as progressive facial hemiatrophy, with extension of the cutaneous lesion to the underlying bone, fascia, and muscle. Patients with *en coup de sabre* or Parry-Romberg syndrome may experience neurologic or ocular symptoms such as headaches, seizures, anterior uveitis, episcleritis, paralytic strabismus, and behavioral or intellectual deterioration.

◉ Look For

The classic morphea lesion is an oval, erythematous, and edematous plaque that extends peripherally to leave a central area of waxy or ivory induration surrounded by a lilac halo (Figs. 4-536 and 4-537). The lesions are asymmetric and exhibit decreased sweat production and hair loss. In dark skin, the initial erythema may be difficult to appreciate, and the halo may be hyperpigmented. Over time, the induration transitions to atrophy with persisting hypopigmentation or hyperpigmentation. Hypopigmentation can be especially distressing for patients with dark skin, since it may be quite noticeable. Morphea-related cutaneous pigment loss in Latin American patients has been described as ill-defined hypopigmented macules and complete depigmentation in sclerotic areas.

In nodular morphea, a subtype of plaque morphea more common in African Americans, red, flesh-colored, or hyperpigmented firm plaques or nodules are found on the chest, back, neck, and proximal extremities. Generalized morphea is characterized by four or more individual plaques larger than 3 cm that involve at least two of the following seven sites: head, neck, right upper extremity, left upper extremity, right lower extremity, and left lower extremity. In a case of generalized morphea in a Japanese patient, the

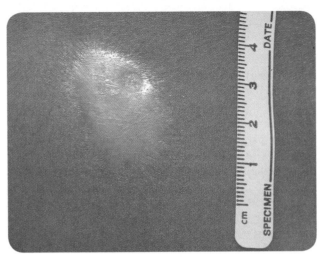

Figure 4-536 A well-demarcated plaque with ivory-white color characteristic of morphea.

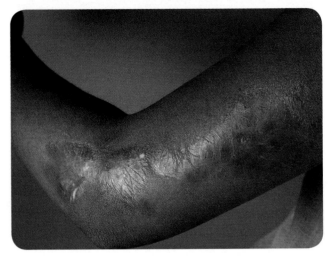

Figure 4-537 Linear atrophic plaque of morphea.

disease presented with dry plaques with a yellowish color. In bullous morphea, there are tense subepidermal bullae. Linear morphea may be located on the trunk, limbs, or head and is characterized by a linear streak of induration that may extend to the underlying muscle and bone. Deep morphea subtypes include morphea profunda and eosinophilic fasciitis. In morphea profunda, the skin feels thickened with inflamed and hyperpigmented plaques, and in eosinophilic fasciitis, extremity edema progresses to skin dimpling, induration, and tightening.

Pediatric Patient Considerations

In disabling pansclerotic morphea of children, a deep morphea variant, sclerotic plaques first appear on the extensor surfaces of the extremities and then spread to involve the entire skin with the exception of the fingertips and toes (Fig. 4-538).

Diagnostic Pearls

- Midforehead atrophy and sclerosis is a common form of localized morphea and is called "coup de sabre" after dueling scars which were common in the eighteenth century (Fig. 4-539).
- Chronic ulcers may be present in pansclerotic morphea. These ulcers have the potential to evolve into squamous cell carcinoma.
- Many patients with morphea have a family history of autoimmune disease. Ask about diseases such as rheumatoid arthritis, systemic lupus erythematosus, psoriasis, vitiligo, thyroiditis, and inflammatory bowel disease.

Pediatric Patient Considerations

It can take over 1 year for a child with morphea to be correctly diagnosed. Consider morphea in any child with circumscribed skin thickening and color change.

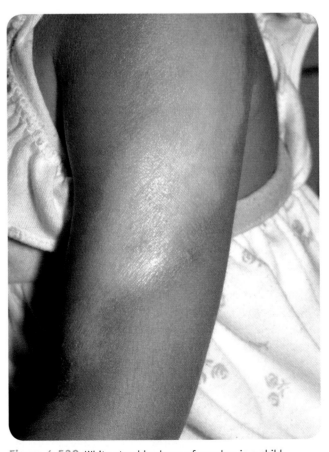

Figure 4-538 White atrophic plaque of morphea in a child.

494

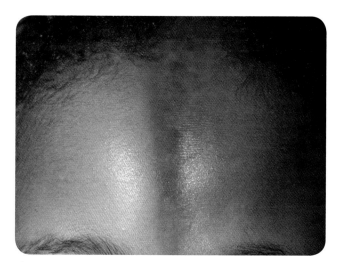

Figure 4-539 Midforehead atrophy and sclerosis and unilateral hyperpigmentation.

?? Differential Diagnosis and Pitfalls

- Acrodermatitis chronica atrophicans
- Amyloidosis
- Carcinoid syndrome
- Chronic graft versus host disease
- Cutaneous metastases
- Dermatofibrosarcoma protuberans
- Drug-induced sclerodermoid lesion
- Keloid or hypertrophic scar
- Lichen sclerosus et atrophicans—often presents with morphea and is considered by some to be a morphea variant
- Lipoatrophy
- Nephrogenic systemic fibrosis
- Panniculitis
- Phenylketonuria
- Porphyria cutanea tarda with sclerodermoid features
- Progeria or Werner syndrome
- Radiation fibrosis
- Reflex sympathetic dystrophy
- Scleredema
- Scleromyxedema
- Stasis dermatitis with fibrosis
- Systemic sclerosis—Look for sclerodactyly, Raynaud phenomenon, and internal organ involvement.

Pediatric Patient Differential Diagnosis

Bullous morphea should be included in the differential of a child presenting with unilateral limb edema. Congenital morphea, while rare, manifests as the linear scleroderma subtype. Congenital morphea is often misdiagnosed as a salmon patch, nevus, or skin infection.

✓ Best Tests

- A skin biopsy, such as a punch biopsy, is the best test to confirm a clinical suspicion of morphea. Active lesions show perivascular and interstitial inflammatory infiltrates with plasma cells, lymphocytes, and eosinophils. The dermis and subcutaneous tissue contain thickened collagen bundles. Skin appendages are atrophied.
- Lab abnormalities are not specific for morphea. However, antinuclear antibodies, anti-dsDNA antibodies, rheumatoid factor, antihistone antibodies, antitopoisomerase II alpha antibodies, anticardiolipin antibodies, and lupus anticoagulant are found in many patients. A patient may also have peripheral eosinophilia, high serum gammaglobulin, increased inflammatory markers, and low serum complement levels.
- Imaging studies such as X-ray, CT, and MRI are used to assess involvement of bones and muscles.
- In Europe, morphea has been reported to be associated with prior *Borrelia* infection. Serologic testing in at-risk populations may be indicated.

Pediatric Patient Considerations

Children with *en coup de sabre* or Parry-Romberg syndrome may exhibit abnormalities on MRI of the brain such as T2 lesions, focal atrophy, and calcifications. Lumbar puncture with CSF analysis may reveal oligoclonal bands and elevated IgG. EEG may demonstrate an epileptiform pattern.

▲▲ Management Pearls

- Patients and families should be reassured that morphea is generally limited to the skin and that the lesions will improve over a few years. Extension and activity of morphea lesions can be monitored with a number of tools such as infrared thermography, laser Doppler flowmetry, and ultrasonography.
- Patients with symptoms of extracutaneous involvement, such as arthralgias, dysphagia, gastroesophageal reflux, dyspnea, and Raynaud phenomenon should be referred to a rheumatologist. In deep morphea, painful flexion contractures, carpal tunnel syndrome, and ulcers may develop. Consider referral to physical therapy, orthopedic surgery, and plastic surgery.

Pediatric Patient Considerations

Children with *en coup de sabre* or Parry-Romberg syndrome, especially those with neurologic or ocular symptoms, should undergo thorough neurologic and ophthalmologic evaluation.

Therapy

The treatment strategy for morphea depends on the stage and subtype of disease. Topical steroids, tacrolimus 0.1% cream, calcipotriol 0.005% cream, and phototherapy work well for patients with plaque morphea where sclerosis is limited to circumscribed areas of the epidermis and dermis. Steroids and tacrolimus may be more effective for erythematous early lesions, while calcipotriol may be more effective for indurated fibrotic lesions. The effectiveness of phototherapy, specifically UVA-1, in dark-skinned individuals is controversial. Some authors insist that phototherapy will not elicit a robust antifibrotic response in dark skin, while others hold that phototherapy is equally efficacious in Fitzpatrick skin types I to V. Phototherapy sessions are administered by a dermatologist, sometimes at a special phototherapy center.

Systemic therapy with methotrexate 15 to 25 mg/wk p.o. and steroids are needed for more extensive cutaneous disease and when the subcutaneous fascia, muscles, and bones are involved, as in generalized morphea, deep morphea, and linear scleroderma. Steroid regimens include prednisolone 5 mg/d p.o. for 2 months, prednisone 1 mg/kg/d p.o. for 3 to 6 months, and methylprednisolone 1 g for 3 d/mo IV for 6 months. Additional systemic agents are the antimalarial drug hydroxychloroquine and the cytotoxic drugs D-penicillamine, cyclosporine, cyclophosphamide, and azathioprine. Such systemic therapy necessitates frequent monitoring of the patient for adverse effects and is usually administered by a dermatologist or a rheumatologist.

There have been a few reports that extracorporeal photophoresis (ECP) may be beneficial to patients with refractory deep or generalized morphea. ECP involves photosensitizing a patient's peripheral white blood cells with 8-methoxypsoralen and then exposing the cells to UVA radiation. The mechanism of action of ECP is not yet fully understood. However, it is hypothesized that ECP triggers an immune response against pathogenic T-cells.

Intralesional triamcinolone 10 mg/mL every 6 weeks for 6 months has been used with modest results in nodular morphea. The chronic ulcers in pansclerotic morphea have been successfully treated with the endothelin receptor antagonist bosentan 4 mg/kg p.o. twice daily for 1 month followed by 4 mg/kg p.o. daily for 7 months.

Pediatric Patient Considerations

Reconstructive surgery with fat transplant is attempted in some children with disfiguring *en coup de sabre*.

Suggested Readings

Bielsa I, Ariza A. Deep morphea. *Semin Cutan Med Surg.* 2007;26:90–95.

Christen-Zaech S, Hakim MD, Afsar FS, et al. Pediatric morphea (localized scleroderma): review of 136 patients. *J Am Acad Dermatol.* 2008;59:385–396.

Falabella R. Pigmentary Disorders in Latin America. *Dermatol Clin.* 2007;25:419–430.

Fett N, Werth VP. Update on morphea: part I. Epidemiology, clinical presentation, and pathogenesis. *J Am Acad Dermatol.* 2011;64(2):217–228; quiz 229–230.

Fett N, Werth VP. Update on morphea: part II. Outcome measures and treatment. *J Am Acad Dermatol.* 2011;64(2):231–242; quiz 243–244.

Jacobe HT, Cayce R, Nguyen J. UVA1 phototherapy is effective in darker skin: A review of 101 patients of Fitzpatrick skin types I-V. *Br J Dermatol.* 2008;159:691–696.

Kawashima H, Watanabe C, Kashiwagi Y, et al. Therapy of childhood generalized morphea: Case reports and reviews of the literature of Japanese cases. *Pediatrics Int.* 2006;48:342–345.

Kister I, Inglese M, Laxer RM, et al. Neurologic manifestations of localized scleroderma: A case report and review of the literature. *Neurology.* 2008;71:1538–1545.

Kreuter A, Altmeyer P, Gambichler T. Treatment of localized scleroderma depends on clinical subtype. *Br J Dermatol.* 2007;156:1362–1365.

Laxer RM, Zulian F. Localized scleroderma. *Curr Opin Rheumatol.* 2006;18:606–613.

Leitenberger JJ, Cayce RL, Haley RW, et al. Distinct autoimmune syndromes in morphea: A review of 245 adult and pediatric cases. *Arch Dermatol.* 2009;145(5):545–550.

Mihas AA, Abou-Assi SG, Heuman DM. Cutae morphea associated with chronic hepatitis C. *J Hepatol.* 2003;39(3):458–459.

Neustadter JH, Samarin F, Carlson KR, et al. Extracorporeal photochemotherapy for generalized deep morphea. *Arch Dermatol.* 2009;145(2):127–130.

Rodriguez-Torres M. Chronic hepatitis C in minority populations. *Curr Hepatitis Rep.* 2008;7:158–163.

Stefanaki C, Stefanaki K, Kontochristopoulos G, et al. Topical tacrolimus 0.1% ointment in the treatment of localized scleroderma. An open label clinical and histological study. *J Dermatol.* 2008;35:712–718.

Wang F, Garza LA, Cho S, et al. Effect of increased pigmentation on the antifibrotic response of human skin to UV-A1 phototherapy. *Arch Dermatol.* 2008;144(7):851–858.

Wriston CC, Rubin AI, Elenitsas R, et al. Nodular scleroderma: A report of 2 cases. *Am J Dermatopathol.* 2008;30(4):385–388.

Zulian F. New developments in localized scleroderma. *Curr Opin Rheumatol.* 2008;20:601–607.

Arthropod Bite or Sting

Mat Davey

■■ Diagnosis Synopsis

Many arthropods bite or sting humans, the cutaneous response to which varies based upon the insect involved and the individual. A bite or sting often results in an inflammatory reaction manifested by localized swelling, redness, burning, pruritus, or pain. Culpable arthropods often include insects (stinging or venomous hymenoptera [bees, wasps, fire ants] and nonvenomous insects [mosquitos, chiggers, fleas, etc.]) as well as ticks, mites, spiders (see Spider Bite for a more detailed discussion), scabies, and pediculosis corporis (body lice). In addition to local skin reactions, arthropods may transmit human illness (including tick bite fever, Lyme disease, Rocky Mountain spotted fever, a variety of encephalitides, and malaria). Venomous bites may trigger systemic toxic or allergic reactions, including anaphylaxis.

◉ Look For

A small central punctum with surrounding erythema and swelling. Vesicles and bullae may develop (Fig. 4-540). Multiple papules and pustules may be seen in fire ant bites. Groupings of linear papules are seen with flea bites (Fig. 4-541). Papular urticarial lesions may be seen with flea bites, chiggers, or bedbugs (Fig. 4-542). Multiple lesions just above the sock line can be due to chigger (harvest mite) bites, which are very common in the southern United States. Papules may be very infiltrated (Fig. 4-543). Tungiasis, found in Africa, India, and Central and South America, is a cutaneous parasitic infestation by the fertilized female sand flea. Look

for a macule that develops into a 3 to 5 mm nodule with a black dot in the center, covered by a white patch, usually on the feet (Fig. 4-544).

Surrounding erythema associated with arthropod bites may be less pronounced in darker skin types. Lesions may resolve with residual postinflammatory pigment changes.

●● Diagnostic Pearls

- Do not discount the possibility of an arthropod bite or sting because other family members or close contacts do not have the same lesions. Some insects will bite one individual preferentially.

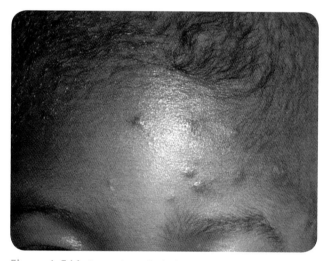

Figure 4-541 Grouped papular lesions are common with arthropod bites.

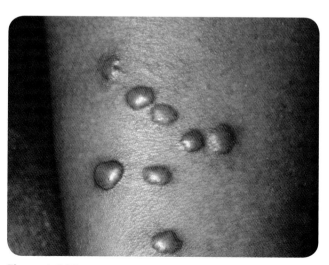

Figure 4-540 Multiple tense bullae from arthropod bites.

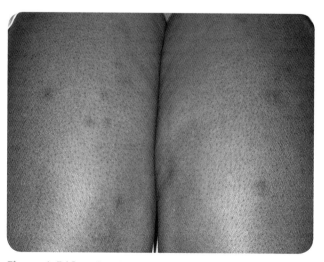

Figure 4-542 Bedbug bites are usually multiple and on the trunk or upper extremities. Three bites may be closely grouped—"breakfast, lunch, and dinner"—but scattered lesions are very frequent.

497

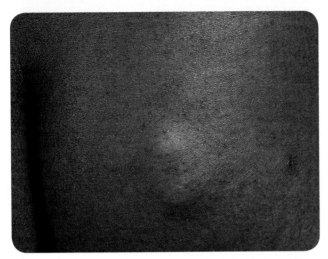

Figure 4-543 Infiltrated papules are often seen in arthropod reactions.

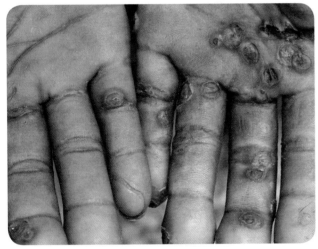

Figure 4-544 Massive infestation of tungiasis in Kilifi, Kenya, mimicking target lesions.

- Bedbugs and fleas often cause several lesions in a row (breakfast, lunch, and dinner) from multiple meal samplings by the insect.

?? Differential Diagnosis and Pitfalls

- Scabies can be identified by microscopic exam of skin scrapings.
- Flea bites, in particular, can cause vesicles and bullae, which may mimic bullous pemphigoid, bullous impetigo, and linear IgA disease.
- Tungiasis is a cutaneous parasitic infestation by the fertilized female sand flea *Tunga penetrans*.
- Folliculitis is often folliculocentric and lacks a central punctum.
- Acne is associated with open and closed comedones.

- Pityriasis lichenoides et varioliformis acuta—central distribution more common than extremities
- Lymphomatoid papulosis
- Bedbug bites

✓ Best Tests

- High index of suspicion or patient recollection of a bite or sting.
- Skin scraping and microscopic examination for scabies mites.
- Recognition of nits and organisms in seams of clothing in pediculosis corporis.
- Although usually unnecessary, biopsy shows a nonspecific superficial and deep, perivascular, and interstitial inflammatory infiltrate with eosinophils or neutrophils. Retained insect parts are occasionally seen.

▲▲ Management Pearls

- Avoid the use of topical diphenhydramine and benzocaine, as they may induce a secondary contact dermatitis.
- Cool compresses and baths are comforting, as are creams with camphor and menthol or topical anesthetics such as pramoxine or lidocaine.
- To reduce insect bites, instruct patients to wear protective shoes and socks and to avoid brightly colored clothing, perfumes, and scented hair and body lotions.
- Other preventative measures include lotions or sprays containing DEET (*N,N*-diethyl-3-methylbenzamide) at 20% to 30% concentration to all exposed skin. Alternatively, picaridin at 7% to 15% concentration may be used in children older than 2 years.
- Consult a veterinarian for eradicating flea infestations in pets. Consult an exterminator for bedbugs or other household infestations.

Therapy

An essential component of therapy is reduction or elimination of further arthropod bites through measures as outlined above. Symptomatic relief can be provided with anti-inflammatory agents and oral antihistamines designed to suppress the inflammatory reaction and itching.

Oral Antihistamines
- Hydroxyzine 25 mg three to four times daily, as needed
- Diphenhydramine hydrochloride 25 to 50 mg every 6 hours, as needed

Nonsedating Antihistamines

- Loratadine 10 mg daily
- Fexofenadine 60 mg twice daily
- Cetirizine hydrochloride 5 or 10 mg nightly

Psychotherapeutic Agents

- Doxepin 25 mg nightly

For lesions on the trunk and extremities, high-potency (classes 1 and 2) topical steroids applied twice daily to individual insect bite reactions can usually control inflammation and itch. These agents should not be used on the face, genitals, or intertriginous areas; low-to-moderate–potency (classes 5 to 7) topical steroids applied twice daily can usually control inflammation and itch in these areas.

For severe anaphylactic reactions, epinephrine and other vasoactive medications, fluids, and systemic glucocorticosteroids are required emergently.

Supportive treatment and hospitalization may be necessary for encephalitis and tick paralysis as well as anaphylaxis.

Other individualized treatment summaries for common bites/stings include:

- Scabies (permethrin)
- Lyme disease (antibiotics [e.g., penicillin, cephalosporin, tetracycline])
- Brown recluse spider bite, spider bite (dapsone, nonsteroidal anti-inflammatory drugs)
- Tungiasis (sterile surgical removal of the flea is the recommended therapy; this can be accomplished with a needle or with a biopsy punch and curette)

Pediatric Patient Considerations

Oral Antihistamines

- Hydroxyzine 2 mg/kg/d total divided every 6 hours in younger children; 10 to 25 mg nightly or three times daily as tolerated for older children

Nonsedating Antihistamines

- Cetirizine hydrochloride 2.5 mg p.o. once to twice daily for children aged 2 to 5 years; 5 or 10 mg nightly for children aged 6 years and older
- Loratadine 5 mg for children aged 2 to 5 years; 10 mg daily for children aged 6 years and older

Low-to-moderate–potency (classes 5 to 7) topical steroids applied twice daily can usually control inflammation and itch.

Suggested Readings

Bircher AJ. Systemic immediate allergic reactions to arthropod stings and bites. *Dermatology.* 2005;210(2):119–127.

James WD, Berger TG, Elston DM, eds. *Andrews' Diseases of the Skin: Clinical Dermatology.* 10th Ed. Philadelphia, PA: Saunders Elsevier; 2006: 455–456.

Katz TM, Miller JH, Hebert AA. Insect repellents: Historical perspectives and new developments. *J Am Acad Dermatol.* 2008585(5):865–871.

Steen CJ, Carbonaro PA, Schwartz RA. Arthropods in dermatology. *J Am Acad Dermatol.* 2004;50:819–842, quiz 842–844.

Steen CJ, Schwartz RA. Arthropod bites and stings. In: Fitzpatrick TB, Wolff K, eds. *Fitzpatrick's Dermatology in General Medicine.* 7th Ed. New York, NY: McGraw-Hill; 2008:2054–2063.

Spider Bite

Lynn McKinley-Grant

 Diagnosis Synopsis

Spiders are members of the Arachnida class, which also includes ticks, mites, and scorpions. The jaws of spiders have fangs that deliver venom via a small hole at the tips. Composition, potency, and clinical effects of venom vary among the different spider species.

Almost all species of spiders are venomous, but only a few dozen can harm humans. Of the few spiders that are of medical importance, envenomation can cause a range of clinical manifestations from skin lesions to systemic illness and in rare cases, even death. Though tarantulas have venom, they usually cause illness from their urticating hairs.

The severity of a spider bite depends on the type of spider, the amount of venom injected, the site of the bite, and the health and age of the patient.

Spiders of medical importance include the following. For more detailed information, refer to VisualDx online.

Widow Spiders

Spiders of the *Latrodectus* genus are found worldwide and have neurotoxic venoms, with alpha-latrotoxin as the major component. The black widow spider, *Lactrodectus mactans*, is the most common widow spider in the United States and is found in woodpiles. Neurotoxic venoms cause systemic symptoms relating to cholinergic and catecholamine excess. The bite is often very painful, and systemic symptoms develop, which include hypertension, tachycardia, palpitations, diaphoresis, anxiety, shortness of breath, hyperthermia or hypothermia, excessive salivation, nausea, vomiting, and severe abdominal pain. The abdominal pain may be misdiagnosed as appendicitis or acute abdomen. The bite may have noticeable fang marks with development of a halolike lesion around the bite. Female black widow spiders can easily be identified by the characteristic red hourglass figure present on their ventral abdomen.

Recluse Spiders

Spiders of the *Loxosceles* genus are found worldwide in temperate and tropical regions. Envenomation can cause local necrosis and, rarely, severe systemic symptoms due to a cytotoxic venom composed of the phospholipase enzyme, sphingomyelinase D. Cytotoxic venoms cause local tissue injury and necrosis. The bite is often initially painless. Pain, swelling, bullae, and ischemia develop minutes to hours later. Lesions may eventually ulcerate and become necrotic and gangrenous. Though systemic toxicity is rare, disseminated intravascular coagulation (DIC) may occur. The brown recluse spider, *Loxosceles recluse,* is regularly and erroneously blamed as the cause of necrotic lesions throughout the

United States, although this spider is most commonly found in the Midwest and Southern states. It can be identified by the characteristic violin-shaped figure spanning its dorsal head and thorax.

Funnel-Web Spiders

In the Pacific Northwest, the hobo spider (*Tegenaria agrestis*), commonly known as the aggressive house spider, is often blamed as the cause of necrotic skin lesions. However, there is only one documented case of hobo spider envenomation causing tissue necrosis. *Atrax/Hadronyche* species in Australia include the most dangerous spider, the Sydney funnel-web spider (*Atrax robustus*). The venom of this spider is neurotoxic, producing severe pain at the bite site and systemic symptoms that can, on occasion, be fatal within minutes.

Tarantulas

Tarantulas, of the family Theraphosidae, have relatively harmless bites. However, they can disperse urticating hairs from their abdomens, resulting in local skin reactions, ocular problems, and allergic rhinitis.

Other Spiders

Other spiders that less commonly cause significant skin irritation or dermal necrosis are as follows:

Yellow sac spiders of the *Cheiracanthium* genus are found in North America, Europe, Africa, Asia, Australia, and the Pacific Islands.

Wolf spiders of the *Lycosa* genus are common spiders found worldwide. Banana spiders of the *Phoneutria* genus, of Central and South America, have extremely potent venom that is neurotoxic and can be lethal.

Six-eyed crab spiders of the *Sicarius* genus are found in Africa and South America and are considered to be extremely venomous but, fortunately, live in remote areas. Their venom is proteolytic.

Look For

Common spider bites usually present with signs of erythema and edema. In darkly pigmented skin erythema can appear as purple, deep red, or sometimes brown-red. A necrotic or dusky center within a red, inflammatory plaque is characteristic.

In brown recluse spider bites, vesicles and bullae can present early. Between 12 and 24 hours after envenomation, a large plaque consisting of erythema, ischemia, and necrosis ("red, white, and blue" sign) develops **(Fig. 4-545)**. Later, these lesions can progress into painful, full-thickness necrotic plaques.

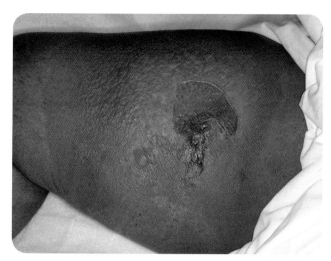

Figure 4-545 Early stage of a brown recluse spider bite with vesiculation and deep erosion and a wide zone of erythema and edema.

Patients with black widow bites have local sweating, piloerection, redness, and mild edema. The systemic symptoms of muscle pain, cramps, abdominal pain, salivation, lacrimation, sweating, and tremors are more prominent than the skin findings.

If the victim brings in the spider, seek out a trained arachnologist or entomologist for accurate identification.

Diagnostic Pearls

- Look closely for two small puncta, the fang marks of the spider.
- Most suspected spider bites seen in the United States turn out to be the result of other causes, most commonly cellulitis or furunculosis. Unless the spider has specifically been identified as the etiology of the symptoms, be cautious about narrowing your differential diagnosis.

?? Differential Diagnosis and Pitfalls

- Acute coronary syndrome
- Acute abdomen:
  - Abdominal aneurysm
  - Acute appendicitis
  - Mesenteric ischemia
  - Ectopic pregnancy
  - Pancreatitis
- Allergic reaction
- Anaphylaxis
- Anxiety
- Caterpillar envenomation
- Cellulitis
- Centipede envenomation

- Contact dermatitis
- Ecthyma
- Ecthyma gangrenosum
- Diabetic ulcer
- Factitial ulcer
- Furuncle (consider methicillin-resistant *Staphylococcus aureus* [MRSA])
- Hymenoptera stings
- Insect bites
- Iritis
- Lyme disease
- Medication-induced drug reactions:
  - Stevens-Johnson syndrome
  - Toxic epidermal necrolysis
- Muscle spasms
- Necrotizing fasciitis
- Priapism
- Pyoderma gangrenosum
- Skin cancer
- Skin infections caused by:
  - Anthrax
  - *Staphylococcus* (particularly community-associated MRSA)
  - *Streptococcus*
  - Sporotrichosis
  - Herpes zoster (shingles)
  - Herpes simplex virus
- Tetanus
- Tularemia
- Uveitis
- Vasculitis such as emboli, ergotism, cryoglobulins

✓ Best Tests

The diagnosis of a spider bite is primarily made on history. There are no tests in widespread clinical use to diagnose spider envenomation.

If systemic involvement due to a brown recluse spider bite is suspected, check for evidence of hemolysis. If systemic involvement is present, serial hemoglobin and plasma-free haptoglobin levels should be followed. Monitor for rhabdomyolysis, renal failure, and DIC.

▲▲ Management Pearls

- Given the difficulty in confirming spider envenomation, always consider other causes of bite wounds, necrotic lesions, and systemic symptoms, and manage them accordingly. Any serous or purulent drainage should be cultured to rule out MRSA infection.
- Most brown spider bites heal in 2 to 3 months without medical treatment.

Therapy

Treatment includes:

- Collection and identification of spider, if possible
- Wound irrigation
- Rest, cold compresses, elevation of the affected extremity
- Symptomatic treatment as indicated
- Tetanus prophylaxis as indicated
- Conservative local debridement of clearly necrotic tissue
- Antivenom as indicated
- Symptomatic treatment as indicated
- For necrotic lesions, treatment with dapsone within the first 36 hours has been advocated by some. However, this remains controversial due to the serious rare side effects of dapsone administration and lack of clear evidence of significant improvement with this therapy.

Suggested Readings

Carbonaro PA, Janniger CK, Schwartz RA. Spider bite reactions. *Cutis.* 1995;56(5):256–259.

Isbister GK, Gray MR. A prospective study of 750 definite spider bites, with expert spider identification. *QJM.* 2002;95(11):723–731.

James WD, Berger TG, Elston DM, eds. Parasitic infestations, stings, and bites. In: *Andrews' Diseases of the Skin: Clinical Dermatology.* 10th Ed. Philadelphia, PA: Saunders Elsevier; 2006:455–456.

Steen CJ, Carbonaro PA, Schwartz RA. Arthropods in dermatology. *J Am Acad Dermatol.* 2004;50(6):819–842, quiz 842–844.

Steen CJ, Schwartz CA. Arthropod bites and stings. In: Fitzpatrick TB, Wolff K, eds. *Fitzpatrick's Dermatology in General Medicine.* 7th Ed. New York, NY: McGraw-Hill; 2008:2054–2063.

Wilson DC, King LE. Spiders and spider bites. *Dermatol Clin.* 1990;8(2): 277–286.

Wilson JR, Hagood CO, Prather ID. Brown recluse spider bites: A complex problem wound. A brief review and case study. *Ostomy Wound Manage.* 2005;51(3):59–66.

Acrochordon

Donna Culton

Diagnosis Synopsis

Acrochordons, also known as skin tags or fibroepithelial polyps, are common benign cutaneous growths. They present as small, flesh-colored or brown, soft papules and are most commonly found in areas of frequent friction such as the eyelids, neck, and axillary and inguinal areas. They are usually asymptomatic but can be irritated by clothing or jewelry. Occasionally, lesions twist upon their own stalk, which leads to strangulation of their blood supply and spontaneous necrosis of the lesion.

Acrochordons are associated with increasing age, pregnancy, diabetes, and obesity. They increase in number in acromegaly and are sometimes associated with acanthosis nigricans. Acrochordons can also be a feature of the autosomal dominantly inherited Birt-Hogg-Dube syndrome. Some early reports suggested that acrochordons may be associated with colonic polyps, but subsequent studies have shown this not to be true, particularly among African Americans and Hispanics. Men and women are affected equally, and there is no difference in prevalence among different ethnicities.

Look For

Look for soft pedunculated (having a stalk) papules, commonly found on the eyelids, neck, groin, and axillae (Figs. 4-546–4-548). They may also occur on the oral, anal, or vulvovaginal mucosa as well (Fig. 4-549). They are often flesh colored or slightly hyperpigmented and range in size from 1 to 6 mm.

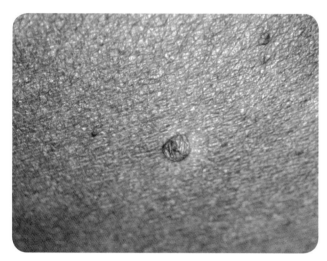

Figure 4-546 Small wide-based acrochordon with surrounding small seborrheic keratosis.

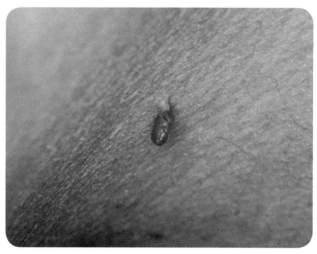

Figure 4-548 Small cylindrical acrochordon darker than surrounding skin.

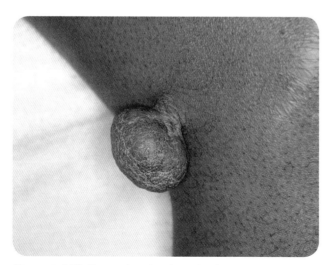

Figure 4-547 Giant pedunculated acrochordon.

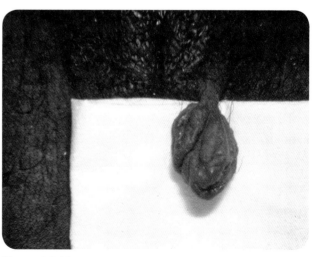

Figure 4-549 Giant acrochordon in vulva.

Diagnostic Pearls

Location in flexural areas can be a good key to the diagnosis. If strangulated, they will occasionally become tender and erythematous, eventually necrosing and falling off spontaneously.

 Differential Diagnosis and Pitfalls

- Seborrheic keratoses
- Dermatosis papulosa nigra
- Verruca vulgaris
- Pedunculated neurofibromas
- In basal cell nevus syndrome, the basal cell carcinomas can be tan to brown and pedunculated, greatly resembling acrochordons.
- Intradermal melanocytic nevus
- Infantile perianal pyramidal protrusions
- Hemorrhoidal tag

✓ **Best Tests**

The diagnosis is clinical. If there is doubt or concern for malignancy, a skin biopsy is diagnostic.

 Management Pearls

Observation is acceptable if the lesion is not irritated or cosmetically a concern for the patient. Patients should be aware that additional lesions are likely to form in sites of frequent friction, even after treatment.

Therapy

If lesions become symptomatic, they can be removed by mechanical snipping (fine iris or Gradle scissors), shave excision, cryotherapy, or electrodesiccation. Smaller lesions can be "snipped" easily without anesthesia, and aluminum chloride or simple pressure will provide hemostasis. Larger lesions may require anesthesia and cauterization.

Suggested Readings

Akhtar AJ, Zhuo J. Non-association between acrochordons and colonic polyps in a minority population. *J Natl Med Assoc.* 2003;95(8):746–749.

Harting M, Hicks MJ, Levy MS. Dermal hypertrophies. In: Wolff K, Goldsmith LA, Katz SI, et al., eds. *Fitzpatrick's Dermatology in General Medicine.* 7th Ed. New York, NY: McGraw-Hill; 2008:554–555.

Yosipovitch G, DeVore A, Dawn A. Obesity and the skin: Skin physiology and skin manifestations of obesity. *J Am Acad Dermatol.* 2007;56(6): 901–916; quiz 917–920.

Calcinosis Cutis

Stephanie Diamantis

▪▪ Diagnosis Synopsis

Calcinosis cutis, or cutaneous calcification, is the deposition of insoluble calcium salts in the skin due to local dysregulation of calcium metabolism. Disorders of calcium metabolism can be broadly categorized into four main groups: dystrophic (most common), metastatic, idiopathic, and iatrogenic. Calcinosis cutis can be viewed as a type of dystrophic calcification, where serum calcium and phosphorus levels are normal, but previously damaged skin leads to altered calcium metabolism and subsequent calcium salt deposition.

Calcinosis cutis is most commonly seen in autoimmune connective tissue diseases, especially in the CREST (calcinosis cutis, Raynaud phenomena, esophageal dysfunction, sclerodactyly, and telangiectasia) form of scleroderma and juvenile dermatomyositis. Approximately 50% to 60% of children with juvenile dermatomyositis will develop calcinosis cutis or some form of cutaneous calcification; about 20% of patients with adult dermatomyositis experience this condition. In addition, affected sites in dermatomyositis and CREST scleroderma differ: knees, elbows, fingers in the former; and hands, upper arms, and bony prominences in the latter. Note, however, that calcinosis cutis can occur anywhere on the body and that local trauma, infections (particularly parasitic), pancreatic disease, lupus profundus, and lymphoma have been associated with calcinosis cutis. Patients with chronic renal disease are also at increased risk of calcinosis cutis because of poor clearance of phosphate that complexes with calcium and deposits in the skin.

The most common clinical presentations include painful, irregularly surfaced nodules. In addition, patients can experience extrusion of chalklike substance from their calcified nodules and secondary infection.

◉ Look For

Lesions are typically small, firm, white-to-yellow papules, plaques, or nodules that may ulcerate and extrude a white chalklike substance (Figs. 4-550–4-552). Lesions typically occur at the tips of fingers and over bony prominences. Calcinosis universalis is the most severe variant, where deposition of calcium salts occurs diffusely along fascial planes. Common locations affected in dermatomyositis include the knees, elbows, and fingers; in scleroderma, the hands, upper arms, tendons, and bony prominences are characteristically affected. An idiopathic variant occurs on the scrotum of otherwise healthy men and presents with nontender, white, firm, papules and nodules.

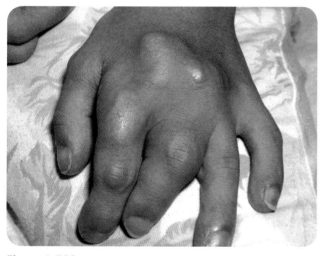

Figure 4-550 Calcinosis cutis in a child with deforming arthritis.

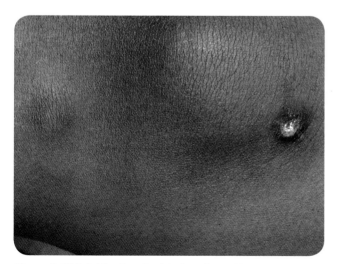

Figure 4-551 Calcinosis cutis with ulceration and hyperpigmentation.

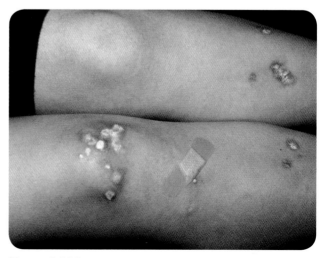

Figure 4-552 Multiple lesions of calcinosis in a diabetic patient (not a general association).

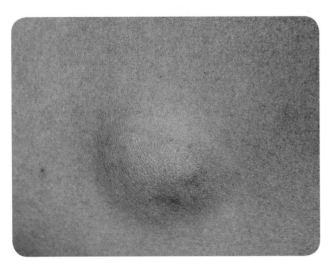

Figure 4-553 Calcinosis cutis can mimic a pilomatricoma.

Diagnostic Pearls

Palpation will demonstrate firm lesions. X-ray will demonstrate characteristic densities.

Differential Diagnosis and Pitfalls

- Gout
- Calcified epidermoid cysts
- Pilomatricoma (Fig. 4-553)
- Milia
- Xanthomas
- Molluscum contagiosum
- Warts
- Osteoma cutis
- Subepidermal calcified nodule (usually solitary; head in children, extremities in adults)
- Scrotal calcinosis (often multiple)
- Pseudoxanthoma elasticum

✓ Best Tests

Histopathologic examination of skin biopsy specimens will be diagnostic, but an underlying cause of the disorder should be sought. Depending on clinical context, systemic evaluation may include the following:

- Calcium, phosphate, parathyroid hormone, vitamin D3 serum levels
- Complete blood count with differential, renal, and liver function studies
- Alkaline phosphatase, lipase, amylase serum levels
- Autoantibodies (ANA, anti-SCL-70, anti-dsDNA, anti-Jo-1) if suspecting autoimmune connective tissue disease
- Serum levels of muscle enzymes including aldolase, creatinine kinase, lactate dehydrogenase if suspecting dermatomyositis
- Soft tissue radiograph to assist in delineating the extent of tissue involvement

Management Pearls

- Consultations are sought on the basis of the underlying disease and may include a nephrologist, hematologist/oncologist, or rheumatologist.
- Consider dietary modifications such as a low phosphate or calcium diet, when appropriate.
- Small lesions can be excised if symptomatic or interfering with patient function. There is a risk that calcification will recur in the surgical scar.

Therapy

Treatment of the underlying disorder is the first line of therapy. Limited cases with a benign etiology can be observed and may heal spontaneously. Appropriate wound care management should be undertaken; skin lesions should be kept clean and antibiotics administered based on culture results.

The vast majority of directed therapies for calcinosis cutis have been described in case reports. The following treatments have been tried with varied success:

- Diltiazem—60 mg p.o. daily initially, slowly increased to 360 mg p.o. daily
- Surgical excision—especially if lesions are painful or interfering with function or cosmesis
- Colchicine—1 mg p.o. daily
- Probenecid—250 mg p.o. daily
- Aluminum hydroxide—320 to 1,800 mg p.o. before every meal
- Intralesional corticosteroids—triamcinolone acetonide 25 mg/mL monthly
- Bisphosphonates

Suggested Readings

Ambler GR, Chaitow J, Rogers M, et al. Rapid improvement of calcinosis in juvenile dermatomyositis with alendronate therapy. *J Rheumatol.* 2005;32(9):1837–1839.

Tourat DM, Sau P. Cutaneous deposition diseases, part II. *J Am Acad Dermatol.* 1998;39(4):527–544.

Walsh JS, Fairly JA. Cutaneous mineralization and ossification. In: Wolff K, Goldsmith LA, Katz SI, Gilchrest BA, Paller AS, Leffell DJ, eds. *Fitzpatrick's Dermatology in General Medicine.* 7th Ed. New York, NY: McGraw Hill; 2008:1293–1297.

Abscess and Abscess of the Newborn

Mat Davey

◼◼ Diagnosis Synopsis

An abscess is a localized inflammatory process in which white blood cells accumulate at a site of infection in the dermis and/or subcutaneous tissue, creating a collection of pus. Commonly associated pathogens include *Staphylococcus aureus*, streptococci, and normal skin flora. Abscesses may arise from infection of surrounding skin appendages, direct inoculation of an injury, or by hematogenous spread. Trauma or any break in the skin barrier predisposes to abscess formation. Individual lesions evolve over days to weeks. They are usually painful/tender, erythematous, warm, and fluctuant masses that are sometimes associated with fever.

Methicillin-resistant *S. aureus* (MRSA)–associated abscesses are becoming increasingly common in the general community. Community-associated MRSA (CA-MRSA) among individuals who lack traditional risk factors for such infections (IV drug use, incarceration, participation in contact sports, etc.) is associated with a unique antibiotic susceptibility profile, and care must be taken to ensure appropriate initial antibiotic coverage.

Pediatric Patient Considerations

Abscess of the newborn—Sites of predilection are around the umbilicus and circumcision sites. Clinically, there is a firm, tender, red nodule that may become fluctuant. Gentle pressure often reveals an opaque white core. Neonatal perianal abscesses (and abscesses in noncutaneous locations) are often associated with chronic granulomatous disease.

◉ Look For

In abscesses, the pus is generally not seen at skin level but may appear as a multiheaded pustule (Figs. 4-554–4-557). Loculations may be present.

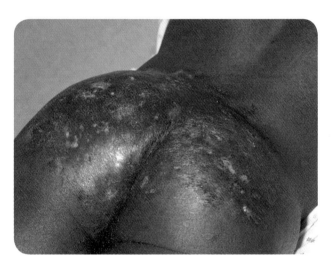

Figure 4-554 Multiple abscesses with sinus tracks on the buttocks.

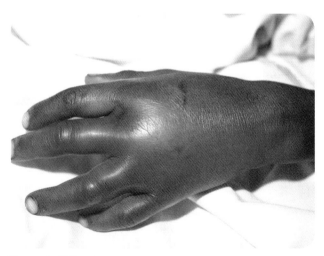

Figure 4-555 Diffuse swelling with abscess of the dorsum of the hand.

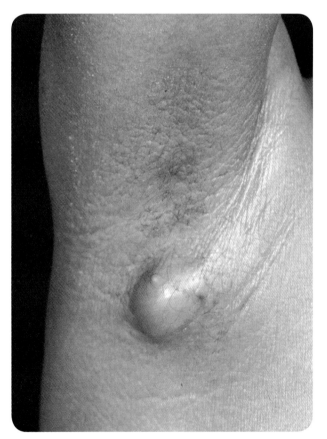

Figure 4-556 Single abscess of axilla; lesions are usually multiple in hidradenitis suppurativa.

507

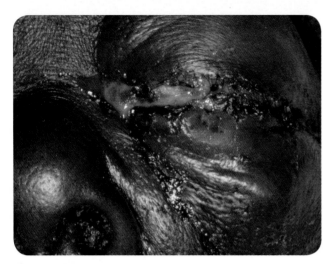

Figure 4-557 Orbital abscess with purulent discharge.

- Gram and fungal stains of exudate or aspirate may yield immediate microbiologic diagnosis. Cultures take a few days (bacterial) to weeks (fungal) to yield results.
- Sensitivities on all cultures should be performed to determine antibiotic resistance.

▲▲▲ Management Pearls

The mainstay of therapy of abscesses is early and adequate drainage. Care must be taken not to incise lesions that are incipient or acutely inflamed. Moist heat with warm saline compresses should be employed until the lesion becomes localized and displays definitive fluctuation. Incision and drainage is carried out with a No. 11 blade. If loculations are present, probing of the abscess may be necessary. Larger cavitations should be packed with iodoform gauze.

In patients with recurrent abscesses, eradication of MRSA nasal carriage may be accomplished by application of mupirocin 2% cream (twice daily for 5 days) to the nares. The combination of rifampin (600 mg daily for 10 days) plus trimethoprim and sulfamethoxazole (TMP/SMX)—one double-strength tab twice daily for 10 days—has also been shown to eradicate colonization.

●● Diagnostic Pearls

In patients who present with multiple abscesses and/or atypical bacterial cultures, evaluation of an underlying immunologic or neutrophil dysfunction (such as hyperimmunoglobulin E syndrome and chronic granulomatous disease) should be pursued.

Multiple abscesses may be seen on the extremities of IV drug abusers.

?? Differential Diagnosis and Pitfalls

Infectious

- Cellulitis or erysipelas
- Cat-scratch disease
- Atypical mycobacterial infections
- Deep fungal infection
- Herpetic whitlow

Noninfectious

- Ruptured subcutaneous cyst
- Gout
- Large dermal nodules of lymphoma/pseudolymphoma may mimic abscesses
- Eosinophilic cellulitis

✓ Best Tests

- The diagnosis is usually clinically evident. If in doubt, needle or incisional aspiration of purulent material may be pursued.

Therapy

Incision and drainage is oftentimes curative; however, antibiotics may be employed, especially if the patient displays any systemic symptoms such as fevers/chills. Antibiotics are also indicated for concomitant cellulitis, multiple lesions, or if the patient is immunosuppressed. Antibiotic coverage must take into account the risk of MRSA. It is helpful to be aware of patterns of antimicrobial resistance within your local community.

In many communities, CA-MRSA is the most likely bacterial isolate from abscesses; therefore, it is now recommended that initial antibiotic therapy cover CA-MRSA until culture data are available. Refer to current CDC guidelines, as treatment recommendations for MRSA are rapidly changing.

Patients exhibiting signs or symptoms of systemic involvement or with rapidly progressing infections or patients with significant comorbidities (e.g., immunosuppression) should be hospitalized for observation, and initiation of antibiotic covering MRSA should be pursued.

In systemically ill patients with atypical bacterial isolates, inpatient empiric IV antibiotics and supportive care must be pursued.

Pediatric Patient Considerations

In the neonatal period, consideration of intravenous antibiotics and acquisition of other cultures (blood and CSF) is mandatory, as the neonate is essentially immunocompromised.

For CA-MRSA coverage, refer to current CDC guidelines, as treatment recommendations are rapidly changing.

Suggested Readings

Cohen PR. Community-acquired methicillin-resistant *Staphylococcus aureus* skin infections: Implications for patients and practioners. *Am J Clin Dermatol.* 2007;8(5):259–270. PubMed ID: 17902728.

Craft NC, Lee PK, Zipoli MT, et al. Superficial cutaneous infections and pyodermas. In: Fitzpatrick TB, Wolff K, eds. *Fitzpatrick's Dermatology in General Medicine.* 7th Ed. New York, NY: McGraw-Hill; 2008:1694–1703.

Daum RS. Clinical practice. Skin and soft-tissue infections caused by methicillin-resistant *Staphylococcus aureus. N Engl J Med.* 2007;357(4): 380–390. PubMed ID: 17652653.

Elston DM. Community-acquired methicillin-resistant *Staphylococcus aureus. J Am Acad Dermatol.* 2007;56(1):1–16; quiz 17–20. PubMed ID: 17190619.

James WD, Berger TG, Elston DM, eds. *Andrews' Diseases of the Skin: Clinical Dermatology.* 10th Ed. Philadelphia, PA: Saunders Elsevier; 2006:251–264.

Majocchi Granuloma

Meaghan Canton Feder

■■ Diagnosis Synopsis

Majocchi granuloma, also known as nodular granulomatous perifolliculitis or fungal folliculitis, is a perifollicular nodular dermatophyte infection. The disease occurs when a dermatophyte invades the hair follicle, causing a granulomatous and suppurative reaction. Majocchi granuloma is most often caused by *Trichophyton rubrum* and less frequently by *Trichophyton mentagrophytes* or *Epidermophyton floccosum*. These are the same fungal species that cause tinea corporis and tinea pedis.

Majocchi granuloma usually occurs on the shins or wrists. It has been seen on the face as a result of shaving, and there have been cases seen on the buttocks and genital area. Risk factors for developing Majocchi granuloma are occlusion of the skin, simple trauma, immunosuppression, and use of topical steroids on unsuspected tinea. The clinical presentation of Majocchi granuloma varies depending on the cause.

Immunocompromised Patient Considerations

In immunocompromised patients, Majocchi granuloma appears deeper and more nodular.

◉ Look For

Lesions can develop on any follicular surface but usually present on the scalp, face, or extremities (Figs. 4-558 and 4-559). They do not affect the palms, soles, or mucous membranes. Majocchi granuloma begins as an annular

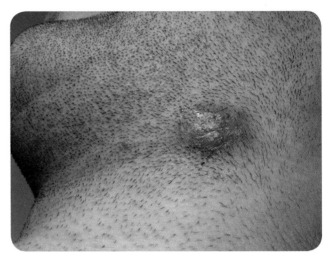

Figure 4-559 Deep *T. rubrum* infection on the neck.

solitary patch or multiple patches with scale and develops into erythematous, scaly, perifollicular papulopustules and nodules. Affected areas may resemble a bacterial furuncle or carbuncle, but there is no pus discharge.

Patients of African descent may have a greater predisposition to developing Majocchi granuloma from a superficial tinea, given the predisposition for pseudofolliculitis from ingrown hairs.

Majocchi granuloma is also more common in women who frequently shave their legs and in those with tinea pedis or onychomycosis.

Immunocompromised Patient Considerations

In immunocompromised patients, Majocchi granuloma appears similar to Kaposi sarcoma.

●● Diagnostic Pearls

When diagnosing Majocchi granuloma, look for a cluster or group of pustules within a plaque. Ask if the patient has already been treated with a topical antifungal; a history of occlusion with bandages or ointments is a predisposing factor. Patients may also have concomitant onychomycosis or tinea pedis.

?? Differential Diagnosis and Pitfalls

- Herpes simplex infections including herpetic folliculitis
- Furunculosis
- Bacterial folliculitis

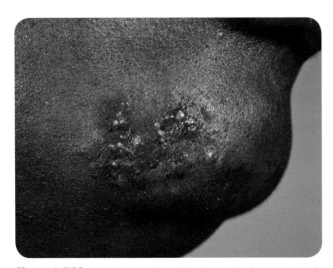

Figure 4-558 Deep dermatophyte infection on the face: an example of Majocchi granuloma.

- Pseudofolliculitis barbae
- Acne keloidalis nuchae
- Lymphocytoma cutis
- Kaposi sarcoma
- Abscess
- Nodular scabies
- Kerion

✓ Best Tests

- Preliminary testing should include a KOH preparation and fungal culture.
- A skin biopsy with fungal stains and tissue culture is the best test, because KOH examination is often negative, especially if a topical antifungal has been used recently.
- Bacterial and viral cultures will rule out bacterial folliculitis and herpes simplex.

▲▲▲ Management Pearls

- Advise patients to abstain from shaving or to shave less frequently, if possible.
- Topical corticosteroids and combination corticosteroid-antifungal preparations should *not* be used.
- Majocchi granuloma typically requires oral antifungal therapy.

Therapy

Systemic antifungal medications are the treatment of choice. Topical agents alone are not effective, as the organism is in the follicles and the perifollicular dermis.

- Terbinafine—250 mg daily for 4 weeks in the immunocompetent
- Itraconazole pulse therapy—200 mg twice daily for 1 week, with 2 weeks off therapy; then, repeat the cycle for a total of three pulses. Itraconazole 200 mg twice daily for 2 to 3 months in the immunocompromised patient
- Griseofulvin—500 mg p.o. twice daily for 4 weeks

Immunocompromised Patient Considerations

- Consider 6 to 8 weeks of terbinafine therapy in the immunocompromised patient.
- Itraconazole 200 mg twice daily for 2 to 3 months in the immunocompromised patient.

Suggested Readings

Chang SE, Lee DK, Choi JH, et al. Majocchi's granuloma of the vulva caused by Trichophyton mentagrophytes. *Mycoses.* 2005;48(6):382–384.

Cho HR, Lee MH, Haw CR. Majocchi's granuloma on the scrotum. *Mycoses.* 2007;50(6):520–522.

Gill M, Sachdeva B, Gill PS, et al. Majocchi's granuloma of the face in an immunocompetent patient. *J Dermatol.* 2007;34(10):702–704.

James WD, Berger TG, Elston DM, eds. Tinea corporis, fungal folliculitis (Majocchi's granuloma) and tinea incognito. In: *Andrews' Disease of the Skin: Clinical Dermatology.* 10th Ed. Philadelphia, PA: Saunders Elsevier; 2006:302–303.

Deep Fungal and Other Infections
Donna Culton • Pooja Sodha • Lynn McKinley-Grant

■■ Diagnosis Synopsis

Deep Fungal Infections

Deep fungal infections represent fungal infections involving the dermis or subcutis. These deeper infections can be divided into subcutaneous and systemic mycoses depending on the extent of infection and the route of inoculation. A common disorder, cat-scratch disease can mimic deep fungal diseases and is discussed in this group. These diseases have to be considered in an immunosuppressed patient.

Subcutaneous Mycoses

Subcutaneous mycoses are infections that result from a penetrating injury that directly inoculates the dermis and/or subcutis with the pathogenic fungi that reside in decaying vegetation, plants, and soil. Lesions most often occur on distal extremities. The lesions tend to be chronic, progressing very slowly within a localized area of the skin. The incubation period is variable but can be quite lengthy. While lymphatic spread may occur in the subcutaneous mycoses, distant involvement does not occur by definition. These infections are most common in the tropics and subtropics. Risk factors include exposure of open skin to soil (occupational, traumatic, etc.) and male sex (5:1, likely related to occupational exposures). Several unique subsets of the disease exist. Sporotrichosis is addressed here. For discussions on other subcutaneous mycoses, for example, mycetoma and chromoblastomycosis, see VisualDx online. (If you are a first-time online user, go to www.essentialdermatology.com/pigmented; if you already have your password set up, go directly to www.visualdx.com/visualdx.)

Sporotrichosis is caused by the dimorphic fungus *Sporothrix schenckii*. The lesions of sporotrichosis most often present on the hand or distal forearm with associated lymphocutaneous or sporotrichoid spread (80% of cases). Other variants include fixed cutaneous lesions, which occur in endemic areas, and disseminated cutaneous disease, which occurs with systemic involvement. The disease is most commonly reported in North and South America and is endemic in the Missouri and Mississippi Valleys. Extracutaneous disease is rare but manifests with osteoarticular involvement in immunocompetent individuals and multisystem involvement in immunocompromised patients.

The organism is present in the soil, plants, and decaying vegetation. Thorny plants, such as barberry and rose bushes, are the most common source of cutaneous inoculation of sporotrichosis, with occupational exposures including farmers, florists, gardeners, and forestry workers. Professional workers in landscaping may be of diverse ethnic and racial backgrounds, and recreational gardeners are all of ethnic and

racial backgrounds and socioeconomic strata. Of all of the deep fungal infections, sporotrichosis is the most commonly occurring in urban areas.

The lesions of sporotrichosis may present in the following four different patterns:

- Lymphocutaneous or sporotrichoid pattern
- Fixed cutaneous
- Multifocal and disseminated cutaneous
- Systemic

Approximately 80% of cases are of the classic lymphocutaneous variety. Fixed cutaneous sporotrichosis occurs in endemic areas, whereas extracutaneous disease is typically due to inhalation or hematogenous spread of the organism, particularly in the immunocompromised. The lesions are papular or nodular, progressively plaquelike, with ulcerations most commonly affecting the face and extremities. Bilateral involvement is uncommon but would suggest infection related to occupation.

Systemic symptoms are rare except in the case of extracutaneous disease, which includes osteoarticular involvement and monoarthritis in immunocompetent individuals and pulmonary, meningeal, and urogenital involvement in patients with decreased immunity. Osteoarticular sporotrichosis is the most common extracutaneous manifestation, occurring in up to 80% of cases. Pulmonary sporotrichosis is associated with alcoholism, tuberculosis, diabetes mellitus, sarcoidosis, and steroid use.

Untreated cutaneous sporotrichosis usually waxes and wanes over months to years without systemic manifestations.

Pediatric Patient Considerations

Sporotrichosis occurs in both children and adults. Children and adolescents are commonly affected on the face.

Systemic Mycoses

Systemic mycoses are disseminated fungal infections that follow primary infection of the respiratory tract. Cutaneous manifestations are rare but can be helpful in diagnosis when they occur. In the developed world, systemic fungal infections are most commonly seen in immunosuppressed patients. Specific pathogenic organisms include the following.

Blastomycosis (Gilchrist disease) is an infection caused by the dimorphic fungus *Blastomyces dermatitidis*, a soil organism endemic to the midwestern, north-central, and southeastern parts of the US in areas bordering the Mississippi and Ohio River basins. Infection manifests as an initial flulike illness with indolent pulmonary infection and variable presence of crusted verrucous or ulcerated skin lesions (approximately 20% of cases). Initial infection can spontaneously resolve (approximately 50% of cases), may progress to localized pulmonary disease, or produce extrapulmonary manifestations after dissemination to other organs, most commonly the skin and bones. There is a higher incidence in African American men (approximately 50% of cases), followed by African American women (approximately 30% of cases). White men and white women have the lowest incidence of the disease (13% and 4%, respectively). Mortality from disseminated disease is higher among African Americans. Primary cutaneous disease is rare (5%).

Coccidioidomycosis, caused by the *Coccidioides* species, is endemic to the southwest United States and Mexico. Following inhalational exposure, 60% of patients are asymptomatic. The remainder of patients develop primary benign pulmonary infection with low-grade fever ("valley fever"), which is occasionally accompanied by erythema nodosum or erythema multiforme (less so in patients of African descent). Most cases of primary pulmonary infection are self-limited; however, a small percentage of patients develop progressive pulmonary infection or extrapulmonary disease. Progression to disseminated disease is severalfold higher in Hispanics, individuals of African descent, and immunosuppressed patients. In disseminated disease, 20% of patients develop cutaneous findings.

Immunocompromised Patient Considerations

Immunocompromised patients are at a significantly increased risk for developing systemic fungal infections. For information about other systemic mycoses (histoplasmosis, cryptococcosis), see VisualDx online.

Cat-Scratch Disease

Cat-scratch disease (subacute regional lymphadenitis) refers to bacterial infection with *Bartonella henselae,* a pleomorphic Gram-negative bacillus transmitted by cat saliva or cat scratch in more than 50% of cases. The infection was first described in 1950, and more than 30 years later, the pathogen was isolated. It is thought that most people carry the infection but never present clinically because they develop immunity, as shown by positive skin test. There are several clinical syndromes associated with *Bartonella* infection, with cat-scratch disease being the most frequent clinical manifestation.

In an analysis of three national databases, the adult incidence was estimated between 0.60 and 0.93 per 100,000 persons discharged from the hospital, with higher incidence in men. A higher incidence was found in children, approximately 2 per 100,000. The incidence among ambulatory patients is estimated to be about 9.3 per 100,000, nearly ten times the number of hospitalized patients, suggesting that the disease is often not recognized. Incidence was lower in African Americans, with 0.53 per 100,000 persons. No ethnic or racial group is naturally immune to this disorder. In the US nationally, incidence was higher in the south and lower in the west. Seasonal variation has been noted with higher incidence in the fall and winter, nearly the last 6 months of the year.

In most cases, it manifests as a primary papulopustular skin lesion and enlarged localized lymph nodes, with a history of cat contact distal to the involved node. Fatigue, low-grade fever, malaise, sore throat, pharyngitis, conjunctivitis, and headache may be present. Following inoculation, incubation period is typically 7 to 12 days for local reaction to surface, with painful nodes appearing up to 4 weeks later. Dermatologic involvement is seen in approximately two thirds of patients and includes evidence of a scratch with or without a papulopustular lesion, a widespread morbilliform eruption, erythema nodosum (warm, erythematous, and painful nodules in lower extremities), erythema multiforme, and/or thrombocytopenic purpura. Splenomegaly, weight loss, parotid swelling, osteomyelitis, hepatitis, or abscesses in the liver or spleen rarely appear. Most patients recover without sequelae.

Immunocompromised Patient Considerations

In immunocompetent patients, the disease is usually benign and self-limited, and most patients recover without sequelae. Atypical presentations include stellate neuroretinitis, hepatosplenomegaly, encephalopathy, persistent fever, osteomyelitis, endocarditis, and the oculoglandular syndrome of Parinaud. Encephalitis may occur in 1% to 7% of cases, typically appearing 2 to 6 weeks after classic cat-scratch disease. In the immunocompromised host, infection with *B. henselae* can manifest in numerous ways, from classic cat-scratch disease to bacillary angiomatosis, peliosis, or sepsis.

Pediatric Patient Considerations

Cat-scratch disease is reportedly more common in children, although diagnosis may be delayed since lesions can go unrecognized.

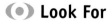 Look For

Deep Fungal Infections

General subcutaneous mycotic infections often start as a dermal nodule that ulcerates. Draining lymphatics can become tender and erythematous with additional lesions developing along the lymphatics.

Sporotrichosis—Painless nodules on distal extremities are most common in the lymphocutaneous form. Initially, an erythematous papule, pustule, or nodule is seen on the distal extremity at the site of inoculation (Figs. 4-560–4-562). New lesions appear proximally along the lymphatics over several weeks. Lesions may eventually ulcerate. Fixed cutaneous lesions are defined by verrucous or gummatous plaques, more commonly on the face, in the absence of lymphangitic spread. Disseminated cutaneous disease occurs in systemic disease with multiple diffusely distributed papules, nodules, ulcers, or plaques.

In systemic forms, ulcerated nodules may develop anywhere on the body or mucous membranes. Extracutaneous involvement occurs by definition, including the lungs, joints, and central nervous system. Immunocompromised patients are susceptible, as in AIDS, corticosteroid use, diabetes mellitus, organ transplantation, alcoholism, and use of immunosuppressive agents.

Histoplasmosis—In acute pulmonary histoplasmosis, look for erythema multiforme or erythema nodosum. In acute disseminated histoplasmosis, look for erythematous papules and umbilicated papules, small nodules, or molluscumlike lesions (Fig. 4-563). Shallow ulcers and crusted papules may develop later. In chronic disseminated histoplasmosis, look for oral ulcers, which are common. Ulcers may also occur anywhere along the gastrointestinal tract

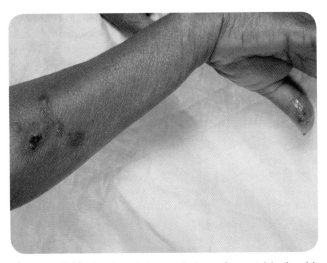

Figure 4-560 Thumb and forearm lesions of sporotrichosis with lymphatic spread.

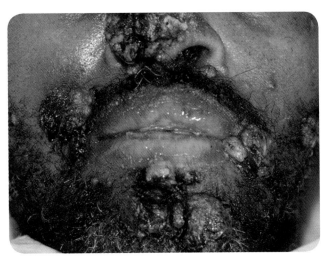

Figure 4-562 Coccidioidomycosis with many disseminated nodules.

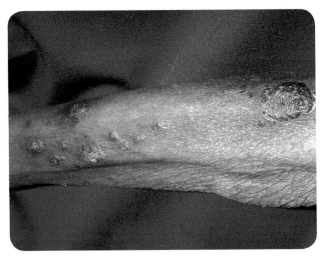

Figure 4-561 Sporotrichosis with large ulceration and multiple papules on the arm.

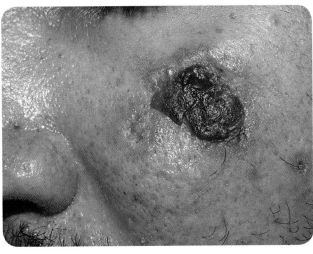

Figure 4-563 Thirty-year-old Latino man with AIDS with a several-month history of crusted lesions with underlying ulcerations due to disseminated histoplasmosis.

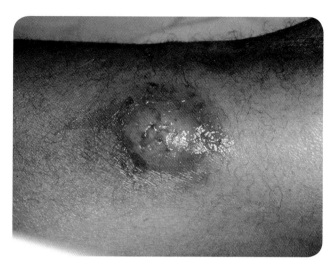

Figure 4-564 Large nodule of blastomycosis with a small ulceration.

from the mouth to the colon. Plaques, nodules, and ulcers of the tongue, buccal mucosa, larynx, or lips may be seen in some patients. In primary cutaneous histoplasmosis, look for an indurated papule or nodule at the trauma site—which may ulcerate and crust—and local lymphadenopathy.

Blastomycosis—Lesions begin as pustules and become shallow ulcers with necrotic edges and granulation tissue at the base (Fig. 4-564). Verrucous skin lesions (found primarily on sun-exposed areas, including the face and extremities) are crusted and have a purplish hue.

Coccidioidomycosis—Primary pulmonary disease is associated with erythema nodosum and erythema multiforme. Disseminated disease presents as verrucous nodules, most commonly on the face especially in those with heavily pigmented skin or immunosuppression (Fig. 4-562).

Cat-Scratch Disease

At the site of inoculation (located on the arm or hand in 50% of cases), look for a 0.5 to 1 cm in diameter lichenoid papule, pustule, nodule, or cluster of tiny nodules appearing nearly 3 to 5 days after inoculation. Evidence of the original abrasion may or may not be present. The papules progress to vesicles and within the first week crust over. If the inoculation site is the conjunctiva, 3 to 5 mm white-yellow granulations on palpebral conjunctiva with tender preauricular or cervical nodes may be seen.

Over the next 1 to 2 weeks, lymphadenopathy appears. Superficial ulcerations, and, occasionally, small coalescent papules in a linear distribution along with the classic regional lymphadenopathy can be seen. Nodes are tender, gradually increasing in size. They often become erythematous and fluctuant. Thirty percent may suppurate spontaneously. In two thirds of patients, the lesion lasts for less than a month, although it may persist for 2 months or more in some cases.

Constitutional symptoms such as mild malaise, fatigue, low-grade fever, and anorexia exist in nearly 75%. Other findings may include conjunctivitis, non-specific exanthem, purpura, or erythema nodosum. Disease resolves with little medical intervention. Prolonged fever may suggest extracutaneous involvement and requires further medical evaluation.

Diagnostic Pearls

Deep Fungal Infections

Sporotrichosis—For lesions presenting with a lymphangitic pattern, a very careful occupational and exposure history is essential.

Histoplasmosis—The skin lesions of histoplasmosis are nonspecific and, thus, make the diagnosis of histoplasmosis difficult by visual exam. Histoplasmosis should be considered in a patient with fever of unknown origin if the patient has traveled to any of the endemic areas or is infected with HIV.

Blastomycosis—Think of this diagnosis in patients with skin nodules or ulcers who live in the endemic regions of the United States, especially when associated with fever or pulmonary symptoms.

Coccidioidomycosis—This diagnosis should be considered in patients with dust exposure, pulmonary symptoms, and verrucous nodules on the face, particularly if they have been in the southwest United States.

Cat-Scratch Disease

- Lymphadenopathy alone is the most common presentation. The axilla is the most common site, followed by the neck, groin, and elbow. The lymphadenopathy is usually unilateral.
- The oculoglandular syndrome of Parinaud refers to granulomatous conjunctivitis and preauricular lymphadenopathy.
- Be sure to get a specific history about exposure to cats, especially kittens. Infection with *B. henselae* has been shown to account for approximately 10% of fevers of unknown origin after EBV infection and osteomyelitis.

Differential Diagnosis and Pitfalls

Deep Fungal Infections

- Atypical mycobacteriosis—in setting of exposure to water containing the organism
- Blastomycosis
- Botryomycosis
- Bromoderma/iododerma
- Cellulitis—has ill-defined erythema but lacks well-formed nodules

515

- Furunculosis—is marked by indurated tender nodules expressing purulent material
- Chromoblastomycosis
- Coccidioidomycosis
- Cryptococcosis
- Cutaneous tuberculosis
- Foreign body granulomas—lack lymphocutaneous spread
- Halogenoderma—will have a history of exposure to iodine or bromine (bromoderma)
- Histoplasmosis
- Leishmaniasis—will have a history of travel to endemic area
- Mycetoma
- *Mycobacterium marinum*
- Nocardiosis
- Panniculitis—characterized by deeper indurated plaques
- Paracoccidioidomycosis
- Pemphigus vegetans
- Psittacosis
- Pyoderma gangrenosum—red- and purple-bordered ulcer with undermined ulcers (sarcoidosis has a sporotrichoid pattern of lesion distribution sometimes)
- Sporotrichosis
- Tularemia—history of exposure to infected animals
- Verrucous carcinoma

Cat-Scratch Disease

- Cutaneous tuberculosis or atypical mycobacterial (i.e., *M. marinum*) infection
- Sarcoidosis
- Sporotrichosis
- Cutaneous T-cell lymphoma
- Toxoplasmosis
- Coccidioidomycosis
- Lymphogranuloma venereum
- Nocardiosis
- Leishmaniasis
- Foreign body granuloma
- Bacillary angiomatosis
- Tularemia
- Brucellosis
- Syphilis
- Cutaneous carcinoma
- Infectious mononucleosis

✓ Best Tests

Deep Fungal Infections

- For any suspected deep fungal infection, a biopsy for histology and for tissue bacterial and fungal culture is essential. Two biopsies are often necessary to yield enough tissue for all testing. Surface swab for culture is often inadequate and, therefore, should be accompanied by the above studies.
- If there is concern for bony involvement, imaging studies should be performed to evaluate for osteomyelitis.

For specific tests and findings, see VisualDx online.

Sporotrichosis—A skin biopsy may not readily show the organisms for sporotrichosis. Fluorescently labeled antibodies can improve visualization of organisms. It is important to rule out mycobacterial and other deep fungal infections with AFB, Gomori methenamine-silver (GMS) stains, and tissue culture.

Histoplasmosis—Note: The laboratory should be informed of the suspicion for histoplasma because the cultures are highly infectious. Skin biopsy reveals small (2 to 4 μm) intracellular yeastlike organisms that must be differentiated from other intracellular organisms. GMS stain may aid in visualization and does not stain nonfungal organisms. In disseminated forms, culture from bone marrow, blood, and sputum is useful. Skin tests have no diagnostic role, as they only indicate prior exposure.

Blastomycosis—Budding yeast forms can be seen in fluids from lesions processed with 10% potassium hydroxide or a fungal stain and cultured. A broad-based bud is a pathognomonic culture finding in blastomycosis. DNA probes can identify *B. dermatitidis*. Culture has a 2- to 4-week incubation period but is considered the gold standard for diagnosis. Serological tests are not useful in diagnosis.

Coccidioidomycosis—On biopsy, spherules in the tissue are approximately 20 μm with a thick refractile wall. Cultures are highly infectious, and lab personnel should be notified. Serologic testing in early disease is most often performed using precipitin, immunodiffusion, ELISA, and latex agglutination with maximal detection between 1 and 2 weeks of infection.

Cat-Scratch Disease

The diagnosis is usually made based upon the clinical history and temporal association with exposure to a cat. It is suggested that the infection typically involves the following criteria: (a) exposure to and contact with a cat, (b) presence of an infection site, (c) positive cat-scratch skin test, (d) lymph node biopsy with characteristic changes, and (e) those changes not being related to other causes of lymphadenopathy. None of these are sufficient for diagnosis in and of themselves. The intradermal skin test is no longer available.

Methods of diagnosis include the following:

- Indirect fluorescent antibody (IFA) assay for *B. henselae*. This test has been reported to have a sensitivity of 88% and a specificity of 94% for cat-scratch disease. Enzyme immunoassay for IgM indicates acute disease. IFA is more frequently used and is considered the most practical diagnostic tool.

- Skin or node biopsies may show pleomorphic Gram-negative bacilli, which are demonstrated on a Warthin-Starry stain.
- Culture of lymph nodes or other tissues are rarely positive and may grow *Afipia felis* in special conditions.
- PCR of pus from inflamed node can be useful particularly for those who do not fit the aforementioned criteria but have lymphadenopathy.

WBC count is normal or only mildly elevated with occasional eosinophilia in 10% to 20% of patients. ESR may be elevated to 40 or 50 mm/h.

▲▲ Management Pearls

Deep Fungal Infections

For most deep fungal infections, but particularly the systemic mycoses, consultation with an infectious disease specialist is necessary, and management and therapy are discussed online.

Sporotrichosis—Local application of heat may help because of the temperature sensitivity of *Sporothrix*.

Histoplasmosis—Chest radiograph may reveal diffuse micronodular pulmonary infiltrates or enlarged mediastinal nodes. Abdominal CT is required to rule out chronic disseminated histoplasmosis and resultant adrenal insufficiency.

Coccidioidomycosis—In patients with the disseminated form, antifungal chemotherapy is essential.

Cat-Scratch Disease

- In some cases, therapeutic lymph node drainage may serve to reduce localized pain and systemic symptoms.
- The disease has a good prognosis and usually self-resolves in 2 to 4 months. It may sometimes persist for longer and should be followed closely if it does. It is also self-limited in the cat, so removal of the pet is not necessary.

Therapy

Deep Fungal Infections

Sporotrichosis—Untreated cutaneous sporotrichosis usually waxes and wanes over months to years without systemic manifestations. Topical therapy is of no value. Localized cutaneous disease (fixed cutaneous or lymphocutaneous) can be treated with:

- Itraconazole 100 to 200 mg p.o. daily for 3 to 6 months is the treatment of choice.
- Oral potassium iodide solution five drops three times daily, gradually increased to 30 to 50 drops three times daily, is also effective but has multiple side effects.
- Terbinafine 500 mg p.o. daily or twice daily

Disseminated cutaneous disease requires amphotericin B IV 0.5 mg/kg/d up to a total of 1 to 2 g.

Histoplasmosis—Primary cutaneous or asymptomatic forms and acute pulmonary forms usually only require supportive therapy. Severe or prolonged cases are usually treated with itraconazole 200 mg daily for 4 to 6 weeks.

Chronic pulmonary and disseminated forms require itraconazole 400 mg/d initially and then 200 mg/d for a total of 6 months. Alternatively, amphotericin B 0.4 to 0.5 mg/kg daily until symptoms subside (usually <500 mg), then switch to itraconazole.

Acute disseminated histoplasmosis requires higher doses (0.7 to 1.0 mg/kg daily) of amphotericin B for the first week, then switch to a lower dose (30 to 35 mg/kg cumulative dose).

Blastomycosis—Amphotericin B is used for complicated and life-threatening infections. For mild to moderate cases without CNS involvement, use oral azoles:

- Itraconazole (200 to 400 mg/d) for 6 months is highly effective for mild to moderately severe infections, especially in adults.
- Fluconazole (400 to 800 mg/d) or ketoconazole (400 to 800 mg/d) can also be used.

In pregnant or immunocompromised patients, use amphotericin B, 1.5 to 2.5 g cumulative dose, followed by itraconazole 200 to 400 mg/d or fluconazole 800 mg/d suppressive therapy. In pediatric patients, use amphotericin B, up to 30 mg/kg cumulative dose or itraconazole 5 mg/kg/d.

Coccidioidomycosis—Amphotericin B, fluconazole 400 to 800 mg/d for at least 12 months. Patients may require suppressive therapy, but this is especially true in HIV patients, where lifetime suppressive dosing of 200 mg/d is necessary. Alternatives include voriconazole, caspofungin, and posaconazole.

Cat-Scratch Disease

Because the disease is usually self-limiting in immunocompetent patients, treatment should be conservative and aimed at ameliorating symptoms. Patients can often be observed until the affected node or nodes involute.

Azithromycin (500 mg on day 1, followed by 250 mg for four more days) is the only antibiotic that has been studied and found effective for treating cat-scratch disease in a randomized, placebo-controlled trial. It should be reserved for patients with systemic symptoms.

(Continued)

In a review of the literature, patients who received any of the following four antibiotics experienced a shorter mean duration of illness:

- Rifampin—10 to 20 mg/kg p.o. daily for 7 to 14 days
- Ciprofloxacin—20 to 30 mg/kg p.o. daily for 7 to 14 days
- Gentamicin—5 to 7.5 mg/kg IV daily divided every 8 hours for 3 days
- Trimethoprim-sulfamethoxazole—dosing based on trimethoprim, 6 to 8 mg/kg p.o. two to three times daily for 7 days

The following three antibiotics have been found to be somewhat efficacious in immunosuppressed patients with cat-scratch disease and its associated conditions:

- Erythromycin—500 mg p.o. four times daily
- Rifampin—as above
- Doxycycline—100 mg p.o. twice daily

Pediatric Patient Considerations

Reports suggest that several oral antibiotics (rifampin, trimethoprim-sulfamethoxazole, cefotaxime, gentamicin, tobramycin, and erythromycin) may be useful in cat-scratch disease, if started early. An infectious disease consultation should be sought for details of treatment for an individual pediatric patient.

Suggested Readings

Carithers HA. Cat-scratch disease: An overview based on a study of 1,200 patients. *Am J Dis Child*. 1985;139:1124–1133.

Florin TA, Zaoutis TE, Zaoutis LB. Beyond cat scratch disease: Widening spectrum of *Bartonella henselae* infection. *Pediatrics*. 2008;121.5: 1413–1425.

Hansmann Y, DeMartino S, Piemont Y, et al. Diagnosis of cat scratch disease with detection of *Bartonella henselae* by PCR: A study of patients with lymph node enlargement. *J Clin Microbiol*. 2005;43.8:3800–3806.

Hay RJ. Deep fungal infections. In: Wolff K, eds. *Fitzpatrick's Dermatology in General Medicine*. 7th Ed. New York, NY: McGraw-Hill; 2008:1831–1844.

Jackson LA, Perkins BA, Wenger JD. Cat scratch disease in the United States: An analysis of three national databases. *Am J Publ Health*. 1993;83.12:1707–1711.

Jacobs RF, Schutze GE. *Bartonella henselae* as a cause of prolonged fever and fever of unknown origin in children. *Clin Infect Dis*. 1998;26:80–84.

Koga T, Matsuda T, Matsumoto T, et al. Therapeutic approaches to subcutaneous mycoses. *Am J Clin Dermatol*. 2003;4(8):537–543.

Laniado-Laborín R. Coccidioidomycosis and other endemic mycoses in Mexico. *Rev Iberoam Micol*. 2007;24(4):249–258.

Lemos LB, Guo M, Baliga M. Blastomycosis: organ involvement and etiologic diagnosis. A review of 123 patients from Mississippi. *Ann Diagn Pathol*. 2000;4(6):391–406.

Lupi O, Tyring SK, McGinnis MR. Tropical dermatology: Fungal tropical diseases. *J Am Acad Dermatol*. 2005;53.6:931–951.

Malatack JJ, Jaffe R. Granulomatous hepatitis in three children due to cat-scratch disease without peripheral adenopathy: An unrecognized cause of fever of unknown origin. *Am J Dis Child*. 1993;147:949–953.

Michel Da Rosa AC, Scroferneker ML, Vettorato R, et al. Epidemiology of sporotrichosis: A study of 304 cases in Brazil. *J Am Acad Dermatol*. 2005;52.3:451–459.

Ramos-e-Silva M, Vasconcelos C, Carneiro S, et al. Sporotrichosis. *Clin Dermatol*. 2007;25:181–187.

Rivitti EA, Aoki V. Deep fungal infections in tropical countries. *Clin Dermatol*. 1999;17(2):171–190; discussion 105–106.

Ware AJ, Cockerell CJ, Skiest DJ, et al. Disseminated sporotrichosis with extensive cutaneous involvement in a patient with AIDS. *J Am Acad Dermatol*. 1999;40.2:350–355.

Cutaneous Leishmaniasis

Pooja Sodha • Lynn McKinley-Grant

▪▪ Diagnosis Synopsis

Cutaneous leishmaniasis results from infection of the skin with obligate intracellular parasites of the *Leishmania* genus. The parasites are transmitted by the bite of infected female phlebotomine sandflies (species in the *Lutzomyia* genus in the New World and in the *Phlebotomus* genus in the Old World). The World Health Organization estimates that 1.5 million new cases of cutaneous leishmaniasis occur each year. Over 90% of the cases occur in the following countries:

- Old World—Afghanistan, Algeria, Iran, Iraq, Saudi Arabia, and Syria
- New World—Brazil and Peru

New World cutaneous leishmaniasis (NWCL), also known as American cutaneous leishmaniasis, chiclero's ulcer, forest yaws, bush yaws, uta, and pian bois, is endemic in some parts of Mexico, Central America, and South America, from northern Argentina to south-central Texas, typically in rural areas. It is not endemic in Uruguay, Chile, or Canada.

Old World cutaneous leishmaniasis (OWCL), also known as Oriental sore, bouton d'Orient, bouton de Crete, bouton d'Alep, bouton de Biskra, Aleppo boil, Baghdad boil, and Delhi boil, is endemic in most countries in southern Europe, Africa (particularly in North and East Africa, with sporadic cases elsewhere), and the Middle East, as well as in parts of the Indian subcontinent, China, and the republics of the former USSR.

However, the geographic areas of acquisition of infection for cases evaluated in the developed world reflect travel and immigration patterns. NWCL is typically a zoonotic disease, with various mammalian reservoir hosts. Humans are incidental hosts of infection. The most common leishmanial species that cause NWCL include those in the *Leishmania mexicana* complex (e.g., *L. mexicana*, *L. amazonensis*) and the *Viannia* subgenus; for example, *L. (V.) braziliensis*, *L. (V.) panamensis*, *L. (V.) guyanensis*. The organisms in the *Viannia* subgenus and *L. amazonensis* may disseminate from the skin to the naso-oropharyngeal mucosa (i.e., cause mucosal leishmaniasis).

OWCL is most commonly caused by infection with *Leishmania major* and *L. tropica*; *L. aethiopica*, *L. infantum*, and *L. donovani* also cause OWCL. The reservoir hosts for the zoonotic *Leishmania* species include dogs, other canines, desert rodents, hyraxes, and gerbils. Infected humans are the reservoir hosts for *L. tropica*, which is anthroponotic and often endemic in urban areas. Recent periods of civil unrest and armed conflicts, with resultant poor sanitation and vector control, are some of the factors associated with ongoing epidemics of OWCL in Afghanistan and Iraq.

The appearance and evolution over time of the skin lesions of OWCL and NWCL can vary widely. Typically, the primary lesions are noted several weeks to months after the sandfly exposure and evolve thereafter, over weeks to months, from papular, to nodular, to ulcerative. Some lesions persist as nodules or plaques. Lymphangitis that ascends the lymphatic chain and lymphadenopathy (sometimes bubonic) can be seen; the latter may precede the presence of skin lesions. Pruritus, pain, and bacterial superinfection may also be present. Systemic symptoms are rarely seen. Ultimately, over months to years, lesions may heal without therapy, leaving hypopigmented, atrophic scars. Reactivation of infection, typically first noted at the margins of scars, can occur months, sometimes years, after clinical resolutions of lesions.

Diffuse cutaneous leishmaniasis (DCL) is a rare variant caused by *L. mexicana*. It occurs in the context of leishmanial-specific anergy and is manifested by disseminated, nonulcerated lesions.

◉ Look For

Initially, look for a smooth (i.e., without scale or crust), erythematous, nonhealing papule or nodule, typically located on exposed parts of the body (e.g., face, ears, arms, lower legs) (Fig. 4-565). The primary lesions usually enlarge slowly and may develop central ulceration (Figs. 4-566 and 4-567). Although lesions may remain small (e.g., up to a few centimeters in diameter), they may gradually enlarge and/or coalesce to become larger, crusted plaques or ulcerations, upwards of 10 cm in diameter. Large plaques usually have central ulceration or crusting with a raised, indurated border.

Multiple primary lesions on one part of the body may be seen; this can result from the probing behavior of sand flies as they attempt to get blood meals. Other variants include the presence of satellite lesions near a primary lesion and lesions that ascend the lymphatic chain.

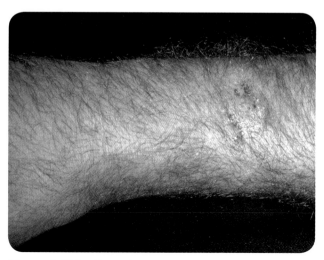

Figure 4-565 Old World Leishmaniasis acquired during military training in the Middle East.

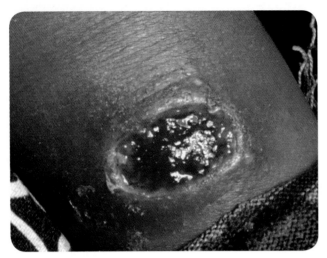

Figure 4-566 Ulceration from Old World Leishmaniasis in a lifelong inhabitant of the region.

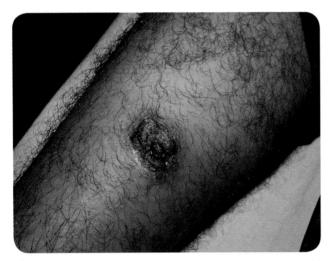

Figure 4-567 Heavily crusted 3-month-old ulcer of New World Leishmaniasis.

In DCL, look for disseminated, nonulcerative plaques and nodules; these can resemble the lesions of lepromatous leprosy.

Diagnostic Pearls

- Persons who had similar exposures to those of the patient may also have developed OCWL and NWCL (e.g., members of a tour group). Therefore, patients should be asked whether other persons had similar exposures and have undiagnosed, persistent skin lesions that should be evaluated for the possibility of either form of cutaneous leishmaniasis.

- Early biopsy of potential lesions is appropriate rather than trials with nonspecific therapy of potential agents.
- Active duty or military personnel returning to their home countries have been a group commonly affected. No racial or ethnic group is naturally immune from infection with these organisms.

?? Differential Diagnosis and Pitfalls

- Tinea corporis
- Sporotrichosis
- Histoplasmosis
- Paracoccidioidomycosis
- Chromomycosis
- Lobomycosis
- Leprosy
- Cutaneous tuberculosis
- Buruli ulcer
- Yaws
- Syphilis
- Myiasis
- Impetigo
- *Mycobacterium marinum* infection
- Infection with other atypical mycobacteria
- Basal cell carcinoma
- Squamous cell carcinoma
- Sarcoidosis
- Foreign body reactions
- Traumatic ulcerations

✓ Best Tests

The most commonly used methods for parasitologic confirmation of the diagnosis include the following:

- Demonstration of amastigotes (the tissue stage of the parasite) by light-microscopic examination of thin smears of tissue scrapings or impression smears of skin (or lymph node) biopsy specimens, or by examination of tissue sections stained with Giemsa or H&E.
- Demonstration of promastigotes (the stage of the parasite found in sandflies and in culture) in cultures of skin (or lymph node) biopsy specimens or tissue aspirates.
- Demonstration of parasite DNA by PCR or other investigational molecular techniques.

The infecting species can be determined by isoenzyme analysis of cultured parasites, molecular methods, or use of monoclonal antibodies.

The currently available serologic tests are not sensitive means of diagnosing cutaneous leishmaniasis.

Management Pearls

Management of each person's case should be individualized in consultation with an expert. In the United States, the CDC provides teleconsultative services, diagnostic testing, and the medication sodium stibogluconate. The lesions should be reexamined 4 to 6 weeks after the end of therapy (earlier, if clinically indicated) and periodically thereafter to determine whether they have resolved and to monitor for relapse (typically first noted at the margins of the scar).

Therapy

Decisions about whether and how to treat OWCL and NWCL should be made in consultation with an expert. First consider whether the patient is at risk for mucosal leishmaniasis. Other important factors include the extent to which the skin lesions are bothersome (e.g., cosmetically or functionally) because of their location (e.g., on the face), number, size, evolution, persistence, or other features (e.g., nodular lymphangitis). In addition, when selecting a medication, consider not only whether the medication is available (e.g., some drugs are not widely available), but also whether data about the effectiveness of that drug for infection with the relevant leishmanial species, in the relevant country, are available. Unfortunately, data are not available about all of the many possible permutations of clinical syndromes, leishmanial species, country, and host factors. Generalizing from data from other settings should be done cautiously and in consultation with an expert. Immunotherapy is considered investigational. The list of possible therapies listed below is not all-inclusive.

First-Line Parenteral
Sodium stibogluconate (available from CDC) or meglumine antimonate (IV or IM)

Alternative Parenteral
Amphotericin B deoxycholate (IV)
Pentamidine (IV or IM)

Oral
Consult an expert.

Topical/Local
Paromomycin (15%) and methylbenzethonium chloride (12%) in soft white paraffin (ointment).

Thermotherapy and cryotherapy may also be effective.

Suggested Readings

Akilov OE, Khachemoune A, Hasan T. Clinical manifestations and classification of Old World cutaneous leishmaniasis. *Int J Dermatol.* 2007;46(2):132–142.

Khatami A, Firooz A, Gorouhi F, et al. Treatment of acute Old World cutaneous leishmaniasis: a systematic review of the randomized controlled trials. *J Am Acad Dermatol.* 2007;57(2):335.e1–29.

Minodier P, Parola P. Cutaneous leishmaniasis treatment. *Travel Med Infect Dis.* 2007;5(3):150–158.

Reithinger R, Dujardin JC, Louzir H, et al. Cutaneous leishmaniasis. *Lancet Infect Dis.* 2007;7(9):581–596.

Schwartz E, Hatz C, Blum J. New world cutaneous leishmaniasis in travelers. *Lancet Infect Dis.* 2006;6(6):342–349.

Scope A, Trau H, Anders G, et al. Experience with New World cutaneous leishmaniasis in travelers. *J Am Acad Dermatol.* 2003;49(4):672–678.

Tuon FF, Amato VS, Graf ME, et al. Treatment of New World cutaneous leishmaniasis--a systematic review with a meta-analysis. *Int J Dermatol.* 2008;47(2):109–124.

Weina PJ, Neafie RC, Wortmann G, et al. Old world leishmaniasis: an emerging infection among deployed US military and civilian workers. *Clin Infect Dis.* 2004;39(11):1674–1680.

Sweet Syndrome (Acute Febrile Neutrophilic Dermatosis)

Laurie Good

◼◼ Diagnosis Synopsis

Sweet syndrome, or acute febrile neutrophilic dermatosis, is an inflammatory disorder manifesting as multiple painful erythematous plaques that are usually associated with fever. The plaques are usually located on the extremities but can also occur on the head, neck, or trunk. The disease may be seen in patients of all ages, but it is more common in women aged between 20 and 60. There is no racial predisposition, and it has been explicitly demonstrated that the clinicopathologic picture in the Indian patient population is consistent with the established disease course.

Although the exact etiology is still unclear, Sweet syndrome has been considered a reactive process and has been associated with a number of inflammatory, infectious, and malignant diseases. These include inflammatory bowel disease, streptococcal pneumonia, and hematologic malignancies (especially myeloid leukemias). It can also occur during pregnancy and with the use of certain drugs (sulfamethoxazole-trimethoprim, minocycline, G-CSF). Most cases are idiopathic or associated with benign conditions; about 15% to 20% are associated with malignancy.

A plethora of reports exist in the Chinese, Korean, and Japanese literature of Sweet syndrome occurring after the use of all-trans retinoic acid (ATRA) for acute promyelocytic leukemia (APL), but interestingly, the incidence of APL has only been shown to be higher in patients of Latino descent thus far. It is unknown whether there is a true genetic predisposition, or if it is related to environmental factors.

While features of the disease are quite distinct, Sweet syndrome is one subtype of the larger category of sterile neutrophilic diseases that includes pyoderma gangrenosum, subcorneal pustular dermatosis, erythema elevatum diutinum, neutrophilic eccrine hidradenitis, leukocytoclastic vasculitis, and others. Sweet syndrome itself frequently includes extracutaneous manifestations. Symptoms such as fever, headaches, myalgias, malaise, and arthralgias are frequently present. Fever often precedes the appearance of lesions. The respiratory system is the most common organ system involved, with cough and infiltrates on chest X-ray. Other sites that may be affected include the gastrointestinal tract, the musculoskeletal system, the kidneys, the heart, and the central nervous system. Conjunctivitis, episcleritis, and oral mucosal lesions have been reported. Sweet syndrome often responds quite well to systemic corticosteroids, but recurrences are common.

Pediatric Patient Considerations

Sweet syndrome occurs in people of all ages, but is reported infrequently in children.

◉ Look For

Deep red, thick, sharply demarcated plaques or nodules that appear vesiculated but have no expressible fluid (Fig. 4-568). The lesions may have pustules within them. The plaques are nonscarring. Ulcers and bullae may occur; however, these lesions are associated more often with underlying malignancy (Figs. 4-569 and 4-570). Subcutaneous forms may mimic erythema nodosum.

The plaques are typically distributed asymmetrically on the extremities, face, neck, and upper trunk. On occasion, lesions may be predominantly distributed over the dorsum

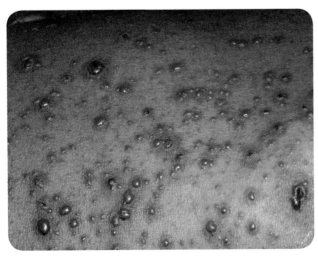

Figure 4-568 Multiple inflammatory papules and cysts in Sweet syndrome.

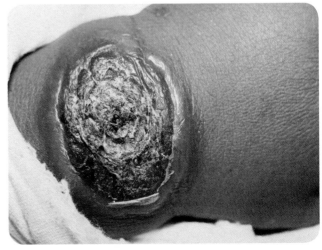

Figure 4-569 Annular ulcerated lesion on wrist of Sweet syndrome with thick central crust.

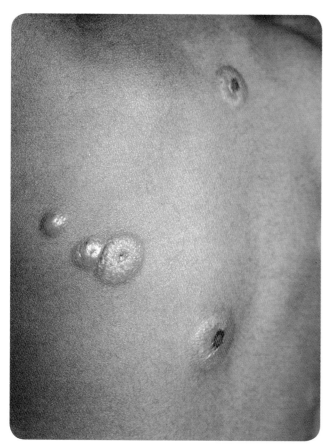

Figure 4-570 Multiple infiltrated nodules, some with small central ulcerations, in Sweet syndrome (same patient as in Fig. 4-569).

of the hands and fingers; some experts consider this to be an anatomically limited subset of Sweet syndrome (neutrophilic dermatosis of the dorsal hands).

Mucosal lesions are infrequent. When present, they usually consist of ulcerations.

Formal diagnosis of Sweet syndrome proceeds from identifying two major and two of four minor diagnostic criteria.

Major Criteria

1. Typical skin lesions—abrupt onset of painful erythematous plaques and nodules
2. Typical histopathology—sterile, dense collections of neutrophils without leukocytoclastic vasculitis

Minor criteria

1. Pyrexia >38°C with constitutional symptoms
2. Excellent response to corticosteroids or potassium iodide
3. Association with an underlying hematologic or visceral malignancy, inflammatory disease, or pregnancy, OR preceded by an upper respiratory or gastrointestinal infection or vaccination

Abnormal laboratory values at presentation (3 of 4): erythrocyte sedimentation rate >20 mm/h; positive C-reactive protein; >8,000 leukocytes; >70% neutrophils.

 Diagnostic Pearls

- Fever often precedes skin lesions.
- Lesions may occur in areas of skin trauma (pathergy). Lesions may form at sites of IV insertion in patients on chemotherapy for hematologic malignancies.
- Oral lesions may occur as well as conjunctivitis and episcleritis.
- Drug-induced Sweet syndrome is defined by lesions with characteristic clinical and histologic morphology, temperature >38°C (100.4°F), and temporal relationship to treatment with a specific drug and resolution subsequent to discontinuation of a suspected drug.
- Neutrophilic eccrine hidradenitis is sometimes seen with chemotherapy and has a neutrophilic infiltrate; it should not be confused with Sweet syndrome.

?? Differential Diagnosis and Pitfalls

- Sweet-like lesions have been seen at sites of erythropoietin injections. Lesions are sometimes mistaken for infiltration of the underlying hematologic malignancy.
- Pyoderma gangrenosum—rolled border around purulent ulcers
- Neutrophilic eccrine hidradenitis
- Bowel-associated dermatosis—arthritis syndrome
- Wells syndrome
- Erythema multiforme—targetoid lesions
- Drug eruption
- Urticarial vasculitis
- Erythema elevatum diutinum—primarily over extensor surfaces
- Cutaneous small vessel vasculitis—palpable purpura
- Behçet disease—associated with oral or genital ulcers
- Bromoderma or iododerma
- Bacterial infections (furunculosis, cellulitis)
- Deep fungal infection
- Erythema nodosum—primarily over the shins
- Atypical mycobacterial infection
- Leishmaniasis—recent travel to endemic areas
- Lymphoma/leukemia cutis
- Metastatic carcinoma

 Best Tests

Skin biopsy is used to confirm the diagnosis and will show a dense neutrophilic infiltrate in the lower dermis.

Consider a medical workup to narrow the differential or elucidate the underlying cause of the condition, such as an infection or hematologic malignancy. Such investigations may include:

- CBC with differential
- Erythrocyte sedimentation rate and/or C-reactive protein level
- Pregnancy test
- Cultures of lesions
- Comprehensive age- and gender-appropriate screening for malignancy
- Chest X-ray
- PET scan, ultrasound, CT or MRI for malignancy
- Bone marrow biopsy

▲▲ Management Pearls

- Consultations with the following specialties may be indicated: dermatology, hematology/oncology.
- If possible, withdraw any suspected triggering medication.

Therapy

- Maximize the treatment of any identified underlying condition.
- Corticosteroids, either systemically (prednisone 0.5 to 1.0 mg/kg p.o. daily and tapered over 4 to 6 weeks) or locally (clobetasol propionate 0.05% twice daily or intralesional injections of triamcinolone 3 to 10 mg/mL) are first-line treatment. In patients receiving oral prednisone, an additional 2 to 3 months of low-dose therapy may be useful to suppress recurrences. Pulsed dosing of intravenous methylprednisolone (up to 1 g daily for 3 to 5 days) is an alternative.

- Topical calcineurin inhibitors (tacrolimus or pimecrolimus) are alternatives to topical steroids in localized disease.
- Oral saturated solution of potassium iodide (SSKI or Lugol solution) is another commonly used agent. Begin SSKI at 5 drops in orange juice three times daily and advance daily 1 drop, as tolerated, to 15 drops three times daily. An alternative is potassiumiodide enteric-coated tablets 900 mg daily. In long-term use, monitor thyroid function.
- Colchicine (0.5 to 0.6 mg p.o. two to three times daily).
- Dapsone (100 to 200 mg p.o. daily), indomethacin (100 to 150 mg p.o. daily), and clofazimine (100 to 200 mg p.o. daily) have also been tried with some success. Doxycycline, cyclosporine, chlorambucil, metronidazole, etretinate, cyclophosphamide, etanercept, and interferon alpha have been used as well. Combination therapy may be useful.

Pediatric Patient Considerations

- Corticosteroids (prednisone 0.5 to 1.0 mg/kg/d) tapered over 4 to 6 weeks, are the treatment of choice.
- Alternatives to oral corticosteroids: oral saturated solution of SSKI, colchicine, dapsone, and clofazimine.

Suggested Readings

Douer D. The epidemiology of acute promyelocytic leukaemia. *Best Prac Res Clin Haematol.* 2003;16(3):357–367.

Li Y-S, Zhao Y-L, Jiang Q-P, et al. Specific chromosome changes and non-occupational exposure to potentially carcinogenic agents in acute leukemia in China. *Leukemia Res.* 1989;13(5):376.

Mahajan VK, Sharma NL, Sharma RC. Sweet's syndrome from an Indian perspective: A report of four cases and review of the literature. *Int J Dermatol.* 2006;45(6):702–708.

Mycobacterium marinum and Other Atypical Mycobacterial Infections

Pooja Sodha • Lynn McKinley-Grant

▪▪ Diagnosis Synopsis

Mycobacterium marinum, first isolated in 1926 and found to be a cause of human infection nearly 25 years later, is an uncommon atypical mycobacterial skin infection contracted from contaminated fish tanks, swimming pools, and, occasionally, ocean or lake water; hence the term fish tank or swimming pool granuloma. This organism has worldwide distribution, associated with aquatic environments. The most common site of infection is aquariums, since increased water disinfection methods have reduced swimming pool infection. Common vectors of human infection include fish, oysters, dolphins, tortoise, snails, and shrimps. Handling of these creatures or working in their environment is a strong clue to possible infection. Estimated incidence of *M. marinum* infection is approximately 0.27 cases per 100,000 inhabitants, though this is likely underreported due to challenges in diagnosis.

The typical skin lesion consists of a pustule or nodule that develops on an exposed extremity 2 to 3 weeks after exposure. Ulcers and proximal lymphatic spread are not commonly found. Since the organism grows best below 33°C and has inhibited growth above 37°C, cooler body extremities are more likely to be involved, and systemic infection is uncommon. Constitutional symptoms are rare, and fever, if present, is typically low-grade.

The disease is usually self-limited, and lesions tend to heal over a period of several months to years if left untreated. Persistent cross-reactivity with PPD is frequently produced. Since there are no clinically pathognomonic features, diagnosis is often delayed, increasing the risk of complications, including systemic infection, osteomyelitis, tenosynovitis, septic arthritis, and infiltrating skin lesions. Complications seem to be more common in women, as the lesions are often misdiagnosed initially as a rheumatological disease and treated with corticosteroids, facilitating spread of the infection.

As an opportunistic infection, minor trauma is a predisposing factor, but there is no reported human transmission. Aquarium enthusiasts are usually not aware of the risk of infection. Because of occupational risks (e.g., to fishermen), men are more commonly affected than women.

A genotypically related but phenotypically distinct relative of *M. marinum*, *M. ulcerans*, has been increasing in prevalence in Australia and West Africa with reports in tropical and subtropical environments. The related disease entity is known as Buruli ulcer, often unrecognized and untreated and occurring near water bodies. The infection is treatable, and often initially manifests as a painless, mobile nodule. Typical presentation is of extensive ulcers on the legs and arms owing to a toxin, mycolactone, which not only drives tissue destruction but also inhibits immune response. Due to the immune suppression, pain and fever are uncommon.

Increased susceptibility in immunocompromised hosts has not been seen.

At least 30 acid-fast bacilli other than those causing tuberculosis and leprosy have been identified. These are known as atypical mycobacteria (ATM). About a dozen of these may cause cutaneous disease; they are found worldwide in water, moist soil, house dust, dairy products, cold-blooded animals, vegetation, and human feces.

The most common of those causing disease in humans (often the immunocompromised) are *M. marinum*, *M. haemophilum*, *M. kansasii*, the rapidly growing members of the *M. fortuitum* complex (*M. fortuitum*, *M. chelonae/abscessus* group, and *M. smegmatis*), and *M. avium intracellulare*. A few other mycobacterial species are rarely reported in HIV-infected patients. These species rarely cause disease in the immunocompetent host.

Infection is acquired by inhalation, ingestion, or percutaneous penetration. Clinical presentation of disease depends upon the species, method of acquisition, and the host's immune state.

Infection presents as pulmonary disease, lymphadenitis, skin and soft tissue infection (the most common presentation in the immunocompetent), or disseminated disease.

Cutaneous lesions may be painful. Patients with pulmonary disease may have a chronic cough and hemoptysis. Those with disseminated disease may present with fatigue, night sweats, and weight loss. Signs of disease include lymphadenopathy, fever, rales, rhonchi, joint edema and erythema, heart murmur, and keratitis or corneal ulceration.

Immunocompromised Patient Considerations

The immunocompromised and the elderly are more at risk. Underlying factors include HIV, autoimmune disease, renal or cardiac transplantation, preceding lung disease, and chemotherapy. Systemic infection has been reported in immunocompromised patients, particularly after organ transplant, with HIV infection, with renal insufficiency, and after prolonged corticosteroid therapy. HIV infection has increased neither the prevalence of the infection nor variation by clinical presentation, course, or outcome.

◉ Look For

A pustule or nodule typically begins distally on an exposed extremity (usually the arm), which can later ulcerate and spread in a lymphangitic (sporotrichoid) fashion up the affected extremity (Fig. 4-571). Clustered plaques or nodules can become verrucous, thus mimicking the lesions of sporotrichosis and may ulcerate (Fig. 4-572). They may also eventually drain pus. Lesions may be painless or painful.

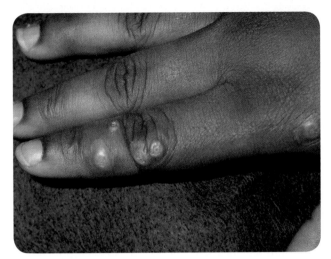

Figure 4-571 *Mycobacterium marinum* infection as firm nodules with a central crust.

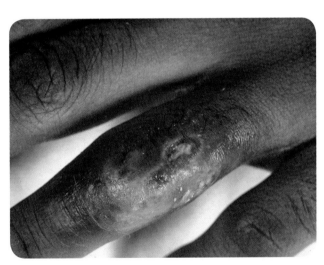

Figure 4-572 Ulcerated nodule caused by *M. marinum*.

Increasing joint stiffening may indicate progressing infection of deeper structures. Twenty percent of cases resemble sporotrichosis, with nodules extending along the lymphatics.

Most often seen on the elbows, knees, feet, and hands.

To guide therapy, clinical presentation has been grouped into three categories:

1. Self-limited verrucous exophytic lesions
2. Subcutaneous granulomas with or without ulceration
3. Infiltrating infection of synovium, tendons, bone

Diagnostic Pearls

- Take a careful history of relevant exposures, including hobbies and domestic animals, as patients may not be aware of known relations. No racial or ethnic group is naturally immune from these infections.

Immunocompromised Patient Considerations

This condition may be seen in an exaggerated fashion in immunosuppressed patients. Bone, synovial, and even systemic involvement may occur.

?? Differential Diagnosis and Pitfalls

- Other infections (sporotrichosis, blastomycosis, coccidioidomycosis, nocardiosis, tularemia, cutaneous tuberculosis, leishmaniasis, and actinomycosis) may have a similar lymphangitic spread from cutaneous inoculation. Exposure and travel history are key for diagnosis.
- The typical pattern of lymphangitic spread can suggest sporotrichosis.
- Sarcoidosis rarely ulcerates or spreads along lymphatics.
- Cellulitis has a background of erythema and a more rapid onset and spread.
- Cutaneous lymphoma may have associated fevers and weight loss.
- Sarcoma may have associated fevers and weight loss.
- Bacterial abscess has an acute onset.
- Pyoderma gangrenosum bleeds easily and appears vascular.
- Vasculitis does not usually have an exophytic growth pattern.
- Superficial thrombophlebitis
- Granuloma annulare rarely ulcerates.
- Hypertrophic lichen planus is highly pruritic and usually located on the shins.
- Foreign body reaction to sea urchin spines or barnacles

✓ Best Tests

- Skin biopsy with tissue culture. The culture results will identify the type of mycobacterium to help direct therapy. Care must be taken to inform the microbiology lab of the suspicion for atypical mycobacteria. Growth occurs on Lowenstein-Jensen slopes at 30°C to 33°C in 14 to 21 days, but may often be negative. Due to the photochromogenicity of the bacteria, colonies will change color from cream to yellow when exposed to light.
- Histological examination using Ziehl-Neelsen staining may reveal inflammatory skin infiltrate, acanthosis, ulceration, and granulomas, the latter of which is encouraging for atypical mycobacterium, but not confirmatory. Acid-fast bacilli may also be identified.
- PCR, due to its rapidity and sensitivity, can be used to detect mycobacterial DNA. However, unlike culture, it

cannot detect antimicrobial sensitivities necessary for optimal treatment.

- Consider imaging studies if tenosynovitis or osteomyelitis is suspected.

▲▲ Management Pearls

- The course is typically that of spontaneous resolution over a period of months to years. The purpose of therapy is to hasten recovery and prevent exacerbation of the disease. Biopsy and culture should be performed prior to commencing antibiotic therapy.
- Due to the temperature sensitivity of the bacteria, heat treatment of the infected area (gloves, hot water, or a heated arm band) has an adjunctive role in therapy. Irradiation has not been shown to be effective.
- Category 1 infections may resolve on their own or with single-agent chemotherapy as directed by culture sensitivities. If the lesion does not resolve, excision biopsy is recommended.
- Category 2 lesions should be excised for histology and empirical therapy initiated. Therapy can be tailored based on culture susceptibilities.
- Category 3 disease is concerning for deep tissue involvement. Tissue debridement with surgical exploration of associated sites of involvement is imperative. IV antibiotic treatment should be initiated. Amputation may be reserved for severe conditions unresponsive to the aforementioned options.

Therapy

Treatment is typically continued for 4 to 6 weeks after clinical resolution. The WHO recommends at least 8 weeks of treatment, and though treatment may rarely last 18 months or more, it averages around 3 months' duration.

Several antibiotic regimens have reported efficacy:

- Clarithromycin (500 mg p.o. twice daily), with ethambutol is a reliable option. Azithromycin may be an appropriate alternative.
- Minocycline or doxycycline therapy (100 mg p.o. twice daily)
- Rifampin (600 mg p.o. daily) plus ethambutol (1.2 g p.o. daily), generally for deep infections/Category 3
- Other effective antibiotics include trimethoprim-sulfamethoxazole, levofloxacin, and ciprofloxacin.

Monotherapy may have slow response, whereas dual therapy may be more effective, but consideration for tolerability/side effects, adherence, and cost is necessary.

Surgical methods (simple excision, incision and drainage, or electrodesiccation and curettage) may be employed for resistant solitary lesions.

Suggested Readings

Aubry A, Chosidow O, Caumes E, et al. Sixty-three cases of *Mycobacterium marinum* infection: Clinical features, treatment, and antibiotic susceptibility of causative isolates. *Arch Intern Med.* 2002;162:1746–1752.

Bhatty MA, Turner DPJ, Chamberlain ST. *Mycobacterium marinum* hand infection: Case reports and review of literature. *Br J Plast Surg.* 2000;53:161–165.

Dodiuk-Gad R, Dyachenko P, Ziv M, et al. Nontuberculous mycobacterial infections of the skin: A retrospective study of 25 cases. *J Am Acad Dermatol.* 2007;57:413–420.

Haddad V Jr, Lupi O, Lonza JP, et al. Tropical dermatology: Marine and aquatic dermatology. *J Am Acad Dermatol.* 2009;61:733–750.

Harris DM, Keating MR. *Mycobacterium marinum*: current recommended pharmacologic therapy. *J Hand Surg.* 2009;34(9):1734–1735.

Imakado S, Kojima Y, Hiyoshi T, et al. Disseminated *Mycobacterium marinum* infection in a patient with diabetic nephropathy. *Diabet Res Clin Pract.* 2009;83:E35–E36.

Loffeld A, Tan C. Fish tank granuloma in renal transplant and diabetic patient. *J Am Acad Dermatol.* 2005;52(Suppl 3):P119.

Pang H-N, Lee JY-L, Puhaindran ME, et al. *Mycobacterium marinum* as a cause of chronic granulomatous tenosynovitis in the hand. *J Infect.* 2007;54:584–588.

Streit M, Bohlen LM, Hunziker T, et al. Disseminated *Mycobacterium marinum* infection with extensive cutaneous eruption and bacteremia in an immunocompromised patient. *Eur J Dermatol.* 2006;16.1:79–83.

Torres F, Hodges T, Zamora MR. *Mycobacterium marinum* infection in a lung transplant recipient. *J Heart Lung Transpl.* 2001;20.4:486–489.

Furuncle and Carbuncle

Mat Davey

■ Diagnosis Synopsis

Furuncles are acute deep hair follicle infections most often associated with *Staphylococcus aureus* infections. Lesions are painful and may occur in crops and be associated with fever.

A carbuncle is the result of several furuncles converging to form a giant cyst with multiple sinuses. Recurrent furunculosis is often associated with nasal colonization of *S. aureus*.

Methicillin-resistant *S. aureus* (MRSA)–associated furunculosis is becoming increasingly common in the general community. Community-associated MRSA (CA-MRSA) among individuals who lack traditional risk factors for such infections (IV drug use, incarceration, participation in contact sports, etc.) is associated with a unique antibiotic susceptibility profile, and care must be taken to ensure appropriate initial antibiotic coverage.

◉ Look For

Furuncles are follicularly based and most often occur on the face, neck, extremities, or anogenital region as a red, tender, hard, or fluctuant mass (Figs. 4-573 and 4-574).

Carbuncles mostly occur at the nape of the neck and present as large, pus-filled plaques or nodules. Other locations of predilection include the posterior trunk and thigh.

●● Diagnostic Pearls

Furuncles caused by CA-MRSA can be necrotic and have been mistaken for spider bites.

With a carbuncle, look for multiheaded boils. The lesion may be fluctuant and is usually painful.

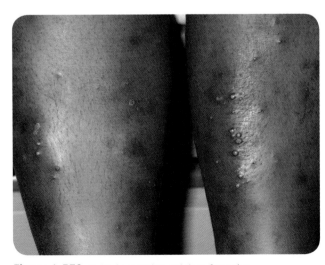

Figure 4-573 Multiple pustules and deep furuncles.

528

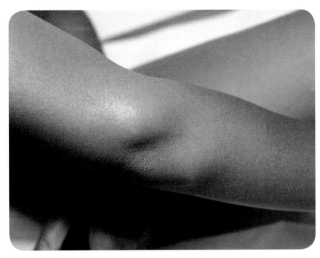

Figure 4-574 Multiple furuncles in a child due to *Staphylococcus*.

?? Differential Diagnosis and Pitfalls

Infectious

- Cellulitis or erysipelas
- Cat-scratch disease
- Atypical mycobacterial infections (*Mycobacterium marinum*)
- Deep fungal infection
- Herpetic whitlow

Noninfectious

- Ruptured subcutaneous cyst
- Gout
- Large dermal nodules of lymphoma/pseudolymphoma may mimic abscesses.
- Eosinophilic cellulitis

✓ Best Tests

- The diagnosis is usually clinically evident. If in doubt, needle or incisional aspiration of purulent material may be pursued.
- Gram and fungal stains of exudate or aspirate may yield immediate microbiologic diagnosis. Cultures take a few days (bacterial) to weeks (fungal) to yield results.
- Sensitivities on all cultures should be performed to determine antibiotic resistance.

▲▲ Management Pearls

- The mainstay of therapy of furuncles and carbuncles is early and adequate drainage. Care must be taken not to incise lesions that are incipient or acutely inflamed. Moist heat with warm saline compresses should be employed until the lesion becomes localized and displays definitive fluctuation. Incision and drainage is carried out with a No. 11 blade. If loculations are present, probing of the abscess may be necessary. Larger cavitations should be packed with iodoform gauze.

- In patients with recurrent furunculosis, eradication of MRSA nasal carriage may be accomplished by application of mupirocin 2% cream (twice daily for 5 days) to the nares. The combination of rifampin (600 mg daily for 10 days) plus trimethoprim and sulfamethoxazole (TMP/SMX)—one double-strength tab twice daily for 10 days—has also been shown to eradicate colonization.

Therapy

Incision and drainage is oftentimes curative; however, antibiotics may be employed, especially if the patient displays any systemic symptoms such as fevers/chills. Antibiotics are also indicated for concomitant cellulitis, multiple lesions, or if the patient is immunosuppressed. Antibiotic coverage must take into account the risk of MRSA. It is helpful to be aware of patterns of antimicrobial resistance within your local community.

In many communities, CA-MRSA is the most likely bacterial isolate; therefore, it is now recommended that initial antibiotic therapy cover CA-MRSA until culture data are available. Refer to current CDC guidelines, as treatment recommendations for MRSA are rapidly changing.

Patients exhibiting signs or symptoms of systemic involvement or with rapidly progressing infections or patients with significant comorbidities (e.g., immunosuppression) should be hospitalized for observation, and initiation of antibiotic covering MRSA should be pursued.

In systemically ill patients with atypical bacterial isolates, inpatient empiric IV antibiotics and supportive care must be pursued.

Pediatric Patient Considerations

In the neonatal period, consideration of intravenous antibiotics and acquisition of other cultures (blood and CSF) is mandatory, as the neonate is essentially immunocompromised.

For MRSA coverage, refer to current CDC guidelines, as treatment recommendations are rapidly changing.

Suggested Readings

Cohen PR. Community-acquired methicillin-resistant Staphylococcus aureus skin infections: Implications for patients and practioners. *Am J Clin Dermatol.* 2007;8(5):259–270. PubMed ID: 17902728.

Craft NC, Lee PK, Zipoli MT, et al. Superficial cutaneous infections and pyodermas. In: Fitzpatrick TB, Wolff K, eds. *Fitzpatrick's Dermatology in General Medicine.* 7th Ed. New York, NY: McGraw-Hill; 2008:1694–1703.

Daum RS. Clinical practice. Skin and soft-tissue infections caused by methicillin-resistant Staphylococcus aureus. *N Engl J Med.* 2007;357(4): 380–390. PubMed ID: 17652653.

Elston DM. Community-acquired methicillin-resistant Staphylococcus aureus. *J Am Acad Dermatol.* 2007;56(1):1–16; quiz 17–20. PubMed ID: 17190619.

James WD, Berger TG, Elston DM, eds. *Andrews' Diseases of the Skin: Clinical Dermatology.* 10th Ed. Philadelphia, PA: Saunders Elsevier; 2006: 251–264.

Pseudofolliculitis Barbae, Tinea Barbae, and Tinea Faciei

Suzanne Berkman

■■ Diagnosis Synopsis

Pseudofolliculitis Barbae

Pseudofolliculitis barbae (PFB) is a chronic inflammatory condition occurring primarily in individuals with tightly coiled hair. It is most common in men of African descent, affecting an estimated 45% to 83% of black patients who shave regularly, followed by those of Hispanic origin. It may also occur in women with hirsutism or who shave the bikini region. PFB is due to extrafollicular or transfollicular ingrown hair penetration resulting in inflammation and a foreign body giant cell reaction surrounding an ingrown hair. A single-nucleotide polymorphism giving rise to a disruptive A1a12Thr substitution in the 1A α-helical segment of the companion layer-specific keratin K6hf may be partially responsible for the phenotypic expression, representing a genetic risk factor for PFB.

Tinea Barbae

Tinea barbae, also known as tinea sycosis or barber's itch, is a rare dermatophytosis affecting the bearded areas of the face and neck. It is often associated with pet or farm animal contact. Two clinical types exist: a deep type due to *Trichophyton mentagrophytes* or *T. verrucosum*, and a superficial type due to *T. violaceum* or *T. rubrum*.

Tinea Faciei

Tinea faciei, also known as tinea faciale, is an uncommon superficial dermatophyte infection occurring in the non-bearded areas of the face. It occurs more commonly in tropical climates. In the United States, it is most commonly caused by *T. tonsurans*, *T. rubrum*, and *Microsporum canis*. Zoophilic dermatophytes, such as *T. verrucosum* and *M. canis*, may also be implicated in association with livestock and pets.

◉ Look For

Pseudofolliculitis Barbae

In PFB, look for multiple, moderately inflammatory lesions concentrated on facial and neck areas with prominent hairs. The mustache area is usually not affected. The eruption is papular and/or pustular, especially in acute lesions, which may bleed easily with shaving (Figs. 4-575–4-577). Hyperpigmentation is common in darker skin types; papules and pustules may resolve with scarring and, in severe cases, large

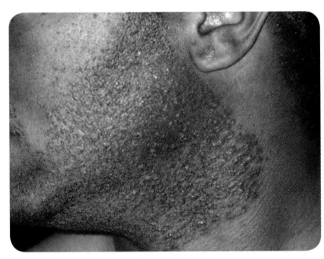

Figure 4-576 Sharply bordered large grouping of PFB papules in the beard region and on the neck.

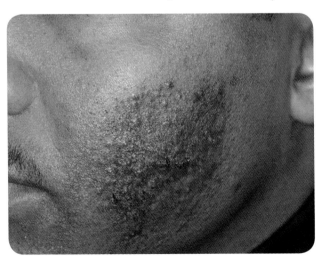

Figure 4-575 Multiple uniform papules without scaling in the beard region in PFB.

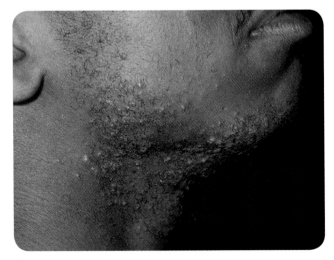

Figure 4-577 PFB with multiple irregular papules and pustules on the face and neck.

530

keloids. In advanced disease, cutaneous grooves containing facial hair are seen.

Tinea Barbae

The deep type of tinea barbae due to zoophilic organisms presents with intense inflammation and multiple follicular pustules (Fig. 4-578). Abscesses and kerionlike swellings may develop. Patients may have constitutional symptoms, including malaise and lymphadenopathy. The superficial type presents with a less inflammatory folliculitis.

Tinea Faciei

Has annular (round) scaly, erythematous plaques on the face or neck. In darker skin types, the erythema may be less conspicuous, but the abundant scale can be seen (Figs. 4-579

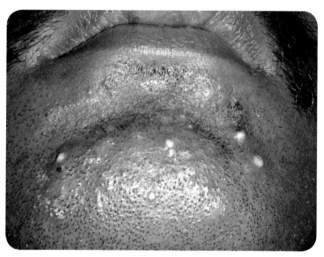

Figure 4-578 Tinea barbae with large pustules and papules and a red serpiginous border in some locations.

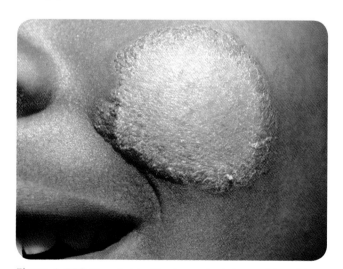

Figure 4-579 Tinea faciei with a large raised plaque with peripheral scale.

and 4-580). Plaques have an active advancing edge with prominent scale with associated fungal hyphae on potassium hydroxide (KOH) examination. The central clearing of the elevated lesions leads to the appearance of annular shape (with a ringlike depressed center); thus the description "ringworm" (a misnomer).

Diagnostic Pearls

Pseudofolliculitis Barbae

Examine hairs with a magnifying glass (for hair curvature); hairs can be removed from the papules with a fine needle or toothpick. Do not pluck these hairs but gently lift the end away from the skin surface.

Tinea Barbae

Tinea barbae can be differentiated from bacterial folliculitis in that it usually spares the upper lip, is often unilateral, and hairs can be removed easily and painlessly.

Tinea Faciei

Tinea faciei is difficult to diagnose clinically and often presents with atypical features. It is known to mimic many skin diseases, especially photosensitive skin disorders, such as lupus erythematosus.

?? Differential Diagnosis and Pitfalls

Pseudofolliculitis Barbae and Tinea Barbae

- Bacterial (staphylococcal) folliculitis
- Acne vulgaris
- Viral infections (herpes simplex or zoster)

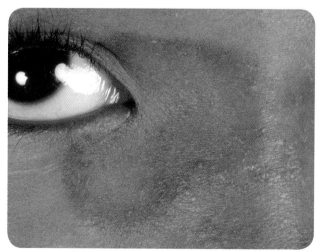

Figure 4-580 Scaling, red, well-demarcated plaque of tinea faciei.

Tinea Faciei

The differential diagnosis for tinea faciei includes the following: seborrheic dermatitis, cutaneous candidiasis, atopic dermatitis, bacterial infections, irritant contact dermatitis, granuloma annulare, systemic lupus erythematosus, discoid lupus erythematosus, bullous lupus erythematosus, drug-induced lupus, perioral dermatitis, pityriasis alba, pityriasis rosea, rosacea, sarcoidosis, *Aspergillus* infections under applied tape in neonates, neonatal lupus erythematosus, and *Demodex* folliculitis.

✓ Best Tests

Pseudofolliculitis Barbae

PFB is a clinical diagnosis.

Tinea Barbae and Tinea Faciei

KOH preparation and a fungal culture should be performed in all cases of possible tinea barbae or faciei. It should be performed at the periphery of lesions, where there are more fungal elements. Culture on Sabouraud agar may identify the causative pathogen. Up to 30% of culture results may be negative. Histopathologic evaluation with hematoxylin and eosin staining and periodic acid-Schiff may establish the diagnosis.

▲▲ Management Pearls

Pseudofolliculitis Barbae

- All treatments for PFB should attempt to eliminate or reduce the foreign body reaction surrounding ingrown hairs. Patient education is essential. Discontinuation of shaving should be encouraged. If patient is able to tolerate, depilatories are preferred. The hair on the face should be as long as tolerable before shaving. The patient should examine the skin prior to shaving to be sure no ends of the hair are growing back into the skin. Any early ingrown hairs should be gently lifted (not plucked) before shaving. Hair should be removed with clean electric clippers when beard hair is as long as socially acceptable.
- If shaving with a razor is preferred, patients should be counseled about proper shaving technique. It is important to wash with an antibacterial cleanser, hydrate the beard area with a moist hot towel, and apply a cream, gel, or foam lubricant. The use of double, triple, and quadruple blade systems, which give very close shaves, should be avoided. A single-edged polymer-coated blade can be used to shave along the grain. After shaving, the patient can use products that calm the skin and prevent infection: topical antibiotics, aftershave soothing gels, Bump Stopper (a sulfur-based product).

Tinea Barbae and Tinea Faciei

Antifungal-corticosteroid preparations are not recommended in the treatment of superficial fungal infections because they may be associated with persistent and recurrent infections. Tinea faciei treated with topical steroids becomes tinea incognito with the loss of its characteristic features.

Therapy

Pseudofolliculitis Barbae

Medical therapy of PFB includes the application of low-potency to midpotency topical steroids in the morning after shaving and topical retinoids at night. Pustular lesions respond to topical and oral antibiotics with anti-inflammatory activity. Benzoyl peroxide 5%-clindamycin 1% gel has been shown to be effective in a double-blind study.

Chemical depilatories (e.g., barium sulfide and calcium thioglycolate) can be used, but these have a high risk of irritant contact dermatitis. Eflornithine hydrochloride cream, which inhibits ornithine decarboxylase, may be used as an adjunct but can cause hair to remain under the skin longer. Salicylic acid chemical peels may be of some benefit in PFB.

Laser hair removal may offer permanent hair reduction and is strongly recommended for PFB. Laser surgery experience with pigmented skin is required. The longer-wavelength lasers, such as the 1,064-nm Nd:YAG or 810-nm diode laser, are more suitable and safer for dark skin types. Laser treatment can significantly reduce both hair and inflammatory papules and pustules.

Tinea Barbae

Oral antifungal agents are required for tinea barbae, in the same doses and duration as for tinea capitis. Topical agents are only helpful as adjunctive therapy. Additional adjunctive measures include shaving/depilation and warm compresses to remove crusts.

- Terbinafine—250 mg p.o. daily for 4 weeks
- Itraconazole —200 mg twice daily for 2 weeks
- Griseofulvin ultramicrosize—330 to 375 mg p.o. twice daily or daily for 4 to 8 weeks

Tinea Faciei

Tinea faciei generally responds well to topical antifungal therapy. Oral antifungal agents may be used for widespread infections. If fungal folliculitis is present, oral medication is required. Infection in pets should be identified and treated, or reinfection is likely.

Limited

Use topical antifungals for 2 to 6 weeks, based on clinical response:

- Terbinafine 1% cream—Apply once to twice daily (7.5, 15 g tubes).
- Clotrimazole 1% cream—Apply twice daily (15, 30, 45, 90 g tubes).

Alternatives

- Econazole cream—Apply once to twice daily (15, 30, 85 g tubes).
- Oxiconazole cream—Apply twice daily (15, 30 g tubes).
- Ketoconazole cream—Apply twice daily (15, 30, 60 g tubes).

Extensive Disease or Disease Unresponsive to Topicals

- Terbinafine—250 mg daily for 2 weeks
- Itraconazole—100 to 200 mg daily for 2 to 4 weeks or 200 mg twice daily for 1 week
- Griseofulvin ultramicrosize—330 to 375 mg daily for 4 to 8 weeks

Pediatric Patient Considerations

Tinea
Topical Antifungals

- Econazole—Apply once to twice daily (15, 30, 85 g tubes).
- Oxiconazole creams—Apply twice daily (15, 30 g tubes).
- Ketoconazole cream—Apply twice daily (15, 30, 60 g tubes).

Over-the-Counter Topical Antifungals

- Terbinafine cream—Apply twice daily (24 g tubes).
- Clotrimazole cream (generic)—Apply twice daily (15, 30 g tubes).

Severe Cases (Older Children)

- Griseofulvin ultramicrosize—5 mg/kg/d for 4 to 6 weeks
- Terbinafine (250 mg/d) for older children weighing over 40 kg
- Alternatives include itraconazole.

Suggested Readings

Bonifaz A, Ramírez-Tamayo T, Saúl A. Tinea barbae (tinea sycosis): Experience with nine cases. *J Dermatol.* 2003;30:898–903.

Bridgeman-Shah S. The medical and surgical therapy of pseudofolliculitis barbae. *Dermatol Ther.* 2004;17:158–163.

Cook-Bolden FE, Barba A, Halder R, et al. Twice-daily applications of benzoyl peroxide 5%/clindamycin 1% gel versus vehicle in the treatment of pseudofolliculitis barbae. *Cutis.* 2004;73:18–24.

Lin RL, Szepietowski JC, Schwartz RA. Tinea faciei, an often deceptive facial eruption. *Int J Dermatol.* 2004;43:437–440.

Meymandi S, Wiseman MC, Crawford RI. Tinea faciei mimicking cutaneous lupus erythematosus: A histopathologic case report. *J Am Acad Dermatol.* 2003;48:S7–S8.

Perry PK, Cook-Bolden FE, Rahman Z, et al. Defining pseudofolliculitis barbae in 2001: A review of the literature and current trends. *J Am Acad Dermatol.* 2002;46:S113–S119.

Quarles FN, Brody H, Johnson BA, et al. Pseudofolliculitis barbae. *Dermatol Ther.* 2007;20:133–136.

Schulze R, Meehan KJ, Lopez A, et al. Low-fluence 1064-nm laser hair reduction for pseudofolliculitis barbae in skin types IV, V, and VI. *Dermatol Surg.* 2009;35:98–107.

Smith EP, Winstanley D, Ross EV. Modified superlong pulse 810 nm diode laser in the treatment of pseudofolliculitis barbae in skin types V and VI. *Dermatol Surg.* 2005;31:297–301.

Facial Dermatitis—Rosacea and Perioral Dermatitis

Pooja Sodha • Lynn McKinley-Grant

■■ Diagnosis Synopsis

Rosacea is a common, chronic inflammatory condition of unknown etiology with a relapsing-remitting course. It presents with facial flushing and localized erythema, telangiectases, papules, and pustules on the nose, cheeks, brow, and chin. There are four main subtypes of the disease: erythematotelangiectatic, papulopustular, phymatous, and ocular rosacea.

Erythematotelangiectatic rosacea has flushing and prolonged erythema and redness of the central portion of the face. Patients often complain of stinging or burning sensations on the skin. This is the most common subtype, accounting for between 72% and 96% of cases.

In papulopustular rosacea, acneiform papules and pustules predominate; there is also erythema and edema of the central face with relative sparing of the periocular areas. In papulopustular rosacea, dramatic swelling can result in lymphedematous changes with solid facial edema or lead to phymatous changes.

In patients with the phymatous subtype of rosacea, chronic inflammation and edema result in marked thickening of the skin with sebaceous hyperplasia, resulting in an enlarged, cobblestoned appearance of affected skin, most commonly on the nose (rhinophyma). Men are more often affected.

Ocular rosacea presents with conjunctivitis, blepharitis, and hyperemia. Patients complain of dry, irritated, itchy eyes. Keratitis, scleritis, and iritis are potential but infrequent complications. The extent of ocular involvement has not been shown to correlate with the severity of cutaneous manifestations. The incidence of eye involvement in rosacea has been estimated between 3% and 58% and may precede cutaneous presentations. Ocular rosacea is more common in individuals of African descent than in whites.

In each of the subtypes, patients typically present with some but not all of the associated findings. In addition, granulomatous rosacea is comprised of papules, nodules, and yellow-brown pustules that are distributed on the central face, eyelids, forehead, cheeks, nasolabial folds, and periocular and perioral regions. It is often described as noninflammatory and may be unilateral. Flushing is less common. African Americans with seborrheic dermatitis who oil their scalp to alleviate the dryness will also apply creams and steroid creams to their midface and may develop granulomatous rosacea.

Rosacea fulminans (pyoderma faciale) refers to the sudden onset of severe facial pustulation with abscess and sinus tract formation, most commonly in young women. Systemic signs and symptoms are present.

The etiology of rosacea is poorly understood, but cutaneous vascular changes and environmental exposures, such as infectious agents, sunlight, and certain foods or drugs, may play a role. Ultraviolet (UV) light exposure has been suggested to play a causative role, since biopsy often shows solar elastosis, but this connection has not been definitively shown. Infectious causes such as *Demodex* mites and *Helicobacter pylori* have been implicated but not proved. Genetic factors are supported by cases of familial rosacea, but the genetics is not clear.

The prevalence of rosacea is estimated to be between 0.09% and 10%, with variations depending on population groups examined. Rosacea is less common in skin types IV to VI than in types I to III possibly because darker skin types are less prone to photodamage, and flushing is harder to visualize.

Erythematotelangiectatic rosacea is the most common subtype independent of age and sex. Rosacea commonly develops in individuals between the ages of 30 and 50. While women tend to present at a younger age than men, overall prevalence is equal in men and women.

Fair-skinned individuals (skin types I to III) with brown hair and blue eyes are primarily affected, though the disease is seen in Mediterranean, Asian, and African skin types as well. In a study of Korean patients with skin types II, III, IV, and V, it was found that a strong correlation existed between erythematotelangiectatic rosacea and ocular disease. Chronic sun exposure, hot baths, exercise, and alcohol ingestion were associated with aggravation of erythematotelangiectatic rosacea in this Asian population.

Since rosacea manifests on the most visible portion of a patient's body, the face, it is important to recognize that this disease can have psychosocial consequences. Some patients experience stressful life events prior to presenting with cutaneous disease. Moreover, rosacea symptoms, such as flushing, and treatment side effects may further limit quality of life.

Perioral dermatitis (including steroid-induced rosacea) is a localized inflammatory disorder of uncertain etiology. It is erythematous papular and pustular eruption with fine scaling, peeling, and microvesicles involving the nasolabial folds, chin, and upper lip with a narrow zone of spared skin adjacent to the vermilion border. It is seen almost exclusively in women between 18 and 40 and in children between 3 and 11 years of age. A number of factors have been implicated, but medications such as topical glucocorticoids (including inhalers) and oral contraceptives are frequent etiologies.

With topical steroid-induced dermatitis, the phenomenon is typically seen in subjects who use the steroid for a primary dermatosis. Because of continued misuse of the topical agent, they are prone to develop symptoms such as erythema, burning, itching, and papulopustular eruption. Sun exposure can worsen symptoms. South Asian cultures often use topical steroids as fairness creams or cosmetic enhancers; so consider this diagnosis in these populations.

Pediatric Patient Considerations

Rosacea and its ocular manifestations are rare in children, but many other associated symptoms such as conjunctivitis, sties, chalazia, and blepharitis are common in children. It has been reported that children who were diagnosed with a stye were more likely to develop rosacea in adulthood, particularly if the diagnosis occurred after age 10.

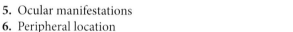 Look For

Rosacea is one of the classic causes of the "red face." Diagnosis is made clinically, as there is no specific laboratory test, using the following guidelines recommended by the Expert Committee (see *J Am Acad Dermatol.* 2002; 46:584–587).

Presence of one or more of the following primary features (Figs. 4-581–4-583):

1. Flushing
2. Nontransient erythema
3. Papules and pustules
4. Telangiectases

May include one or more of the following secondary features:

1. Burning or stinging
2. Plaque
3. Dry appearance
4. Edema
5. Ocular manifestations
6. Peripheral location
7. Phymatous changes

Common features of rosacea subtypes:

- Erythematotelangiectatic—flushing and persistent central facial erythema with or without telangiectasia
- Papulopustular—persistent central facial erythema with transient, central facial papules or pustules or both
- Phymatous—thickening skin, irregular surface nodularities, and enlargement. May occur on the nose, chin, forehead, cheeks, or ears
- Granulomatous variant—noninflammatory; hard; brown, yellow, or red cutaneous papules; or nodules of uniform size

Extrafacial involvement is rare, but the disease may involve the neck and superior chest.

Rosacea fulminans presents with pustules, nodules, and abscesses with sinus tract formation.

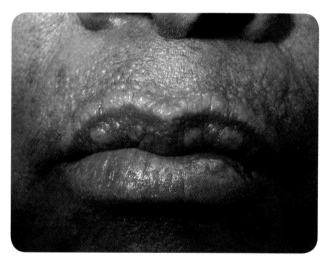

Figure 4-582 Granulomatous rosacea on upper lip and vermilion border in granulomatous rosacea.

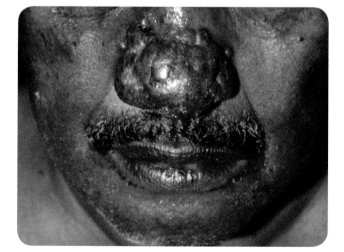

Figure 4-581 Rosacea with multiple nose papules and nodules requires biopsy to exclude sarcoidosis.

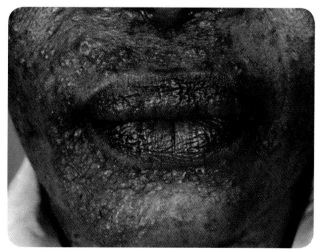

Figure 4-583 Multiple, very inflammatory papules associated with rosacea.

Perioral dermatitis presents as monomorphous red papules, both grouped and individual, on the chin, lips, and nasolabial folds. There may be pustules, and there may be associated scaling and erythema. On occasion, lesions are periocular but characteristically spare the skin immediately adjacent to the vermilion border. In African Americans, pustules can predominate. There may be associated scaling and pigmented plaques that appear as seborrheic dermatitis, atopic dermatitis, or postinflammatory hyperpigmentation.

- Rosacea patients do not have comedones, which are frequently seen in acne.
- Seborrheic dermatitis is commonly observed in patients who also have rosacea.
- Perioral dermatitis is differentiated from rosacea based on the absence of flushing and telangiectases. Perioral dermatitis also tends to occur in a younger age group. Perioral dermatitis in patients of African decent can appear pustular like acne. It may also cause postinflammatory hyperpigmentation or hypopigmentation (Figs. 4-584–4-588).

Diagnostic Pearls

- Ask the patient about ocular symptoms; many patients experience a gritty sensation in their eyes and have evidence of conjunctivitis, episcleritis, iritis, and keratitis. Further evaluation by an ophthalmologist may be useful.

?? Differential Diagnosis and Pitfalls

Erythematotelangiectatic Rosacea

- Menopause, "hot flashes"
- Carcinoid syndrome

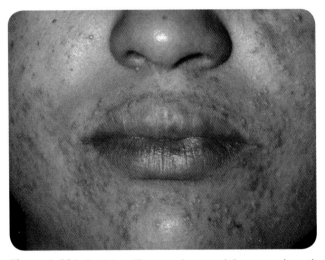

Figure 4-584 Multiple uniform papules around the nose and mouth suggest perioral dermatitis.

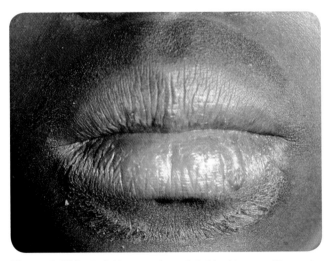

Figure 4-586 Lip licking must be excluded in this case with a perioral distribution.

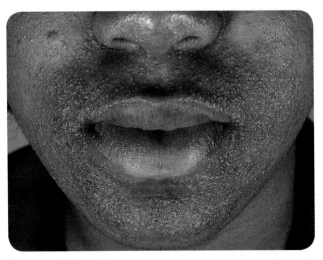

Figure 4-585 Multiple closely grouped papules around the mouth with minimum redness suggest perioral dermatitis.

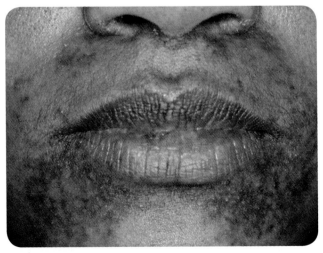

Figure 4-587 Perioral dermatitis frequently leads to hyperpigmented lesions in darker skin types.

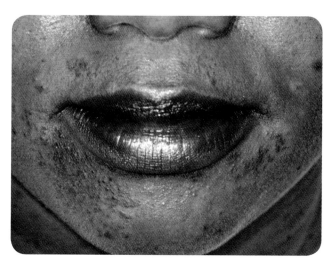

Figure 4-588 Typical papules of perioral dermatitis limited to perioral location; there is often an uninvolved region close to the vermilion borders.

- Pheochromocytoma
- Medullary thyroid carcinoma and VIPoma
- Lupus erythematosus
- Seborrheic dermatitis
- Photodermatitis—Expect to see photodistribution.
- Mastocytosis

Papulopustular Rosacea

- Acne vulgaris
- Perioral dermatitis (periorificial dermatitis)—This is also a clinical diagnosis based on uniformity of papules and characteristic distributions.
- Bromoderma
- Folliculitis
- Gram-negative folliculitis
- Sarcoidosis
- Demodicidosis
- Pyoderma faciale

Perioral Dermatitis

- Rosacea
- Granulomatous periorificial dermatitis
- Lupus miliaris disseminata faciei
- Seborrheic dermatitis
- Atopic dermatitis
- Contact dermatitis
- Gram-negative folliculitis
- Acne

✓ Best Tests

- This is a clinical diagnosis. A skin biopsy could be suggestive of the diagnosis but is not confirmatory.

- Serology to rule out lupus erythematosus with other symptoms

▲▲ Management Pearls

- In severe cases, use of both an oral and topical therapy is often warranted.
- Advise patients to avoid triggers that aggravate vasodilation (e.g., coffee, tea, hot drinks in general, spicy foods, chocolate, and alcohol). Encourage the use of sunscreens and sun-protective clothing.
- Patients with long-standing or severe rosacea should be seen by an ophthalmologist.
- If the perioral dermatitis was triggered by the use of mid-potency or high-potency topical steroids (as in steroid rosacea), then use low-potency class 6 or 7 steroids to taper because the disorder will flare if corticosteroids are discontinued abruptly. Patients must be warned that their skin will likely flare before it improves after the topical steroid is stopped.
- Postinflammatory hyperpigmentation is the most disturbing feature of rosacea to the patient with pigmented skin. Treatment may require combination with hydroquinones and other skin lighteners.

Therapy

Conservative Therapy

- Appropriate use of broad-spectrum sunscreens and sun avoidance are also important. Unfortunately, certain preservative ingredients can be particularly irritating and further complicate erythema. Silicones, as in dimethicone or cyclomethicone, are noncomedogenic and nonirritating and can be found in certain brands. Zinc oxide and titanium oxide are best tolerated and provide optimum coverage against UVA and UVB.
- Facial cleansers should be soap free. Avoid astringents, toners, and menthol- and camphor-containing products.
- Camouflage make-up and concealers with green- or yellow-based preparations are helpful in masking underlying redness. These should also contain silicones. Powder base is best.

Topical Therapies

There are many topical medications that are reported to be effective in the treatment of rosacea. These topical agents are most effective in papulopustular rosacea. Only specific metronidazole preparations and 15% azelaic acid gel have an FDA indication for rosacea.

(Continued)

Topical therapies for rosacea include the following:

- Metronidazole cream, gel (Pregnancy category B)
- Sodium sulfacetamide lotion, wash (Pregnancy category C; contraindicated in those with sulfonamide allergy)
- Azelaic acid 15% gel (Pregnancy category B)
- Erythromycin and clindamycin lotion, solution (Pregnancy category B)
- Benzoyl peroxide 5% to 10% cream, lotion, gel, or wash (Pregnancy category C; use with caution in those with sensitive skin but otherwise very efficient therapy)
- Calcineurin inhibitors such as tacrolimus ointment and pimecrolimus cream
- Tretinoin cream, gel (Pregnancy class C)

Systemic Therapies

Tetracyclines are a mainstay of therapy in rosacea and are first line: tetracycline 500 to 1,000 mg twice daily OR doxycycline 100 to 200 mg daily OR minocycline 50 mg twice daily for at least 2 to 3 months, then taper to one pill daily. Oral erythromycin is also a good choice: 250 to 500 mg twice daily. Low-dose doxycycline (20 mg twice daily or 40 mg slow release form daily) has also shown effectiveness for rosacea.

Alternative Regimens

- Oral metronidazole 200 mg twice daily
- Azithromycin 250 to 500 mg daily three time weekly
- Isotretinoin is also effective in treating severe papulopustular rosacea and rosacea fulminans.

Therapies aimed at specific disease manifestations and subtypes include the following:

- Telangiectases/erythematotelangiectasia rosacea—vascular lasers (pulsed dye, potassium-titanyl-phosphate [KTP], etc.), intense pulsed light therapy, camouflage cosmetics
- Flushing—clonidine 0.05 mg twice daily (appropriate for alcohol-induced rosacea flushing, but no general flushing associated with disease). *Note*: the following treatments are appropriate when the physician is experienced with these agents—naloxone (as there may be relation to opioid signaling pathways), intense pulsed light, pulsed dye laser, beta-blockers (nadolol 40 mg daily)
- Rhinophyma—surgical paring/sculpting, electrosurgery, and laser (argon, carbon dioxide, Nd:YAG [neodymium-yttrium-aluminum-garnet])
- Rosacea fulminans—prednisolone 1 mg/kg daily is usually required while isotretinoin is being initiated and then tapered over several weeks. Isotretinoin therapy is continued for several months.

In dark skin, risk of laser therapy often involves dyschromia (hyperpigmentation or hypopigmentation). Nd-YAG coupled with cooling regimens reduces papule eruption. Skin pretreated with topical retinoids often has more postlaser erythema.

In patients with a history of steroid-induced dermatitis, topical corticosteroids should be discontinued with tapering as necessary. Topical tacrolimus ointment 0.1% has been shown to be beneficial in these patients.

Topical and oral antibiotics may also be used. These are of particular value in patients with no history of topical steroid use.

Topical Antibiotics

- Topical erythromycin solution applied to affected area twice daily
- Topical metronidazole (0.75% gel) applied to affected area twice daily
- Topical azelaic acid (20% cream) applied to affected area twice daily
- Topical clindamycin lotion applied to the affected area twice daily

Oral Antibiotics

- Tetracycline 500 mg p.o. twice daily for 1 month, then taper to once daily for 2 weeks
- Doxycycline 100 mg p.o. twice daily for 1 month, then taper slowly over several weeks
- Erythromycin 333 mg p.o. every 8 hours

Treatment is often required for several months.

Suggested Readings

Alster TS, Lupton JR. Prevention and treatment of side effects and complications of cutaneous laser resurfacing. *Plast Reconstruct Surg.* 2002;109.1:308–316.

Askoy B, Altaykan-Hapa A, Egemen D, et al. The impact of rosacea on quality of life: Effects of demographic and clinical characteristics and various treatment modalities. *Br J Dermatol.* 2010;163(4):719–725.

Bae YI, Yun S-J, Lee J-B, et al. Clinical evaluation of 168 korean patients with rosacea: The sun exposure correlates with the erythematotelangiectatic subtype. *Ann Dermatol.* 2009;21.3:243–249.

Bamford JTM, Gessery CE, Renier CM, et al. Childhood stye and adult rosacea. *J Am Acad Dermatol.* 2006;55:951–955.

Coley MK, Alexis AF. Managing common dermatoses in skin of color. *Semin Cutan Med Surg.* 2009;28:63–70.

Crawford GH, Pelle MT, James WD. Rosacea: I. Etiology, pathogenesis, and subtype classification. *J Am Acad Dermatol.* 2004;51:327–341.

Kyriakis KP, Palamaras I, Terzoudi S, et al. Epidemiologic aspects of rosacea. *J Am Acad Dermatol*. 2005;53.5:918–920.

McAleer MA, Fitzpatrick P, Powell FC. Papulopustular rosacea: Prevalence and relationship to photodamage. *J Am Acad Dermatol*. 2010;63:33–39.

Pelle MT, Crawford GH, James WD. Rosacea: II. Therapy. *J Am Acad Dermatol*. 2004;51:499–512.

Utas S, Ozbakir O, Turasan A, et al. *Helicobacter pylori* eradication treatment reduces the severity of rosacea. *J Am Acad Dermatol*. 1999;40: 433–435.

Wilkin J, Dahl M, Detmar M, et al. Standard classification of rosacea: Report of the national rosacea society expert committee on the classification and staging of rosacea. *J Am Acad Dermatol*. 2002;46.4:584–587.

Acne

Mat Davey

Diagnosis Synopsis

Acne, or acne vulgaris, is an extremely common, usually self-limited chronic inflammatory condition of the pilosebaceous unit, which typically begins at puberty as a result of androgen stimulation of the pilosebaceous unit and changes in the keratinization at the follicular orifice. Acne can last through the teenage years into adulthood. Clinical manifestations range widely from a mild comedonal form to a severe inflammatory nodular variant known as acne conglobata. There is no ethnic predilection, although nodulocystic acne has been reported to be more common in white men than in men of African descent. Family history of severe acne, while nonspecific, is often helpful in predicting disease course.

Multiple acne variants exist. Acne fulminans is the most severe form of nodulocystic acne and is associated with fever and peripheral leukocytosis. Acne excoriée, an uncommon variant seen mostly among young women, consists of extensive neurotic excoriations and may suggest underlying depression, anxiety, or a personality disorder. Neonatal acne occurs in infants at approximately 2 weeks of age and spontaneously resolves in the first few months. It is characterized by inflamed papules in the absence of comedones and is thought by many to be a variant of benign cephalic pustulosis; it has been attributed to overgrowth of *Malassezia* species. Infantile acne occurs later, at 3 to 6 months of age, and is associated with comedones. Etiology is postulated to be secondary to hormonal imbalances, an immature adrenal gland with elevated dehydroepiandrosterone (DHEA) and elevated luteinizing hormone (LH), often noted in infant boys.

Medication and systemic disease can result in acneiform eruptions. Steroid acne, also known as steroid folliculitis, follows exposure to topical or systemic glucocorticoids. In contrast to acne vulgaris, this eruption appears mainly on the trunk and upper arms, and it lacks comedones. Other medications commonly associated with acneiform eruptions include anabolic steroids, phenytoin, lithium, isoniazid, halogenated compounds, and epidermal growth factor receptor inhibitors.

Look For

Open comedones (blackheads), closed comedones (whiteheads), and erythematous papules and pustules. Nodules and cysts can result in pitted or hypertrophic scars. In adult women, deeper-seated, tender, red papules are common along the jawline. Acne most frequently targets the face, neck, upper trunk, and upper arms (Figs. 4-589–4-594).

In darker-skinned individuals, open and closed comedones are subtle in comparison to white skin. Look for

hyperpigmented and red/brown papules and pustules. Prolonged hyperpigmentation after resolution of acute acne lesions commonly occurs.

Patients with acne fulminans are febrile with systemic complaints, which may include polyarthralgia, myalgias, malaise, anorexia, and weight loss. Tender spleen, arthralgia, and bone pain from aseptic osteolysis have been reported.

Medication-induced acneiform eruptions often present on the trunk, shoulders, and upper arms. The eruption typically consists of monomorphous, small papules and pustules, all in the same stage of development (Fig. 4-595). Comedones are uncommon.

Pediatric Patient Considerations

In neonatal acne, small inflamed papules and pustules occur primarily on the cheeks (Figs. 4-596–4-598). Comedones are rare. In infantile acne, inflammatory papules, pustules, and open and closed comedones occur primarily on the cheeks.

Diagnostic Pearls

- In adult women, touching, rubbing, and overcleansing the face may exacerbate acne. In men, acne tends to be more severe on the trunk. Consider external agents such as oils from hair preparations (pomade acne), grease from working in fast-food restaurants, occlusion from sports equipment, etc., all of which can exacerbate acne. Medications (e.g., progesterone-only birth control, steroids, some anticonvulsants, lithium, isoniazid) may aggravate acne.

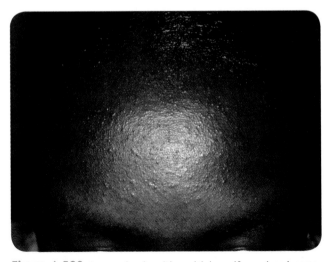

Figure 4-589 Acne vulgaris with multiple uniform closed comedones on the forehead.

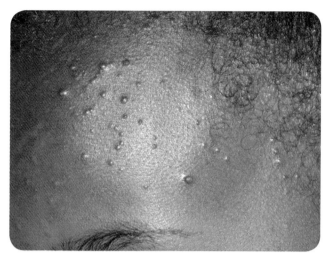

Figure 4-590 Acne vulgaris with multiple closed comedones on the forehead.

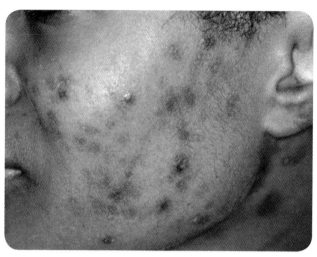

Figure 4-591 Acne vulgaris in deeply pigmented skin is frequently hyperpigmented.

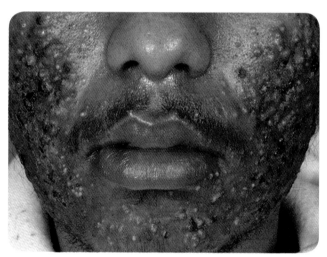

Figure 4-592 Bilateral keloidal scarring associated with acne vulgaris.

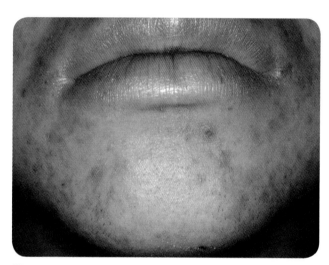

Figure 4-593 Acne with excoriations and hyperpigmentation.

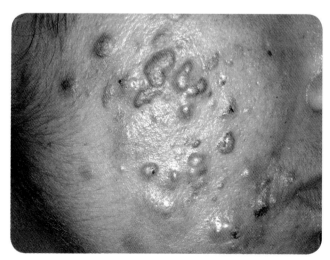

Figure 4-594 Acne with deep and raised inflammatory nodules and cysts.

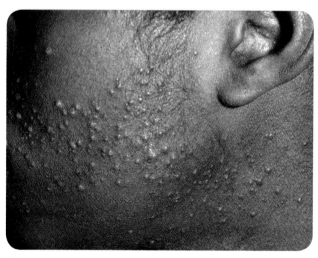

Figure 4-595 Steroid acne with multiple papules and small cysts associated with systemic corticosteroid therapy.

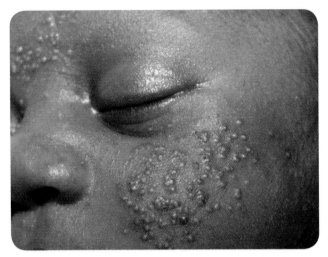

Figure 4-596 Neonatal acne (benign cephalic pustulosis) with multiple uniform red papules.

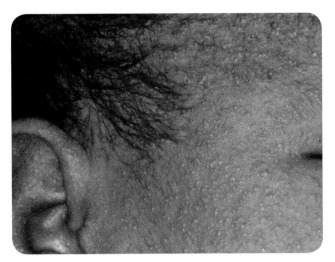

Figure 4-598 Regular papules of infantile acne.

- In women, if there is a perioral predilection, this may represent perioral dermatitis, not acne.
- In patients with acne excoriée, refer to a mental health professional if there is suspicion of an underlying psychiatric illness.

?? Differential Diagnosis and Pitfalls

- Perioral dermatitis
- Milia
- Folliculitis
- *Malassezia* folliculitis
- Flat warts
- Molluscum contagiosum
- Rosacea
- Sebaceous hyperplasia
- Benign appendageal lesions—for example, syringomas
- Angiofibromas in tuberous sclerosis
- Steatocystoma multiplex

Pediatric Patient Differential Diagnosis

- Miliaria rubra and pustulosa
- Milia
- Congenital candidiasis
- Eosinophilic pustular folliculitis
- Folliculitis
- Scabies
- Keratosis pilaris
- Nevus comedonicus
- Erythema toxicum neonatorum

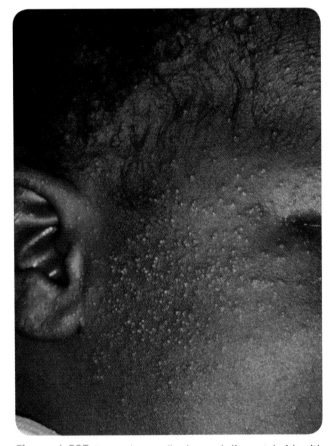

Figure 4-597 Neonatal acne (benign cephalic pustulosis) with multiple small uniform closed comedones.

- A history of initial success with treatment followed by worsening of acne in patients treated with topical or systemic antibiotics may be a sign of Gram-negative folliculitis.
- Congenital adrenal hyperplasia, polycystic ovarian syndrome, and certain other endocrine disorders that cause hyperandrogenism may predispose to the development of acne.

542

✓ Best Tests

Acne is typically a clinical diagnosis, although a skin biopsy will define the process if there is any doubt. An assessment of acne severity is necessary for choosing the appropriate therapy. If acne is not responding to traditional therapy, consider obtaining skin and nasal swabs to exclude Gram-negative folliculitis.

If the clinical scenario warrants (poor response to therapy, hirsutism, irregular menses, etc.), check sex hormone levels: testosterone, sex hormone-binding globulin, follicle-stimulating hormone, LH, prolactin, and DHEA. Late-onset congenital adrenal hyperplasia can be screened for, using 9:00 AM levels of cortisol and 17-α-hydroxyprogesterone.

In patients with symptoms of acne fulminans, a CBC with differential may show leukocytosis to 30,000 with a shift toward polymorphonuclear leukocytes, elevated erythrocyte sedimentation rate, and anemia. There may be proteinuria. Radiographic studies may reveal the presence of osteolytic lesions in areas of bone tenderness. Blood cultures are usually found to be sterile.

▲▲ Management Pearls

- Acne often resolves after the teenage years. Severe cases of nodulocystic acne will require more aggressive treatment. Acne needs consistent, regular care administered over months. Make sure the patient has the correct expectation and applies topical medication to the entire area of potential acne involvement, not just on individual lesions. Topical combination products with a topical antibiotic and benzoyl peroxide, if tolerated, are preferable to antibiotic preparations alone, as they may discourage the development of antibiotic resistance and enhance compliance.
- In darkly pigmented individuals, postinflammatory hyperpigmentation from acne can persist for months to years. Advise patients that the pigment is usually in the epidermis and therefore has more of a chance of resolving with bleaching creams. Distinguish the drugs used for treating acne from those used for treating the pigmentation, and explain that the latter will resolve more slowly.
- If there are cysts and scarring, consider timely referral to a dermatologist for isotretinoin therapy and to minimize permanent scarring. Referral to a dermatologist who regularly prescribes this medication is recommended, as a systematized method for monitoring patients for side effects and pregnancy avoidance in women are essential. Isotretinoin is teratogenic, and every effort must be made to monitor and manage these patients appropriately.
- In acne fulminans, oral glucocorticoids are usually essential for control of the severe inflammatory response. Isotretinoin is also of benefit in some cases (although oral glucocorticoids must first be administered to prevent explosive flares and should be tapered slowly to avoid flares). Topical antibiotics are unhelpful in acne fulminans.

- In patients with acne excoriée, explain to the patients, in detail, how the lesions are produced. Explain to the patients that excoriated lesions are more likely to scar than acne lesions. If acne is clear and excoriated lesions persist, referral to a psychiatrist may be helpful if the condition is severe enough or if it is felt there is an underlying psychological disorder.

Pediatric Patient Considerations

- Parents should be reassured that the vast majority of neonatal acne and benign cephalic pustulosis are non-scarring and self-limited. In infantile acne, scarring may occur, even in patients with mild disease.
- An endocrinology referral is appropriate for patients with severe or persistent neonatal acne. Additionally, a careful physical exam looking for signs of virilization and growth charts should be followed every 4 to 6 months to rule out evolving pathology in severely affected patients.

Therapy

For mild comedonal acne (whiteheads and blackheads predominate), use a topical retinoid:

- Tretinoin 0.025% to 0.1% nightly
- Adapalene 0.1% to 0.3% nightly
- Tazarotene 0.05% to 0.1% once daily

For mild papular or pustular acne, use or add a topical antibiotic/benzoyl peroxide combination:

- Erythromycin/benzoyl peroxide gel
- 1% clindamycin/5% benzoyl peroxide gel
- Benzoyl peroxide gels can also be used without combination with an antibiotic: 2.5%, 4%, 5%, or 10% gel depending on skin dryness. (Use milder strengths when the skin is dry and higher concentrations on very oily skin.)

Topical antibiotics alone can be less costly than antibiotic-benzoyl peroxide combination products. To reduce the emergence of antibiotic resistance, they are best used with a benzoyl peroxide product. Examples are clindamycin 1% solution, erythromycin 2% gel or solution, erythromycin 2% ointment (well tolerated by those with easily irritated skin) and sodium sulfacetamide 10% with 5% sulfur.

Many exfoliant agents are available over the counter with sulfur, salicylic acid, or resorcinol; they are less effective than retinoids and, while sometimes helpful for mild acne, can add an irritant factor if used in addition to the above prescription agents.

(Continued)

When there are inflammatory papules or deeper-seated lesions, use or add an oral medication:

- Tetracycline 500 mg twice daily, doxycycline 100 mg twice daily, or minocycline 100 mg twice daily.
  - Caution the patient regarding photosensitivity while taking tetracyclines, and advise patients to use sunscreens (SPF 30) when anticipating sun exposure.
- Trimethoprim-sulfamethoxazole has also been used and is particularly useful if Gram-negative organisms evolve.

For acne control in women, estrogen-containing oral conceptives are often used, as is spironolactone (100 to 200 mg/d), particularly in hirsute women with acne.

Note: Patients taking spironolactone will need their serum electrolytes monitored and should avoid becoming pregnant.

Isotretinoin should be considered in cases of severe acne or moderate acne that has failed more conservative measures. Due to the drug's teratogenicity, patients and prescribers are required to be registered with the iPLEDGE program. Female patients should use two forms of birth control while taking isotretinoin and for 30 days after treatment has ended. Patients are usually started on a dose of 0.5 mg/kg/d, which is increased to 1 mg/kg/d after 1 month. Blood work is required before and after the course of treatment.

In acne fulminans, systemic glucocorticoids and isotretinoin with adjunctive oral antibiotics are the standard of therapy. Intralesional steroids and dapsone therapy may also be effective in some cases.

- Recommended dosages: 0.5 to 1 mg/kg/d of prednisone (usually 20 to 60 mg/d), tapered over 6 weeks. Isotretinoin 0.25 mg/kg/d can be initiated after the prednisone has controlled the severe inflammation (usually after 3 weeks) and increased to 1 mg/kg/d for a total course of 20 weeks.
- Oral antibiotics with tetracycline as per above.
- Dapsone at 100 mg/d can be considered as an alternative therapy.
  - **Note:** Be sure to check glucose-6-phosphate dehydrogenase level prior to administering dapsone.

Other acne treatment modalities:

- Sub-purpuric pulsed dye laser
- Red (660 nm) and blue (415 nm) light therapy

Pediatric Patient Considerations

Antibiotics in tetracycline class (tetracycline, doxycycline, minocycline) should not be used in children younger than 9 years.

Most cases of neonatal acne (and benign cephalic pustulosis) are mild and will resolve within 3 months without treatment. At most, parents should wash the child's face daily with a gentle soap or cleanser and water. Occlusive baby oils and lotions should be avoided on the face, as they may exacerbate the disease. For more moderate cases, one should attempt to distinguish between neonatal acne and benign cephalic pustulosis before beginning therapy:

- Neonatal acne can usually be managed with 2.5% to 5% benzoyl peroxide cream, topical clindamycin 1% cream, topical erythromycin 2% cream, or tretinoin 0.025% cream every other day to daily if there is no irritation. More severe cases require oral erythromycin to prevent scarring.
- Benign cephalic pustulosis is managed with either topical antifungal agents (ketoconazole cream) or hydrocortisone 1% to 2.5% cream twice daily as needed for flares.

In patients with infantile acne, mild disease can be controlled similarly to neonatal acne with benzoyl peroxide, topical retinoids, and/or topical antibiotics.

Suggested Readings

Campbell JL. A comparative review of the efficacy and tolerability of retinoid-containing combination regimens for the treatment of acne vulgaris. *J Drugs Dermatol.* 2007;6(6):625–629.

Haider A, Shaw JC. Treatment of acne vulgaris. *JAMA.* 2004;292(6): 726–735.

James WD, Berger TG, Elston DM, eds. *Andrews' Diseases of the Skin: Clinical Dermatology.* 10th Ed. Philadelphia, PA: Saunders Elsevier; 2006:231–245.

Thiboutot DM. Overview of acne and its treatment. *Cutis.* 2008;81 (1 Suppl):3–7.

Zaenglein AL, Graber EM, Thiboutot DM, et al. Acne vulgaris and acneiform eruptions. In: Fitzpatrick TB, Wolff K, eds. *Fitzpatrick's Dermatology in General Medicine.* 7th Ed. New York, NY: McGraw-Hill; 2008:690–703.

Milia

Jennifer Alston DeSimone

Diagnosis Synopsis

Milia (singular, milium) are minute epidermoid cysts (also known as infundibular cysts) that present as small white or yellow papules, usually on the face. They are typically smaller than 3 mm in diameter. Primary milia affect 40% to 50% of newborns but may be found in patients of all ages. Secondary milia often occur after cosmetic procedures (dermabrasion, chemical peels, ablative laser therapy) or trauma, or in conjunction with a number of blistering disorders. Milia have also been known to occur in areas of topical steroid-induced atrophy. Persistent or widespread milia are associated with a number of blistering diseases, including porphyria cutanea tarda, and subepidermal blistering diseases, such as forms of epidermolysis bullosa and cicatricial pemphigoid and even, at times, bullous pemphigoid. There is no predilection for either sex or for any ethnicity. Patients with skin types IV through VI tend to be more likely to develop milia as sequelae of chemical peels.

Pediatric Patient Considerations

Primary milia are extremely common on the face of newborns and usually resolve spontaneously by the end of the first month of life.

Secondary milia occur after injury to the skin, such as from burns or subepidermal blistering disorders (e.g., dystrophic forms of epidermolysis bullosa) (Fig. 4-599).

Look For

White to yellow 1- to 2-mm papules typically seen on the cheeks and eyelids and also commonly on the nose and chin areas (Fig. 4-600). Milia are also well documented as occurring on genital skin.

Milia en plaque has recently been described and refers to a rare entity with multiple milia within an erythematous, edematous plaque. It most commonly occurs in the postauricular area but may be found anterior to the ear.

Milia may persist for months or years, and in darker skin types overlying hyperpigmentation may develop in chronic lesions. The lesions may appear as dark brown translucent papules.

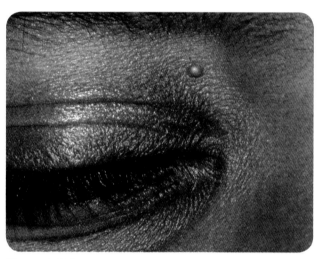

Figure 4-600 Single milium as a white noninflamed papule in a common location around the eye.

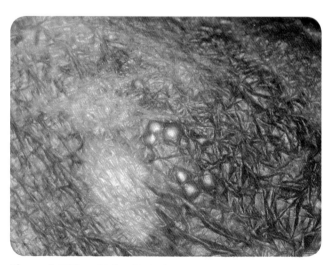

Figure 4-599 Multiple milia in damaged skin.

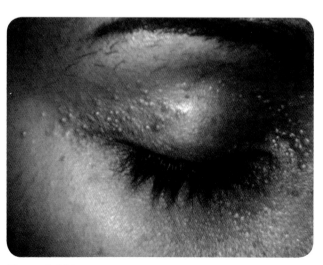

Figure 4-601 Multiple milia in child.

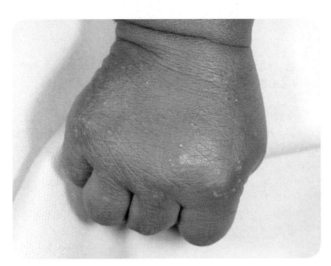

Figure 4-602 Multiple milia due to trauma in a premature infant.

Pediatric Patient Considerations

Milia are firm 1- to 2-mm white, pearly papules (Figs. 4-601 and 4-602). Primary milia appear predominantly on the face of newborns but may affect the trunk, genitalia, and extremities as well. Secondary milia occur within areas of chronic skin injury.

Diagnostic Pearls

- Milia may be a sign that there is a subepidermal bullous disease such as porphyria cutanea tarda or epidermolysis bullosa acquisita if present on the hands. Ask the patient about preceding lesions.
- Take a thorough history including inquiries about previous laser treatments or chemical peels.

Pediatric Patient Considerations

Milia that are widespread, in unusual locations, or persist over several months should alert one to the possibility of an associated syndrome (Marie-Unna hypotrichosis, Bazex-Dupré-Christol disease, or orofacial-digital syndrome type 1).

?? Differential Diagnosis and Pitfalls

- Closed comedones
- Pustular acne
- Molluscum contagiosum
- Sebaceous hyperplasia
- Sebaceoma
- Syringomas
- Lichen nitidus
- Eruptive vellus hair cyst
- Nevus comedonicus

✓ Best Tests

Milia are diagnosed clinically. A No. 11 blade or a 27-gauge needle may be used to make a 0.5-mm incision in the lesion, and pressure with a comedone extractor will remove the keratinous debris.

▲▲ Management Pearls

- Treatment of milia is identical to the diagnostic procedure. Using a No. 11 blade or a 27-gauge needle, make a 0.5-mm incision into the lesion and express the keratinous debris with a comedone extractor.
- It is important to avoid unnecessary trauma to the skin that may result in postinflammatory pigmentation in darker skin types.

Therapy

Milia do not require treatment. For patients who request it, the extraction technique described above is appropriate if there are only a few lesions.

Suggested Readings

Gass JK, Todd PM, Rytina E. Generalized granuloma annulare in a photosensitive distribution resolving with scarring and milia formation. *Clin Exp Dermatol.* 2009;34(5):e53–e55. Epub 2009 May 5.

Nanda A, Kaur S, Bhakoo ON, et al. Survey of cutaneous lesions in Indian newborns. *Pediatr Dermatol.* 1989;6(1):39–42.

Park JH, Choi YD, Kim SW, et al. Effectiveness of modified phenol peel (Exoderm) on facial wrinkles, acne scars and other skin problems of Asian patients. *J Dermatol.* 2007;34(1):17–24.

Pierce HE, Brown LA. Laminar dermal reticulotomy and chemical face peeling in the black patient. *J Dermatol Surg Oncol.* 1986;12(1):69–72.

Acne Keloidalis Nuchae

Sridhar Dronavalli

■■ Diagnosis Synopsis

Acne keloidalis nuchae (AKN), or folliculitis keloidalis, is a chronic inflammatory disease in which keloidlike papules, plaques, and pustules occur at the nape of the neck and on the occipital scalp. Inflammation of the hair follicle and fibrosis of the tissue typically result in scarring, including scarring alopecia. The condition is often painful and disfiguring. The etiology is idiopathic, although lesions are often associated with friction from shirt collars, football or military helmets, trauma from shaving or short haircuts, chronic bacterial infection, or an autoimmune process.

Keloids at other locations or having a family history of keloids are not features of the disease. The overwhelming majority of patients with AKN are young adult African American or Hispanic men, especially those with coarse, curly hair. Women are rarely affected unless they shave their hair at the nape of the neck. AKN is rare in prepubertal children.

Look For

AKN starts as follicular papules and pustules on the superior back, nape of the neck, and the occipital scalp (Figs. 4-603–4-606). The papules and pustules may coalesce as they partially heal to form keloidlike firm plaques. Scarring alopecia and subcutaneous abscesses with draining sinuses may be present.

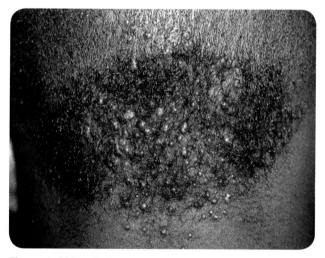

Figure 4-603 Multiple small skin-colored papules of acne keloidalis nuchae on the lower scalp and upper neck.

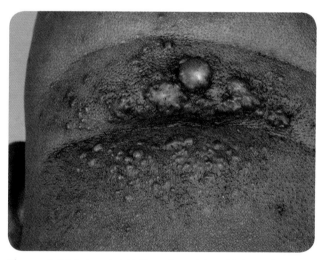

Figure 4-604 Acne keloidalis nuchae with multiple small papules and some larger papules.

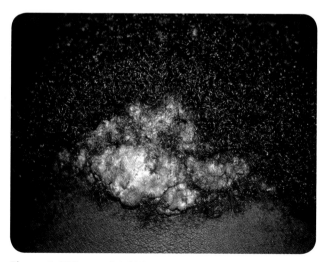

Figure 4-605 Large keloidal areas are not uncommon in acne keloidalis nuchae.

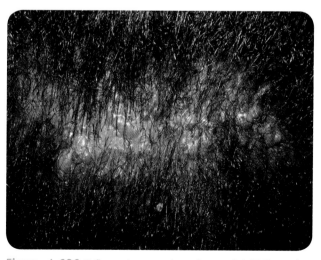

Figure 4-606 Inflammatory papules of acne keloidalis nuchae (same patient as in Fig. 4-605).

Diagnostic Pearls

Comedones (such as in cases of acne) are not present. Early lesions have a follicular distribution. Patients frequently have a history of sports helmet use or occupational headgear that presses on the affected sites.

 Differential Diagnosis and Pitfalls

- Sarcoidosis—can present with keloidlike papules in this area
- Tinea capitis/kerion—a dermatophyte infection commonly seen in children
- Folliculitis—may affect other hair-bearing areas of the body
- Dissecting cellulitis of the scalp—frequently involves the vertex in addition to the occiput
- Hidradenitis suppurativa—usually located in axillary, inguinal, or anogenital areas
- Acne vulgaris—look for comedones
- Keloids
- Nevus sebaceus
- Pseudofolliculitis barbae

✓ **Best Tests**

The diagnosis may be made clinically, as the presence of papules, pustules, and scar formation at the occiput of an African American man is virtually pathognomonic, but a definitive diagnosis can only be made by deep biopsy (below the level of the follicular bulbs and scar tissue). A biopsy is indicated only if the presentation is atypical.

Obtain a bacterial culture with sensitivities from any pustular or draining lesions. This will help identify infected lesions and exclude other diagnoses (e.g., *Staphylococcus aureus* folliculitis).

 Management Pearls

- Discourage skin picking and wearing shirts with tight collars. Athletes who frequently wear helmets should ensure that they fit properly.

- Hair must be grown out several millimeters before cutting, and there should never be close shaves. In fact, shaving the area is not recommended.
- Referral to the dermatologist
- Aggressive treatment with topical or oral antibiotics is important to prevent further scarring.

Therapy

Topical Therapies
Clindamycin 1% gel should be applied twice daily to pustular, crusted, or draining lesions. A combination of tretinoin cream and a potent topical steroid may improve symptoms and flatten lesions. Intralesional triamcinolone acetonide (10 to 40 mg/mL) is another alternative. Patients should be warned that the injected areas may become hypopigmented.

Systemic Therapies
Tetracyclines are useful for treating active inflammation uncontrolled by topical therapies. Isotretinoin has also resulted in improvement in some patients.

Surgical Treatments
Surgical excision of larger keloidal lesions results in impressive cosmetic results. After excision, patients should have intralesional triamcinolone injections every 2 to 3 weeks. In addition, carbon dioxide or Nd:YAG laser treatments have also had promising results.

Suggested Readings

Gloster HM. The surgical management of extensive cases of acne keloidalis nuchae. *Arch Dermatol*. 2000;136(11):1376–1379.

James WD, Berger TG, Elston DM, eds. Diseases of the skin appendages. In: *Andrews' Disease of the Skin: Clinical Dermatology*. 10th Ed. Philadephia, PA: Saunders Elsevier; 2006:749–781.

Kelly P. Folliculitis and the follicular occlusion tetrad. In: Bolognia JL, Jorizzo JL, Rapini RR, eds. *Dermatology*. 2nd Ed. New York, NY: Mosby; 2008:553–566.

Quarles FN, Brody H, Badreshia S, et al. Acne keloidalis nuchae. *Dermatol Therap*. 2007;20(3):128–132.

Shah GK. Efficacy of diode laser for treating acne keloidalis nuchae. *Ind J Dermatol Venereol Leprol*. 2005;71(1):31–34.

Aphthous Ulcers

Donna Culton

■■ Diagnosis Synopsis

Aphthous ulcers (aphthae or canker sores) are recurrent, painful ulcers that occur on mucous membranes, with the mouth being the most typical site of involvement. They are quite common, affecting approximately 25% of the general population. The etiology of aphthae is not completely understood, but some studies suggest that dysregulated Th1-type immune responses with increased TNF-alpha may play a role.

Aphthous ulcers are divided into three morphologic types: minor, major, and herpetiform. Minor aphthae (80% of cases) present as single or multiple lesions that are <1.0 cm in size and associated with mild pain. They often heal within 1 to 2 weeks. Major aphthae (Sutton disease, 10% of cases) are deep ulcers ranging in size from 1 to 3 cm and associated with significant pain. They heal within 2 to 6 weeks and often heal with scarring. Herpetiform aphthae (10% of cases) present as multiple small ulcerations ranging from 1 to 3 mm with a clinical course similar to minor aphthae.

Patients typically suffer from recurrent bouts of aphthous ulcers (recurrent aphthous stomatitis or aphthosis). Simple aphthosis is characterized by minor aphthae that occur intermittently with disease-free intervals ranging from weeks to months. These patients tend to be young and otherwise healthy, with lesions limited to the mouth. Complex aphthosis is marked by near-constant presence of three or more minor aphthae or major aphthae. These patients often have underlying diseases such as HIV, gluten-sensitive enteropathy, inflammatory bowel disease, or others.

Recurrent aphthous stomatitis is more common in women, in patients younger than 40, in nonsmokers, and in people of higher socioeconomic status. Prevalence seems to be higher in whites compared to other ethnicities.

Onset tends to be in adolescence, and there is often an associated family history of oral ulcerations. New lesions are precipitated by oral trauma, stress, and smoking cessation. Other inciting factors include spicy foods, citrus fruits, and hormonal changes in women.

Pediatric Patient Considerations

Onset is typically during adolescence but frequently persists into adulthood.

Immunocompromised Patient Considerations

Immunocompromised patients may be more susceptible to complex aphthosis.

◉ Look For

Look for painful craterlike or "punched-out," shallow ulcers on the nonkeratinized mucosa of the lips, buccal mucosa, and tongue (Figs. 4-607 and 4-608) Although they can occur on the gingiva, there is a predilection for mucosal surfaces that are not bound down. The ulcers tend to be round or oval with a gray, white, or yellow base and an erythematous halo (Fig. 4-609). Minor aphthae tend to be smaller than 1 cm, while major aphthae can range from 1 to 3 cm. Herpetiform aphthae tend to be multiple.

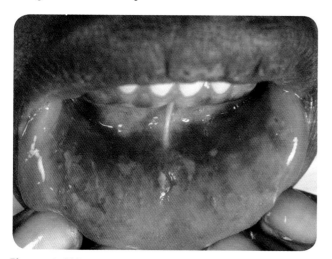

Figure 4-607 Aphthous ulcers with multiple small erosions and ulcers on the inner lower lip.

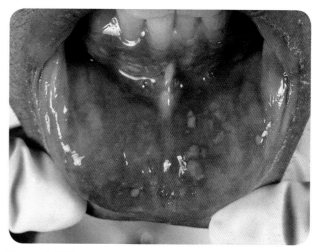

Figure 4-608 Aphthous ulcers with multiple small erosions on the inner lower lip.

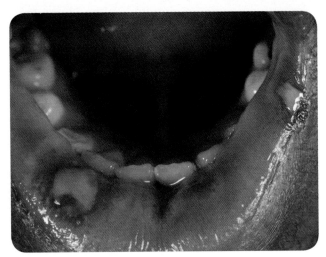

Figure 4-609 Aphthous ulcer with opaque center and red border on the buccal mucosa.

Diagnostic Pearls

- Aphthouslike ulcers are morphologically indistinguishable from aphthous ulcers but are associated with more systemic diseases, such as Behçet disease, systemic lupus erythematosus, AIDS, and inflammatory bowel disease, among others. A thorough review of systems should be conducted to evaluate for underlying systemic disease.
- Aphthous ulcers should occur at different sites with each recurrence, compared to the ulcerations of herpes simplex virus (HSV) infection.

?? Differential Diagnosis and Pitfalls

Diseases with Oral Ulcerations Clinically Distinguishable From Aphthae

- Hand-foot-and-mouth disease usually has skin lesions.
- Herpangina is characteristically located on the soft palate and adjacent mucosa.
- Chemotherapy-induced lesions
- Erosive lichen planus
- Pemphigus
- Cicatricial pemphigoid
- Dermatitis herpetiformis
- Chronic ulcerative stomatitis
- Herpes zoster
- Varicella
- HSV, including primary herpes gingivostomatitis
- Chemical burn (e.g., from holding aspirin near the mucosa)
- Oral candidiasis—typically painless
- Erythema multiforme

- Squamous cell carcinoma
- Drug induced (nonsteroidal anti-inflammatory agents, beta-blockers, nicorandil, alendronate, and ddC [zalcitabine]).

Systemic Diseases with Aphthouslike Ulcerations

- Behçet disease
- Inflammatory bowel disease
- HIV
- Celiac disease—gluten-sensitive enteropathy
- Systemic lupus erythematosus
- Hematinic deficiencies—iron, zinc, folate, vitamins B_1, B_2, B_6, B_{12}
- Cyclic neutropenia
- Sweet syndrome
- FAPA syndrome (*f*ever, *a*phthae, *p*haryngitis, cervical *a*denitis)
- MAGIC syndrome (*m*outh *a*nd *g*enital ulcers with *i*nflamed *c*artilage)

Immunocompromised Patient Differential Diagnosis

- The nucleoside reverse transcriptase inhibitor used to treat HIV, ddC (zalcitabine), may cause aphthouslike ulcerations of the oropharynx and esophagus.
- Cytomegalovirus infections

✓ Best Tests

Aphthous stomatitis is a clinical diagnosis. Histology is usually nonspecific, but biopsy can be helpful in ruling out other causes of oral ulcers. Consider the following tests: vitamin B_{12}, serum folate, zinc, iron, and ferritin. Biopsy of oral ulcerations lasting longer than 3 weeks is necessary to exclude malignancy. Direct immunofluorescence should be performed if pemphigus is suspected. Consider HSV PCR or Tzanck smear for ulcerations recurring at the same anatomic site.

▲▲ Management Pearls

While simple aphthosis does not require additional workup, patients diagnosed with complex aphthosis should be evaluated for an underlying cause, as aphthouslike ulcers can be associated with deficiencies in iron, zinc, folate, and B_{12}. Aphthouslike ulcers are also seen in Behçet disease, systemic lupus erythematosus, AIDS, inflammatory bowel disease, and other systemic illnesses, and a thorough review of systems should be conducted in all patients presenting with oral ulcerations.

Therapy

Most patients with simple aphthosis can be treated successfully with topical agents. The goals are symptomatic relief and accelerated ulcer healing. Systemic treatments should be reserved for severe cases. Any underlying vitamin or mineral deficiencies should be corrected.

Counsel the patient regarding trigger avoidance. Inciting factors include emotional stress, oral trauma from sharp or hard foods, and menstruation. Acidic foods and beverages increase ulcer pain.

Limited data support the use of toothpastes free of the detergent sodium lauryl sulfate to decrease frequency of attacks of recurrent aphthous stomatitis. Chlorhexidine-containing mouthwashes may also decrease frequency of attacks.

Patient-Directed Treatments to Palliate Symptoms From Aphthae
- Topical local anesthetics—lidocaine, benzocaine, or dyclonine (some over the counter) available in a variety of preparations designed for oral use
- Anesthetic mouthwashes combining aluminum and magnesium hydroxide, lidocaine, and diphenhydramine
- Sucralfate
- Oral nonsteroidal analgesics
- Opioid analgesics in severe cases

Patient-Directed Topical Treatments to Accelerate Healing of Aphthae (Best Used at Earliest Onset of a New Ulceration)
- Topical corticosteroids (e.g., triamcinolone, halobetasol, clobetasol) available in gels or oral preparations such as carboxymethylcellulose base—applied two to four times daily
- Diclofenac in hyaluronic acid—single treatment
- Amlexanox 5% oral paste four times daily for 5 days
- Oral suspensions of tetracyclines, used for anti-inflammatory effect. Data support the use of tetracycline, doxycycline, and minocycline, though topical forms are not widely available. A 250-mg capsule of tetracycline may be dissolved in a tablespoon of water and swished around the mouth for 5 minutes three to four times daily

- Hyaluronic acid 0.2% twice daily for 2 weeks
- 5-Aminosalicylic acid 5% cream three times daily

Clinician-Directed Treatment for Individual Stubborn or Severe Aphthae
- Chemical cautery with silver nitrate 1% to 2%
- Chemical cautery with 50% sulfonated phenolics in 30% sulfuric acid (also available in applicators intended for patient-directed use)
- Intralesional injection with triamcinolone acetonide 5 to 10 mg/mL

Systemic Treatments for Severe Cases or Patients Prone to Severe Recurrences
- Prednisone 10 to 20 mg/d for 5 to 7 days, or other oral corticosteroids
- Colchicine 0.6 mg two to three times daily
- Pentoxifylline 400 mg three times daily
- Doxycycline 20 mg two times daily
- Methotrexate 7.5 to 20 mg weekly
- Dapsone 100 mg daily
- Thalidomide 50 to 300 mg/d—a known teratogen with a special access program for the drug in all patients
- Azathioprine 50 to 150 mg/d
- Cyclosporine A 3 to 6 mg/kg daily
- Biologic anti-TNF-alpha agents (e.g., etanercept, infliximab, adalimumab) have demonstrated efficacy in case reports.
- Other systemic therapies include levamisole, alkylating agents, and antimetabolites.

Combination therapy should be considered when a single agent does not suffice.

Suggested Readings

Mirowski GW, Parker ER. Disorders of the oral and genital integument. In: Wolff K, Goldsmith LA, Katz SI, Gilchrest BA, Paller AS, Leffell DJ, eds. *Fitzpatrick's Dermatology in General Medicine.* 7th Ed. New York, NY: McGraw-Hill; 2008:645–647.

Porter S, Scully C. Aphthous ulcers (recurrent). *Clin Evid.* 2005;(13):1687–1694.

Scully C. Aphthous ulceration. *N Engl J Med.* 2006;355(2):165–172.

Oral Candidiasis (Thrush) and Periodontal Disease

Laurie Good

■■ Diagnosis Synopsis

Oral candidiasis, also known as moniliasis or thrush, is a common yeast infection of the oral mucosal membranes typically caused by overgrowth of *Candida albicans*. *Candida* frequently affects immunocompromised individuals such as those receiving immunosuppressive agents (e.g., systemic or inhaled corticosteroids, chemotherapy) as well as patients with diabetes mellitus, HIV, and AIDS. It is common during infancy when the immune system and immune responses are developing. Frequent or chronic antibiotic use disrupts the normal oral flora and will also predispose normal individuals, as well as immunosuppressed patients, to oral candidiasis. Other conditions that may predispose to periodontal disease include hyposalivation states leading to dry mouth (post–head and neck radiation, anticholinergic medications) and wearing dentures that do not adequately support the oral musculature. Additionally, people with normal age-related facial sagging causing drooping of the corners of the mouth and pooling of saliva are also susceptible.

Periodontal disease can lead to the loss of teeth, which drives denture usage in developed countries. Although dentures are less commonly available in the developing world, risk factors for periodontal disease are worthy of mention, as ethnicity and cultural practices influence disparities in prevalence worldwide. Periodontal disease (chronic inflammation) also puts one at greater risk for cardiovascular disease.

One global epidemiologic study demonstrated that the highest prevalence of periodontal disease exists in Africans, followed by Latin Americans, then Asians, and lastly whites. There are genetic predispositions to the dental plaque microorganisms as well as environmental factors at play, the roles of which are still being defined. For example, betel quid (betel nut) chewing is practiced across Asia, and preliminary research suggests there could be a periodontal health risk associated with chewing. Although studies from Papua New Guinea indicate it is protective against caries, due to the encasing of the teeth by the betel nut dye, there are oral lesions associated with chewing. However, oral candidiasis has not been shown to be among them.

A study that examined salivary flow and pH in protein energy–malnourished Haitian children found that, although pH was not statistically significantly different, salivary flow was significantly diminished in malnourished children. Delayed exfoliation and eruption of primary and permanent teeth as well as higher rates of dental caries and poorer periodontal status in permanent dentition have also been associated with protein energy malnutrition in studies in Peru and Haiti. According to a study in Uganda, 28% of school attendees 12 to 25 years of age had early-onset periodontitis, although the predisposing factors for such a high prevalence have yet to be elucidated. In Sudan, a comparative study found evidence that African tribe ethnicity, compared to Afro-Arab tribe ethnicity, was a risk factor for aggressive periodontal disease.

Oral lesions are present in roughly 30% of individuals who are HIV-positive, with oral candidiasis being the most common form. It is unclear if racial or ethnic differences exist with regard to the prevalence of oral candidiasis in certain patient subgroups, such as the HIV-positive population. It is clear, however, that race and ethnicity play a large role in the access to care, as studies have demonstrated that African Americans and Hispanics with HIV-related oral lesions in the United States are less likely to seek medical care for such lesions. In Brazil, lower socioeconomic status was associated with higher prevalence of pseudomembranous oral candidiasis.

Pediatric Patient Considerations

Thrush is common in the neonate. It can be picked up from the mother during vaginal delivery or acquired as a newborn through antibiotic usage by baby or mother. As the baby's immune system matures, the baby will be less susceptible to oral *Candida* infections. Often, oral candidiasis is asymptomatic and need not be treated. At other times, it can cause irritability during breastfeeding and should be treated.

Oral candidiasis is the most common oral lesion in perinatally affected HIV-positive children and adolescents.

Immunocompromised Patient Considerations

All states of immunocompromise, such as being on immunosuppressives or having diabetes or AIDS, render one susceptible to oral candidiasis. *C. albicans* is common in patients who are HIV positive.

Recently *C. dubliniensis* has been differentiated from *C. albicans* and is now recognized as an important emerging pathogen in the HIV-infected population as well, though its virulence is less than that of *C. albicans*. Studies have shown carriage in the HIV-positive population in Venezuela, South Africa, and Italy, and it is likely to be an important consideration in antifungal resistance worldwide, as reduced azole susceptibility has been demonstrated. In Venezuelan isolates of *C. dubliniensis*, 19% demonstrated resistance to fluconazole. There does not seem to be a difference in carriage rates of *C. dubliniensis* based on race.

A small Hong Kong study in ethnic Chinese showed a lower prevalence of oral candidiasis compared to a

Western population of HIV-positive individuals. It is possible that geographic, ethnic, and racial factors predispose some, while protecting others, from certain oral lesions such as candidiasis. In contrast to the ethnic Chinese population, a Pan-American study examined data from HIV-positive populations in Argentina, Brazil, Chile, Mexico, Peru, the United States, Uruguay, and the English Caribbean and showed oral candidiasis to be the most common oral manifestation in HIV-positive individuals in these countries; this mirrors findings based on the US HIV-positive population. Similarly, a large study in Thailand demonstrated oral candidiasis as the most frequent oral manifestation among patients who had contracted HIV through heterosexual activity or intravenous drug use. No difference was seen in the prevalence of oral candidiasis based on routes of HIV transmission.

Risk factors for oral candidiasis in the HIV-positive population include antiviral combination therapy, low CD4 count (<200 cells/μL), and current smoking. One study in Thailand also found male gender as a risk factor for developing oral lesions, the most common of which was oral candidiasis, in an HIV-positive setting, as women were less likely to have oral lesions than men.

⦿ Look For

There are three main clinical forms of candidiasis that exist:

- Pseudomembranous (thrush) is the most common—curdy white papules and plaques that wipe off with some difficulty, leaving a raw, bleeding surface. Any mucosal surface may be involved (Figs. 4-610–4-613).
- Atrophic/erythematous form—This occurs more commonly than thrush in HIV-infected individuals and appears red, atrophic, and eroded (Fig. 4-614). It also

often occurs underneath dentures (also called denture sore mouth) and on the dorsum of the tongue. When it occurs at the corners of the mouth, it is called angular cheilitis (perlèche).
- Hyperplastic form (less common)—white papules and plaques that do not wipe off, are often indistinguishable from leukoplakia, and are often associated with mucocutaneous disease

Hands should be examined for evidence of *Candida* infection (Fig. 4-615).

Median rhomboid glossitis is a form of chronic oral candidiasis that presents as an ovoid or rhomboidal area in the midline of the tongue just anterior to the circumvallate papillae. In AIDS patients in Brazil, the most common clinical form was found to be pseudomembranous, followed by erythematous and then angular cheilitis oral candidiasis. This finding was corroborated by a study in Ugandan AIDS

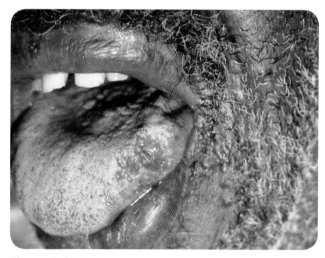

Figure 4-611 Plaques of *Candida* on the lateral margins of the tongue and the corner of the mouth.

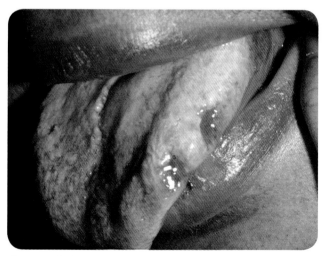

Figure 4-610 Thrush in an older child with lateral tongue erosions.

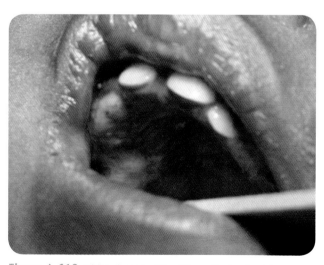

Figure 4-612 White plaques of *Candida* on the hard palate.

553

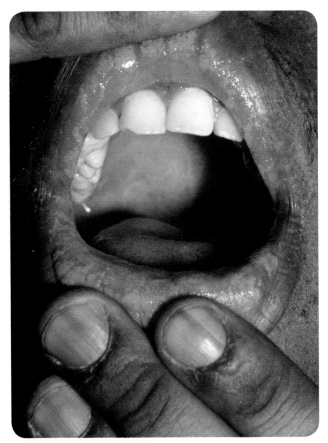

Figure 4-613 Multiple white plaques on lips and adjacent buccal mucosa with *Candida* infection.

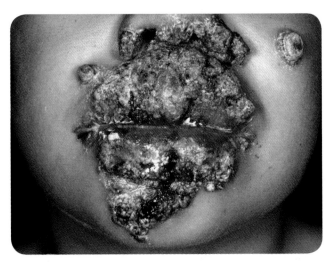

Figure 4-614 Candidiasis associated with immunosuppression and extensive scale crust.

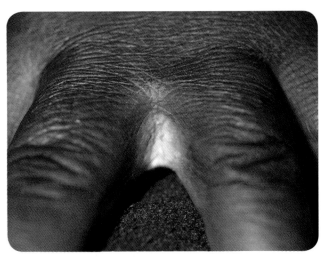

Figure 4-615 Candidal intertrigo of hand with white plaque (erosio interdigitalis blastomycetica).

patients. In Brazilian patients, the most common anatomical location for oral candidiasis lesions of all clinical forms was the tongue.

Pediatric Patient Considerations

Look for whitish plaques or cottage cheese–like spots on the tongue/mouth/cheeks of a baby who is fussy during breastfeeding. In a nursing infant, lesions can be difficult to distinguish from milk residue after feeding. However, a cotton swab or wet washcloth can easily remove milk from an infant's mouth, whereas thrush will not wipe away.

Diagnostic Pearls

Dentures and malocclusion can predispose to candidiasis. Candidiasis beneath dentures can present as redness and soreness of the palate with few organisms on KOH prep.

?? Differential Diagnosis and Pitfalls

- Oral hairy leukoplakia—an HIV-associated disease, often with an associated secondary candidal infection; most common on the lateral borders of the tongue; often (but not always) in a bilateral and symmetric distribution
- Chronic bite injury—usually painless with a gelatinous, shaggy consistency
- Leukoplakia
- Erythroplakia
- Hypersensitivity reaction to denture base material
- Lichen planus—usually reticulated and erythematous rather than plaquelike
- Geographic tongue
- Diphtheria—The membrane is often associated with hemorrhagic crusts around the mouth and nares.
- Hairy tongue

✓ Best Tests

- Scrape white plaques with a tongue blade, apply to glass slide, and stain with KOH. Look for budding yeast forms and nonseptate hyphae (pseudohyphae).
- Cultures are not recommended because 20% of the population is a carrier.

Immunocompromised Patient Considerations

In immunocompromised patients, culture for speciation is important because some species (e.g., *C. tropicalis*, *C. dubliniensis*) may be resistant to standard therapy.

▲▲▲ Management Pearls

- One dose of oral fluconazole 200 mg may be curative, especially in those patients in whom antibiotic usage has allowed *Candida* overgrowth. Regular use (e.g., once weekly) may be necessary for those with predisposing conditions.
- If using nystatin (see below), make sure that the patient removes any dentures before using the rinse to make sure that the nystatin contacts the infected mucosa under the denture.
- Also, dentures need to be treated to kill yeast they may be harboring.
- If possible, discontinue the antibiotic and/or immunosuppressive agent.
- Voriconazole, both peroral and parenteral formulations, and parenteral caspofungin are new agents effective against resistant *Candida* species.

Pediatric Patient Considerations

A breastfeeding baby with oral candidiasis will likely pass the yeast back and forth between his/her mouth and the mother's nipples. Thus, both mother and infant should be treated to clear the infection.

Therapy

Nystatin rinse (1:100,000 IU/mL)—Swish and spit out 5 mL three to four times daily. Be careful about using this in patients with dry mouths (especially patients who have received head and neck radiation), because nystatin contains sucrose and can aggravate a tendency to develop caries in these patients.

Clotrimazole troches—10 mg troche five times daily for 2 weeks. This does not work well if the mouth is dry, since saliva is necessary for the troches to dissolve.

One dose of oral fluconazole 200 mg may be curative, especially in those patients in whom antibiotic usage has allowed *Candida* overgrowth. Regular use (e.g., once weekly) may be necessary for those with predisposing conditions.

Nystatin and triamcinolone cream or topical ketoconazole ointment for corners of mouth—Apply three times daily.

Alternative therapies and complementary medicines, including various aromatherapies and essential oils, are commonly employed in other countries for their antifungal properties. In Japan, commonly used treatments for fungal infections include lemongrass (*Cymbopogon citratus*) essential oil and citral, which is an active component of lemongrass. Both have demonstrated antifungal properties against *C. albicans* in studies examining essential oils for this purpose. Interestingly, a Brazilian study of anticandidal properties of essential oils found that fluconazole-resistant strains of *C. albicans* and *C. dubliniensis* were more susceptible to certain oils, namely Mexican oregano, oregano, thyme, and ginger essential oil, than fluconazole-sensitive *Candida*. Oregano was found to have the greatest level of efficiency in controlling candidal species, but several essential oils showed fungicidal and fungistatic properties against *C. albicans* and *C. dubliniensis*. Studies in other parts of the world have had similar findings. Additionally, a study using clinical candidiasis isolates in Portugal demonstrated strong antifungal activity in clove oil and its major component, eugenol, especially in fluconazole-resistant strains.

Pediatric Patient Considerations

Thrush in newborns is common and often causes no symptoms and can resolve on its own. If symptomatic, however, nystatin suspension can be prescribed for the baby and nystatin cream for the breastfeeding mother.

Nystatin Suspension (100,000 U/mL)
Premature/low-birth-weight infants—1 mL p.o. four times daily. Give 0.5 mL in each side of mouth; continue use for 48 hour after resolution of symptoms.

Infants—2 mL p.o. four times daily. Give 1 mL in each side of mouth; continue use for 48 hour after resolution of symptoms.

Children—4 to 6 mL p.o. four times daily. Give 2 to 3 mL in each side of mouth; continue use for 48 hour after resolution of symptoms.

Breastfeeding Mother
Nystatin cream (100,000 U/g cream)—Apply to nipples two to three times per day.

Immunocompromised Patient Considerations

A Chinese herbal medicine, xiaomi granules, was studied in 40 HIV-positive Chinese patients with oral candidiasis. The efficacy was 90% with an 11% relapse rate. This was more effective than anticandine, which was used in the control group. Traditional herbal medications, when tested for efficacy and safety, have an important role in the treatment of modern-day illness. Because they have firm roots in various cultures, patients may often be more open to herbal treatments.

Suggested Readings

Albandar JM, Tinoco EMB. Global epidemiology of periodontal diseases in children and young persons. *Periodontology*. 2000;29(1):153–176.

Albandar JM. Global risk factors and risk indicators for periodontal diseases. *Periodontol 2000*. 2002;29:177–206.

Elamin AM, Skaug N, Ali RW, et al. Ethnic disparities in the prevalence of periodontitis among high school students in Sudan. *J Periodontol*. 2010. [Epub ahead of print].

Gabler IG, Barbosa AC, Velela RR, et al. Incidence and anatomic localization of oral candidiasis in patients with AIDS hospitalized in a public hospital in Belo Horizonte, MG, Brazil. *J Appl Oral Sci*. 2008;16(4):247–250.

Gaitán-Cepeda LA, Domínguez-Sánchez A, Pavía-Ruz N, et al. Oral lesions in HIV+/AIDS Adolescents perinatally infected undergoing HAART. *Med Oral Patol Oral Cir Bucal*. 2010. [Epub ahead of print].

Mascarenhas AK, Smith SR. Factors associated with utilization of care for oral lesions in HIV disease. *Oral Surg Oral Med Oral Pathol Oral Radiol Endodontol*. 1999;87(6):708–713.

Nittayananta W, Chanowanna N, Sripatanakul S, et al. Risk factors associated with oral lesions in HIV-infected heterosexual people and intravenous drug users in Thailand. *J Oral Pathol Med*. 2001;30(4):224–230.

Noce CW, Ferreira SM, Silva Júnior A, et al. Association between socioeconomic status and HIV-associated oral lesions in Rio de Janeiro from 1997 to 2004. *Braz Oral Res*. 2009;23(2):149–154.

Pinto E, Vale-Silva L, Cavaleiro C, et al. Antifungal activity of the clove essential oil from Syzygium aromaticum on *Candida, Aspergillus* and dermatophyte species. *J Med Microbiol*. 2009;58(11):1454–1462.

Psoter W, Gebrian B, Prophete S, et al. Effect of early childhood malnutrition on tooth eruption in Haitian adolescents. *Community Dent Oral Epidemiol*. 2008;36(2):179–189.

Psoter WJ, Spielman AL, Gebrian B, et al. Effect of childhood malnutrition on salivary flow and pH. *Arch Oral Biol*. 2008;53(3):231–237. Epub 2007 Nov 5.

Reichart PA, Khongkhunthian P, Samaranayake LP, et al. Oral *Candida* species and betel quid-associated oral lesions in Padaung women of Northern Thailand. *Mycoses*. 2005;48(2):132–136.

Reichart PA, Schmidtberg W, Samaranayake LP, et al. Betel quid-associated oral lesions and oral *Candida* species in a female Cambodian cohort. *J Oral Pathol Med*. 2002;31(8):468–472.

Russell SL, Psoter WJ, Jean-Charles G, et al. Protein-energy malnutrition during early childhood and periodontal disease in the permanent dentition of Haitian adolescents aged 12-19 years: A retrospective cohort study. *Int J Paediatr Dent*. 2010;20(3):222–229.

Tirwomwe JF, Rwenyonyi CM, Muwazi LM, et al. Oral manifestations of HIV/AIDS in clients attending TASO clinics in Uganda. *Clin Oral Investig*. 2007;11(3):289–292.

Tsang PCS, Samaranayake LP. Oral manifestations of HIV infection in a group of predominantly ethnic Chinese. *J Oral Pathol Med*. 1999;28:122–127.

Orofacial Herpes

Kamilah Dixon • Lynn McKinley-Grant

◼◼ Diagnosis Synopsis

Orofacial herpes, or oral herpes, is an infection of the oral mucosa caused by herpes simplex viruses. Herpes simplex virus type 1 (HSV-1) causes the majority of cases of oral herpes. This infection is extremely common and it is estimated that up to 90% of people will be infected with the HSV-1 virus in their lifetime. HSV-1 is spread through contact with oral secretions, and like HSV-2, can be spread even during episode-free periods (asymptomatic shedding).

A primary infection presents with a prodromal period, including burning, tingling, and localized pain in the orofacial area. Subsequently, small vesicles form and then rupture, leaving small, tender ulcerations in and around the oral mucosa. These ulcers will crust and heal without scarring. The initial infection will usually resolve within 10 to 14 days in immunocompetent individuals.

Recurrent infections are marked by shorter duration and severity. Only 15% to 40% of the affected population will experience recurrent symptoms of oral herpes. These symptoms are usually preceded by a prodrome of localized pain, burning, or tingling at the affected site. This is followed by the appearance of small vesicles that rupture to form tender erosions. Like the primary infection, these erosions will crust over and heal without scarring. Recurrent herpes simplex is a common precipitator of erythema multiforme minor.

Pediatric Patient Considerations

Childhood infection is common via child-to-child contact or kissing by a parent.

◉ Look For

- Small, tender, grouped vesicles or erosions on an erythematous base that resolve without scarring (Fig. 4-616)
- Vesicles at the vermilion border may show umbilication before they are denuded or crusted (Fig. 4-616)

In the oral cavity, look for painful yellow ulcers on the mucosa involving any site but in particular the gingiva, dorsum of tongue, and buccal and labial mucosa. Ulcers are usually 2 to 4 mm in diameter but may coalesce to form larger, irregularly shaped ulcers with scalloped borders. It is rare to see intact blisters in the oral cavity. Primary and recurrent HSV infections are associated with the development of erythema multiforme.

Disseminated lesions occur in those with underlying skin diseases such as atopic dermatitis and those who are immunosuppressed (Fig. 4-617).

◉◉ Diagnostic Pearls

- Be aware of grouped vesicles or erosions that have a recurrent nature and resolve without scarring. These are the hallmark signs of herpes simplex infections.
- Herpes simplex can occur anywhere on the skin. In dental or health personnel who are exposed to oral lesions or bitten, a herpetic whitlow may occur, which is painful swelling of the distal finger with opaque grey epidermis and only subtle evidence of discrete vesicles.

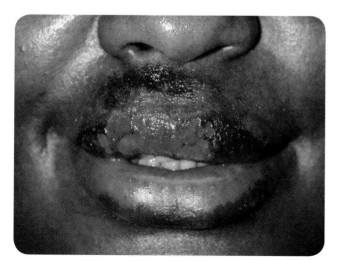

Figure 4-616 Herpes simplex with opaque vesicles on the upper lip and vermilion border.

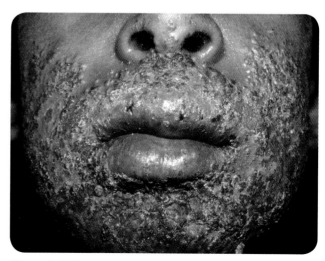

Figure 4-617 Disseminated herpes simplex with crusts and erosions.

557

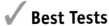 Differential Diagnosis and Pitfalls

- Varicella infection
- Hand-foot-and-mouth disease
- Herpangina
- Erythema multiforme
- Pemphigus vulgaris
- Intraoral herpes zoster
- Acute necrotizing ulcerative gingivitis

Best Tests

In patients with lesions:

- Viral isolation in tissue culture is the gold standard. This must be done in patients with active lesions, preferably 2 to 7 days within the episode to ensure proper visualization.
- Tzanck smear
- Direct fluorescence antigen testing
- PCR-based clinical assays

In patients without lesions:

- Type-specific serology tests

▲▲▲ Management Pearls

- There is currently no vaccine for herpes simplex infections. With this in mind, it is most important to prevent the initial infection and to control the subsequent outbreaks.
- In patients with orofacial herpes, care should be taken to ensure that others do not have contact with active lesions. It is important that the patients keep the erosions clean to avoid bacterial infection. Along with suppressive treatment, it is important to consider the stigma associated with herpes infections and to provide support to patients when they discover that they have the infection.

Therapy

Topical and systemic medications are available for the treatment of orofacial herpes. While the topical medication may be more useful in initial outbreaks to help relieve pain, they are less effective than systemic medications to prevent further outbreaks.

Topical Medications
Use one of the following:

- Penciclovir 1% cream—Apply to affected area every 2 hours for 4 days.

- Acyclovir 5% ointment—Apply to affected area every 3 hours, six times a day for 7 days.
- Docosanol 10% cream—Apply to affected area five times a day until healed.

Systemic Medications
Use one of the following:

- Valacyclovir, 500 mg, 2 g orally at first prodrome, and 2 g orally 12 hours later
- Famciclovir, 250 mg, 500 mg orally at first prodrome, two times per day for 5 to 10 days

Immunocompromised Patient Considerations

Systemic medication used in immunocompromised patients with mucocutaneous HSV infection:

- Foscarnet—40 mg/kg every 8 hours for 2 to 3 weeks

Pediatric Patient Considerations

The first episode:

- Acyclovir 20 mg/kg/d divided into five doses for a total of 7 days

Dosing recommendations vary for recurrent episodes. For patients who suffer from frequent recurrences, daily dosing may be necessary.

- Valacyclovir is approved for use in children over the age of 12.
- Famciclovir is *not* approved for use in children.
- If secondary bacterial infection is suspected, a culture should be taken and the choice of oral antibiotic should be based on the results.

Suggested Reading

Fatahzadeh M, Schwartz RA. Human herpes simplex virus infections: Epidemiology, pathogenesis, symptomatology, diagnosis and management. *J Am Acad Dermatol.* 2007;57(5):737–763.

Leukoplakia, Oral Squamous Cell Carcinoma, and Hairy Leukoplakia

Stephanie Diamantis

◼◼ Diagnosis Synopsis

Leukoplakia

Leukoplakia refers to a white plaque found on a mucosal site. It is a common finding that can be a precursor of mucosal squamous cell carcinoma (SCC). Malignant transformation of intraoral leukoplakia ranges from 6% to 10%, with an increased risk if red lesions are present (erythroleukoplakia). Premalignant leukoplakia may have areas of ulceration or erosion and will show cellular atypia upon histologic examination. Leukoplakia is more common in smokers and is frequently seen in association with pipe smoking or chewing tobacco. It can also result from mechanical irritation by ill-fitting dentures (benign form secondary to chronic irritation). Leukoplakia is most commonly found in middle-aged or elderly men. Leukoplakia in women can also involve the vulva, usually in obese postmenopausal women.

Clinically, the lesions are white and glistening but may be thick and elevated. Typical locations include the lips, gums, buccal mucosa, and lateral edges of the tongue.

Oral Squamous Cell Carcinoma

Oral SCC is a malignancy of surface oral epithelium origin. Chronic UV light exposure is responsible for SCC occurring on the vermilion zone of the lips, overwhelmingly the lower lip. These are typically fair-skinned individuals. In the United States, approximately 80% of intraoral SCC is related to cigarette smoking, with or without alcohol abuse; alcohol plays a synergistic role in the development of oral SCC.

Most patients are between the ages of 50 and 70 at the time of diagnosis, although patients as young as 20 may be affected. Men are affected twice as frequently as women. Oral SCC is generally asymptomatic in its early stages. Eventually patients will complain of tenderness or pain associated with the lesion. Depending on the location and size of the lesion, dysphagia or dysphonia may be present.

Systemic signs and symptoms are usually not evident until the later stages of disease, and manifestations would include cachexia. Increased risk of developing oral SCC has been described in immunosuppressed patients, including HIV-infected patients and transplant recipients.

The principal risk factor in the United States is cigarette smoking, usually in combination with alcohol abuse.

Oral SCC generally begins as a red or white patch that evolves into an infiltrative ulceration or exophytic mass over a period of months to years in most cases.

Hairy Leukoplakia

Hairy leukoplakia is a benign mucosal disorder caused by Epstein-Barr virus (EBV) infection and is almost always noted in immunocompromised patients. It was first described in HIV-infected patients but is also noted in patients after organ transplantation. They are asymptomatic and do not scrape off although they may be associated with a concomitant candidal infection. Lesions develop over weeks and months.

◉ Look For

Leukoplakia

White plaques overlying any mucosal surface, but often located on the buccal mucosa or tongue (Figs. 4-618 and 4-619). Lesions are adherent to underlying mucosa.

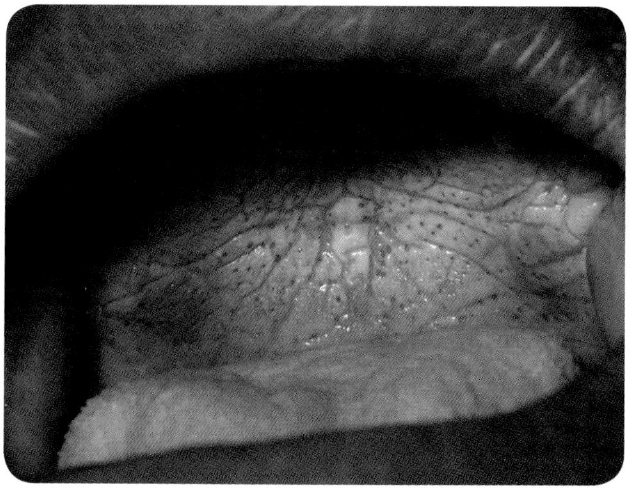

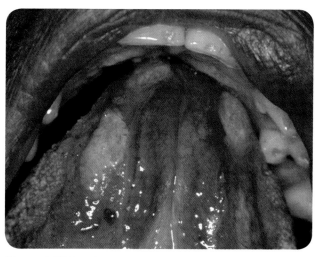

Figure 4-618 Nicotine stomatitis with diffuse hyperkeratosis of hard palate with two hyperpigmented macules.

Figure 4-619 Leukoplakia and erosions on the tongue.

Oral Squamous Cell Carcinoma

Look for a firm mass with an irregular erythematous and/or keratotic (white) surface that is usually ulcerated (Fig. 4-620). Some lesions have an endophytic growth pattern. The favored locations include the vermilion zone of the lower lip, the lateral or ventral tongue, the floor of the mouth, and the lateral soft palate. Gingival carcinomas are seen occasionally, and these are more frequently seen in women who have none of the traditional risk factors for oral cancer. Sometimes gingival carcinomas may clinically mimic the inflammatory hyperplastic changes seen with chronic periodontitis. Verrucous carcinoma is a rare, well-differentiated variety of SCC that tends to spread laterally as a warty-surfaced white plaque affecting the hard palate, alveolar mucosa, or buccal mucosa of an elderly person.

Hairy Leukoplakia

Look for painless white plaques, often on the lateral border of the tongue and often bilateral in distribution (Fig. 4-621). Some lesions occur on the buccal mucosa. Early lesions may be milky white and subtle. They become increasingly more prominent, whiter, and more shaggy ("more hairy") as they mature and may form thick matted plaques.

 Diagnostic Pearls

Leukoplakia

There are hereditary syndromes with benign intraoral lesions such as white sponge nevus that often begin in childhood or adolescence.

Oral Squamous Cell Carcinoma

Any ulceration or mass with an uneven surface and firm consistency that develops in a high-risk site for oral cancer should be viewed with suspicion, particularly if it has been present for at least 2 weeks with no sign of healing after potentially contributing local factors (sharp broken teeth, for example) have been eliminated.

Hairy Leukoplakia

The presence of bilateral slightly shaggy painless white plaques on the lateral border of the tongue in an immunocompromised patient is strongly suggestive of hairy leukoplakia.

 Differential Diagnosis and Pitfalls

Leukoplakia

- Oral hairy leukoplakia—most frequently seen in HIV and AIDS patients. Look for painless white plaques, often on the lateral border of the tongue and often bilateral in distribution. Early lesions may be milky white and subtle. They become increasingly more prominent, whiter, and more shaggy ("more hairy") as they mature and may form thick matted plaques. Lesions are not removed by gentle scraping as are those of candidiasis (thrush).
- Irritation (e.g., from chewing, smoking, snuff use) or from cheek chewing.
- SCC—Look for a firm mass with an irregular erythematous and/or keratotic (white) surface that is usually ulcerated. Some lesions have an endophytic growth pattern. The favored locations include the vermilion zone of the lower lip, the lateral or ventral tongue, the floor of the mouth, and the lateral soft palate.
- Lichen planus
- Lupus erythematosus
- Candidiasis
- Lichen sclerosus

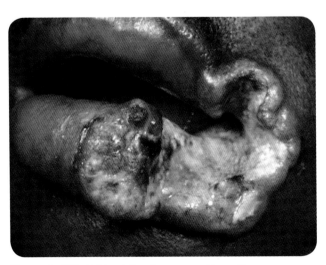

Figure 4-620 SCC involving the upper and lower lips.

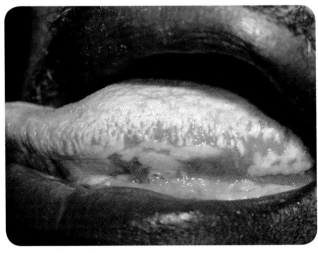

Figure 4-621 Multiple plaques of oral hairy leukoplakia, especially on the tongue margins.

- Leukoedema—normal variant of buccal mucosa; very common in darkly pigmented individuals. The white pattern decreases with stretching of the mucosa compared with the striae of lichen planus or leukoplakia.
- Syphilis
- Psoriasis
- Pityriasis rubra pilaris
- White sponge nevus

Oral Squamous Cell Carcinoma

- Actinic cheilitis—This represents a premalignant process of the vermilion zone of the lower lip, and some degree of epithelial dysplasia is present in these lesions. Biopsy is often necessary to distinguish between this condition and SCC of the vermilion zone of the lower lip.
- Lichen planus
- Condyloma
- Secondary syphilis
- Verrucous carcinoma
- Proliferative verrucous leukoplakia
- Nonspecific ulcer—Usually these have surrounding keratosis (white), the borders of which tend to blend with the adjacent mucosa, as opposed to leukoplakia, which usually has sharply demarcated borders.
- Pyogenic granuloma—This lesion usually grows more rapidly than SCC, and it is usually more sharply demarcated.
- Amelanotic melanoma—This very rare intraoral lesion usually grows more rapidly than SCC but could appear clinically identical.
- Specific (TB; deep fungal) infection—Systemic signs and symptoms would probably be present with these specific infections, although, clinically, the lesions could appear identical to SCC.
- Lymphoma—Lymphomas tend to evolve in the deeper soft tissues, but with ulceration of the overlying epithelium, they can mimic SCC.
- Malignant salivary gland tumor—As with lymphoma, these lesions tend to develop in the deeper soft tissues. Overlying ulceration is not unusual, however, and the result could mimic oral SCC.
- Wegener granulomatosis—Epistaxis and evidence of systemic involvement could be present with Wegener granulomatosis.
- Crohn disease—Oral manifestations of Crohn disease include ill-defined ulcerations with an irregular surface that could mimic SCC. Gastrointestinal symptoms may be present, but the oral lesions are sometimes the initial manifestation of Crohn disease.

Hairy Leukoplakia

- Chronic cheek chewing—This may appear as painless, shaggy white plaques that are bilateral; the buccal mucosa may also be involved. Patients are not usually immuno-compromised, although they may coincidentally be so. A biopsy distinguishes between the two.
- Candidiasis—This may appear similar but tends not to be bilaterally symmetrical and not to primarily affect the lateral tongue. The plaques scrape off with some difficulty, leaving a raw, bleeding surface. Often, papules will be present elsewhere on the oral mucosa.
- Hairy tongue (overgrowth and retention of filiform papillae)—This generally involves the dorsum of the tongue only, where filiform papillae are located.
- Leukoplakia, especially proliferative verrucous leukoplakia—This may be white and rough-looking but usually does not have a symmetric distribution. The plaques are usually denser.
- Lichen planus—This is often white and bilaterally located in a symmetric fashion, but it is usually associated with pain, sensitivity, and reticulations.
- White sponge nevus—This is an uncommon developmental mucosal disorder and may involve the tongue bilaterally but will usually also involve the buccal mucosa and other mucosal sites. These do not usually have a shaggy appearance.

 Best Tests

-

Leukoplakia

- Biopsy is recommended to rule out SCC, especially if erythema or erosions are present within the lesion.
- Any ulceration or mass with an uneven surface and firm consistency that develops in a high-risk site for oral cancer should be viewed with suspicion, particularly if it has been present for at least 2 weeks with no sign of healing after potentially contributing local factors (e.g., sharp broken teeth) have been eliminated.

Oral Squamous Cell Carcinoma

Biopsy of the lesion will demonstrate characteristic histopathologic features of SCC.

Hairy Leukoplakia

Biopsy establishes the diagnosis. Immunohistochemistry is usually required to identify the EBV.

 Management Pearls

Leukoplakia

Treatment is dependent upon the specific diagnosis. The patient should be monitored with future visits and additional biopsies if there is a consideration of early SCC.

Oral Squamous Cell Carcinoma

Oral SCC has a higher likelihood of metastasis compared to cutaneous SCC. Refer these patients to a head and neck oncology specialist.

Hairy Leukoplakia

If there is candidal colonization, treatment with topical antifungal agents will reduce the whiteness and thickness of the lesion but not resolve it entirely. Treatment with antiretroviral therapy in the HIV patients will generally resolve the lesion.

Therapy

Leukoplakia

Cessation of tobacco use is essential, as is avoidance of local trauma. Proper dental care is advised.

If the lesion is premalignant, ensure complete removal. Effective techniques have included excision, CO_2 laser, fulguration, and cryotherapy. Medical therapies have not been successful in preventing malignant transformation, and frequent relapses are seen with these treatments.

Oral Squamous Cell Carcinoma

Complete excision or radiation therapy of smaller lesions is indicated. Staging is essential to select the most appropriate surgical approach and the necessity for node dissection. For patients who are not surgical candidates, radiation therapy is a reasonable alternative.

Hairy Leukoplakia

No treatment is necessary except for antifungal therapy if colonized by *Candida*.

Suggested Readings

Bsoul SA, Huber MA, Terezhalmy GT. Squamous cell carcinoma of the oral tissues: A comprehensive review for oral healthcare providers. *J Contemp Dent Pract.* 2005;6(4):1–16.

Campana JP, Meyers AD. The surgical management of oral cancer. *Otolaryngol Clin North Am.* 2006;39(2):331–348.

Gangadharan P, Paymaster JC. Leukoplakia—an epidemiologic study of 1504 cases observed at the Tata Memorial Hospital, Bombay, India. *Br J Cancer.* 1971;25(4):657–668.

Husak R, Garbe C, Orfanos CE. Oral hairy leukoplakia in 71 HIV-seropositive patients: Clinical symptoms, relation to immunologic status, and prognostic significance. *J Am Acad Dermatol.* 1996;35(6):928–934.

James WD, Berger TG, Elston DM, eds. Disorders of the mucous membranes. In: *Andrews' Diseases of the Skin: Clinical Dermatology.* 10th Ed. Philadelphia, PA: Elsevier; 2006:804–806.

Konkimalla VB, Suhas VL, Chandra NR, et al. Diagnosis and therapy of oral squamous cell carcinoma. *Expert Rev Anticancer Ther.* 2007;7(3):317–329.

Lodi G, Sardella A, Bez C, et al. Systematic review of randomized trials for the treatment of oral leukoplakia. *J Dent Educ.* 2002;66(8):896–902.

Martin JL. Leukoedema: A review of the literature. *J Natl Med Assoc.* 1992;84(11):938–940.

Montes DM, Schmidt BL. Oral maxillary squamous cell carcinoma: Management of the clinically negative neck. *J Oral Maxillofac Surg.* 2008;66(4):762–766.

Palme CE, Gullane PJ, Gilbert RW. Current treatment options in squamous cell carcinoma of the oral cavity. *Surg Oncol Clin N Am.* 2004;13(1):47–70.

Prince S, Bailey BM. Squamous carcinoma of the tongue: Review. *Br J Oral Maxillofac Surg.* 1999;37(3):164–174.

Resnick L, Herbst JS, Raab-Traub N. Oral hairy leukoplakia. *J Am Acad Dermatol.* 1990;22(6 Pt 2):1278–1282.

Sciubba JJ. Opportunistic oral infections in the immunosuppressed patient: Oral hairy leukoplakia and oral candidiasis. *Adv Dent Res.* 1996;10(1):69–72.

Sciubba JJ. Oral cancer. The importance of early diagnosis and treatment. *Am J Clin Dermatol.* 2001;2(4):239–251.

Tenzer JA, Sugarman HM, Britton JC. Squamous cell carcinoma of the gingiva found in a patient with AIDS. *J Am Dent Assoc.* 1992;123(12):65–67.

Thomas G, Hashibe M, Jacob BJ, et al. Risk factors for multiple oral premalignant lesions. *Int J Cancer.* 2003;107(2):285–291.

Triantos D, Porter SR, Scully C, et al. Oral hairy leukoplakia: Clinicopathologic features, pathogenesis, diagnosis, and clinical significance. *Clin Infect Dis.* 1997;25(6):1392–1396.

Onychomycosis

Stephanie Diamantis

■■ Diagnosis Synopsis

Onychomycosis refers to fungal infection of the nail plate. Four patterns of involvement have been described: distal lateral subungual onychomycosis (DLSO), white superficial onychomycosis (WSO), proximal subungual onychomycosis (PSO), and *Candida* onychomycosis. Dermatophytes (especially *Trichophyton rubrum* and *Trichophyton mentagrophytes*) are the most common cause of onychomycosis.

Predisposing factors include male sex, older age, diabetes, immune suppression, hyperhidrosis, poor peripheral circulation, trauma, and nail dystrophy. Toenails are more frequently affected.

DLSO, the most common form, begins with fungal invasion of the hyponychium and spreads proximally along the nail bed and the lateral nail grooves. In Western countries, DLSO is mainly due to *T. rubrum*.

WSO involves only the nail plate and presents with porcelain-white discoloration and crumbling on the surface of the nail plate. The most common causative organism is *T. mentagrophytes*.

PSO is caused by invasion of the proximal nail fold, with spread to the newly formed nail plate. A variant, proximal white subungual onychomycosis (PWSO) is seen in patients with AIDS and is caused by *T. rubrum*. The finding of PWSO should prompt the practitioner to obtain HIV serologies.

True nail invasion by *Candida* is seen almost exclusively in chronic mucocutaneous candidiasis. Nail bed yellowing and thickening is accompanied by swelling of the nail folds.

◉ Look For

DLSO—Toenails are more frequently affected than fingernails; if fingernails are involved, it is almost always in association with toenail disease. Nails show yellowish-white discoloration, nail thickening, subungual hyperkeratosis, and onycholysis (lifting of the nail plate from the nail bed) (Figs. 4-622 and 4-623).

WSO—Milky-white discoloration and crumbling of the nail plate, with plaster-like consistency.

PSO—Discoloration is noted at the proximal aspect of the nail plate; onychomadesis (separation of the nail plate from the proximal side) may occur (Fig. 4-624).

In the setting of onychomycosis secondary to a dermatophyte, there is frequently concomitant tinea pedis (marked

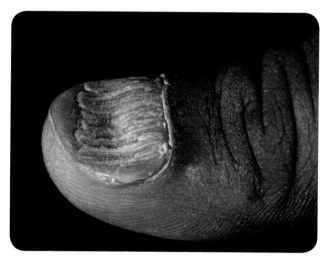

Figure 4-623 Roughness and spooning of the thumbnail from dermatophyte infection.

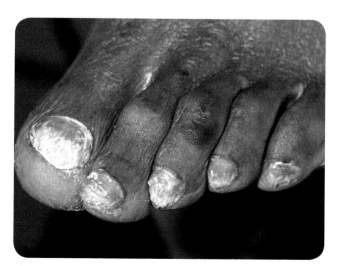

Figure 4-622 Onychomycosis with varying degrees of destruction of the nail plate.

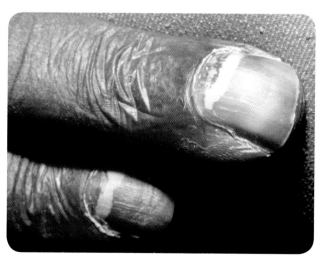

Figure 4-624 Proximal subungual onychomycosis due to *T. rubrum* manifested by a dense white transverse band.

by scaly erythematous patches in the web spaces of the toes and on the soles or sides of the feet). Maceration of the web spaces may lead to painful fissures and secondary bacterial infection. Infection with *T. mentagrophytes* var. *interdigitale* may show bullae. There may also be concomitant tinea corporis or tinea capitis.

Diagnostic Pearls

- Onychomycosis is usually asymmetrical, involving one to three nails of only one hand or foot. In case of symmetrical involvement of all the nails, an alternative diagnosis or immunodeficiency should be considered.
- Always check the skin, particularly the feet and scalp, for coexistent dermatophyte infection, and screen family members.
- Apparent SWO caused by *T. rubrum* should raise concern for possible HIV/AIDS.

?? Differential Diagnosis and Pitfalls

- Psoriasis—may also see splinter hemorrhages, oil spots, onycholysis, random pitting in the nail plate
- Lichen planus—pterygium most common
- Twenty-nail dystrophy or trachyonychia
- Pachyonychia congenita

✓ Best Tests

- Laboratory confirmation with direct microscopy (KOH) and/or fungal culture. Material should be collected from nail clippings and subungual debris (undersurface of the nail plate).
- Direct microscopy using KOH is the most inexpensive method and has a sensitivity of approximately 80% but cannot identify the specific genus or species of fungus.
- Fungal culture allows for identification of a viable, specific pathogen but has a sensitivity of only 50% to 70% and may show false-positive results due to contamination.
- Histopathology with a periodic acid-Schiff (PAS) stain is the most sensitive method, though it cannot identify viable or specific pathogens. Histopathology is generally reserved for cases in which direct microscopy and culture have failed to confirm infection.

▲▲ Management Pearls

- A patient should never be treated with systemic antifungal agents without confirmed infection based on direct microscopy, fungal culture, or histopathology because of the cost and potential morbidity associated with systemic antifungal agents.
- Measurement of the distance from proximal nail fold to proximal edge of onycholysis will monitor response to treatment.

Therapy

Oral antifungal treatments offer the best mycologic cure rates in documented dermatophyte infections. Antifungal medications itraconazole and terbinafine have better cure and relapse rates than griseofulvin for onychomycosis. Moreover, the duration of treatment is shorter (2 to 5 months). Clinical trials show that itraconazole and terbinafine appear to be safe and effective. Continuous or pulsed regimens are equally effective. If continuous treatment is the goal, duration of therapy is 6 weeks for fingernails and 12 weeks for toenails. Accepted treatment regimens are as follows:

- Terbinafine 250 mg by mouth daily for 6 to 12 weeks
- Itraconazole 200 mg by mouth daily for 6 to 12 weeks
- Pulsed itraconazole 400 mg by mouth daily for 1 week each month (continued for 2 months for fingernails and 3 months for toenails)

Monitoring of hepatic parameters is recommended when using the above systemic therapies.

Other Medications

Fluconazole is fungistatic against dermatophytes, *Candida*, and some nondermatophyte molds and can be given as weekly intermittent therapy (150 to 400 mg weekly for 12 weeks for fingernails, 26 weeks for toenails).

Topical therapy has a role in patients with mild infections or those who do not desire or cannot tolerate systemic therapy. Ciclopirox 8% nail lacquer alone requires daily application for 9 to 12 months. Topical 40% urea ointment/cream under occlusion is a useful adjunct to either topical or oral antifungal agents.

Mechanical debridement with total or partial surgical nail avulsion is also effective.

Suggested Readings

Billstein S, Kianifard F, Justice A. Terbinafine vs. placebo for onychomycosis in black patients. *Int J Dermatol.* 1999;38:377–379.

Sobera JO, Elewski BE. Onychomycosis. In: Scher RK, Daniel CR III, eds. *Nails: Diagnosis, Therapy, Surgery.* 3rd Ed. Philadelphia, PA: Elsevier; 2005:123–131.

Zaias N, Rebell G. The successful treatment of Trichophyton rubrum nail bed (distal subungual) onychomycosis with intermittent pulse-dosed terbinafine. *Arch Dermatol.* 2004;140(6):691–695.

Paronychia

Stephanie Diamantis

■■ Diagnosis Synopsis

Paronychia is a term that describes inflammation and swelling of periungual soft tissues. There are two types of paronychia: acute and chronic. Paronychia can also be drug induced. Patients often report pain in association with paronychia, particularly in the acute form. Nail dystrophy is more common with chronic paronychia. No ethnic predilection has been documented.

Acute paronychia occurs rapidly and is associated with redness, pain, and, in the case of infection, purulent drainage. Acute paronychia is often bacterial in nature and most commonly caused by *Staphylococcus aureus*. This condition tends to occur in individuals exposed to hand trauma or chronic moisture. Paronychia may also originate from a break in the epidermis (hangnail, foreign body, etc.). The skin and soft tissue of the nail fold(s) will be red, swollen, and tender and can evolve into an abscess if not treated. Inflammation may move under the nail plate leading to an onychomadesis (proximal separation of the nail plate from the nail bed). Paronychia may result in more serious infections such as felons (whitlow, or pyogenic infection of distal digit), osteomyelitis, and septic tenosynovitis.

Chronic paronychia lasts for more than 6 weeks, results in loss of the cuticle, and can have nail dystrophy. The initial insult is often traumatic or irritant and compromises the barrier between the nail plate and nail fold (e.g., repeated immersions in water, thumb sucking, or overzealous manicuring). The dominant hand is often the one affected, which supports a traumatic or contact etiology. The condition is frequently seen in diabetics as well as those who frequently have their hands in water, such as cooks, homemakers, dishwashers, bartenders, laundry workers, etc. Individuals affected by inflammatory dermatoses such as eczematous dermatitis

and other diseases that can cause lifting of the nail plate from the nail bed (onycholysis) are at an increased risk. *Candida* can often be found in fungal culture obtained from chronic paronychia, although the exact role (superinfection vs. primary pathogen) is not known.

While infectious causes are more common, there are several reports of paronychia caused by medications. Reported medications include retinoids, lamivudine, cyclosporine, indinavir, azidothymidine (AZT), cephalexin, sulfonamides, cetuximab, gefitinib, fluorouracil (5-FU), methotrexate, and docetaxel. The paronychia coincides with the start of the drug and can present as acute or chronic, depending on the length of duration. The paronychia usually resolves once the medication is discontinued.

Look For

Swelling and erythema of the tissues surrounding the nail unit (Fig. 4-625). Pus may also be present, and lesions are usually tender (Figs. 4-626 and 4-627). Onycholysis and cuticle loss are also seen. Distortion of the nail plate is not uncommon if inflammation is chronic in nature (Fig. 4-628). Acute paronychia usually involves only one digit that is often significantly inflamed.

Diagnostic Pearls

- Chronic paronychia can cause transverse ridging of the nail plates and loss of the cuticle. There is no subungual debris as in nail psoriasis or onychomycosis.
- Patients whose occupations require them to have their hands in contact with water for extended periods of

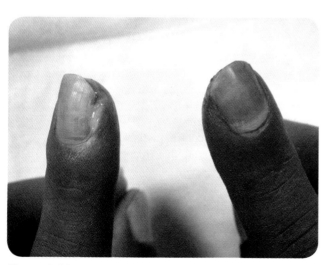
Figure 4-625 Acute paronychia may have visible pus.

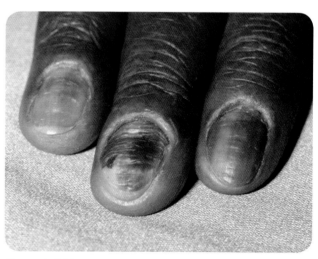
Figure 4-626 Chronic nail fold swelling and nail ridging characteristic of chronic paronychia.

565

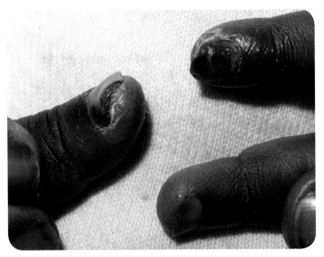

Figure 4-627 Chronic *Candida* paronychia in a child due to finger sucking.

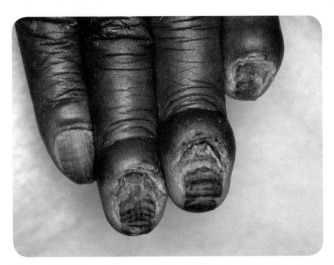

Figure 4-628 Massive paronychia and nail plate destruction due to *Candida* infection.

time (e.g., bartenders, florists, cleaners, dishwashers) are particularly susceptible to paronychia, as are the immunocompromised.

- Suspicion for drug-induced paronychia should be considered if history is consistent.

?? Differential Diagnosis and Pitfalls

Acute Paronychia

- Pustular psoriasis
- Reactive arthritis (Reiter syndrome)
- Onychomycosis
- Herpetic whitlow
- Syphilitic chancre
- Acropustulosis continua
- Ingrown nail
- Allergic contact dermatitis
- Irritant dermatitis
- Fixed drug eruption

Chronic Paronychia

- Contact dermatitis
- Atopic dermatitis
- Irritant dermatitis (e.g., thumb sucking, constant wetting)
- Occupational paronychia (foreign bodies, e.g., hairs, bristles)
- Parasitic infection of the paronychia (*Tunga penetrans*)
- Drug-induced paronychia
- Dermatologic diseases (psoriasis, lichen planus, atopic dermatitis, contact dermatitis)

- Systemic diseases (yellow nail syndrome, acrodermatitis, sarcoidosis)
- Tumors (exostosis, metastasis, melanoma)
- Self-induced (onychophagia, onychotillomania)

✓ Best Tests

Diagnosis of acute and chronic paronychia is usually clinical. To differentiate among different causes of paronychia, a Gram stain and culture of any purulent material should be undertaken. Microscopic examination with potassium hydroxide (KOH) may show yeast forms or hyphae if *Candida* or a fungal etiology is suspected. A Tzanck smear may be helpful if herpetic whitlow is suspected. Thorough history will aid in diagnosing drug-induced paronychia.

▲▲ Management Pearls

- Manage environmental factors. Patients should be instructed to avoid trauma to the nails (cease nail biting, etc.) and to wear gloves during prolonged contact with water. Keeping the affected area dry is essential. Encourage avoidance of thumb sucking in children. Discourage overzealous manicuring.
- Optimize glycemic control in diabetics.
- For drug-induced paronychia, stopping the medication is the most important step in managing these patients. Application of a steroid and possibly a topical antibiotic can help alleviate the inflammation and help prevent secondary infection.
- Imaging should be considered in patients unresponsive to treatment to evaluate for underlying osteomyelitis or malignancy.

Therapy

Acute Paronychia

If acute paronychia does not respond within 48 hours, it should be treated surgically to prevent damage to the nail matrix.

Medical Approach

- Soaks three to four times a day with warm water and disinfectant solution (e.g., chlorhexidine).
- Systemic antibiotics with staphylococcal coverage are recommended following culture. First-line antibiotics include the cephalosporin family (cephalexin 250 to 500 mg by mouth four times daily). Amoxicillin/clavulanic acid (500 to 875 mg p.o. every 12 hours for adults) or clindamycin (150 to 450 mg p.o. every 6 to 8 hours for adults) are also effective. Antibiotics should be continued for 1 week after clinical infection resolves.

Surgical Approach

Any collection of purulent material should be drained. Paronychia that worsens or fails to respond to conservative medical management may benefit from a surgical approach. Under a proximal digital block, the nail plate is detached from the proximal nail fold with a small, blunt instrument (dental spatula, Freer elevator). The proximal third of the nail can then be excised with scissors and the pus evacuated. The abscess cavity should be irrigated and packed and the patient placed on systemic antibiotics. Packing can be removed after 2 days and warm soaks begun. More advanced paronychia will require incision and drainage under a proximal digital block. With a no. 11 or 15 blade, a longitudinal incision is made in the nail fold to the base of the nail and the eponychium elevated to drain the pus. The proximal third of the nail is removed and the abscess cavity treated as above.

Chronic Paronychia

Initial approach should be to minimize or eliminate causative or exacerbating factors (e.g., contactants, irritants, exposure to water). Avoid physical trauma to cuticles. Patients should be instructed to wear protective gloves and prevent hands from chapping or drying.

Midpotency to high-potency corticosteroids are the mainstay of therapy and should be applied twice daily until the cuticle has regrown. Topical antifungals (e.g., clotrimazole, ciclopirox) are helpful as drying and antiyeast agents. Oral antibiotics (e.g., cephalosporins) are not routinely used for the chronic condition but may be helpful in acute exacerbations of chronic paronychia. In more resistant cases, patients may need systemic antifungal agents: fluconazole (100 mg daily for 14 days), itraconazole (200 mg twice daily for 1 week of each of 3 months) or terbinafine (250 mg daily for 3 months).

Surgical therapy (e.g., excision of proximal nail fold) may be indicated if paronychia is resistant to other therapies.

Drug-Induced Paronychia

Discontinue the offending drug, if possible.

Suggested Readings

Chow E, Goh CL. Epidemiology of chronic paronychia in a skin hospital in Singapore. *Int J Dermatol.* 1991;30(11):795–798.

Daniel CR III. Simple chronic paronychia. In: Scher RK, Daniel CR III, eds. *Nails: Diagnosis, Therapy, Surgery.* 3rd Ed. Philadelphia, PA: Elsevier; 2005:99–103.

Pseudomonas Nail Infection

Stephanie Diamantis

Diagnosis Synopsis

The "green nail syndrome" is characterized by the following clinical triad:

- Green discoloration of the nail plate
- Paronychia
- Distolateral onycholysis

Exposure to a moist environment or frequent soaps/detergents, trauma, onychotillomania (compulsive manipulation or pulling out of the nails), and associated nail diseases such as psoriasis may promote infection by *Pseudomonas*. *Pseudomonas* species can colonize any area (distal, lateral, proximal) of the nail plate where there is onycholysis. The subsequent pigmentation varies both with the species involved and with the composition of the pigments produced. The greenish hue varies from light green to deep, dark green. *Pseudomonas* species produce a number of diffusible pigments such as pyocyanin (dark green) and fluorescein (yellow-green). Both are soluble in water; the former is also soluble in chloroform.

The main complaint of patients is the green discoloration of the nails. Patients must avoid excessive exposure to moist environments, or they will have a high rate of recolonization even after treatment.

Look For

Lifting of the nail plate from the nail bed (onycholysis) and green-black or green-blue discoloration of the nail (Fig. 4-629).

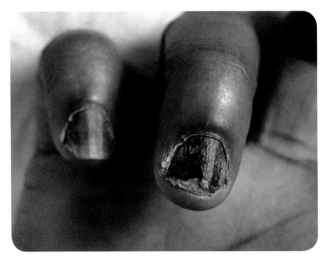

Figure 4-629 Green-black nail plate caused by *Pseudomonas* infection.

Diagnostic Pearls

Usually only one or two nails are affected, and there is little periungual inflammation and no discomfort. Color change may appear in discrete horizontal bands, as activity of infection varies in the proximal nail fold.

Differential Diagnosis and Pitfalls

- Subungual hematoma
- Melanonychia
- Melanocytic nevus
- Melanoma
- Psoriasis
- Infection of nail plate with other organisms: dermatophyte, *Proteus mirabilis*, *Aspergillus*, *Candida*, *Fusarium*

Best Tests

Gram stain and culture of the nail plate or any obtainable exudates may be performed.

Management Pearls

- The most important method for preventing future infection is to protect the hands/nails from water by using vinyl gloves. Be sure the patient turns the gloves inside out after use to prevent the growth of the organism in the gloves.
- Other predisposing factors, such as trauma and underlying nail disease (psoriasis, etc.), should be minimized whenever possible. Nails should be kept clipped short.

Therapy

Trim the nail plate and follow with local therapy (e.g., topical gentamicin, 15% sulfacetamide, chloramphenicol ophthalmic solution) three times daily, typically for 1 to 4 months. Soaking in 1% acetic acid twice daily may help as well.

Note: It will take several months for the discoloration to grow out with the nail plate.

Suggested Readings

Agger WA, Mardan A. *Pseudomonas aeruginosa* infections of intact skin. *Clin Infect Dis.* 1995;20(2):302–308.

Elewski BE. Bacterial infection in a patient with onychomycosis. *J Am Acad Dermatol.* 1997;37(3 Pt 1):493–494.

LeFeber WP, Golitz LE. Green foot. *Pediatr Dermatol.* 1984;2(1):38–40.

Maes M, Richert B, de la Brassinne M. Green nail syndrome or chloronychia. *Rev Med Liege.* 2002;57(4):233–235.

Mermel LA, McKay M, Dempsey J, et al. Pseudomonas surgical-site infections linked to a healthcare worker with onychomycosis. *Infect Control Hosp Epidemiol.* 2003;24(10):749–752.

Sakata S, Howard A. Pseudomonas chloronychia in a patient with nail psoriasis. *Med J Aust.* 2007;186(8):424.

Shellow WV, Koplon BS. Green striped nails: chromonychia due to *Pseudomonas aeruginosa. Arch Dermatol.* 1968;97(2):149–153.

Swartz MN. Gram-negative coccal and bacillary infections. In: Fitzpatrick TB, Wolff K, eds. *Fitzpatrick's Dermatology in General Medicine.* 7th Ed. New York, NY: McGraw-Hill; 2008:1735–1739.

Winslow EH, Jacobson AF. Can a fashion statement harm the patient? Long and artificial nails may cause nosocomial infections. *Am J Nurs.* 2000;100(9):63–65.

Juvenile Plantar Dermatosis

Randa Khoury

■■ Diagnosis Synopsis

Juvenile plantar dermatosis is a localized scaling and fissuring dermatitis of the plantar surface seen in prepubertal and early teenage children. The condition is more frequent in atopic children. It is thought to be caused by repeated maceration followed by drying, inducing impairment of the superficial epidermis.

◉ Look For

Taut shiny-appearing plantar skin with accentuation of the skin folds (Fig. 4-630). Fissures can be prominent. Although sweating can be marked, the skin feels dry and scaly. Flares are episodic and last 1 to 2 weeks.

●● Diagnostic Pearls

Note that in juvenile plantar dermatosis, the great toe, ball of the foot, and heel are most often involved. Interdigital and arch areas are usually spared. Patients often pick at the scale and cause painful wounds.

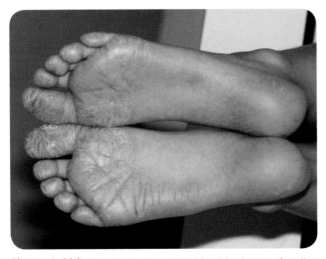

Figure 4-630 Juvenile plantar dermatitis with plaques of scaling and erythema.

?? Differential Diagnosis and Pitfalls

- When limited to the feet, all efforts to exclude a bullous dermatophyte infection should be made.
- Tinea pedis may present similarly to juvenile plantar dermatosis, but can be easily differentiated by demonstrating fungal elements using a KOH preparation from scale.
- Dyshidrotic dermatitis
- Allergic contact dermatitis reaction to shoes more commonly involves the dorsal surface of the foot.
- Psoriasis can also affect the bilateral soles. Additional pertinent skin and nail findings can help make this diagnosis.
- Pitted keratolysis
- Keratoderma often involves the palms as well, and patients may report a family history of similar findings.

✓ Best Tests

Juvenile plantar dermatitis is a clinical diagnosis. Rule out dermatophytosis with a KOH examination of the scale.

▲▲ Management Pearls

Encourage patients to use a different pair of shoes on alternating days to allow the shoes to dry out.

Therapy

Avoid excessive moisture and maceration followed by complete drying. Encourage use of foot powders, thick absorbent or moisture-wicking socks, and absorbent insoles. White petrolatum or urea-containing preparations (Carmol) may be helpful to repair barrier function of epidermis.

Suggested Readings

Guenst BJ. Common pediatric foot dermatoses. *J Pediatr Health Care*. 1999;13(2)68–71.

Lemont H, Pearl B. Juvenile plantar dermatosis. *J Am Podiatr Med Assoc*. 1992;82(3):167–169.

Palmoplantar Keratoderma

Stephanie Diamantis

■■ Diagnosis Synopsis

Palmoplantar keratoderma (PPK) is thickening of the palms and/or soles that cannot be attributed to friction alone. Cases are either inherited or acquired. Heritable PPKs are identified by the presence of a family history and childhood onset; they may manifest in isolation, as the defining feature of a syndrome, or as a minor aspect of a syndrome (e.g., congenital ichthyoses, Darier disease).

Hereditary PPKs are approached and classified by the pattern of hyperkeratosis: diffuse, focal (often occurring over weight-bearing areas), or punctate.

- Diffuse hereditary PPK
  - Vorner (epidermolytic) PPK and Unna-Thost (non-epidermolytic) PPK are the result of keratin mutations and show waxy or verrucous, white-yellow, symmetric hyperkeratosis.
  - Mal de Meleda is a rare diffuse hereditary PPK associated with *SLURP1* gene mutations and features stocking-glove distribution of hyperkeratosis with malodor and nail changes.
  - Vohwinkel syndrome (mutilating PPK) has two variants: the classic form associated with deafness and mutations of the connexin gene *GJB2*; and the loricrin variant associated with loricrin mutations and ichthyosis. The PPK shows a diffuse honeycomb pattern. Additional features include starfish-shaped keratotic plaques on dorsal hands, feet, elbows, and knees as well as constricting digital bands termed "pseudo-ainhum," which may progress to autoamputation (Fig. 4-631). This condition is more common in whites and in women.

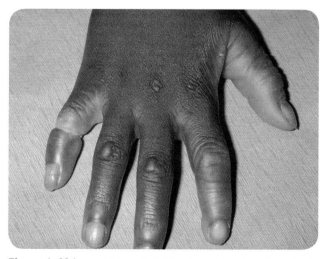

Figure 4-631 Constricting digital bands and dorsal hand papules in keratosis palmaris plantaris resembling Vohwinkel syndrome.

- Papillon-Lefèvre syndrome is associated with mutations in the gene that encodes cathepsin C and demonstrates diffuse PPK, periodontal disease with loss of teeth, and frequent cutaneous and systemic pyogenic infections.
  - Other diffuse hereditary PPKs include Greither syndrome, Bart-Pumphrey syndrome (PPK with knuckle pads, leukonychia, and deafness), Huriez syndrome (PPK with scleroatrophy), Clouston syndrome (hidrotic ectodermal dysplasia), Olmsted syndrome (mutilating PPK with periorificial plaques), diffuse nonepidermolytic PPK with sensorineural deafness, and Naxos disease (diffuse nonepidermolytic PPK with wooly hair and cardiomyopathy).
- Focal hereditary PPK
  - Isolated focal PPKs (striate PPKs) are due to autosomal dominant mutations in genes encoding desmosomal proteins. Lesions favor pressure points on feet and may present as linear plaques on hands.
  - Howel-Evans syndrome is associated with mutations in the TOC gene, focal weight-bearing area plantar hyperkeratosis, milder palm involvement, and development of esophageal carcinoma.
  - Richner-Hanhart syndrome is associated with mutations in the gene that encodes tyrosine aminotransferase. Accumulation of tyrosine leads to focal (or diffuse) hyperkeratotic plaques on the hands, feet, elbows, and knees; corneal inflammation/ulceration; and mental retardation in some cases. Diets low in phenylalanine and tyrosine may prevent complications.
  - Focal PPK may also be seen in pachyonychia congenita type I and type II (syndromes with nail, skin, teeth, and eye anomalies) as well as Carvajal syndrome (striate focal epidermolytic PPK with wooly hair and dilated cardiomyopathy).
- Punctate hereditary PPK or keratosis punctata (may not appear until adolescence or after)
  - Punctate PPKs are characterized by autosomal dominant inheritance and multiple firm 2- to 8-mm papules on the palms and soles. A pattern with lesions favoring palmar creases has been identified in patients of African descent.
  - Focal acral hyperkeratosis and acrokeratoelastoidosis present as 2- to 4-mm papules (some umbilicated) at the marginal borders of hands and feet.

Acquired PPKs occur later in life and have no associated family history. They may be subdivided as follows:

- Keratoderma climactericum—seen in menopausal women, often associated with obesity or hypertension; pressure points on the soles of the feet are affected first
- Infectious PPK—associated with dermatophytosis, leprosy, HIV, syphilis, crusted scabies, and human papillomavirus infections

- Chemical-/drug-induced PPK—associated with exposure to arsenic, halogenated aromatic chemicals such as dioxin, venlafaxine, verapamil, hydroxyurea, etodolac, quinacrine, proguanil, methyldopa, practolol, doxorubicin, bleomycin, hydroxyurea, imatinib, capecitabine, tegafur, lithium, gold, and mexiletine
- Dermatosis-related PPK—may be associated with atopic and contact dermatitis, psoriasis, reactive arthritis (keratoderma blennorrhagicum), lichen planus, lichen nitidus, lupus erythematosus, and pityriasis rubra pilaris
- PPK as a feature of systemic disease—hypothyroidism, myxedema, diabetes mellitus, and chronic lymphedema
- Malnutrition-associated PPK
- Aquagenic keratoderma—most often affects palms in patients in the second decade of life. Symptoms develop within 5 minutes of immersion in water. May be a marker for cystic fibrosis.
- Paraneoplastic PPK—Acrokeratosis paraneoplastica of Bazex is associated with squamous cell carcinoma of the upper GI tract, and "tripe palm" is associated with pulmonary or gastric malignancies. Other malignancies with associated paraneoplastic PPK include breast, bladder, and skin malignancies; myeloma; mycosis fungoides (cutaneous T-cell lymphoma); and Sézary syndrome.
- Idiopathic PPK—a diagnosis of exclusion

(◉) Look For

Thickening of the palms and/or soles with variable areas affected (Fig. 4-632). Sometimes, there is platelike scale or confluent, brown-to-yellow thickening. Patterns include diffuse, focal, and punctate. In the focal variants, the areas of hyperkeratosis can be very well defined.

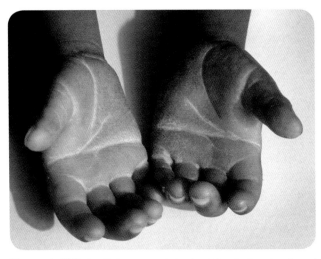

Figure 4-632 Familial autosomal dominant keratosis palmaris and plantaris.

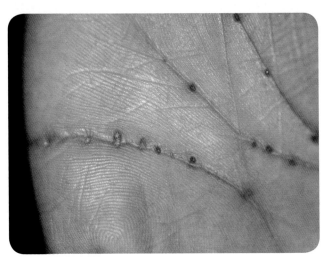

Figure 4-633 Typical well-defined painful punctate depressions in the palm creases of PPK.

Lesions that extend beyond the plantar or palmar skin may occur. These are referred to as "transgrediens."

In keratosis punctata, look for 2- to 4-mm keratotic depressions on the palms and soles (Fig. 4-633). A variant favoring the creases of the palms is commonly seen in patients of African descent and can be somewhat painful.

●● Diagnostic Pearls

- Assessment begins by characterizing cases as inherited or acquired.
- Hereditary PPK cases are initially evaluated by pattern (diffuse, focal, or punctuate), by the presence or absence of transgrediens, accompanying symptoms, and family history.
- Acquired cases should be evaluated with history and physical examination attuned to the list provided in the synopsis section. If no diagnosis is evident, limited diagnostic testing is indicated, including fungal scrapings, chest radiograph, thyroid-stimulating hormone, complete blood count, antinuclear antibody, rapid plasma reagin, HIV, and purified protein derivative. If the cause remains obscure after these tests, an age- and sex-appropriate search for malignancy is indicated, including CT scans of the chest/abdomen/pelvis, upper and lower gastrointestinal tract endoscopy, and cystoscopy. Only if these are negative should the designation of idiopathic PPK be assigned.
- Aquagenic keratoderma may be a marker for cystic fibrosis.
- Symmetry is usual, and asymmetric changes should prompt consideration of infectious or dermatosis-related PPK.
- Patients of African decent can present with small hyperkeratotic plugs in the large creases of palms and fingers (punctate keratosis of palmar creases). Fifty percent of

black patients aged older than 50 will have punctate keratosis of the palmar or finger creases. These lesions may be tender and painful when performing manual labor. Both idiopathic and inherited cases exist.

?? Differential Diagnosis and Pitfalls

Acquired Conditions That May Have PPK as a Feature

- Psoriasis
- Atopic dermatitis
- Dyshidrotic eczema
- Contact dermatitis
- Pityriasis rubra pilaris
- Reactive arthritis
- Acrodermatitis paraneoplastica of Bazex
- Tinea pedis/manuum
- Arsenical exposure
- Acanthosis nigricans (tripe palms are associated)
- Acquired ichthyosis associated with a malignancy
- Cutaneous T-cell lymphoma
- Lymphedema
- Secondary syphilis

Additional Inherited Conditions That May Have PPK as a Feature (See "Diagnosis Synopsis" for Inherited Conditions in Which PPK Predominates)

- Congenital ichthyoses
- Erythrokeratodermas
- Ectodermal dysplasias
- Dyskeratosis congenita
- Darier disease
- Basal cell nevus syndrome
- Incontinentia pigmenti
- Epidermolysis bullosa simplex
- Kindler syndrome
- Naegeli-Franceschetti-Jadassohn syndrome

PPK may occasionally be confused with pitted keratolysis, corns and callosities, or warts. Pitted keratolysis is a superficial cutaneous infection caused by the bacterium *Micrococcus sedentarius* or *Corynebacterium* sp. It is differentiated by the crateriform coalescing pits on the pressure-bearing areas of the foot.

✓ Best Tests

- Biopsy can usually differentiate warts from PPK but is often not helpful in defining the underlying cause of an acquired keratoderma. In hereditary cases, however, the presence or absence of epidermolysis on histopathology may narrow the differential diagnosis.
- Scrape any scaly lesions and examine under the microscope with KOH 20% to rule out a fungal infection. Dermatophytosis may be the cause of PPK or a treatable complication of a PPK.
- Consider thyroid function testing if the clinical scenario warrants, as cases of PPK associated with myxedema have been reported.
- Genetic testing may be an option in inherited cases.

▲▲ Management Pearls

- Saline soaks and the paring down of hyperkeratotic areas are important adjunctive treatments.
- Keratolytics are the mainstay of therapy.
- Referral to a dermatologist or podiatrist may be helpful in management of palmar and plantar hyperkeratosis. Consider referral to a geneticist in hereditary forms of PPK. Certain syndromes have an increased risk of malignancy and need ongoing evaluation by a specialist.

Therapy

Treat any identifiable underlying condition (e.g., infection, malignancy, dermatosis, hypothyroidism), or stop any causative agents (e.g., drug).

Topical keratolytics are the mainstay of treatment. Examples include 5% to 10% salicylic acid, 10% lactic acid, 10% to 40% propylene glycol, or a 10% to 40% urea cream applied once or twice daily to thickened skin. Overnight occlusion may enhance the results.

Topical retinoids are also efficacious, but their use may be limited by irritation: tretinoin 0.1% gel or 0.1% cream nightly. Systemic retinoids (isotretinoin 1 mg/kg daily, acitretin 25 to 50 mg daily) should be considered second-line and require careful monitoring for toxicities.

Alternative therapies that have demonstrated some efficacy include:

- Surgical excision and grafting
- Manual paring of hyperkeratosis
- Topical calcipotriol
- Topical corticosteroids
- Topical psoralen plus UVA (PUVA), sometimes combined with acitretin or isotretinoin
- Dermabrasion
- Carbon dioxide laser
- Transplantation of normal body epidermis to the affected volar skin (Fig. 4-634).

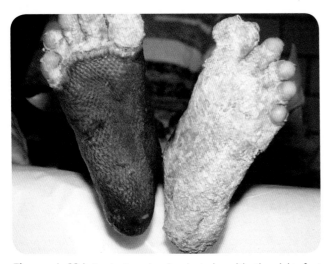

Figure 4-634 Keratosis palmaris plantaris, with the right foot treated by autotransplantation of general body skin that has retained its pigmentation.

Suggested Readings

James WD, Berger TG, Elston DM, eds. Pityriasis rosea, pityriasis rubra pilaris, and other papulosquamous and hyperkeratotic diseases. In: *Andrews' Diseases of the Skin: Clinical Dermatology*. 10th Ed. Philadelphia, PA: Elsevier; 2006:211–215.

Patel S, Zirwas M, English JC III. Acquired palmoplantar keratoderma. *Am J Clin Dermatol*. 2007;8(1):1–11.

Ratnavel RC, Griffiths WA. The inherited palmoplantar keratodermas. *Br J Dermatol*. 1997;137(4):485–490.

Spitz JL. Disorders of cornification. In: *Genodermatoses: A Clinical Guide to Genetic Skin Disorders*. 2nd Ed. Philadelphia, PA: Lippincott Williams &Wilkins; 2005:2–54.

Tinea Pedis
Stephanie Diamantis

■■ Diagnosis Synopsis

Tinea pedis is a localized inflammatory reaction to a fungal infection of the foot. The most common species of dermatophyte responsible are *Trichophyton rubrum*, *Trichophyton mentagrophytes*, and *Epidermophyton floccosum*. The condition causes dry scales on the feet and maceration between the toes and, in some cases, leads to destruction of the nail plate (onychomycosis). Factors leading to this infection include high levels of humidity, occlusive footwear, and the use of communal pools or baths. Athletes are at increased risk. Hyperhidrosis (increased sweating) can predispose to tinea pedis. Tinea pedis may lead to a secondary (Gram-negative) bacterial infection, especially in diabetic patients. Tinea pedis is more common in men. There is no ethnic predilection, and prevalence of the condition increases with age.

Tinea pedis can have different clinical presentations. Generally, dermatophytes (especially *T. rubrum*) present with red, scaly, moccasinlike plaques. Other variants include bullous tinea or interdigital tinea (athlete's foot).

A dermatophytid reaction (also called the "id reaction"), a hypersensitivity reaction, on the palms may occur in cases of bullous tinea pedis. This condition mimics dyshidrotic dermatitis in that both can demonstrate papules, vesicles, and, occasionally, pustules on the palms and lateral aspects of the fingers. The lesions on the hands do not contain fungi. The exact pathogenesis of this reaction is unknown, but it will clear with adequate treatment of the dermatophyte infection.

◉ Look For

Scaly, erythematous plaques on the dorsum of the foot, with a prominent "active" border. Hyperpigmentation may be present and lesions can extend to the dorsum of the foot or the Achilles tendon (Fig. 4-635). Plantar surfaces tend to have a powdery, white scale, sometimes in a "moccasin" distribution (i.e., the entire plantar foot and 2 to 3 cm surrounding the bottom). Web space involvement (the fourth web space is the most common) usually consists of white and macerated skin and may represent a mixed infection with bacteria (Fig. 4-636). Fissuring may occur.

Bullous tinea pedis is an uncommon variant, usually resulting from infection with *T. mentagrophytes* (Fig. 4-637). Acute ulcerative and vesiculobullous types are rarely seen in children.

Concomitant onychomycosis and/or tinea manuum (the two-foot-one-hand syndrome, named for two infected feet plus one hand) may be present (Fig. 4-638).

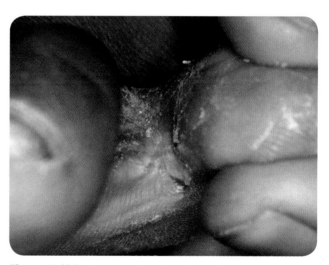
Figure 4-636 Dermatophyte with scaling in the toe web.

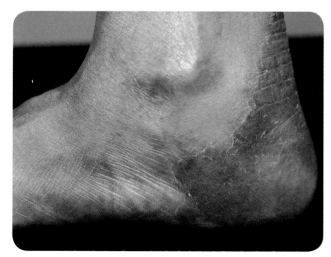
Figure 4-635 Sharply bordered hyperpigmented plaque of tinea pedis.

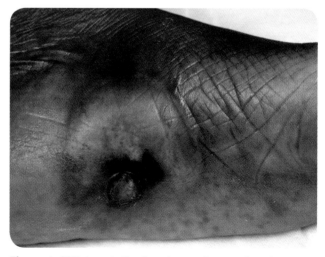
Figure 4-637 Large bullae from dermatophyte on the sole.

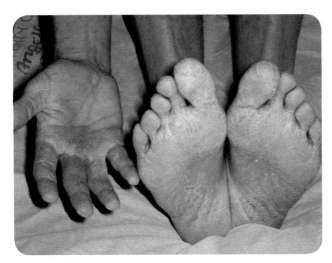

Figure 4-638 Dermatophyte infection often has scaling of both feet and one hand.

Diagnostic Pearls

- Dermatophytosis that has been treated with topical steroids can demonstrate the absence of redness and minimal scaling despite impressive fungal infection (tinea incognito). If the skin scraping is negative in a lesion that has been treated with steroids, the lesion is probably *not* fungal in etiology.
- Use a Wood light to rule out toe web erythrasma by looking for a pink to red fluorescence.
- Intertriginous tinea pedis often involves the third and fourth web spaces of the foot, unlike atopic dermatitis, which favors the first and second web spaces.
- Evaluation of toenails may reveal coexistent onychomycosis with thickening, whitening, or onycholysis.
- Tinea pedis is especially common among athletes. Pruritus may be severe.

Differential Diagnosis and Pitfalls

- Erythrasma— typically hyperkeratotic but can be erosive
- Maceration with mixed bacteria
- Candidiasis
- Contact dermatitis
- Psoriasis—sometimes may be limited to soles or may present in a palmoplantar distribution
- Erythema multiforme
- Dyshidrosis (also called dyshidrotic eczema or pompholyx)
- Pityriasis rubra pilaris
- Secondary syphilis
- Pitted keratolysis
- Juvenile plantar dermatosis
- Keratoderma

Bullous tinea pedis may be confused with friction blisters or autoimmune blistering disorders.

✓ Best Tests

- A KOH test should be performed in any patient in whom tinea pedis is suspected. If bacterial coinfection is suspected (pustules, crust, or significant inflammation), a bacterial culture should also be sent.
- To perform a KOH examination, scrape the scaly "active" border with a scalpel blade or the edge of a glass slide. If there are vesicles or bullae present, scrape the underside of the vesicle roof. Direct a drop of 10% to 20% KOH (potassium hydroxide) solution onto the slide followed by application of the coverslip. Apply gentle heat to break down scales. Under the microscope, observe for branching or curving fungal hyphae crossing cell borders.
- A fungal culture will allow species determination, but it will take several weeks.

▲▲ Management Pearls

- Small, localized lesions can be treated topically. Extensive disease may require oral antifungal agents. In persons with recurrent disease, regular use of a topical antifungal powder may be preventative.
- Encourage patients to wear protective footwear in communal bathing/swimming areas and to limit the use of highly occlusive footwear. Cotton socks are preferred, and these should be changed frequently when there is excessive perspiration. Dry the feet and interdigital spaces completely before putting on clean socks.
- Old footwear can be a source of reinfection. It is advisable to treat potentially contaminated shoes with an antifungal powder or spray (such as miconazole or tolnaftate).
- Patients with severe interdigital maceration may benefit from the use of a topical astringent such as aluminum acetate soaks combined with topical antifungals and topical gentamicin ointment to cover for Gram-negative bacterial superinfection.
- If nail involvement is present, prolonged therapy with an oral agent provides the best chance for clearance.

Therapy

Tinea pedis can often be treated with a topical antifungal cream. More extensive or complicated infections (e.g., bullous tinea pedis, tinea pedis with onychomycosis, infection in immunocompromised patients) may require systemic treatment.

Topical Antifungals

- Use topical antifungals twice daily for 2 to 6 weeks, based on clinical response.
- Examples are terbinafine 1% cream; econazole 1% cream; oxiconazole 1% cream; ciclopirox 0.77% cream, gel, or lotion; ketoconazole 2% cream; naftifine 1% cream; or butenafine 1% cream.

Note that treatments listed above are effective in the treatment of tinea pedis. To avoid recurrence, topical antifungals should be applied in the web spaces and to the soles, including approximately 2 cm of unaffected skin in the treatment area. Treatment should be continued for at least a week past the point of clinical clearing.

Allylamines (e.g., terbinafine, naftifine) are highly active against dermatophytes and are fungicidal.

Azoles (e.g., oxiconazole, clotrimazole, miconazole, econazole) have a broad spectrum of activity but are fungistatic.

Ciclopirox is among the few antifungal agents that also have antibacterial activity, which may be useful if bacterial superinfection is suspected.

Topical corticosteroids are generally not indicated, though certain authors have suggested their concomitant use with antifungals when pruritus is intense. Topical steroids should be discontinued when symptoms are relieved.

Patients with hyperkeratotic tinea pedis may benefit from a keratolytic agent such as salicylic acid or urea creams and lotions.

Extensive Disease or Disease Unresponsive to Topical Agents

- Terbinafine—250 mg daily for 2 weeks
- Itraconazole—100 to 200 mg daily for 2 to 4 weeks or 200 mg twice daily for 1 week
- Griseofulvin ultramicrosize 330 to 750 mg daily for 4 to 8 weeks
- Fluconazole—150 mg weekly for 4 weeks

Systemic antifungals are contraindicated in patients with liver disease and can cause liver failure and death, even in healthy patients. Monitoring of liver enzymes is recommended. Drug interactions are very common with systemic antifungals. If simultaneous treatment of onychomycosis is a goal, longer treatment courses than those listed here are required, but pulsed dosing of 1 week per month should be considered.

Topical antibacterials (especially those with Gram-negative coverage) may be necessary if bacterial coinfection is present. Oral antibiotics are rarely necessary.

Suggested Readings

Erbagci Z. Topical therapy for dermatophytoses: should corticosteroids be included? *Am J Clin Dermatol.* 2004;5(6):375–384.

Gupta AK, Cooper EA. Update in antifungal therapy of dermatophytosis. *Mycopathologica.* 2008;166:353–367.

Havlickova B, Czaika VA, Friedrich M. Epidemiological trends in skin mycoses worldwide. *Mycoses.* 2008;51(Suppl 4);2–15.

James WD, Berger TG, Elston DM, eds. Diseases resulting from fungi and yeasts. In: *Andrews' Diseases of the Skin: Clinical Dermatology.* 10th Ed. Philadelphia, PA: Elsevier; 2006:303–305.

Plantar Warts, Corns (Clavi), and Calluses

Arden Fredeking

■■ Diagnosis Synopsis

Plantar Wart

Plantar warts (verruca plantaris) are caused by the human papillomavirus (HPV), most frequently HPV types 1, 2, and 4. Plantar warts are hyperkeratotic papules that often favor pressure points such as the ball of the foot and under the metatarsal heads, but they may develop anywhere else on the sole and without the association of pressure. Multiple adjacent warts frequently fuse to form one large plaque, called a mosaic wart, which appears as a well-demarcated calluslike plaque on the sole of the foot with scattered central black dots. Normal dermatoglyphics are disrupted. Lesions are often asymptomatic, but a callus overlying the wart on pressure points may lead to pain with pressure or walking. They are frequently transmitted person-to-person through exposure to the virus on locker room floors, public showers, and pool areas. They are slightly more common in women, young children, and immunocompromised patients.

Corn and Callus

Corns (clavi) are keratinous thickenings of the skin of the toes that are caused by repeated friction or pressure to the area. The base of the corn is seen on the surface of the skin while the apex points inward, causing discomfort. Corns are classified as either hard or soft, depending upon their location and appearance. Hard corns typically affect the tops of the toes and are composed of a dense core that presses on sensory nerves, causing extreme pain. Soft corns, which are a source of infection in diabetic patients, occur between the toes and are continuously softened by sweat. These usually appear macerated and white.

Factors that can lead to and exacerbate corns include ill-fitting shoes, not wearing shoes, the bunching up of socks, bony prominences in the feet or other faulty foot mechanics, and repetitive physical activities that stress the skin.

A callus is a thickening of the epidermis that occurs in response to excessive, repeated shear or friction forces, commonly due to constant rubbing of the skin. Calluses are similar to corns, but calluses occur when abnormal forces are exerted over a larger area. Certain deformities of the feet, such as crookedness of the toes, may predispose to the development of calluses. Calluses may cause pain, typically a burning sensation. Excessive weight bearing and certain types of shoes are often contributing factors.

In 784 multicultural including Hispanic, non-Hispanic white, African American, and Puerto Rican men and women, over half had corns or calluses; Thickened toenails, cracks and fissures, maceration and ulcers or lacerations were more common in men, whereas corns and calluses were more common in women. Women's footwear is often suggested as the reason. Increasing height of heels increases the pressure placed on the balls of the feet. African Americans had a significantly higher prevalence of corns and calluses followed by non-Hispanic whites, and finally Puerto Ricans. This could be secondary to different rates of chronic conditions such as vascular disease, diabetes (diabetic neuropathy), and obesity. Bunions, inflammation, and thickening of the first metatarsal joint of the big toe were not reported before the introduction of western footwear.

◉ Look For

Plantar Wart

Flat, hyperkeratotic, skin-colored papules studded with pinpoint hemorrhage and often associated with overlying callus on the plantar surface of the foot (Figs. 4-639 and 4-640).

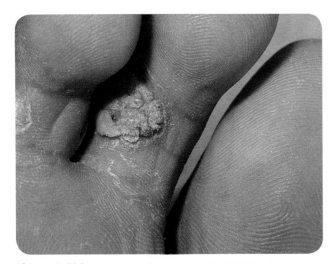

Figure 4-639 Plantar wart in a patient with HIV infection.

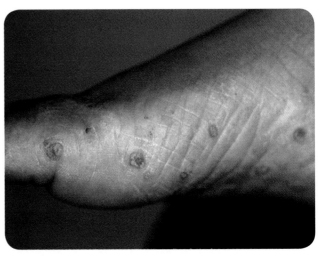

Figure 4-640 Multiple plantar warts in a pregnant woman.

Occasionally, several lesions can merge and form one large mosaic wart. Some plantar warts are inverted secondary to pressure.

Corn and Callus

Soft corns—well-circumscribed thickenings and conical, macerated papules between the toes (Fig. 4-641).

Hard corns—typically affect the tops of the toes or the side of the fifth toe and appear like calluses. They can also appear on top of the foot and even on the sole, anywhere friction occurs. They are dry and often have a waxy or transparent appearance.

Calluses—most frequently located on the feet and sometimes on the hands. They usually are located next to over bony prominences (Fig. 4-642).

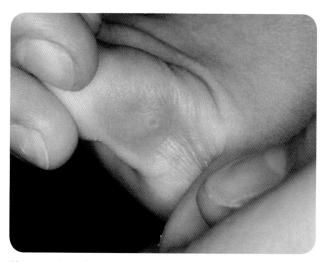

Figure 4-641 Corn on the inner surface of the toe with a prominent central core.

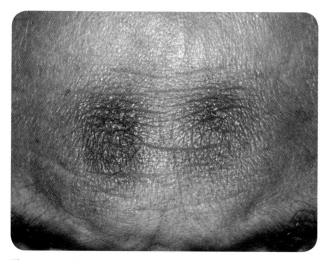

Figure 4-642 Forehead callus associated with frequent contact with a prayer rug.

 Diagnostic Pearls

Plantar Wart

Tiny black or red dots within the lesion are characteristic of warts and represent thrombosed capillaries. These are best visualized by removing the surface of the wart with a no. 15 surgical blade. Plantar warts also cause an interruption in the normal skin lines (dermatoglyphics).

Corn and Callus

The small, dark, hemorrhagic foci seen in warts are absent in corns and calluses.

?? Differential Diagnosis and Pitfalls

Plantar Wart

- A corn is a painful hyperkeratotic lesion with a central core that lacks the pinpoint thrombosed capillaries and retains normal skin dermatoglyphics. Corns occur in sites of pressure and repeated friction.
- Foreign body reaction may have a history of trauma or inoculation.
- Acquired digital fibrokeratoma tends to have a smoother and more pedunculated appearance with a collarette of normal skin.
- Squamous cell carcinoma (SCC) can arise in preexisting warts and may be recalcitrant to therapy.
- If the patient has recently traveled to a tropical area, consider tungiasis (infestation with a burrowing flea into the sole of the foot). Look for a firm, white papule with a central black dot.

Corn and Callus

- Soft corns may be mistaken for tinea pedis or psoriasis.
- Hard corns may be mistaken for the following:
  - Warts
  - Calluses—lack the dense core found in corns
  - Porokeratosis plantaris discreta
  - Eccrine poromas
  - Foreign body reaction
  - Palmoplantar keratoderma

✓ Best Tests

Plantar Wart

This is usually a clinical diagnosis; however, biopsy is confirmatory if the diagnosis is in doubt.

Lesions that are resistant to therapy should be biopsied to rule out SCC.

Corn and Callus

This is a clinical diagnosis based on morphology, symptoms, and location.

Plain films of the feet in a weight-bearing position may help identify bony protuberances.

Pediatric Patient Considerations

This is usually a clinical diagnosis. If necessary, a skin biopsy should reveal characteristic histopathological findings.

▲▲ Management Pearls

Plantar Wart

- Plantar warts can remit spontaneously. Therefore, medical intervention is usually instituted for cosmetic reasons, if the wart is painful, and in immunosuppressed patients to decrease the spread of new lesions.
- Aggressive at-home therapy with 40% salicylic acid plaster, available over the counter (OTC), applied daily or twice daily and occluded with strong adhesive tape (e.g., duct tape). Have the patient pare the wart down with a file or a pumice stone between applications of each patch.
- Given the risk of scarring, surgical removal should be limited to only special cases.
- Remind the patient he or she will need multiple treatments and that plantar warts tend to recur. Advise the use of shower shoes or sandals in public locker rooms and showers.

Corn and Callus

- Make sure that shoes fit properly. There should be plenty of room in the toe box. Orthotic insoles may be necessary. Special corn pads are commercially available to redistribute the pressure over bony prominences. For interdigital soft corns, the web space can be padded with spacers specifically designed for this purpose.
- Patients with recurrent or recalcitrant corns may require referral to a podiatrist or orthopedic surgeon for surgical correction of bony abnormalities.

Pediatric Patient Considerations

If treatment is pursued, combination therapy is usually necessary.

Therapy

Plantar Wart

Be sure to pare the wart down before cryosurgery or application of any topical therapy to improve the chance of treatment success.

Warts are benign and usually self-limited. Therefore, it is reasonable to not treat them. Patients often request treatment, however, in which case therapeutic options include the following:

- Destructive therapy: 40% salicylic acid plasters/ointments (OTC) with strong adhesive tape as described above. Can leave on for 2 to 4 days, followed by paring or pumice stone. Alternatives include silver nitrate and glutaraldehyde solution.
- Cryotherapy using liquid nitrogen applied for 5 seconds with one to three freeze/thaw cycles. Trichloroacetic acid (TCA) or monochloroacetic acid under occlusion for 48 to 72 hours. Electrodesiccation and CO_2 laser therapy should be used with caution to avoid scarring.
- Topical medications: 5-fluorouracil (1% or 5% cream) applied once or twice daily; or imiquimod 5% cream can be applied three to five times per week for 6 weeks or longer until lesions disappear. Irritation of the lesions is expected. Tretinoin 0.1% cream or gel once or twice daily as tolerated. Tretinoin can be combined with imiquimod as well. Occlusion of any topical therapy for plantar warts should improve efficacy.
- Intralesional immunotherapy: topical diphenylcyclopropenone, topical squaric acid, intralesional candida antigen, mumps antigen, and trichophyton antigens can sensitize patients to HPV. Intralesional interferon alfa 2b 1 mL of 1 million IU three times a week for 3 weeks.
- Intralesional chemotherapy: intralesional bleomycin 0.5 U/mL with no more than 3 mL injected at one time. (Use with caution because scarring and neuropathy can result.)

Be careful when treating not to induce a scar on the bottom of the foot, because this may be uncomfortable with ambulation.

Corn

Instruct the patient on conservative measures, such as attention to foot hygiene, padding, and properly fitting footwear, as above.

Pare down the corn with a no. 15 blade, and remove the central core of the lesion. Alternatively, the patient can soak corns in warm water and file down with an emery board or pumice stone. OTC salicylic acid creams or lotions (Compound W, Dr. Scholl's Corn Removers) applied daily for 4 to 6 weeks can be effective.

Callus

Pare the callus with a scalpel; unlike a corn, it does not have a central core.

Salicylic acid and TCA and aggressive paring should be used with caution in neuropathy and diabetics.

Pediatric Patient Considerations

Warts

As warts in young children may resolve spontaneously, reassurance alone is an option for asymptomatic warts. Plantar warts are typically more refractory to treatment than common warts.

For symptomatic warts, aggressive home therapy with 40% salicylic acid plaster (Mediplast) applied daily and taped on with strong tape (e.g., duct tape). Have the parent soak, then pare down the wart between applications of each patch. Diligent treatment is necessary, as larger lesions will often take up to 16 weeks to resolve.

Destructive therapies should be reserved for patients able to tolerate associated pain. These therapies include cryosurgery (liquid nitrogen), laser therapy, or treatment

with acids such as bichloroacetic acid or TCA. Make sure to pare the wart down before cryosurgery or application of any topical therapy to improve the chance of treatment success. These treatments, spaced 3 to 4 weeks apart, can be combined with home application of salicylic acid to speed resolution.

Corn and Callus

See above.

Suggested Readings

Bae JM, Kang H, Kim HO, et al. Differential diagnosis of plantar wart from corn, callus and healed wart with the aid of dermoscopy. *Br J Dermatol.* 2009;160(1):220–222.

Dunn JE, Link CL, Felson, et al. Prevalence of foot and ankle conditions in a multiethnic community sample of older adults. *Am J Epidemiol.* 2004;159(5):491–498.

Gupta AK. Single-blind, randomized, controlled trial to evaluate the efficacy and safety of photodynamic therapy using aminolevulinic acid versusliquid nitrogen cryotherapy in the management of verrucae plantaris. *J Am Acad Dermatol.* 2004;50(3):111.

Holder B, Ravishankar J, Lynfield Y. Recalcitrant plantar wart or squamous cell carcinoma? *J Am Acad Dermatol.* 2004;50(3):128.

Houseman T, Jorizzo J. Anecdotal reports of 3 cases illustrating a spectrum of resistant common warts treated with cryotherapy followed by topical imiquimod and salicylic acid. *J Am Acad of Dermatol.* 2002;47(50):217–220.

Salk R, Grogan K, Chang T. Crossover study of 5% 5-fluorouracil cream under tape occlusion in patients who failed tape occlusion alone for the treatment of plantar warts. *J Am Acad Dermatol.* 2005;52(3):131.

Dyshidrotic Dermatitis and Palmoplantar Pustulosis

Randa Khoury

■■ Diagnosis Synopsis

Eruptions on the palms and soles can frequently be distinguished from one another by their appearance and patient age.

Dyshidrotic Dermatitis

Dyshidrotic dermatitis (dyshidrotic eczema, pompholyx) is generally defined as a recurrent vesicular eruption limited to the hands (most often the sides of the digits) and sometimes the feet. The etiology is unknown; no causal relationship with sweating has been shown. The lesions are extremely pruritic, and the condition often presents episodically, more commonly in warm weather. Dyshidrotic eczema has been associated with contact irritants and allergens, atopic dermatitis, dermatophyte and bacterial infections, hyperhidrosis, hot weather, and emotional stress. Some cases spontaneously resolve. There is no gender predilection. Treatment is aimed at symptomatic relief and control of vesiculation.

Pediatric Patient Considerations

Dyshidrotic dermatitis is rare in younger children and is generally seen after the age of 10.

Palmoplantar Pustulosis

Palmoplantar pustulosis is a chronic eruption of the palms and soles composed of sterile vesicles and pustules. It is symmetric in distribution, often accompanied by painful fissuring, and is most commonly seen in women aged between 40 and 60. It often resolves spontaneously, and systemic symptoms are usually absent. The pathogenesis is not well understood. It is primarily a diagnosis of exclusion when the clinical exam does not suggest the diagnosis of dermatitis or psoriasis. Risk factors include focal infection, stress, and smoking. Only a minority of patients demonstrate classic plaque psoriasis elsewhere. Associated diseases include thyroid disease, sterile inflammatory bone lesions (part of the SAPHO syndrome: synovitis, acne, pustulosis, hyperostosis, and osteitis), psoriasis, and diabetes mellitus.

◉ Look For

Dyshidrotic Dermatitis

In dyshidrotic dermatitis, look for small, tense, clear, fluid-filled blisters at the lateral aspects of the digits (Fig. 4-643). The vesicles are deep seated in appearance (often referred to as "tapioca pudding" lesions; in dark skin, tapioca pudding

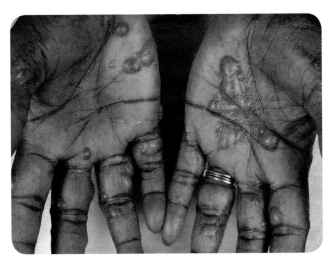

Figure 4-643 Dyshidrotic dermatitis with vesicles and lichenification on the palms and interdigitally. Vesicles on the lateral surface of the digits suggest dyshidrosis but contact dermatitis must be excluded.

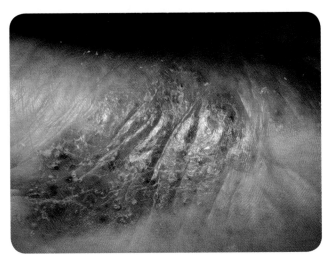

Figure 4-644 Palmoplantar pustulosis with grouped and crusted lesions.

lesions can be reddish-brown/hemorrhagic) and may converge to form bullae. In severe cases, lesions can become large and extend to the palmar surfaces. Interdigital maceration may be present. Once vesicles rupture, thin, scaly papules and plaques can form. The presence of scale can make it difficult to see the primary deep-seated vesicles that are the hallmark of dyshidrotic dermatitis. Patients with longstanding disease may have nail changes (transverse ridges, thickening, pitting).

Palmoplantar Pustulosis

With palmoplantar pustulosis, look for deep-seated vesicles, pustules, and papules on the palms, often with surrounding erythema and scale (Fig. 4-644). There are often yellow-brown macules with the pustules.

Diagnostic Pearls

Dyshidrotic Dermatitis

When dyshidrotic dermatitis is limited to the feet, all efforts to exclude dermatophyte infection should be made. Scraping the undersurface of the roof of bullae can often lead to a positive fungal scraping and culture, while studies of other portions of the lesions may be negative.

Palmoplantar Pustulosis

When considering palmoplantar pustulosis, look for subtle signs of psoriasis, such as nail pitting or scale on the scalp, umbilicus, or gluteal cleft. Also, assess for other manifestations of SAPHO syndrome (synovitis, acne, pustulosis, hyperostosis, and osteitis).

 Differential Diagnosis and Pitfalls

Dyshidrotic Dermatitis

- When limited to the feet, all efforts to exclude a bullous dermatophyte infection should be made.
- Distinguishing idiopathic dyshidrotic dermatitis from allergic contact dermatitis can be difficult, although contact dermatitis often involves the dorsum of the hand. An extensive history of environmental exposure should be gathered when a vesicular hand rash is present.
- Palmoplantar pustulosis
- Dermatophyte infection (e.g., tinea pedis and/or manuum)—pruritic, erythematous, and scaly; KOH+
- Herpetic whitlow
- Pustular psoriasis
- Scabies—look for burrows in web spaces of the fingers. Not restricted to palms and soles.
- Epidermolysis bullosa simplex
- Porphyria cutanea tarda
- Hand-foot-and-mouth disease causes cutaneous oval-shaped vesicles as well as concomitant oral mucosal vesicles or erosions.
- Zoster

Pediatric Patient Differential Diagnosis

Also include:
- Bullous impetigo
- Infantile acropustulosis

Palmoplantar Pustulosis

- Pustular psoriasis has a widespread distribution, not restricted to palms and soles; acute eruption of sterile pustules resolving within days.
- Dyshidrotic eczema has deep-seated vesicles of the palms and is intensely pruritic.
- Tinea pedis (or manus) is pruritic, erythematous, and scaly; KOH+.
- Infected atopic dermatitis will not be restricted to palms and soles; patient usually carries history of the diagnosis. Perform culture when in doubt.
- Scabies is associated with superficial vesicles, pustules, and burrows; often has coexistent lesions on the wrists, waist, and axillae; and is diffusely pruritic.
- Reiter syndrome
- Epidermolysis bullosa simplex
- Herpes simplex virus infection

 Best Tests

Dyshidrotic Dermatitis

Dyshidrotic dermatitis is usually a clinical diagnosis. Biopsy is confirmatory but does not help establish the etiology.

Palmoplantar Pustulosis

Palmoplantar pustulosis is a clinical diagnosis of exclusion. Thyroid function and glucose tolerance testing as well as screening for arthropathy should be considered.

Further testing may be done to rule out other conditions:

- Patch testing (allergic contact dermatitis)
- KOH preparation of scrapings (dermatophyte)
- Bacterial culture (bacterial infection)
- Biopsy for direct immunofluorescence (bullous pemphigoid)

▲▲ Management Pearls

Dyshidrotic Dermatitis

- To manage vesicles and bullae, use compresses (Burow solution). Drain large bullae, leaving the roof intact. Symptomatic relief of pruritus can be obtained with lotions or creams containing pramoxine, camphor, or menthol. Systemic antihistamines may also help. Removal of any irritating agents and classes 2 and 3 steroids with or without occlusive vinyl gloves are the mainstays of treatment.

- A brief course of oral prednisone may be necessary, but patients often cannot tolerate being tapered off this therapy. Likewise, monthly triamcinolone 40 IM injections are not recommended because of long-term side effects and possible aseptic necrosis of the hip.

Pediatric Patient Considerations

- Warm saline compresses may be soothing and induce drainage of vesicles.
- Parents should be educated that dyshidrotic dermatitis is a chronic relapsing disease and that current therapies ameliorate but do not cure the dermatitis.
- Avoiding wet work, using soft soaps, and application of moisturizers immediately after washing are all helpful.
- Although not caused by sweating, topical aluminum chloride is helpful in some instances.
- Oral steroids should be considered only in recalcitrant, severe cases. Patch testing for the presence of a contact allergy should be considered.

Palmoplantar Pustulosis

- With palmoplantar pustulosis, educate the patient about realistic expectations, and explain that this disease can be particularly difficult to treat. Advise smoking cessation in all patients who smoke.
- There has been an association of palmoplantar pustulosis and smoking. With the well-documented prevalence of tobacco abuse in minority communities, screening for lifestyle habits may be important in management.

Therapy

Dyshidrotic Dermatitis

For dyshidrotic dermatitis, conservative measures as above, plus a high- or midpotency topical steroid initially (classes 2 and 3)

Note: Topical steroids may cause hypopigmentation, which is particularly noticeable on heavily pigmented skin types.

High-potency Topical Corticosteroids (Class 2)
- Fluocinonide cream, ointment—apply twice daily (15, 30, 60, 120 g)
- Desoximetasone cream, ointment—apply twice daily (15, 60, 120 g)
- Halcinonide cream, ointment—apply twice daily (15, 60, 240 g)
- Clobetasol cream, ointment—apply twice daily
- Amcinonide ointment—apply twice daily (15, 30, 60 g)

Midpotency Topical Corticosteroids (Classes 3 and 4)
- Triamcinolone cream, ointment—apply twice daily (15, 30, 60, 120, 240 g)
- Mometasone cream, ointment—apply twice daily (15, 45 g)
- Fluocinolone ointment, cream—apply twice daily (15, 30, 60 g)

If dyshidrotic dermatitis is severe, use a superpotent topical steroid for a short 2-week course, and schedule close follow-up (class 1):
- Clobetasol 0.05% cream—apply twice daily (15, 30, 45 g)
- Betamethasone 0.05% cream—apply twice daily (15, 30, 45 g)
- Diflorasone 0.05% cream—apply twice daily (15, 30, 60 g)
- Halobetasol cream—apply twice daily (15, 50 g)

Beware of skin atrophy with potent and superpotent steroids!

Topical tacrolimus 0.1% ointment twice daily can be used alone or in combination with topical corticosteroids.

Severe cases can be treated with short courses of prednisone, beginning with 0.5 mg/kg each morning with gradual taper over 2 weeks, but beware of the difficulty tapering these patients. Chronic, severe disease can be treated with topical PUVA (psoralen and UVA phototherapy administered by a dermatologist) or other systemic immunosuppressives (including azathioprine, methotrexate).

Botulinum toxin injections have also been used in refractory cases.

Palmoplantar Pustulosis

For mild cases of palmoplantar pustulosis, high-potency topical steroids (see above) under occlusion can be tried first.

For severe or recalcitrant cases of palmoplantar pustulosis, systemic retinoids, tetracycline, and PUVA are the treatments of choice.

- Acitretin—0.5 mg/kg p.o. daily or 25 mg p.o. daily
- Isotretinoin—40 to 80 mg p.o. daily
- Methotrexate—2.5 to 20 mg p.o. weekly
- Tetracycline—250 mg p.o. twice daily
- Topical hand and foot PUVA—10 to 40 mg p.o. daily two to three times a week

Cyclosporine (2.5 to 5 mg/kg/d) is considered second-line therapy due to its significant side-effect profile.

Suggested Readings

Doshi DN, Kimball AB. Vesicular palmoplantar eczema. In: Fitzpatrick TB, Wolff K, eds. *Fitzpatrick's Dermatology in General Medicine*. 7th Ed. New York, NY: McGraw-Hill; 2008:162–167.

Guenst BJ. Common pediatric foot dermatoses. *J Pediatr Health Care*. 1999;13(2):68–71.

Lemont H, Pearl B. Juvenile plantar dermatosis. *J Am Podiatr Med Assoc*. 1992;82(3):167–169.

Lofgren SM, Warshaw EM. Dyshidrosis: epidemiology, clinical characteristics, and therapy. *Dermatitis*. 2006;17(4):165–181.

Marsland AM, Chalmers RJ, Hollis S, et al. Interventions for chronic palmoplantar pustulosis. *Cochrane Database Syst Rev*. 2006;(1):CD001433.

O'Doherty CJ, MacIntyre C. Palmoplantar pustulosis and smoking. *Br Med J*. 291(6499):861–864 (1985).

Warshaw EM. Therapeutic options for chronic hand dermatitis. *Dermatol Ther*. 2004;17(3):240–250.

Diagnosis Synopsis

Blistering distal dactylitis, a variant of cellulitis, is an acute superficial infection of the anterior fat pad of the finger, usually caused by group A streptococci (*Streptococcus pyogenes*) or *Staphylococcus aureus*. Occasionally, lesions may occur on the proximal digit or palmar surface. School-aged children are most commonly affected, but it may occur in any age group.

Look For

Look for a purulent vesicle or bulla (1 to 2 cm in size) on an erythematous base affecting the palmar pad at the tip of the digit or, rarely, the proximal digit or palm (Fig. 4-645). Involvement of a toe has also been described.

Diagnostic Pearls

The blister usually occurs on the volar fat pad.

?? Differential Diagnosis and Pitfalls

- Herpetic whitlow—usually a single digit, painful, opaque lesion with suggestion of underlining grouped vesicles (Fig. 4-646).
- Paronychia
- Friction blister
- Brucellosis (rare)

✓ Best Tests

Gram stain and culture of the blister fluid. Gram stain will reveal Gram-positive cocci in chains or clusters.

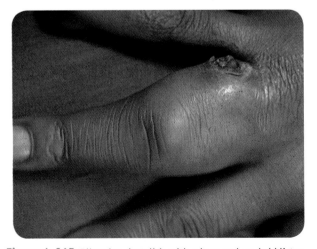

Figure 4-645 Blistering dactylitis with edema and eroded blister.

586

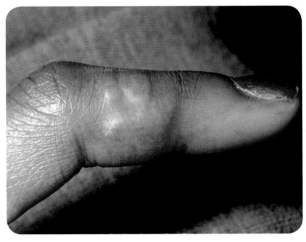

Figure 4-646 Herpetic whitlow with a deep vesicular lesion on the middle phalanx; it more typically presents on the distal phalanx.

▲▲ Management Pearls

For prevention of future lesions, antibacterial soap should be used to cleanse the body. The patient and all household members should be treated with mupirocin (topically) to the nasal passages to reduce carriage of both group A streptococci and *S. aureus*. Or consider obtaining a nasopharyngeal swab for bacteriology.

Therapy

Incision and drainage along with a 10-day course of oral antibiotics as follows.

If the organism is unknown:

- Cephalexin: 25 to 50 mg/kg/d p.o. divided four times daily, not to exceed 4 g/d

For penicillin- and cephalosporin-allergic patients:

- Erythromycin: 30 to 50 mg/kg/d p.o. divided four times daily
- Clindamycin: 15 mg/kg/d p.o. divided four times daily

Suggested Readings

Bernard P. Management of common bacterial infections in the skin. *Curr Opin Infect Dis.* 2008;21(2):122–128.

Craft NC, Lee PK, Zipoli MT, et al. Superficial cutaneous infections and pyodermas. In: Fitzpatrick TB, Wolff K, eds. *Fitzpatrick's Dermatology in General Medicine.* 7th Ed. New York, NY: McGraw-Hill; 2008:1694–1703.

James WD, Berger TG, Elston DM, eds. *Andrews' Diseases of the Skin: Clinical Dermatology.* 10th Ed. Philadelphia, PA: Saunders Elsevier; 2006:251–264.

Genital Candidiasis

Kamilah Dixon • Lynn McKinley-Grant

■■ Diagnosis Synopsis

Candidiasis is one of the most common fungal infections worldwide and is most commonly caused by *Candida albicans* of the skin, genitals, or oral mucosa and can result in systemic infection. Candidiasis of the genitals includes vulvovaginal candidiasis, male genital candidiasis, and balanitis. While candidiasis can occur in both immunocompetent and immunocompromised individuals, those with recurrent candidal infections should be considered for immunological investigations after "ping-pong" infection between sexual partners, a common reason for recurrent disease, is excluded.

- Vulvovaginal candidiasis—This is the second most common cause of vaginitis and close to 75% of healthy women will have at least one episode of vulvovaginal candidiasis in their lifetime. While *C. albicans* is the cause of most candidiasis, *C. glabrata* has increased in prevalence, possibly due to the overuse of over-the-counter antifungal treatments. Vulvovaginal candidiasis begins with attachment of *C. albicans* to the vaginal epithelial wall and subsequent colonization throughout the vagina. Some women may be completely asymptomatic, while others will have severe pruritus and irritation. While most infections are uncomplicated and limited, some women experience recurrent vulvovaginal candidiasis (four or more episodes in a given year) without an obvious explanation.
- Male genital candidiasis—Like vulvovaginitis, this is most commonly caused by a *C. albicans*. Men with candidal infections most often present with complaints of pruritus and erythema of the shaft of the penis, glans penis, and inguinal folds; or with pustules or eroding papules in the same locations.
- Balanitis—This infection of the glans penis that causes inflammation and erythema. 11% of patients in STD clinics present with balanitis. It is most often caused by Candida species but is also associated with *Streptococcus*, *Neisseria gonorrhea*, *Trichomonas vaginalis*, and *Gardnerella vaginalis*. Occurring along with balanitis, patients often report inflammation of the prepuce or balanoposthitis. The major risk factors for balanitis are an uncircumcised penis, diabetes, and being immunocompromised.

Obesity is associated with candidal infections, with up to 23% of obese subjects in a French study presenting with candidal infections. Along with comorbidities of diabetes and cardiovascular diseases, these infections are found because of increased skin folds causing pressure abrasions and providing a moist environment for fungal growth.

Uncircumcised males are at an increased risk of developing genital candidiasis and balanitis. The infection is related to poor hygiene and the retention of candida within the foreskin, which provides a moist environment for growth.

The use of feminine cleansing products alone has not been proven to cause vulvovaginal candidiasis, but if these practices cause hypersensitivity reactions or local inflammation, patients can be more susceptible to candidal infections.

Immunocompromised Patient Considerations

Immunocompromised patients include those with diabetes, HIV, systemic lupus erythematosus (SLE), being treated with corticosteroids, obesity, and those being treated with chemotherapy. Since many patients will first present with candidal infections while the underlying cause of their immunocompromised state is undiscovered (e.g., HIV infection), a consideration of the underlying condition is important.

Diabetes is often recognized as a risk factor for candidal infections because of the decreased vascularity and increase in blood glucose, which provides an excellent growth media for *Candida*, and candidal infections are often a presenting sign of previously undetected diabetes. Excellent glucose control will decrease the rates of candidiasis. There is an increased prevalence of diabetes in African American, Hispanic, Asian, and Native Americans. The National Diabetes Information Clearinghouse declared that in 2007, 7.5% of Asian Americans, 10.4% of Hispanics, 11.8% of African Americans, and 14.2% of Native Americans had diabetes.

Patients with HIV may first present with mucocutaneous candidal infections or genital candidiasis. The highest rates of HIV are in sub-Saharan Africa with 22.4 million people infected. East and southeast Asia come second with 3.8 million people infected. Within the United States, African Americans make up 51% of the prevalence of HIV. Many of these patients initially presented with candidiasis of unknown origin.

Patients with autoimmune conditions and being treated with corticosteroids and other immunosuppressives are at an increased risk for having candidal infections.

◉ Look For

Vulvovaginal

- Thick, white to yellow discharge from the vagina best visualized under speculum exam.

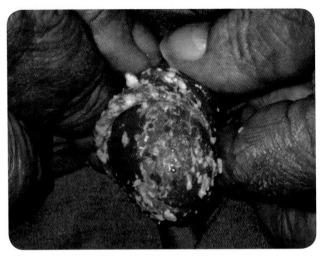

Figure 4-647 Red erosions and thick white exudate in penile candidiasis.

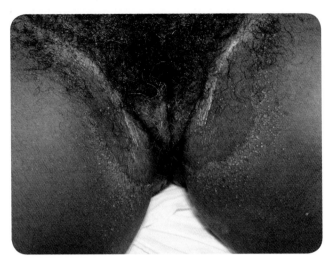

Figure 4-649 Candidal intertrigo with satellite pustules; erythema may be difficult to see in very heavily pigmented skin.

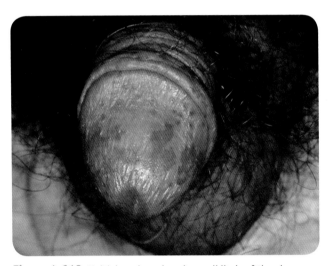

Figure 4-648 Multiple red erosions in candidiasis of the glans.

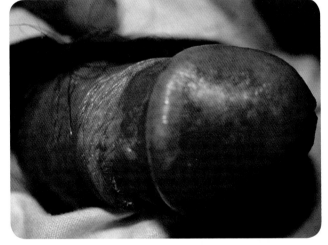

Figure 4-650 Balanitis with erythema; biopsies to exclude carcinoma *in situ* and Zoon disease are necessary with persistent undiagnosed balanitis in an adult.

- The surrounding labia majora and minora may present with diffuse erythema, swelling, fissures, excoriations and pruritus.
- Some patients may present with an eczematous-like rash on the labia majora.

Male Genital

- Patients will present with erythema and eroding papules in affected areas, which may include the shaft of the penis, glans, scrotum and inguinal folds (Figs. 4-647–4-649).
- Patients may also have white, scaly patches.

Balanitis

- Areas of marked erythema on the glans penis (Fig. 4-650).
- Some patients may present with papules and eroded pustules.

Diagnostic Pearls

Vulvovaginal

- It is common after treatment with broad-spectrum antibiotics.
- Patients may report pruritus, dysuria, dyspareunia, and a proper speculum exam and workup should be performed to rule out other diagnoses including gonorrhea and chlamydia culture, HIV test, and RPR test.

Male Genital

- Immunocompromised patients with genital erythema, pruritus, and eroding papules are likely to have a candidal infection.

Balanitis

- Itchiness and burning of the glans is common as is difficulty retracting the foreskin.
- Urethral discharge is inconsistent with the presentation of balanitis.
- Patients who are uncircumcised are at a greater risk of having balanitis.

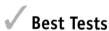 **Differential Diagnosis and Pitfalls**

Vulvovaginal

- Bacterial vaginosis
- *T. vaginalis*
- Contact or irritant dermatitis
- Lichen sclerosis
- Psoriasis
- Bullous diseases

Male Genital and Balanitis

- Allergic or irritant contact dermatitis (condoms, catheter, lubricants, cleansers)
- Fixed drug eruption
- Psoriasis
- Lichen planus
- Zoon balanitis (plasma cell balanitis)
- Nonspecific balanitis
- Reactive arthritis (formerly "Reiter syndrome")
- Erythroplasia of Queyrat and squamous cell carcinoma
- Herpes simplex virus
- Pemphigus vulgaris
- Lichen sclerosus
- Reactive arthritis with balanitis circinata

✓ Best Tests

Vulvovaginal

- A wet mount of the vaginal discharge with 10% KOH to look for pseudohyphae and budding yeasts.
- A pH test should be in the normal range for women with vulvovaginal candidiasis. If the pH is higher than 4.5, other infections should be suspected.

Male Genital

- A wet mount of discharge from a lesion with 10% KOH to look for pseudohyphae and budding yeasts.

Balanitis

- Generally, this is a clinical diagnosis based on a thorough history and physical exam.

- Cultures of the affected area can be collected and tested for bacteria and fungal species.

 Management Pearls

Vulvovaginal

- Not all patients will be symptomatic; the best test is a wet mount of vaginal secretions.
- Patients should be encouraged to come to their doctor when they have any vaginal symptoms to avoid incorrect treatment.
- Pregnant patients and those who use oral contraceptives are at an increased risk of developing vulvovaginal candidiasis.

Male Genital and Balanitis

- Patient education on proper hygiene in uncircumcised populations will help decrease these infections.
- Patients should also be advised that their sexual partners should be treated for candidal infection to decrease reinfection rates.

Therapy

With all genital candidiasis, it is important to treat the underlying cause of immunosuppression as well as the infection.

Vulvovaginal
- Fluconazole—150 mg oral tablet for 1 day
- Clotrimazole—1% cream 5 g daily for 7 days, 2% cream 5 g daily for 3 days; 100 mg vaginal suppository for 7 days, 200 mg vaginal suppository for 3 days, or 500 mg vaginal suppository for 1 day

Male Genital
- Vinegar soaks (one half teaspoon of vinegar per 8 oz glass of water twice a day), followed by a mixture of 1% hydrocortisone in miconazole cream
- Econazole cream, apply twice daily for 10 days
- Miconazole cream, apply twice daily for 10 days
- Clotrimazole, apply twice daily for 10 days
- Oral fluconazole (single dose of 100 to 200 mg) can be used for cases that are refractory to local therapy.
- Be sure to examine sexual partners and treat if necessary.

(Continued)

Balanitis

- Temporary relief for nonspecific balanitis can be achieved with improved personal hygiene. Try daily foreskin retraction and cleansing with warm water.
- Vinegar and water soaks (one half teaspoon of vinegar per 8 oz glass of water) or saline soaks are alternatives.
- Avoid any other cosmetic or lotion products.
- If symptoms persist after 2 to 3 weeks, add application of low-to-medium–potency topical steroid only until improved. An ointment base is usually better tolerated. Do not continue long-term topical corticosteroid use (i.e., more than 2 to 3 weeks).
  - Low-potency topical corticosteroids (classes 6 and 7)—twice daily
  - Midpotency topical corticosteroids (classes 3 to 5)—twice daily
- Topical tacrolimus 0.1% ointment applied twice daily is another option.

Further treatments that can be tried include:

- High-potency topical corticosteroids (if lower-potency formulations fail first) for very short periods (3 to 4 days)

Suggested Readings

AIDS epidemic update 2009. UNAIDS. WHO. http://data.unaids.org/pub/Report/2009/JC1700_Epi_Update_2009_en.pdf

Goswami D, Goswami R, Banerjiee U, et al. Pattern of *Candida* species isolated from patients with diabetes mellitus and vulvovaginal candidiasis and their response to single dose oral fluconazole therapy. *J Infect.* 2006;52(2):111–117.

Kang I, Park SH. Infectious complications in SLE after immunosuppressive therapies. *Curr Opin Rheumatol.* 2003;15(5):528–534.

Lisboa C, Ferreira A, Resende C, et al. Infectious balanoposthitis: management, clinical and laboratory features. *Int J Dermatol.* 2009;48:121–124.

Marot-Leblond A, Nail-Bilaud S, Pilon F, et al. Efficient diagnosis of vulvovaginal candidiasis by used of a new rapid immunochromatography test. *J Clin Microbiol.* 2009;47(12):3821–3825.

National Diabetes Statistics 2007. National Diabetes Information Clearinghouse, http://diabetes.niddk.nih.gov/DM/PUBS/statistics/#allages

Nyirjesy P. Vulvovaginal candidiasis and bacterial vaginosis. *Infect Dis Clin N Am.* 2008;22(4):637–652, vi.

Scheinfeld N. Obesity and dermatology. *Clin Dermatol.* 2004;22(4):303–309.

Sobel J. Vulvovaginal. *Lancet.* 2007 candidiasis; 369(9577):1961–1971.

Condyloma Acuminatum (Genital Wart, HPV)

Mat Davey

▪▪ Diagnosis Synopsis

Condylomata acuminata, or genital warts, are caused by human papillomavirus (HPV), a DNA virus of which there are over 200 genotypes. Approximately 90% of condylomata acuminata are related to HPV types 6 and 11. Genital warts are the most common of sexually transmitted diseases and should be considered in the differential diagnosis of patients presenting with genital papules.

The virus can remain latent in skin cells without any visible sign of infection. Subclinical infection is common and carries both infection and oncogenic potential. The highest prevalence rates occur in sexually active young adults, but do not discount this diagnosis in older individuals. HPV infection is more common and severe in patients with various immunologic deficiencies. Most lesions are asymptomatic, although pruritus and bleeding may occur. Recurrent disease is common.

The significant public health problem posed by genital HPV infection lies in the oncogenic potential of the virus. Subtypes 16, 18, 31, and many others predispose infected individuals to the development of cancer of the cervix and squamous cell carcinoma (SCC) of the anogenital area.

Pediatric Patient Considerations

Genital warts in children often represent common warts transmitted to the genital skin. While sexual abuse should always be considered, the majority of cases in children aged younger than 4 years represent other modes of transmission, such as autoinoculation from other involved sites or perinatal transmission. The virus can remain latent in skin cells without any visible sign of infection.

Abuse affects children of all ages and backgrounds and, if suspected, needs appropriate referral.

◉ Look For

Small 1 to 2 mm or larger white, gray, or skin-colored warty papules on the genitals, crural folds, perineum, and/or perianal skin (Figs. 4-651–4-655). Common areas of involvement include the penile glans and the shaft in men, and the vulvovaginal and the cervical areas in woman (Fig. 4-656). Sometimes, there may be giant cauliflower-like lesions. In incompletely keratinized surfaces, like the vulva or under the foreskin, the papules will have a smoother surface. Search carefully for simultaneously involved multiple sites. Presence of external condylomata in both men and women warrants a thorough search for cervical, urethral, and anal lesions.

●● Diagnostic Pearls

Recurrence rates and risk of oncogenic progression are highest among patients with immunologic deficiencies.

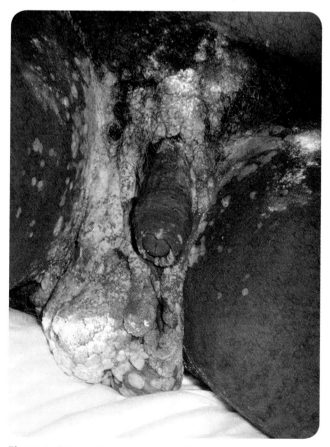

Figure 4-651 Confluent crural warts with relative sparing of the penis.

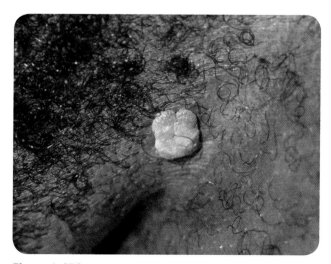

Figure 4-652 Pedunculated wart at the base of the penis.

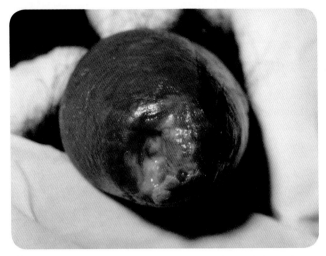

Figure 4-653 Preputial wart with massive edema of the uncircumcised foreskin.

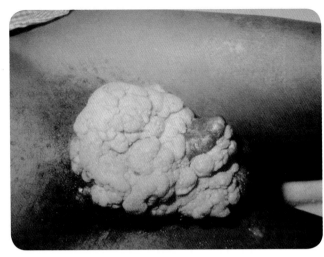

Figure 4-655 Envelopment of the scrotum, penis, and pubic regions by massive verrucous genital warts.

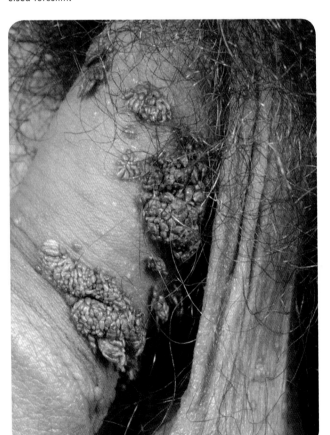

Figure 4-654 Genital warts enveloping the penile shaft with linear papules and plaques.

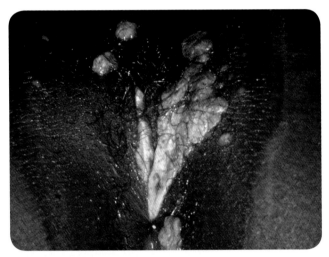

Figure 4-656 Verrucous labial and pubic genital warts.

?? Differential Diagnosis and Pitfalls

- Bowenoid papulosis
- SCC
- Condyloma latum (associated with syphilis)
- Seborrheic keratoses
- Lichen nitidus
- Pearly penile papules
- Sebaceous glands
- Acrochordons (skin tags)
- Lichen planus
- Nevi (moles)
- Papillae
- Fordyce spots
- Molluscum contagiosum

Pediatric Patient Considerations

Ask parents for history of genital and nongenital warts. Ask mothers for a history of preceding abnormal PAP smears prior to delivery of child.

✓ Best Tests

- Per the CDC, diagnosis of genital warts is made by visual inspection and may be confirmed by biopsy. Biopsy is needed only under certain circumstances (e.g., if the diagnosis is uncertain, the lesions do not respond to standard therapy, the disease worsens during therapy, the patient is immunocompromised, or the warts are pigmented, indurated, fixed, bleeding, or ulcerated).
- The acetowhitening test involves the application of diluted acetic acid solution (3% to 5%) to genital tissue for 5 to 10 minutes before clinical examination. The solution whitens the warts, making it easier to visualize and focus treatment.
- Per the CDC, no data support the use of HPV nucleic acid tests in the routine diagnosis or management of visible genital warts. Presently, there is no evidence for performing HPV DNA typing.

▲▲ Management Pearls

- The wart virus persists and is often present beyond the clinically visible borders of the lesions. This must be considered during destructive therapies. Lesions frequently recur, requiring vigilant surveillance.
- Other concomitant sexually transmitted diseases should be considered. Patients should be checked for immunodeficiency when there is severe involvement.
- Sexual partners of patients should be evaluated for disease, and female patients and partners should have regular PAP smears indefinitely.
- Patients should be advised that using condoms cannot completely protect them from HPV because vaginal or anal penetration does not need to occur to contract the virus.
- Consultations with specialists in gynecology, urology, or general or colorectal surgery may be needed.
- Gardasil (http://www.gardasil.com/) is a vaccine that protects against 4 strains of HPV (types 6, 11, 16, and 18), which cause 70% of cervical cancers and 90% of genital warts. In 2006, the FDA licensed this vaccine for use in girls/women of ages 9 to 26.
- Warts may increase during pregnancy, and podophyllin drugs are contraindicated in pregnancy.

Therapy

CDC-Recommended Regimens for External Genital Warts

Patient-applied options include the following:

- Podofilox 0.5% solution or gel—Patients should apply podofilox solution with a cotton swab, or podofilox gel with a finger, to visible genital warts twice daily for 3 days, followed by 4 days of no therapy. This cycle may be repeated, as necessary, for up to 4 cycles.

- Imiquimod 5% cream—Patients should apply imiquimod cream once daily at bedtime, three times a week for up to 16 weeks.
  - The treatment area should be washed with soap and water 6 to 10 hours after the application. The safety of imiquimod during pregnancy has not been established.

Provider-administered:

- Cryotherapy with liquid nitrogen or cryoprobe—Repeat application every few weeks.
- Podophyllin resin 10% to 25% in a compound tincture of benzoin. This treatment can be repeated weekly, if necessary.
- Trichloroacetic acid (TCA) or bichloracetic acid 80% to 90%. This treatment can be repeated weekly, if necessary.
- Surgical removal by scissor excision, shave excision, curettage, or electrosurgery.

CDC-Recommended Alternative Regimens
Intralesional interferon

OR

Laser surgery

Per the CDC, many persons with warts on the anal mucosa also have warts on the rectal mucosa, so persons with anal warts can benefit from an inspection of the rectal mucosa by digital examination or anoscopy. Warts on the rectal mucosa should be managed in consultation with a specialist.

Pediatric Patient Considerations

Currently available treatments for visible genital warts include cryotherapy, podophyllin resin, podophyllotoxin, TCA, interferon, carbon dioxide laser, and surgical excision.

Imiquimod, an immune response mediator, is approved for use in patients with genital warts aged 12 years or older.

Condyloma may spontaneously regress, so active surveillance is also an option.

Suggested Readings

Androphy EJ, Lowy DR. Warts. In: Fitzpatrick TB, Wolff K, eds. *Fitzpatrick's Dermatology in General Medicine*. 7th Ed. New York, NY: McGraw-Hill; 2008:1914–1922.

Centers for Disease Control and Prevention. Sexually Transmitted Diseases: Treatment Guidelines 2006, http://www.cdc.gov/STD/treatment/2006/genital-warts.htm. Reviewed April 12, 2007. Accessed May 2010.

Huang CM. Human papillomavirus and vaccination. *Mayo Clin Proc*. 2008;83(6):701–706.

James WD, Berger TG, Elston DM, eds. *Andrews' Diseases of the Skin: Clinical Dermatology*. 10th Ed. Philadelphia, PA: Saunders Elsevier; 2006:407–411.

Jayasinghe Y, Garland SM. Genital warts in children: What do they mean? *Arch Dis Child*. 2006;91(8):696–700.

O'Mahony C. Genital warts: Current and future management options. *Am J Clin Dermatol*. 2005;6(4):239–243.

Angiokeratoma of Scrotum

Lynn McKinley-Grant

■■ Diagnosis Synopsis

Angiokeratomas of the scrotum (Fordyce angiokeratoma) are benign, often asymptomatic, 2 to 5 mm, warty or smooth-topped, red to violaceous papules composed of dilated dermal capillaries. The pathophysiology is unknown; they may be caused by increased venous pressure due to their occasional association with vascular conditions such as varicoceles. The lesions may bleed spontaneously or with slight trauma, which is distressing to patients.

As the name implies, the condition is more common in men, although angiokeratomas occur on the inner thighs, lower abdomen, and on the vulva in women. Prevalence data indicates that the condition is more common in whites and the Japanese, and that incidence increases with advancing age.

◉ Look For

Very deep red to purple-black papules that are 2 to 5 mm in diameter. The color has occasionally been described as blue or black (Fig. 4-657). Lesions are most often multiple. There may be a superficial wart-like appearance to some lesions. Lesions are compressible, but the purple to deep red color will persist.

The scrotum is the most common site, but lesions may also be seen on the inner thighs, lower abdomen, or the vulva of women.

●● Diagnostic Pearls

- Fabry lesions are smaller and appear at an earlier age. Patients with Fabry disease may also report limb pain, history of renal or cardiac disease, and decreased sweating.

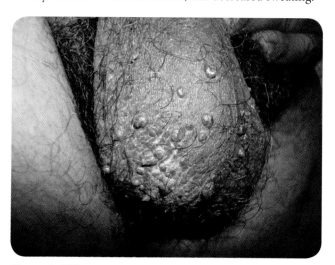

Figure 4-657 Large angiokeratomas of the scrotum; the lesions can vary in size.

- The scrotum may appear red in half of the patients with angiokeratoma of the scrotum. The scrotum is not tender or edematous; it is red in color due to a background of telangiectasia. This asymptomatic redness may be the presenting factor for many patients.

?? Differential Diagnosis and Pitfalls

- Angiokeratoma corporis diffusum (Fabry disease)
- Hereditary hemorrhagic telangiectasia
- Genital warts (condyloma acuminatum)
- Melanoma
- Melanocytic nevi
- Cherry hemangiomas

✓ Best Tests

- Skin biopsy will confirm the clinical impression but is often not necessary.
- Examination with a hand lens or dermatoscope may help to distinguish a vascular from a melanocytic lesion.

▲▲ Management Pearls

Lesions do not have to be treated, but symptomatic, bleeding lesions can easily be treated by electrodesiccation.

Therapy

No treatment is necessary other than reassurance. If treatment is desired, however, cryotherapy, electrocautery, and laser therapy have all demonstrated success in clearing the lesions. Excision is impractical in cases where there are many lesions.

Lasers that have reportedly achieved success with single treatments include the 578-nm copper laser, the argon laser, and the 532-nm KTP laser.

Suggested Readings

Lapidoth M, Ad-El D, David M, et al. Treatment of angiokeratoma of Fordyce with pulsed dye laser. *Dermatol Surg.* 2006;32(9):1147–1150.

Miller C, James WD. Angiokeratoma of Fordyce as a cause of red scrotum. *Cutis.* 2002;69(1):50–51.

Occella C, Bleidl D, Rampini P, et al. Argon laser treatment of cutaneous multiple angiokeratomas. *Dermatol Surg.* 1995;21(2):170–172.

Trickett R, Dowd H. Angiokeratoma of the scrotum: A case of scrotal bleeding. *Emerg Med J.* 2006;23(10):e57.

Diaper Dermatitis—Irritant and Candida-associated

Chris G. Adigun

■■ Diagnosis Synopsis

Diaper dermatitis (DD) includes irritant diaper dermatitis (IDD), which typically occurs in the moist, occlusive environment provided by the diaper, and very rare variants of IDD: pseudoverrucous papules and nodules, granuloma gluteale infantum, and Jacquet erosive DD. Pre-existing IDD may be secondarily infected by *Candida* spp., leading to the development of candidal diaper dermatitis (CDD).

IDD is the most common form of DD and is associated with occlusion, moisture, warmth, urine, feces, and friction produced by diapers. Once the skin barrier is compromised, secondary factors, such as urinary ammonia, increased urine pH, fecal proteases and lipases, *Candida albicans*, bacterial overgrowth, and detergent soaps, exacerbate the dermatitis. IDD, a very common therapeutic challenge, is seen in 25% of children wearing diapers. Despite superabsorbent and breathable disposable diapers, it is still a common occurrence.

Wet diapers increase hydration and maceration of the stratum corneum, and this impairs barrier function, enhances epidermal penetration by irritants and microbes, and increases frictional trauma. Friction plays a large role as well and IDD is most commonly distributed in areas with the greatest skin-to-diaper contact. Mechanical trauma disrupts the macerated stratum corneum and exacerbates barrier dysfunction. Bacterial ureases in the stool degrade the urea found in urine, releasing ammonia and increasing the local pH. Fecal lipases and proteases are activated by the increased pH, causing further irritation and disruption of the epidermal barrier. Urinary ammonia on its own does not irritate intact skin, but enhances the IDD process by increasing the local pH. The warm, humid, and high-pH environment is the ideal milieu for microbial proliferation.

Diarrhea from viral infections, antibiotics, and laxatives accelerates the development of IDD. Diarrhea contained and occluded by a diaper can cause severe IDD with bullae and erosions.

Circumstances predisposed to IDD increases the risk of developing CDD since sufficient moisture in the diaper area allows *C. albicans* to proliferate and invade the stratum corneum. CDD is the second-most-common type of DD, and it may occur in infants of any gestational age or birth weight. The rule of thumb in the treatment of IDD is that if the DD has not improved after 3 days of therapy, it is likely secondarily infected with *Candida*.

The greatest risk factor for the development of candidal dermatitis is pre-existing irritant dermatitis. *Candida* from intestinal flora frequently contaminates a pre-existing irritant dermatitis that has been present for more than 3 days. Recent antibiotic use is also a risk factor for CDD. One of the most common antibiotics used in infants, amoxicillin,

increases the density of *C. albicans* on perineal skin by more than 14-fold.

DD may affect any age group where diapers are used including elderly or infirm adults with thin, aging skin. Pseudoverrucous papules and nodules may occur in the diaper and perianal areas of patients of any age with a predisposition to prolonged wetness, such as children or adults who wear diapers due to chronic urinary incontinence.

Granuloma gluteale infantum presents with violaceous papules and nodules in the diaper area in the setting of IDD. Potential risk factors for this condition include previous treatment with topical steroids, coexisting candidal infection, and the use of occlusive plastic covers. Granuloma gluteale infantum will eventually resolve over weeks to months and may leave residual scarring.

Jacquet erosive DD is characterized by punched-out ulcerations with heaped-up borders. Risk factors for the development of this syndrome include frequent liquid stools (such as a diarrheal syndrome), poor hygiene, infrequent diaper changes, or use of occlusive plastic diapers.

◉ Look For

Irritant Diaper Dermatitis

IDD presents as confluent erythema covering areas in greatest contact with the diaper (i.e., the convexities of the buttocks, lower abdomen, medial thighs, mons pubis, scrotum, and labia majora) (Figs. 4-658–4-660). Early or mild disease may manifest only as perianal erythema. More severe cases appear glazed and have edema and erythematous papules in the involved skin. A wrinkled surface and postinflammatory hyperpigmentation may develop as the inflammation resolves.

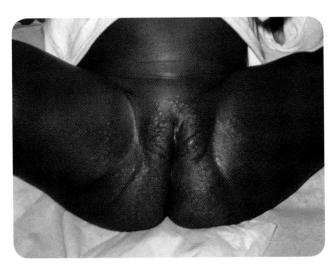

Figure 4-658 IDD commonly involves the vulva.

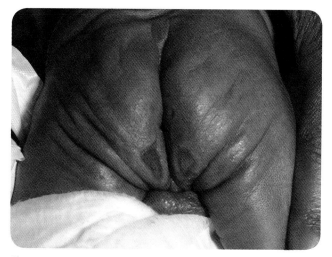

Figure 4-659 Erosions can be part of severe DD.

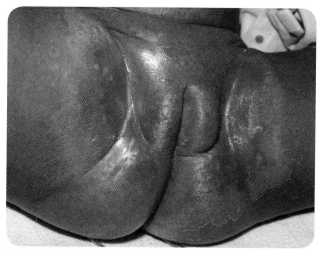

Figure 4-661 Candidiasis with peripheral *Candida* folliculitis.

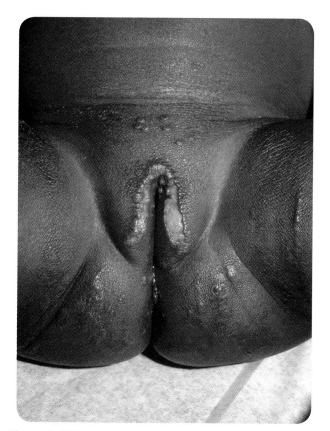

Figure 4-660 Papular lesions along the diaper margins and on the vulva with IDD.

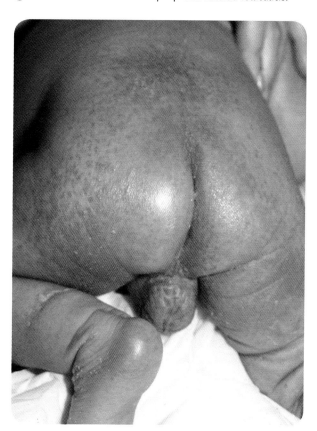

Figure 4-662 CDD commonly involves the scrotum.

Alternative presentations of IDD may include bandlike erythema and maceration along the diaper margins (tidewater mark dermatitis). Jacquet erosive DD presents with severe dermatitis with punched-out ulcerations. Granuloma gluteale infantum presents with reddish-purplish nodules of different sizes (0.5 to 3.0 cm), occurring on the convexities of the diaper area in 2- to 9-month-old infants. It arises within pre-existing DD.

Candida-associated Dermatitis

Classically, CDD presents as a sharply demarcated, beefy-red diaper area (Figs. 4-661 and 4-662). Satellite pustular lesions are characteristic. Most commonly, there is diffuse erythema with peripheral scale, or pink, scaly papules that coalesce into plaques. These erythematous, moist papules, patches, and plaques tend to involve body folds as well as convex surfaces. The skin folds and the entire scrotum or labia may be confluently involved.

In severe cases, there may be large erosions within the diaper area or there may be psoriasiform skin lesions on the trunk and extremities, known as "CDD with psoriasiform IDD."

Diagnostic Pearls

- In IDD, sparing of the skin folds is often seen.
- In contrast, peripheral papulopustules ("satellite pustules") and involvement of the deep skin folds are highly suggestive of CDD. Candidiasis should be strongly considered in any IDD that does not respond to standard therapies.
- A recent history of antibiotic use is highly suggestive of CDD.

?? Differential Diagnosis and Pitfalls

- DD often coexists with and exacerbates other dermatoses, and the presence of another dermatosis does not exclude concurrent IDD.
- Complications of IDD include Jacquet erosive DD, granuloma gluteale infantum, and pseudoverrucous papules. Any DD that persists longer than 72 hours is likely secondarily infected with *Candida*.

Diaper-induced or Exacerbated Dermatoses

- Allergic contact dermatitis—This should be in the differential diagnosis, especially in refractory cases. An allergen in the diaper may be the culprit. There are data showing that some patients have demonstrated allergic contact dermatitis in response to the various blue, pink, and green dyes in diapers.
- Miliaria rubra
- Infantile granular parakeratosis

Dermatoses Unrelated to the Presence of a Diaper

- Seborrheic dermatitis
- Atopic dermatitis
- Psoriasis—When candidiasis involves the genitalia, lesions are confluent, as opposed to psoriasis, in which lesions are more localized and sharply demarcated.
- Bullous impetigo
- Acrodermatitis enteropathica
- Scabies
- Hand-foot-and-mouth disease

- Herpes simplex infections
- Cystic fibrosis
- Langerhans cell histiocytosis—Skin biopsy is indicated to rule out Langerhans cell histiocytosis if nonhealing erosions or petechiae are seen in the diaper area.
- Lichen sclerosus
- Kawasaki disease
- Perianal streptococcal dermatitis
- Congenital syphilis
- Kawasaki disease
- Lichen sclerosus

✓ Best Tests

This is a clinical diagnosis. Perform a potassium hydroxide (KOH) preparation and fungal cultures (Sabouraud medium is usually positive by 3 days) for secondary candidal infection.

▲▲ Management Pearls

- IDD is frequently superinfected with *C. albicans*; consider adding anticandidal agents when the rash is severe, there are coexistent pustules, or the response to therapy takes longer than 3 days. If the dermatitis is unresponsive to concurrent treatment of IDD and CDD, other diagnoses should be considered.
- Parents should be reassured that DD is not the result of improper or negligent care of the infant and is an almost inevitable consequence of diapering and that there are numerous treatment strategies to treat the condition.
- CDD will quickly recur if concurrent IDD is not treated simultaneously. Therefore, diligent application of barrier creams with each diaper change helps improve the barrier function of the skin. In addition, in order to successfully clear CDD, infants with CDD should be examined for coexisting oral candidiasis (thrush).
- Additionally, parents should be advised to use high-quality disposable diapers, and if they continue to prefer cloth diapers, then these should be changed immediately when soiled (every 1 to 2 hours). However, even with frequent diaper changes, IDD may still readily occur in the setting of cloth diaper use. Cloth diapers should not be recommended for patients with DD.
- Breathable disposable diapers decreases DD compared to infants wearing standard nonbreathable disposable diapers.
- A common misconception is that baby wipes contribute to DD.
- Corticosteroids in the diaper area should be used with caution. Mid- to high- potency topical steroids should never be used in this circumstance.

- Parents should be counseled that even after the IDD or CDD has been treated, postinflammatory hyperpigmentation may persist. This condition is far more common and persistent in darker skin types. However, if the child developed granuloma gluteale infantum, the scarring that results may leave permanent hyperpigmentation.

Therapy

Application of a suitable barrier cream is the cornerstone of prevention and treatment of IDD. It is important that the barrier cream adheres to the affected skin.

Diapers should be changed immediately after urinating or defecating (usually hourly for neonates and every 3 to 4 hours for infants). Infants with diarrhea will require more frequent diaper changes. More generous-fitting diapers (by 1 to 2 sizes) are preferable to tight-fitting diapers.

Improving the Skin Barrier
Thick ointments and pastes, such as petrolatum and zinc oxide preparations, should be applied with every diaper change.

- Avoid harsh soaps and alcohol and instead use plain water or unscented diaper wipes.
- Avoid scrubbing, and instead use mineral oil or petroleum jelly on a cotton ball to remove thick pastes and dried feces.
- Pat the diaper area dry instead of rubbing.
- Avoid using hair dryers in the diaper area.
- Topical barrier should be applied liberally, like "cake icing."
- Suggested barrier creams: Desitin, Balmex, and others that contain zinc oxide as an active ingredient.

Reducing Inflammation
A short course of a mild topical corticosteroid is frequently necessary in moderate-to-severe IDD. Mid-to-high potency corticosteroids should never be used in the diaper area. Suggest application of low-potency topical steroid ointments, such as 1% hydrocortisone, 0.05% alclometasone dipropionate, or 0.05% desonide ointment twice daily for inflamed areas. Alternatively, consider tacrolimus ointment twice daily for inflamed areas, but note that this is an off-label use.

Treating Candidal Diaper Dermatitis
CDD is treated topically with either nystatin; an azole antifungal (e.g., clotrimazole, miconazole, econazole); or ciclopirox twice daily for 2 to 3 weeks, or until 1 week after the rash has cleared.

If thrush is also present, oral nystatin suspension should be applied to the mucosa dosed at 1 mL four times daily until 2 to 3 days after resolution.

Although many studies have investigated their efficacy in CDD, many antifungal agents are not FDA-approved in infancy. FDA-approved topical antifungals in infancy include nystatin and miconazole.

Suggested Readings

Akin F, Spraker M, Aly R, et al. Effects of breathable disposable diapers: Reduced prevalence of Candida and common diaper dermatitis. *Pediatr Dermatol.* 2001;18(4):282–290.

Alberta L, Sweeney SM, Wiss K. Diaper dye dermatitis. *Pediatrics.* 2005; 116(3):e450–e452.

Atherton DJ. A review of the pathophysiology, prevention and treatment of irritant diaper dermatitis. *Curr Med Res Opin.* 2004;20(5):645–649.

Baldwin S, Odio MR, Haines SL, et al. Skin benefits from continuous topical administration of a zinc oxide/petrolatum formulation by a novel disposable diaper. *J Eur Acad Dermatol Venereol.* 2001;15(Suppl 1):5–11.

Concannon P, Gisoldi E, Phillips S, et al. Diaper dermatitis: A therapeutic dilemma. Results of a double-blind placebo controlled trial of miconazole nitrate 0.25%. *Pediatr Dermatol.* 2001;18(2):149–155.

Fiorillo L. Therapy of pediatric genital diseases. *Dermatol Ther.* 2004; 17(1):117–128.

Guin JD, Kincannon J, Church FL. Baby-wipe dermatitis: Preservative-induced hand eczema in parents and persons using moist towelettes. *Am J Contact Dermat.* 2001;12(4):189–192.

Humphrey S, Bergman JN, Au S. Practical management strategies for diaper dermatitis. *Skin Therapy Lett.* 2006;11(7):1–6. Review.

Kazaks EL, Lane AT. Diaper dermatitis. *Pediatr Clin North Am.* 2000; 47(4):909–919.

Robson KJ, Maughan JA, Purcell SD, et al. Erosive papulonodular dermatosis associated with topical benzocaine: A report of two cases and evidence that granuloma gluteale, pseudoverrucous papules, and Jacquet's erosive dermatitis are a disease spectrum. *J Am Acad Dermatol.* 2006;55 (5 Suppl):S74–S80. Epub 2006 Sep 1.

Runeman B. Skin interaction with absorbent hygiene products. *Clin Dermatol.* 2008;26(1):45–51.

Shin HT. Diaper dermatitis that does not quit. *Dermatol Ther.* 2005;18(2): 124–135.

Visscher M, Odio M, Taylor T, et al. Skin care in the NICU patient: Effects of wipes versus cloth and water on stratum corneum integrity. *Neonatology.* 200929;96(4):226–234.

Lichen Sclerosus et Atrophicus

Stephanie Diamantis

◼◼ Diagnosis Synopsis

Lichen sclerosus (lichen sclerosus et atrophicus) is a chronic dermatosis of unknown etiology characterized by an initial short inflammatory phase followed by chronic scarring and skin atrophy. Lichen sclerosus is primarily a disease of anogenital skin in both males and females of all ethnicities but is more common in females, with two peaks in age distribution: prepubertal children and postmenopausal women. Lichen sclerosus remains one of the most common causes of chronic vulvar pruritus in adult females. Girls may present with urinary or bowel symptoms (i.e., constipation secondary to perianal involvement). The majority of cases of male genital lichen sclerosus occur in uncircumcised men.

Clinically, over 85% of lesions are found on anogenital skin. Anogenital lichen sclerosus usually presents as dry, tender, and severely pruritic, white plaques with epidermal atrophy resembling scarring. Plaques can progress to cause functional impairment, most commonly phimosis in males and sclerosis of the vaginal introitus in females.

Lichen sclerosus on nongenital skin is frequently asymptomatic but can be pruritic. Extragenital lichen sclerosus most commonly presents as ivory-colored, atrophic, scarlike plaques with follicular accentuation on the neck, shoulders, back, and upper extremities. It also has a predilection for sites of previous trauma (Koebner phenomenon).

In Europe, some cases of lichen sclerosus are thought to be late cutaneous sequelae of *Borrelia afzelii* or *Borrelia garinii* infection, and treatment with antibiotics has improved the condition. Autoimmune diseases such as vitiligo, alopecia areata, thyroid disease, and pernicious anemia disproportionately affect women with lichen sclerosus.

Lesions of lichen sclerosus should be treated. Squamous cell carcinoma can arise in genital lesions, and there may be complications related to genital scarring—including dyspareunia, urinary obstruction, ulceration, painful erection, and phimosis. Extragenital lesions may cause psychosocial distress secondary to cosmesis and chronic pruritus.

Synonyms of lichen sclerosus are kraurosis vulvae (lichen sclerosus of the vulva) and balanitis xerotica obliterans (lichen sclerosus of the penis).

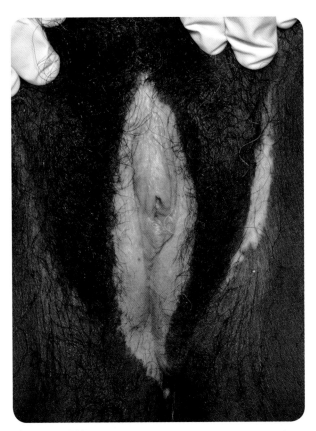

Figure 4-663 Lichen sclerosus with vulva depigmentation and inguinal depigmentation.

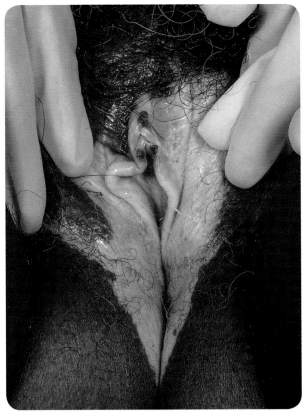

Figure 4-664 Foci of normal pigmentation may be present in a typical lesion of lichen sclerosus.

600

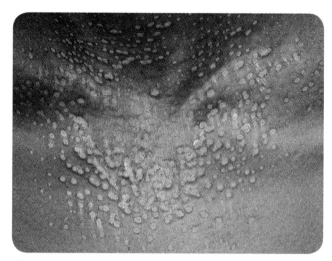

Figure 4-665 Lichen sclerosus infrequently has shiny smooth hypopigmented papules on the general body skin.

Look For

Initial lesions of lichen sclerosus are flat, ivory-white plaques surrounded by a red-, purple-, or violet-colored border (Figs. 4-663 and 4-664). Over time, the lesions become sclerotic and atrophied (fine wrinkling of the epidermis) and develop a shiny, porcelain-like appearance. Telangiectases/purpura and follicular plugs may be present in chronic lesions. Usual locations include the genitalia, perineum, or perianal skin. Itching is generally severe.

In females, an "hourglass" or "figure-of-eight" pattern may be seen surrounding the perivaginal and perianal areas. When inflammation is severe, ulcerations/erosions and bullae can be seen. Female genital lesions may eventually obliterate the labia minora and narrow the introitus.

Male genital lesions are often confined to the glans and the prepuce. Often, the presenting lesion is a sclerotic band or ring at the edge of the prepuce. Untreated disease can progress to phimosis and urethral stricture.

Extragenital lesions most commonly occur on the back and the shoulders and often begin as white, polygonal papules that coalesce into plaques (Fig. 4-665). Oral lichen sclerosus is rare. It presents as bluish-white papules on the buccal mucosa that evolve into scarlike plaques or superficial erosions.

Diagnostic Pearls

- Lesions are not unusual in childhood (Fig. 4-666). When on the genitals, purpura may also be present, and caretakers of affected individuals must consider abuse.
- The Koebner phenomenon has been described in this condition, with lesions being found in surgical and burn scars and areas subject to trauma.

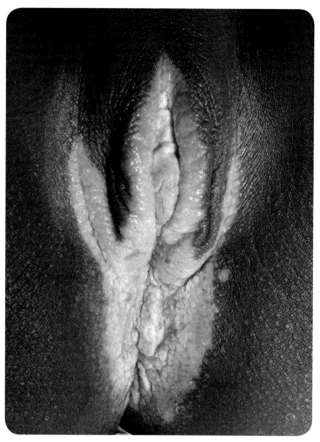

Figure 4-666 Lichen sclerosus is frequently seen in childhood in this characteristic location.

- Multiple features of lichen sclerosus (atrophy, purpura, fissures, and telangiectases) are often concentrated at the clitoral hood.

Differential Diagnosis and Pitfalls

- Morphea (localized scleroderma)—often overlaps with lichen sclerosus
- Abuse should always be considered in individuals with scarlike lesions of the anogenital area. Sexual abuse may present with disrupted hymen, additional sexually transmitted diseases, purpura, and bruising outside of atrophic areas. Note that a diagnosis of lichen sclerosus does not exclude concomitant sexual abuse, and social work should investigate when suspicion is high.
- Scar
- Sclerosing basal cell carcinoma
- Chronic radiation dermatitis
- Vitiligo—lacks signs of atrophy
- Idiopathic guttate hypomelanosis
- Bowen disease/erythroplasia of Queyrat
- Anetoderma
- Atrophoderma of Pasini and Pierini

- Extramammary Paget disease
- Erosive lichen planus—vaginal and cervical mucosa can be involved
- Cutaneous candidiasis—can see erosions, satellite lesions
- Irritant or contact dermatitis
- Bacterial vaginosis—vulvar pruritus, but no other specific vulvar cutaneous findings
- Trauma (straddle injury)—no atrophy, consistent history

✓ Best Tests

Skin biopsy will confirm the clinical suspicion.

▲▲ Management Pearls

- The treatment of choice for lichen sclerosus is a high-potency (class 1) topical steroid. Patients should be followed regularly to monitor for the correct use of the medication.
- Affected patients should be referred to a dermatologist, and a gynecologist or urologist if the situation warrants (i.e., for management of genitourinary complications). Uncircumcised males with lichen sclerosus may benefit from circumcision.
- Patients should be monitored for malignant change in lesions of genital lichen sclerosus.

Therapy

Superpotent (class 1) topical steroids, such as clobetasol propionate 0.05% cream, are the universally accepted treatment for lichen sclerosus. Steroids are applied one to three times daily until skin thickening and symptoms subside. Use is gradually tapered to less frequent applications and to less potent formulations. In general, use of a more potent steroid applied sparingly is preferred to daily use of a weaker steroid. Continued use of these medications may cause atrophy, making close clinical follow-up essential.

Topical immunomodulators (tacrolimus 0.1% ointment) are another alternative for patients, usually reserved for those who cannot tolerate or do not respond to topical steroids. These medications do not increase the risk for iatrogenic cutaneous atrophy. Theoretically, there is the potential for an increased risk of malignancy with chronic use of the calcineurin inhibitors. Because malignancies have been reported to develop within lesions of lichen sclerosus, calcineurin inhibitors are generally not used as chronic therapy.

Topical and oral retinoids or calcipotriene are additional treatment alternatives to employ if steroids are only partially effective. Extragenital lesions may respond to UVA1 light or PUVA (psoralen plus UVA), potassium *p*-aminobenzoic acid, or antimalarials, but controlled studies are lacking.

Various supportive measures may be needed:

- Stool softeners when there is painful defecation
- Avoidance of local irritants and use of soap substitutes
- Education and/or counseling regarding impact on sexual functioning

Topical testosterone has been shown to be ineffective in this condition and is no longer recommended.

Suggested Readings

Ballester I, Banuls J, Perez-Crespo M, et al. Extragenital bullous lichen sclerosus atrophicus. *Dermatol Online J.* 2009;15(1):6.

Cooper SM, Ali I, Baldo M, et al. The association of lichen sclerosus and erosive lichen planus of the vulva with autoimmune disease. *Arch Dermatol.* 2008;144(11):1432–1435.

Cooper SM, Gao XH, Powell JJ, et al. Does treatment of vulvar lichen sclerosus influence its prognosis? *Arch Dermatol.* 2004;140:702–706.

James WD, Berger TG, Elston DM, eds. Lichen planus and related conditions. In: *Andrews' Diseases of the Skin: Clinical Dermatology.* 10th Ed. Philadelphia, PA: Elsevier; 2006:227–229.

Tinea Cruris

Lynn McKinley-Grant

■■ Diagnosis Synopsis

Tinea cruris (jock itch) is a superficial fungal infection of the skin most commonly caused by *Trichophyton rubrum* or other dermatophytes. Tinea cruris manifests as a symmetric erythematous rash in the inner thighs and the crural folds. It rarely spreads to the penis, but if it does, it will be found only at the base of the penis. It is often spread to the groin from fungal infection of the feet (tinea pedis).

Tinea cruris is usually associated with pruritus and is more common in postpubertal males. People at higher risk include those who have diabetes mellitus, are obese, have recently visited a tropical climate, wear tight-fitting or wet clothes (including bathing suits) for extended periods, share clothing with others, or participate in sports.

Immunocompromised Patient Considerations

In the immunocompromised patient, pruritus may be absent. There is an increased risk of all dermatophyte infections (tinea pedis, cruris, corporis, faciale, as well as Majocchi granuloma) in the immunocompromised.

◉ Look For

Look for circular or annular, deep red to dark brown, scaly plaques extending from the inguinal creases, down the medial thigh, and all around the pubic area and buttocks (Fig. 4-667). The plaques usually have a sharply demarcated

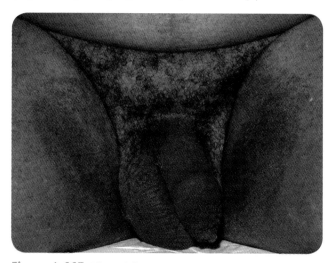

Figure 4-667 Bilateral fungal infection of the groin with some peripheral scale; the genitals are usually spared in dermatophyte infection and involved in *Candida* infections of the groin.

edge. Plaques are described as having an active border, meaning that the advancing edge of the plaque has a prominent scale containing fungal hyphae. The border may be slightly raised and have a red or purple-red color. The area affected may be moist and exudative in acute infections and dry in chronic infections. Chronic infections may result in either hyperpigmentation or hypopigmentation, even after resolution.

Immunocompromised Patient Considerations

In the immunocompromised patient, infection can be quite extensive. Tinea cruris may extend well beyond the typical crural or intragluteal distribution to involve the trunk or the lower extremities. Plaques may show only well-demarcated hyperkeratosis as opposed to the typical annular pattern.

●● Diagnostic Pearls

In fungal lesions that have been treated with topical steroids, the redness can be absent, and minimal scaling may be present while the lesion is loaded with fungi. If the scraping is negative in a lesion that has not been treated, the lesion is probably *not* fungal in etiology.

?? Differential Diagnosis and Pitfalls

- Psoriasis
- Intertrigo
- Lichen simplex chronicus
- Allergic contact dermatitis
- Irritant contact dermatitis
- Cutaneous candidiasis—often beefy red with satellite lesions
- Erythrasma—tan/brown with slight scaling and no active border
- Familial benign pemphigus (Hailey-Hailey disease)
- Folliculitis
- Bowen disease
- Extramammary Paget disease
- Glucagonoma syndrome

✓ Best Tests

Scrape the scaly, active border with a scalpel blade or the edge of a glass slide. Collect scale on a slide and coverslip. Direct a drop of 10% KOH (potassium hydroxide) to the edge of the coverslip, or put a drop of the KOH on the scales before covering with the coverslip. Wait for about 5 minutes, then examine with the microscope. Observe for branching or curving fungal hyphae, which cross the keratin cell borders.

 Management Pearls

Treat all active areas of infection simultaneously to prevent reinfection of the groin from other body sites. Treat clinically affected areas and a 2-cm margin of healthy-appearing skin, and continue to treat for 1 week after clinical resolution. Also, advise drying the inguinal folds completely after bathing. Explain to the patient that permanent cure is rare, but proper treatment results in excellent control that will, however, require periodic retreatment.

Therapy

Limited, localized disease should be treated topically. Allylamines (e.g., terbinafine, naftifine) and imidazoles (e.g., clotrimazole) are the mainstays of therapy. Allylamines may require shorter courses, but imidazoles are less expensive.

Use topical antifungals for 1 to 6 weeks, based on clinical response:

- Terbinafine 1% cream or spray—apply once to twice daily
- Clotrimazole 1% cream—apply twice daily
- Econazole 1% cream—apply once to twice daily
- Oxiconazole 1% cream—apply twice daily
- Ciclopirox 0.77% cream, gel, or lotion—apply twice daily
- Ketoconazole 2% cream—apply once to twice daily
- Miconazole 2% cream—apply twice daily
- Naftifine 1% cream—apply once to twice daily
- Butenafine 1% cream—apply once to twice daily

Topical corticosteroids by themselves or in combination with antifungals are generally not indicated and are absolutely contraindicated in immunosuppressed patients. Use of corticosteroid-antifungal combinations in cases of diagnostic uncertainty may lead to persistent fungal infections and is not recommended.

Extensive disease, particularly when other body parts are involved, may require weeks of oral antifungal agents:

- Terbinafine—250 mg once a day for 2 to 4 weeks
- Itraconazole—100 to 200 mg twice a day for 1 week

- Fluconazole—150 to 300 mg once a week for 2 to 4 weeks
- Griseofulvin ultramicrosize—5 mg/kg/d for 4 to 8 weeks (generally reserved for severe cases)

Systemic antifungals are contraindicated in patients with liver disease; monitoring of liver enzymes is generally recommended.

Immunocompromised Patient Considerations

Localized disease may still be treated topically in immunocompromised patients.

Extensive disease may require longer courses of systemic antifungals than are used in immunocompetent patients:

- Terbinafine—250 mg/d for 2 to 6 weeks, depending on response
- Itraconazole—200 mg twice daily for 2 to 6 weeks, depending on response
- Griseofulvin ultramicrosize—5 mg/kg/d for 4 to 8 weeks

Avoid topical corticosteroids in immunocompromised patients.

Suggested Readings

Drake LA, Dinehart SM, Farmer ER, et al. Guidelines of care for superficial mycotic infections of the skin: tinea corporis, tinea cruris, tinea faciei, tinea manuum, and tinea pedis. Guidelines/Outcomes Committee. American Academy of Dermatology. *J Am Acad Dermatol.* 1996;34(2 Pt 1): 282–286.

Gupta AK, Chaudhry M, Elewski B. Tinea corporis, tinea cruris, tinea nigra, and piedra. *Dermatol Clin.* 2003;21(3):395–400, v.

Gupta AK, Cooper EA. Update in antifungal therapy of dermatophytosis. *Mycopathologia.* 2008;166(5–6):353–367.

Kyle AA, Dahl MV. Topical therapy for fungal infections. *Am J Clin Dermatol.* 2004;5(6):443–451.

Lebwohl M, Elewski B, Eisen D, et al. Efficacy and safety of terbinafine 1% solution in the treatment of interdigital tinea pedis and tinea corporis or tinea cruris. *Cutis.* 2001;67(3):261–266.

van Heerden JS, Vismer HF. Tinea corporis/cruris: new treatment options. *Dermatology.* 1997;194(Suppl 1):14–18.

Verma S, Heffernan MP. Superficial fungal infection: dermatophytosis, onychomycosis, tinea nigra, piedra. In: Fitzpatrick TB, Wolff K, eds. *Fitzpatrick's Dermatology in General Medicine.* 7th Ed. New York, NY: McGraw-Hill; 2008:1815.

Pediculosis Pubis (Pubic Lice)

Aída Lugo-Somolinos

■■ Diagnosis Synopsis

Pediculosis pubis (pubic lice, crabs) is a highly contagious sexually transmitted parasitic infestation with the pubic, or crab, louse, *Pthirus pubis*. Disease is most often spread from person to person by close physical contact, but it may occasionally be spread by fomites such as clothing or linens. Lice feed on human blood several times daily. The bites of the lice are usually painless, but patients often experience intense pruritus. The itching is the result of a reaction to the saliva and/or an anticoagulant injected into the skin by the louse as it feeds. The eggs (nits) are cemented to hair shafts with chitin and are difficult to remove. Lice hatch in approximately 6 to 10 days. Pubic lice are more common in sexually active individuals. In addition to the pubic hair, infestation may involve perianal skin, the axillae, and, rarely, the eyelashes, eyebrows, or chest and facial hair. Patients of African descent are less likely to be infected than whites, but when they are, they may have scalp infestation. Treatment is aimed at eliminating lice via the use of medications and environmental control measures, including treatment of all close contacts.

Pediatric Patient Considerations

Children are most commonly affected with head lice, not pubic lice. Eyelash infection by *P. pubis* is more common in children.

◉ Look For

Look for lice and nits in the pubic hair (Fig. 4-668). They are also occasionally found on eyelashes, eyebrows, facial hair, body hair, or scalp. The lice are approximately 1 mm in diameter and may be tightly adherent to hair shafts. They may be mistaken for crusts or hair casts when attached near the ostia, or openings, of hair follicles.

Inguinal lymph node swelling may be seen.

Erythematous macules or papules may appear at feeding sites after hours or days, and acute wheals may be seen as an immediate reaction. Erythema is often perifollicular. In patients with longstanding infection, *maculae ceruleae* (bluish-gray macules) may form at feeding sites. These may be more difficult to observe in patients with darker skin color.

●● Diagnostic Pearls

- Itching is the main symptom.
- Nits fluoresce under Wood light.

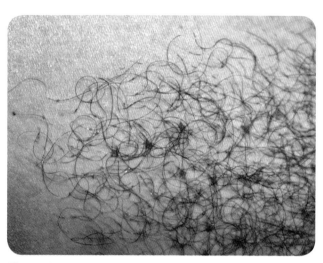

Figure 4-668 Multiple pubic lice may be mistaken for small brown papules, although lice move.

?? Differential Diagnosis and Pitfalls

- Trichorrhexis nodosa
- White piedra
- Peripilar hair casts may be mistaken for nits
- Bites from other insects
- Scabies
- Impetigo
- Other causes of anogenital itch, including tinea cruris, contact dermatitis, and candidiasis

✓ Best Tests

Demonstration of the insect or the nit (from a hair visually or under the microscope) is diagnostic. A magnification glass or a Wood lamp may facilitate the diagnosis.

▲▲ Management Pearls

- The CDC recommends that sex partners within the previous month be treated for pubic lice. Patients should avoid sexual contact with their sex partner(s) until patients and partners have been treated and re-evaluated to rule out persistent disease. Patients should be evaluated and treated for other sexually transmitted diseases. Patients should be aware that condoms do not prevent transmission.
- All potential fomites should be discarded or laundered in hot water and dried on the highest heat. Dry cleaning may also be used. Items that are not easily washed can be sealed

605

in airtight plastic bags for 12 to 14 days. Soak combs and brushes in very hot water for a minimum of 5 minutes. Vacuum the carpets and furniture within the home.

- Shaving the involved area(s) may help eradicate the lice; however, this is not acceptable to many patients.

Precautions: Standard and Contact. (Isolate patient, wear gloves and a gown, limit patient transport, and avoid sharing patient-care equipment.)

Therapy

CDC-Recommended Regimens
Permethrin 1% cream rinse applied to affected areas and washed off after 10 minutes

OR

Pyrethrins with piperonyl butoxide applied to the affected area and washed off after 10 minutes (do not use in those with ragweed or turpentine allergy)

CDC-Recommended Alternative Regimens
Malathion 0.5% lotion applied for 8 to 12 hours and washed off

OR

Ivermectin 250 μg/kg orally, repeated in 2 weeks

Use only aqueous preparations. For all topical preparations, rectal hair treatment is necessary to ensure complete eradication. Hairy individuals should treat their thighs, trunk, and axillary hair.

Infestation of the eyelashes can be treated with ophthalmic petroleum jelly applications twice daily for 2 weeks. Alternatively, nits and lice can be removed with forceps.

Treat any secondarily infected lesions with an appropriate topical or systemic antibiotic.

Additional Information from the CDC
Reported resistance to pediculicides has been increasing and is widespread. Malathion may be used when treatment failure is believed to have occurred because of resistance. The odor and long duration of application for malathion make it a less attractive alternative than the recommended pediculicides. Ivermectin has been successfully used to treat lice but has only been evaluated in small studies.

Lindane is not recommended as first-line therapy because of toxicity. It should only be used as an alternative because of inability to tolerate other therapies or if other therapies have failed. Lindane toxicity, as indicated by seizure and aplastic anemia, has not been reported when treatment was limited to the recommended 4-minute period. Permethrin has less potential for toxicity than lindane.

Suggested Readings

Centers for Disease Control and Prevention. Sexually Transmitted Diseases: Treatment Guidelines 2006, http://www.cdc.gov/STD/treatment/2006/ectoparasitic.htm. Reviewed April 12, 2007. Accessed May 2010.

Chapel TA, Katta T, Kuszmar T, et al. Pediculosis pubis in a clinic for treatment of sexually transmitted diseases. *Sex Transm Dis.* 1979;6(4):257–260.

Short SL, Stockman DL, Wolinsky SM, et al. Comparative rates of sexually transmitted diseases among heterosexual men, homosexual men, and heterosexual women. *Sex Transm Dis.* 1984;11(4):271–274.

Stone SP, Goldfarb JN, Bacelieri RE. Scabies, other mites, and pediculosis. In: Wolff K, Goldsmith LA, et al., eds. *Fitzpatricks Dermatology in General Medicine.* 7th Ed. New York, NY: McGraw Hill; 2008:2029–2037.

Primary Syphilis and Other Sexually Transmitted Diseases

Stephanie Diamantis

◼◼ Diagnosis Synopsis

Primary Syphilis

Syphilis is a sexually transmitted infection (STI) caused by the bacterium *Treponema pallidum* (a spirochete) and is characterized by a chronic intermittent clinical course. *T. pallidum* is transmitted person to person via direct contact and may enter through skin or mucous membranes. *T. pallidum* can also cross the placenta and infect an unborn child, resulting in congenital syphilis.

In the primary stage of syphilis, a painless ulceration, or chancre, typically appears 18 to 21 days after initial infection with syphilis (direct inoculation). In women, the genital chancre is difficult to observe because of its location in the vagina or on the cervix. In men, the chancre is easily seen on the frenulum or on the coronal sulcus of the penis. In both sexes, 15% to 30% of lesions go unnoticed. Chancres vary from a few millimeters to several centimeters. They have an incubation period of 10 to 90 days (average: 21 days). All patients with primary syphilis will go on to develop secondary syphilis if the condition is left untreated.

According to the Centers for Disease Control and Prevention (CDC), over 36,000 cases of syphilis were reported in the United States in 2006. Between 2005 and 2006, the number of primary and secondary syphilis cases increased by 11.8%. Sixty-four percent of syphilis cases were among men who have sex with men. An increased incidence of syphilis in the United States has been observed in African American and Hispanic individuals, sex workers, individuals who sexually expose themselves to sex workers, and individuals with a history of other STIs and/or HIV. The incidence rate among non-Hispanic African Americans remains 50 times higher than for non-Hispanic whites. The presence of other concomitant STIs is common, particularly chancroid and herpes simplex virus (HSV).

Note: See Secondary, Tertiary, and Congenital Syphilis for information on other stages.

Lymphogranuloma Venereum

Lymphogranuloma venereum (LGV) is an uncommon sexually transmitted disease caused by the obligate intracellular bacteria *Chlamydia trachomatis*. It is worldwide in distribution but more commonly seen in tropical and subtropical countries.

There are three distinct stages in the course of the disease. In the first stage, after a 3- to 30-day incubation period, a small painless papule or pustule develops that may erode to form an ulceration. This lesion is often asymptomatic and heals without scarring within 1 week.

The second or inguinal stage begins 2 to 6 weeks after the primary lesion and consists of painful inflammation of the inguinal and/or femoral lymph nodes. There may be prominent systemic symptoms of fever, chills, and malaise.

The third stage of disease is called the genitoanorectal syndrome. In women in particular, it may present after asymptomatic first and second stages. Patients initially present in the third stage with proctocolitis, followed by perirectal abscesses, strictures, fistulas, and rectal stenosis.

Chancroid and granuloma inguinale, very rare in primary care practices, are discussed in the differential diagnosis section. For discussion of other chlamydial infections, refer to VisualDx online.

◉ Look For

Primary Syphilis

Painless indurated ulcer (chancre) with raised/rolled border, clean base, and little exudate (Figs. 4-669–4-671). Common locations include the vagina, cervix, penis (coronal sulcus, sides of frenum), anus, lips, and inside of the mouth (related to unprotected oral sex). The primary chancre typically lasts 3 to 6 weeks. The typical chancre is similar in appearance in dark and light skin types. Unilateral regional lymphadenopathy is nontender and firm.

Lymphogranuloma Venereum

Asymptomatic genital ulceration with mucopurulent cervical/urethral discharge and subsequent development of painful, fluctuant lymphadenopathy. The painful lymph nodes

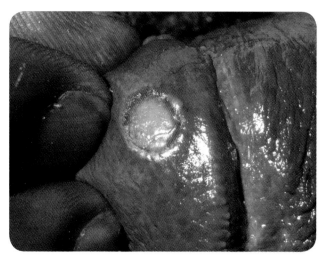

Figure 4-669 Sharply bordered "clean" ulcer on the glans is characteristic of syphilis.

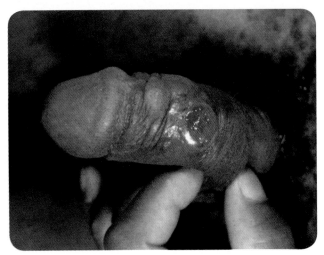

Figure 4-670 Cleanly bordered ulcer on the penile shaft is common in syphilis.

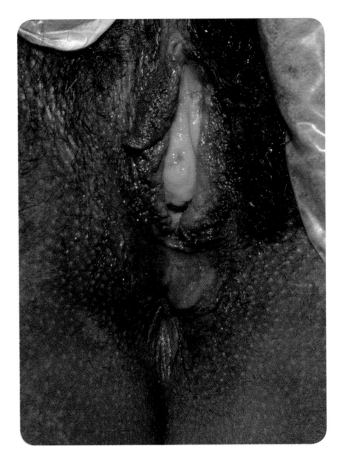

Figure 4-671 Sharply bordered ulcer of primary syphilis on the perineum.

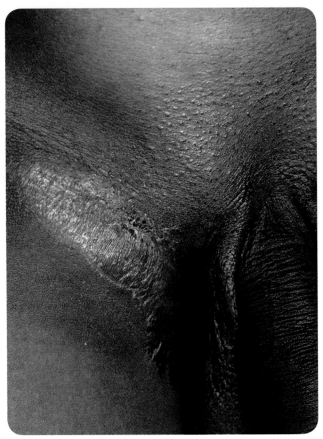

Figure 4-672 Lymphogranuloma venereum with groove sign of swelling above and below the inguinal fold.

Diagnostic Pearls

Primary Syphilis

Chancre is a painless, solitary ulcer with a clean base and an indurated, smooth, firm border.

Differential Diagnosis and Pitfalls

Primary Syphilis

All patients with a genital ulcer should have serologic testing for syphilis. The following differential will be focused on the chancre of primary syphilis.

Infectious

- Genital HSV—look for multiple small vesicles on an erythematous base; usually painful; check Tzanck smear, PCR, and viral culture
- Chancroid (*Haemophilus ducreyi*)—multiple nonindurated ulcers with irregular, ragged, undermined edges; very painful (Fig. 4-673); do Gram stain and culture on selective media for *H. ducreyi*

are known as buboes, and they become fluctuant and rupture. Chronic sinus tract infections may develop. The "groove sign" that results from enlargement of the inguinal nodes above and the femoral nodes below Poupart ligament is seen in one-third of patients (Fig. 4-672).

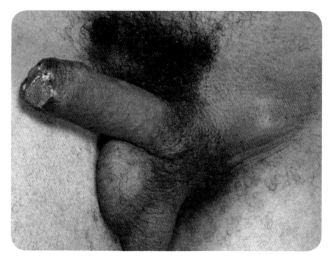

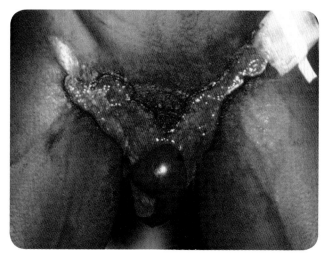

Figure 4-673 Irregular chancroid ulcer of the penis with enlarged warm inguinal lymph node.

Figure 4-674 Bilateral ulcers and penile edema in granuloma inguinale.

- Lymphogranuloma venereum (LGV, *C. trachomatis* serovars L1-L3)—ulcers usually not observed but can have small, shallow, painless ulcer; do serologic testing for LGV
- Granuloma inguinale (*Klebsiella granulomatis*)—painless, extensive, and progressive; looks like granulation tissue (Fig. 4-674); do tissue biopsy

Noninfectious

- Fixed drug eruption—red-brown papules or annular plaques that are commonly on the penis; can progress to bullae and erosions mimicking syphilis
- Behçet disease—Do tissue biopsy if suspecting this diagnosis, and look for recurrent oral ulceration, recurrent genital ulceration, and ocular abnormalities.
- Ulcerative genital carcinoma (i.e., squamous cell carcinoma)—Do a tissue biopsy.
- Genital trauma
- Contact dermatitis
- Apthous ulcers
- Sarcoidosis

Lymphogranuloma Venereum

- Cellulitis/superinfected erosions
- Abscess
- HSV or herpes zoster
- Chancroid
- Granuloma inguinale
- Carcinoma—squamous cell, basal cell, etc.
- Behçet disease
- Syphilis
- Fournier or gas gangrene
- Hidradenitis suppurativa
- Pyoderma gangrenosum
- Ecthyma gangrenosum

✓ Best Tests

Primary Syphilis

The diagnosis of syphilis includes the following strategies:

- Direct visualization of *T. pallidum* via dark-field microscopy
- Direct detection of the bacterial DNA via PCR (useful in genital ulcerations)
- Serologic antibody tests (nonspecific and treponemal specific)

Nontreponemal tests (detection of antibodies to cardiolipin):

- Venereal Disease Research Laboratory (VDRL)
- Rapid plasma reagin (RPR or STS)
- Titers correlate with disease activity; useful in screening and monitoring treatment
- False positives due to pregnancy, lupus erythematosus, lymphoma, antiphospholipid syndrome, cirrhosis, vaccinations, drug abuse, and infectious diseases

Treponemal-specific tests (to be performed when nontreponemal test is reactive):

- Microhemagglutination assay for *T. pallidum* (MTA-TP)
- Fluorescent treponemal antibody absorption test (FTA-ABS)
- Captia enzyme-linked immunosorbent assay
- Not reactive in early primary syphilis
- Will remain positive forever, so not useful for monitoring response to treatment
- False positives in HIV infection, autoimmune diseases, and additional bacteria from treponeme and spirochete families

Note that an early primary lesion (<1 to 2 weeks) must be evaluated by dark-field examination or direct immunofluorescent microscopy of the spirochete (recall that primary lesion occurs *prior* to hematogenous dissemination, so serology will be negative in early primary syphilis).

Do not perform a dark-field examination on oral lesions because nonpathogenic spirochetes are present in normal oral flora.

Patients with very high antibody titers may have a false-negative test, but serial dilutions will correct for this (prozone phenomenon).

Lymphogranuloma Venereum

A definitive diagnosis of LGV can be made with isolation of the organism (from the ulcer or lymph node) on culture and cell typing of the isolate, but recovery of the organism is generally <30%. The diagnosis often rests on serologic testing utilizing complement fixation. Complement fixation antibody titers are usually positive within 2 weeks of disease onset.

Management Pearls

Primary Syphilis

- All patients diagnosed with syphilis should be screened for HIV infection and, if negative, should be retested 3 months later. Syphilis patients with HIV infection can be recalcitrant to therapy and require close follow-up.
- Management of sex partners—Persons exposed to an infected sexual partner within 90 days preceding the diagnosis of primary, secondary, or early latent syphilis may also be infected, irrespective of serologic results; such persons should be treated presumptively.
- Per the CDC, post treatment, repeat nontreponemal serology to ensure fourfold decrease in titer. Check VDRL or RPR every 3 months for the first year and every 6 months for the second year and then yearly thereafter. A fourfold increase in titer indicates reinfection or treatment failure.

Therapy

Syphilis
General
- Penicillin G, IM or IV, for all stages of syphilis remains the gold standard.
- Type of preparation, dosage, and length of treatment depend on stage and clinical manifestations.

Primary, Secondary, Early Latent (<1 year) Infection
Adults
- Benzathine penicillin G—2.4 million units IM, single dose
- Penicillin-allergic patients—doxycycline 100 mg orally twice daily for 14 days
- Patients with penicillin allergy whose compliance with therapy or follow-up cannot be ensured should be desensitized and treated with benzathine penicillin.

Pregnancy
- Treatment during pregnancy is dictated by the penicillin schedule that is appropriate for the given stage of syphilis.
- Note that no alternative exists for penicillin. If the patient has a history of penicillin allergy, she should undergo desensitization.

Lymphogranuloma Venereum
Because this is an STI, screening for other STIs such as gonorrhea, syphilis, HIV, hepatitis, and *Chlamydia* should be considered. Strictures are irreversible. Massive scarring and deformity may require surgery.

Persons who have had sexual contact with a patient who has LGV within the 60 days before onset of the patient's symptoms should be examined, tested for urethral or cervical chlamydial infection, and treated with a standard chlamydia regimen (azithromycin 1 g p.o. once or doxycycline 100 mg p.o. twice a day for 7 days). The optimum contact interval is unknown; some specialists use longer contact intervals.

Suggested Readings

Centers for Disease Control and Prevention. Sexually Transmitted Diseases: Treatment Guidelines 2006, http://www.cdc.gov/std/treatment/2006/genital-ulcers.htm. Reviewed April 12, 2007. Accessed May 2010.

Dourmishev LA, Dourmishev AL. Syphilis: uncommon presentations in adults. *Clin Dermatol.* 2005;23(6):555–564.

James WD, Berger TG, Elston DM, eds. Syphilis, yaws, bejel, and pinta. In: *Andrews' Diseases of the Skin: Clinical Dermatology.* 10th Ed. Philadelphia, PA: Elsevier; 2006:352–364.

Lautenschlager S. Cutaneous manifestations of syphilis: recognition and management. *Am J Clin Dermatol.* 2006;7(5):291–304.

Newman LM, Berman SM. Epidemiology of STD disparities in African American communities. *Sex Transm Dis.* 2008;35(12 Suppl):S4–S12.

Diagnosis Synopsis

Genital herpes has been recorded as the most common cause of genital ulcerations in the United States. Herpes simplex virus type 2 (HSV-2) is the most common strain associated with genital infections, but HSV-1 also contributes to the pathogenesis of genital herpes. This said, it is important to perform a thorough history and exam in order to rule out other potential diagnoses. Most cases of genital herpes are unrecognized, which contributes to the spread of this infection. The risk factors for genital herpes include female gender, non-white ethnicity, low socioeconomic status, older age, prior infection with a sexually transmitted disease, a higher number of lifetime sexual partners, and early age of first sexual intercourse.

Genital herpes is spread through contact with genital secretions of affected individuals. Infected individuals will experience their first outbreak 5 to 7 days after exposure. Primary infections can include a prodromal period of burning, tingling, and localized pain followed by systemic symptoms of fever, headache, and myalgia. The local symptoms include initial tenderness of the affected areas, leading to the appearance of variously sized vesicles that have an erythematous base.

In females, this may occur in the labia minora, introitus, and urethral meatus. In males, it is seen on the shaft and glans of the penis. Other affected areas can include the buttocks, perineum, and thighs. A few days after the appearance of the vesicles, they erupt, leaving small, tender erosions that eventually crust over and heal without scarring. Because of tender lesions, dysuria is a common complaint of affected individuals. The primary infection may last 2 to 6 weeks; subsequent reactivation episodes are classically shorter in duration and severity, typically lasting less than a week.

The phenomenon of asymptomatic shedding has been addressed in recent literature that suggests that the spread of genital herpes can occur during the silent episodes of the disease. This is problematic because it makes the control of new cases extremely difficult and requires that individuals know their status to prevent new infections in sexual partners.

Pediatric Patient Considerations

When children have documented genital herpes simplex infection, strong consideration of sexual abuse is warranted.

Look For

Small, tender, grouped vesicles or erosions on an erythematous base that can resolve with or without scarring (Figs. 4-675 and 4-676). In more deeply pigmented skin, there can be hypopigmentation, hyperpigmentation, and keloidal scarring.

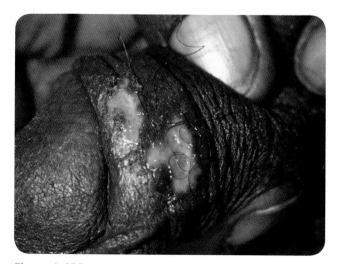

Figure 4-675 Deep, grouped herpes simplex ulcers.

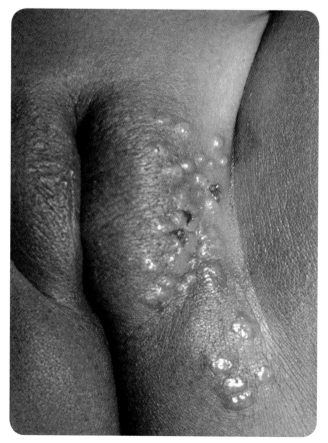

Figure 4-676 Two-year-old patient with primary herpes simplex.

Diagnostic Pearls

Be aware of grouped vesicles or erosions that have a recurrent nature and resolve without scarring. These are the hallmark signs of herpes simplex infections and should be suspected in patients who are in the high-risk categories for having herpes simplex infections including female patients, non-white patients, and patients who have had many sexual partners and/or an early first sexual intercourse experience.

 Differential Diagnosis and Pitfalls

- Herpes zoster (shingles)
- Fixed drug eruption
- Syphilis
- Chancroid
- Trauma
- Behçet disease
- *Candida*
- Pyoderma
- Erosive lichen planus

✓ Best Tests

In patients with lesions:

- Viral isolation in tissue culture is the gold standard. This must be done in patients with active lesions, preferably 2 to 7 days within the episode to ensure proper visualization.
- Tzanck smear
- Direct fluorescence antigen testing
- PCR-based clinical assays

In patients without lesions:

- Type-specific serology tests

 Management Pearls

- There is currently no cure available for herpes simplex infections. With this in mind, it is most important to prevent the initial infection and to control the subsequent outbreaks.
- In patients with genital herpes, barrier methods (condoms) should be advocated to prevent asymptomatic shedding of the virus. It is also important that the patients keep the erosions clean to avoid bacterial infection. Along with suppressive treatment, it is important to consider the stigma associated with herpes infections and to provide support to patients when they discover they have the infection.

Therapy

Initial Infection
One of the following should be administered:

- Acyclovir—200 mg orally five times a day for 10 days
- Acyclovir—400 mg orally three times a day for 10 days
- Famciclovir—250 mg orally three times a day for 7 to 10 days
- Valacyclovir—1,000 mg orally twice a day for 7 to 10 days

Episodic Infection
One of the following should be administered:

- Acyclovir—400 mg orally three times a day for 5 days
- Acyclovir—800 mg orally two times a day for 5 days
- Acyclovir—800 mg orally three times a day for 2 days
- Valacyclovir—500 mg orally two times a day for 3 days
- Valacyclovir—1,000 mg orally once a day for 5 days
- Famciclovir—125 mg orally two times a day for 5 days
- Famciclovir—1,000 mg orally twice a day for 1 day

Suppressive Therapy
One of the following should be administered:

- Acyclovir—400 mg orally twice a day
- Famciclovir—250 mg orally two times a day
- Valacyclovir—500 mg orally once a day
- Valacyclovir—1,000 mg orally once a day

Immunocompromised Patient Considerations

Suppressive Therapy in HIV-Infected Individuals
One of the following should be administered:

- Acyclovir—400 to 800 mg orally two to three times daily
- Famciclovir—500 mg orally twice daily
- Valacyclovir—500 mg orally twice daily

Episodic Therapy in HIV-Infected Individuals
One of the following should be administered:

- Acyclovir—400 mg orally three times daily for 5 to 10 days
- Famciclovir—500 mg orally twice daily for 5 to 10 days
- Valacyclovir—1.0 g orally twice daily for 5 to 10 days

Pediatric Patient Considerations

Limited data are available on the use of acyclovir in children aged younger than 2 years. However, no unusual toxicities have been observed in these children in doses up to 80 mg/kg/d. The safety and efficacy of valacyclovir and famciclovir have not been established in children aged up to 18 years.

- First episode of genital HSV (children weighing more than 40 kg): acyclovir—400 mg p.o. three times daily for 7 to 10 days
- Chronic suppression (children weighing more than 40 kg): acyclovir—400 mg p.o. twice daily

Suggested Readings

Fatahzadeh M, Schwartz RA. Human herpes simplex virus infections: epidemiology, pathogenesis, symptomatology, diagnosis and management. *J Am Acad Dermatol*. 2007;57(5):737–763.

Gupta R, Warren T, Wald A. Genital herpes. *Lancet*. 2007;370.

Money D, Steben M. SOGC clinical practice guidelines: Genital herpes: gynaecological aspects. *Int J Gyn Obs*. 2009;104(2):162–166.

Sizemore JM, Lakeman F, Whitley R, et al. The spectrum of genital herpes simplex virus infection in men attending a sexually transmitted disease clinic. *J Infect Dis*. 2006;193(7):905–911.

Workowski KA, Berman SM. Centers for Disease Control and Prevention. Sexually transmitted diseases treatment guidelines. *Clin Infect Dis*. 2007;44(Suppl 3):S73–S76.

A Practical Approach to Patients with Hair Problems

Lynn McKinley-Grant

"Hair brings one's self-image into focus; it is vanity's proving ground. Hair is terribly personal, a tangle of mysterious prejudices."

—Shana Alexander

Hair is important in defining who a person is, their sex, their racial identification, their ethnic identification, and in many cultures their status and role in the culture. Hair styles are reflective of cultures, socioeconomic backgrounds, and the style of the time. All mammals have hair, and they can be identified by the type and location of the hair. Men and women who have too much or too little in the wrong distribution can be mistaken for the opposite sex. The pattern of growth of hair is a reflection on the patients overall health, and changes in the pattern can reflect scalp diseases and systemic diseases. When a patient is seeking care or advice for a hair problem from a *physician*, the patient is seeing the hair problem as a medical problem, not a cosmetic concern.

The structure of hair is different among different groups. The overall density (hairs per square centimeter) of hair is lower in patients of African descent than in whites or Asians. The hair shaft of patients of African descent is elliptical or flattened in cross section and spiraled or tightly curled in tertiary structure, and the hair follicle is curved, making the hair brittle and giving it a curlier and fuzzier appearance. In the African American community, this hair is referred to as "nappy" hair; however, it is offensive to the patient of African descent for the physician to use the term "nappy." Asian hair is round in cross section and larger in diameter than hair in other groups, with a greater density of hair follicles.

The most common hair complaint is hair loss. We have been struck that many hair complaints are from patients who have thick, luxuriant hair—hair that could pass for normal—when they seek medical attention. The amount of hair lost is relative, though, to what they had originally, and the physician must never minimize the significance of the hair loss.

Patients of a racial or ethnic group other than the physician's are sometimes concerned that a physician of a different background will not be knowledgeable about hair characteristics in their ethnic group and the hair grooming and cosmetic practices commonly used. To establish the patient's trust, the physician must be familiar with the common disorders of hair and have a plan to decide when a biopsy is necessary and useful, and which laboratory tests will aid them in planning therapies and giving useful advice. The physician must make decisions based on the answers received when asking the patient to describe their hair grooming practices; it is important for the physician to repeat the answer back to the patient with an understanding that will fit with medicine and allow the physician to treat the patient.

For over 100 years, the differential diagnosis of hair problems has had an early branching point distinguishing alopecias that scar the scalp from those that do not. Making an error in this early branch point may make establishing the correct diagnosis very difficult. Knowing something about the diseases in each category helps guide the diagnostic paradigm.

Nonscarring alopecias are important because some are easily reversible—like telogen effluvium—and others, like androgenetic alopecias, require lifelong drugs or surgical procedures. Our experience has led us to be most concerned about undiagnosed tinea capitis due to *Trichophyton tonsurans* and telogen effluvium due to thyroid increased or decreased function and iron deficiency without profound anemia. Other tests—for example, of reproductive hormones—should be ordered in conjunction with experts familiar with those tests and their associated disorders. Examination of the hair microscopically—both the shaft and the roots—gives valuable diagnostic information.

Many nonscarring alopecias are due to excessive cosmetic treatments of the hair that can be detected microscopically. Patients are often very reluctant to modify these treatments and often think that the hair salon operator knows best.

Scarring alopecias need treatments to ameliorate progression and also may require surgical transplantations. Scarring alopecia requires a biopsy to establish an etiology. Biopsies can be examined using transverse or longitudinal sections; use of a dermatopathologist experienced with these techniques is recommended.

All forms of alopecia affect the psyche of the patients, and the psyche must be addressed by frank discussions,

Nonscarring Alopecias	Scarring Alopecias
Tinea capitis	Central centrifugal cicatrical alopecia
Trichorrhexis nodosa	Traction alopecia
Telogen effluvium	Folliculitis decalvans
Alopecia areata	Frontal fibrosing alopecia
Male and female pattern alopecia	Kerion
	Halo scalp ring
	Nevus sebaceous
	Aplasia cutis congenita

introduction to support groups, and the use of hair replacement therapies such as falls and wigs.

Individual diseases are discussed in detail on the following pages and on VisualDx online, and the most common forms of scarring and nonscarring alopecia are listed above. Practical approach to hair care of people of African descent:

1. Washing routine is not daily but usually once a week or once every 2 weeks, frequently at a beauty salon. Prescription medications must match this pattern of washing, and patients will get better results if they wash more frequently.

2. Instruct patients not to brush their hair but to use a wide-tooth comb.

3. Instruct patients to sleep on a silk pillow case.

4. The change in texture between new growth and relaxed hair can be one of the major causes of breakage.

5. Patients should not let the stylist put braids in so tightly that they get a headache, as they will lose hair this way.

Nonscarring Alopecia

Ivy Lee • Morgana Colombo • Jennifer Alston DeSimone •
Sridhar Dronavalli • Lynn McKinley-Grant

■■ Diagnosis Synopsis

Tinea Capitis

Tinea capitis is also known as "scalp ringworm." It is an infection caused by dermatophyte species of fungi, most often those of the genera *Trichophyton* and *Microsporum*. The most common causative species in the United States is *Trichophyton tonsurans*. The condition manifests as numerous scaly lesions and patches of broken hair on the scalp. Lesions may suppurate and evolve into kerions. The severity of the disease depends on the organism and the host immune response. Two patterns of infections are recognized: ectothrix and endothrix. An ectothrix infection involves both the inside and outside of the hair shaft, while an endothrix infection involves only the inside. Infections of either type may be anthropophilic (spread from person to person) or zoophilic (spread from a nonhuman species to humans).

Tinea capitis is most commonly encountered in children and occurs in epidemics on all continents, but it is also seen in adults. In older adults or those from outside the United States, unusual dermatophytes may be present. In African Americans, it can be masked and worsened by the hairstyling practice of oiling a dry scalp and the longer intervals of shampooing. Systemic antifungal agents are required for treatment.

Trichorrhexis Nodosa

Trichorrhexis nodosa is a congenital, familial, or acquired disorder of the hair shaft, resulting in characteristic fractured and easily broken hair. In trichorrhexis nodosa, there is damage to the hair cuticle, leading to a frayed microscopic appearance. Proximal acquired trichorrhexis is seen more often in children of African descent and may be related to straightening, perms, combing, and other hair care practices. Distal trichorrhexis is also caused by repeated trauma and is more frequently seen in whites and Asians.

Telogen Effluvium

Telogen effluvium is a nonscarring alopecia resulting from a shift in the hair growth cycle, resulting in excessive hair shedding. At any given time, approximately 90% of normal scalp hair is in anagen (growth) phase and 10% is in telogen (shedding) phase. In telogen effluvium, there is an increase in the percentage of follicles in the telogen phase of the hair growth cycle to >20%. This premature transition of hair follicles to telogen phase may occur in response to acute physical or psychological stress, thyroid disease, hormonal changes including pregnancy, or drugs (beta-blockers and other hypertensive drugs, statins, diabetic drugs, chemotherapeutic agents). Telogen effluvium is the most common alopecia associated with systemic illness. Other causes include iron deficiency and extreme dieting with rapid weight loss. If a sentinel event is identified, it usually precedes the clinically evident telogen effluvium by 3 to 4 months. Many cases of telogen effluvium appear to be idiopathic with no identifiable precipitating factor.

Telogen effluvium primarily affects women of all races and ethnicities and usually occurs in the fourth to the seventh decades of life. Patients present complaining of a sudden increase in hair shedding from the root. Women often describe hair falling out in the shower or during combing or styling. The hair loss occurs uniformly over the entire scalp, and patients do not complain of associated stinging or pruritus. Hair loss usually exceeds 150 hairs daily and may continue for 6 to 12 months. A chronic variant does exist in which the telogen effluvium persists indefinitely.

Alopecia Areata

Alopecia areata is an autoimmune disease of the hair follicle resulting in nonscarring hair loss. Most cases are limited to one or two small patches of alopecia, but in severe cases all scalp hair is lost (alopecia totalis) or all body hair is lost (alopecia universalis). Hair loss can also occur along the sides and back of the scalp (ophiasis), or on the frontal and the vertex areas (sisaipho). Hair in most patients will spontaneously regrow, though recurrences are common. Alopecia areata is seen equally in both sexes and in patients of all ages and ethnicities, with no increased incidence in any particular race. The prevalence is estimated at 0.1% to 0.2% of the US population. There is an increased incidence of alopecia areata in patients with Down syndrome. There is also an association with other autoimmune diseases, particularly thyroid disease, vitiligo, and collagen vascular diseases. Patients with alopecia areata are also more likely to have atopy, and its presence is felt to be a poor prognostic indicator for alopecia areata.

Pediatric Patient Considerations

Alopecia areata is more commonly seen in the first three decades of life.

Male and Female Pattern Alopecia

Male and female pattern hair loss, also referred to as "androgenetic alopecia," is a common androgen-driven hereditary disorder typically seen as patterned hair loss affecting many men and women. It is characterized by miniaturization of terminal hairs in affected areas of the central scalp. There is a gradual conversion of terminal hairs into indeterminate and finally vellus hairs. The frequency and severity increase with age in both sexes. Women are less affected than men. The hair loss onset peaks in the fourth decade in males. In females, there are two peaks of onset: third and fifth decades. The incidence is highest in white men, followed by men of Asian and African descent.

(◉) Look For

Tinea Capitis

Scaly annular patches of alopecia, often with broken hairs (Fig. 4-677). The lesions may contain erythematous papules or pustules, which may be crusted and inflamed. In darker skin types, erythema may be less prominent, while scaling and pustules may be more prominent. Tinea capitis may manifest as diffuse scaling and mimic seborrheic dermatitis.

Kerion, boggy thick plaques often studded with pustules and broken hairs, is a more severe manifestation and is more commonly seen in children of African descent.

Favus, thick yellow crusts composed of hyphae and skin debris (scutula), is the most severe form of tinea capitis.

Both kerion formation and favus may result in scarring alopecia.

There may be associated neck and postauricular lymphadenopathy and pruritus.

Trichorrhexis Nodosa

Small, whitish nodules of the hair shaft (Fig. 4-678). Microscopically, look for the appearance of two straw brooms interlocking to form a nodule of the shaft.

Telogen Effluvium

In the evaluation of hair loss, a complete and detailed history is critical to making the correct diagnosis. Examination of the scalp reveals a diffuse, uniformly decreased hair density (Figs. 4-679 and 4-680). Follicular ostia are intact, and there

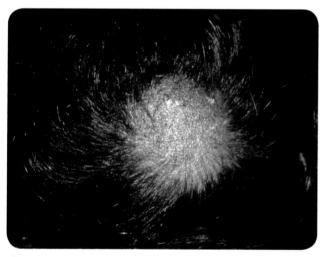

Figure 4-677 Broken-off hairs causing the "black dot" pattern of *Trichophyton tonsurans* infection.

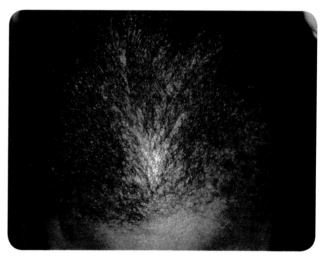

Figure 4-679 Telogen effluvium with diffuse hair loss.

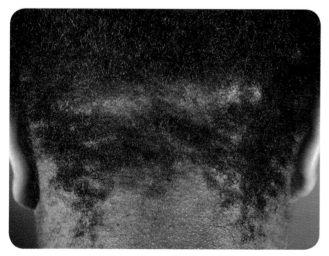

Figure 4-678 Trauma-induced trichorrhexis nodosa.

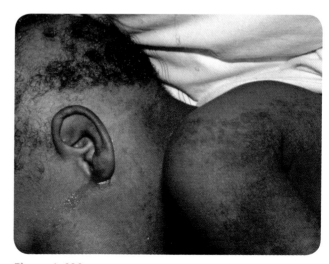

Figure 4-680 Amoxicillin-induced alopecia and exanthem.

is no associated follicular erythema or scale. A pull test performed by applying gentle traction will reveal >10 club hairs. Club hairs are identified as full-length hair shafts with a beaded follicle attached at the proximal end. Telogen effluvium involves terminal hairs of the scalp, and loss of body hair is rare.

Alopecia Areata

Alopecia areata usually presents as round, patchy areas of nonscarring hair loss (Figs. 4-681 and 4-682). Although it usually affects the scalp, the condition can also target the eyebrows, eyelashes, beard, and other body sites (Fig. 4-683). Hairs that grow back are often hypopigmented, temporarily or permanently. This hypopigmentation is not seen in other forms of alopecia.

Regular pitting of the fingernails often occurs with this disease.

Male and Female Pattern Alopecia

Carefully examine with a magnifying glass to see progressive miniaturization of hair in areas of alopecia. Follicles are intact.

In men, hair loss can begin at the anterior hairline with bilateral temporal recession and move posteriorly, or it can present with thinning at the vertex of the scalp (Fig. 4-684). Males of African, Asian, and Native American backgrounds have a decreased frequency of frontal hair loss and less extensive hair loss compared to whites.

In women, the classically described pattern involves central hair thinning of the crown with preservation of the frontal hairline (Fig. 4-685). A male pattern hair loss with frontal or bilateral temporal recession can also be seen. More recently, a third pattern of increased hair loss toward the front of the scalp with encroachment or breach of the

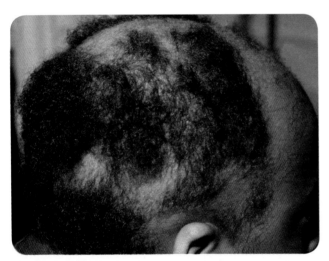

Figure 4-681 Multiple locations of alopecia areata.

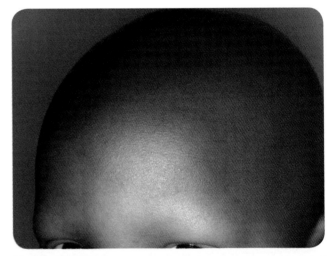

Figure 4-683 Alopecia universalis with entire scalp involved and missing eyebrows.

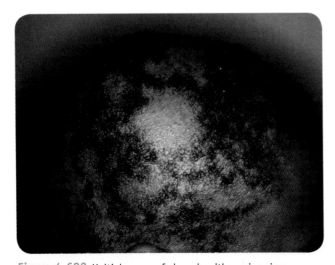

Figure 4-682 Multiple areas of alopecia with varying sizes.

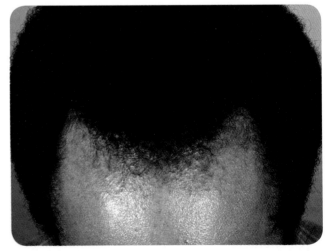

Figure 4-684 Early male pattern hair loss with bilateral temporal recession.

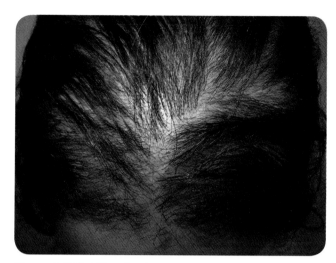

Figure 4-685 Diffuse female pattern alopecia.

frontal hairline, also termed "Christmas tree" pattern, has been described. Women with pattern hair loss usually do not develop true baldness in affected areas as do males.

Women with male or female pattern alopecia must be examined for acne, hirsutism, irregular menses, and other signs of endocrine disorders. When there are suspicions of increased androgen levels, reasonable initial-level screening tests can include serum-free testosterone, DHEAS. Further workups should be done in conjunction with a reproductive endocrinologist.

Diagnostic Pearls

Tinea Capitis

- The tiny black dots on the scalp ("black dot tinea capitis") represent broken-off hairs caused by endothrix infection. The infected stubs of hair remain visible in the follicular orifices.
- *Trichophyton tonsurans*-involved hairs do not fluoresce under a Wood lamp. Animal ringworms (such as *Microsporum canis*) do fluoresce yellow-green.
- The disease may be endemic in families, with adults as asymptomatic carriers.

Trichorrhexis Nodosa

Hair is much more susceptible to trauma when it is wet. The vigorous drying of hair with a towel is a frequent cause of this abnormality.

Telogen Effluvium

The pull test is invaluable. Identification of multiple club hairs is highly suggestive of telogen effluvium. Take a

thorough drug history, as many medications can induce telogen effluvium.

Alopecia Areata

- Scalp burning with or without slight erythema can accompany the lesions. Exclamation point hairs with a tapering base and a ragged proximal portion are diagnostic of the disease. They are frequently at the border of the lesions and can be seen with the aid of a magnifying glass.
- A positive pull test from the periphery of a patch of hair loss indicates that the disease is active and additional hair loss can be expected.

Male and Female Pattern Alopecia

- Male pattern alopecia may be precipitated, or hastened, by other forms of hair loss such as chemotherapy-induced hair loss. Older literature suggests pattern hair loss is less common in individuals of African descent.
- All females with pattern hair loss should have basic blood work including TSH, ferritin, and hematocrit/hemoglobin to rule out underlying thyroid disease or iron deficiency, both of which can lead to telogen effluvium and may mimic pattern hair loss.
- In females, signs or symptoms of hyperandrogenism should also be looked for, such as the following: hirsutism, moderate-to-severe or treatment refractory acne, irregular menses, infertility, acanthosis nigricans, and/or galactorrhea. Females with hyperandrogenic state will usually present with a male pattern hair with bilateral temporal/frontal recession.
- If a hyperandrogenic state is suspected, further evaluation is warranted and should include the following: free and total testosterone, DHEAS, and prolactin. If testosterone is >2.5 times normal, or >200 ng/dL, or DHEAS is >2 times normal, or >700 ng/dL in premenopausal women or >400 ng/dL in postmenopausal women, a workup for a tumor with radiographic tests should be undertaken.

?? Differential Diagnosis and Pitfalls

Tinea Capitis

- Seborrheic dermatitis
- Atopic dermatitis
- Alopecia areata
- Psoriasis
- Secondary syphilis
- Impetigo
- Folliculitis
- Folliculitis decalvans
- Dissecting cellulitis

- Pediculosis
- Traction alopecia
- Systemic lupus erythematosus
- Trichotillomania

Trichorrhexis Nodosa

- In very young children, consider a metabolic disorder such as argininosuccinic aciduria, citrullinemia, or Menkes kinky hair syndrome.
- Trichorrhexis invaginata
- Pediculosis capitis

Telogen Effluvium

- Alopecia areata/totalis—localized patches of alopecia
- Androgenetic alopecia—slow, gradual onset; localized to classic male and female pattern distributions
- Chemical damage—from permanent solutions and heat styling; the hair shafts are broken and are of heterogeneous lengths
- Systemic lupus
- Seborrheic dermatitis—erythema; greasy yellow scale throughout the scalp and often involving the nasolabial folds
- Trichotillomania—broken hairs of varying lengths; shaved test patches will regrow immediately, as the patient cannot grasp the short hairs to pull them out

Alopecia Areata

- Trichotillomania—presents with broken hairs with varying lengths
- Telogen effluvium—presents with diffuse loss of large clumps of hair
- Tinea capitis—presents with erythema and scale; diagnose with KOH prep or fungal culture
- Syphilis—presents with ragged patches of hair loss; diagnose with RPR
- Scarring alopecia—presents with loss of follicular ostia
- Androgenetic alopecia—presents with decreased density of hair in male or female pattern

Male and Female Pattern Alopecia

Other causes of nonscarring alopecia should be considered if the hair loss does not fit the typical frontal/temporal or vertex pattern of hair loss.

- Alopecia areata
- Drug-related alopecia
- Telogen effluvium
- Anagen effluvium
- Tinea capitis
- Trichotillomania

✓ Best Tests

Tinea Capitis

- Examine a KOH preparation of infected, plucked hairs or skin scrapings under the microscope. Hairs may be removed with forceps or by rubbing the area with a toothbrush or moist gauze. Firm scraping with the edge of a glass slide may dislodge small, broken hairs for exam.
- *Trichophyton tonsurans*-involved hairs do not fluoresce with a Wood lamp. Animal ringworms (such as *M. canis*) do fluoresce.
- Fungal culture of hairs or biopsy will provide speciation but will take several weeks. Cultures can be obtained by moistening a sterile cotton swab and vigorously rubbing it over affected areas of the scalp.

Trichorrhexis Nodosa

Examination of the hair shaft under the light microscope will reveal damaged hair cuticle; look for the appearance of two straw brooms interlocking to form a nodule of the shaft.

Telogen Effluvium

A careful history will guide the laboratory workup. When acute illness, profound psychological stress, postpartum status, or sudden weight loss is not present, a standard panel of alopecia laboratory studies is indicated and includes the following:

- TSH, free T4, total T3
- CBC, serum iron, ferritin, total iron binding capacity
- ANA

If the diagnosis remains in question, a scalp biopsy is performed to provide histopathological diagnostic information.

Alopecia Areata

- This diagnosis can usually be made clinically.
- Scalp biopsy is diagnostic in equivocal cases.
- If the clinical situation warrants, tests for associated conditions and other autoimmune diseases may be necessary. Thyroid function tests may be useful to screen for thyroid disease, and ANA can be used to screen for collagen vascular diseases and HBA1C for diabetes.

Male and Female Pattern Alopecia

This is a clinical diagnosis most easily confirmed by the specific pattern of hair loss. Take a family history and use the above management. If there is any doubt, a scalp biopsy would be helpful.

▲▲ Management Pearls

Tinea Capitis

- Because fungal organisms invade the follicle where topical therapy is ineffective, dermatophytosis of the scalp needs to be treated with oral agents.
- Griseofulvin and terbinafine are equally effective in treating tinea capitis due to *Trichophyton* infections. Griseofulvin is fungistatic, requires an 8-week treatment duration, and is poorly absorbed; therefore, advise the patient to take it along with fatty food to enhance absorption. Terbinafine is fungicidal and requires a 4-week treatment duration. The shorter regimen may help in increasing patient compliance and decreasing resistance secondary to early termination of therapy. There is no significant difference in tolerability or adverse effects between griseofulvin and terbinafine.
- Griseofulvin is the treatment of choice in *Microsporum* infections.
- To prevent reinfection and spread of the infection:
  - Patients with ringworm should not use another person's hat, comb, or brush, nor should anyone else use their hat(s) or hair-grooming utensils. Patients should wear a cap if sitting in high-back chairs and should have their own pillowcase.
  - Adjunctive use of a selenium sulfide shampoo or ketoconazole shampoo two or three times a week may reduce the risk of spreading the infection. These shampoos make the hair difficult to comb and cause breakage; thus in patients of African descent, a hair conditioner must be used in conjunction to decrease hair fragility.

Trichorrhexis Nodosa

Advise the patient to wear loose-fitting hats (tight-fitting hats can cause further damage) to protect the hair from prolonged or intense exposure to the sun and to minimize exposing the hair to salt water.

Telogen Effluvium

- Reassurance is the most important step in management. The overwhelming majority of women with telogen effluvium recover within 1 year. Counsel your patients that they will not go bald. It is highly unusual for a woman to lose more than 50% of her hair from telogen effluvium. In women with the chronic variant, the prognosis is the same and patients should be encouraged that they will not progress to baldness.
- Recognize that a telogen effluvium may unmask androgenetic alopecia, and that these two diagnoses may occur simultaneously.

Alopecia Areata

It is important to help the patient understand the nature of the disease. In most cases, hair will spontaneously regrow, though there is a chance of recurrences. The condition is benign but can be psychosocially devastating to the patient or family; therefore, treatment is best made on a case-by-case basis. Support groups, wigs, hats, caps, and scarves are important options for some patients.

Male and Female Pattern Alopecia

- Patient should be advised that the hair loss is nonscarring, so there is a population of cells that can grow and enlarge the hair.
- Currently, finasteride 1 mg and minoxidil topical solution (2% or 5%) or 5% foam are FDA-approved for the treatment of male pattern hair loss.
- Two percent minoxidil solution is FDA-approved for females with pattern hair loss. Five percent topical minoxidil is safe for use in females and better results may be achieved with it; however, it has a higher incidence of facial hypertrichosis. The foam formulation has the advantage of decreased spillage of product outside scalp and has less irritation potential.
- Treatment should be continued for at least 12 months before making a decision about efficacy, although benefits may be seen sooner. If these treatments are discontinued, the extent of loss will rapidly progress to where it would have been had treatment not been initiated.
- Patients should avoid hair care products likely to damage scalp/hair. This is particularly important in African-American females.
- Treat all other underlying causes of hair loss such as seborrheic dermatitis.

Therapy

Tinea Capitis
Preferred Treatment
- Griseofulvin ultra-microsize—375 mg daily for 4 to 8 weeks
- Terbinafine (approved in 2007 for tinea capitis)—250 mg daily for 4 weeks

(Continued)

Pediatric Patient Considerations

- Griseofulvin ultramicrosize—5 to 10 mg/kg/d for 4 to 8 weeks
- Terbinafine—62.5 mg daily (weight < 20 kg), 125 mg daily (20 to 40 kg), or 250 mg daily (>40 kg)

There are limited data on the efficacy and the safety of ketoconazole and itraconazole in children.

Trichorrhexis Nodosa

In acquired forms, minimize damage to the hair shaft. Advise the patient to avoid processes that are traumatizing to the hair, including brushing of the hair, and to shampoo only when necessary, using a mild and creamy shampoo as well as conditioner.

Telogen Effluvium

Therapy is directed at the underlying cause of the telogen effluvium. Infections, psychological stress, and endocrinopathies must be treated appropriately. Regarding iron deficiency, the literature shows that, in individuals without iron deficiency anemia who have serum ferritin levels less than 40 ng/mL, iron supplementation to a level of 70 ng/mL or higher may bring clinical improvement. Standard ferrous sulfate tablets may be prescribed to these patients at a dose of 325 mg by mouth twice daily for 6 weeks. Biotin is a safe therapy that has been used to enhance hair and nail growth. The low risk and the possible benefit make a several-month trial appropriate in those patients who need to feel all safe therapies have been tried.

Alopecia Areata

Counsel carefully before attempting treatment. Patients with limited areas of loss in regions of no cosmetic importance are often best left untreated because spontaneous regrowth often occurs within a year. Treatments may stimulate hair growth, but there is no evidence that the natural course of disease is altered.

Very limited mild alopecia areata and children with alopecia areata are often treated with topical mid–high-potency steroids. Greater extent of disease (totalis, universalis) confers a worse prognosis.

Mild-to-moderate alopecia areata (<25% involvement) can be treated with intralesional corticosteroids to speed regrowth: triamcinolone acetonide aqueous suspension (5 to 10 mg/mL) injected just beneath the dermis in per 0.1-mL injection (maximum 3 mL per monthly visit). Repeat at 4 to 6 week intervals. Adverse effects including pain during injection and atrophy are generally temporary.

There are non–FDA-approved therapies being used including topical immunotherapy with diphencyprone to induce a contact dermatitis. A 2% lotion is applied initially to a small area of alopecia to incite an allergic contact reaction. Subsequent weekly applications to larger areas of alopecia should be at more dilute concentrations (0.001% to 0.1%) that maintain a tolerable level of pruritus and erythema.

For extensive disease, consider PUVA or topical steroids plus minoxidil (each applied twice daily). The efficacy of each is debated. Systemic corticosteroids may offer short-term help, but they have no long-term benefit and should be considered cautiously.

Male and Female Pattern Alopecia

Hairpieces and certain hair weaving techniques are an alternative to medical or surgical intervention.

Topical Therapy
- Minoxidil 5% or 2% solution or 5% foam applied to scalp twice daily.

Systemic Therapy
- Finasteride: 1 mg daily. *Note*: finasteride should not be administered to women.

Antiandrogenic treatments such as oral contraceptive pills and/or spironolactone can be used in females with pattern hair loss, particularly if there's evidence of a hyperandrogenic state.

Scalp reduction or hair transplantation surgeries are effective surgical procedures that should be performed by a qualified dermatologic surgeon or plastic surgeon.

Suggested Readings

Alkhalifah A, Alsantali A, Wang E, et al. Alopecia areata update: Part 1. Clinical picture, histopathology, and pathogenesis. *J Am Acad Dermatol.* 2010;62(2):177–188.

Alkhalifah A, Alsantali A, Wang E, et al. Alopecia areata update: Part 2. Treatment. *J Am Acad Dermatol.* 2010;62(2):191–202.

Andrews M, Burns M. Common tinea infections in children. *Am Fam Physician.* 2008;77(10):1415–1420.

Burkhart CG, Burkhart CN. Trichorrhexis nodosa revisited. *Skinmed.* 2007;6(2):57–58. PubMed Id: 17342017.

Camacho-Martínez F. Localized trichorrhexis nodosa. *J Am Acad Dermatol.* 1989;20(4):696–697. PubMed Id: 2715420.

Gonzalez U, Seaton T, Bergus G, et al. Systemic antifungal therapy for tinea capitis in children (Review). *Cochrane Database Syst Rev.* 2007;4. Art No: CD004685.

Hordinsky MK. Alopecias. In: Bolognia JL, Jorizzo JL, Rapini RR, eds. *Dermatology.* 2nd Ed. New York, NY: Mosby, 2008:1033–1050.

Hordisnky MK, Roberts JL, Stough D, et al. Evaluation and treatment of male and female pattern hair loss. *J Am Acad Dermatol.* 2005;52:301–311.

James WD, Berger TG, Elston DM, eds. Diseases of the skin appendages. In: *Andrews' Diseases of the Skin: Clinical Dermatology.* 10th Ed. 2006; 749–781.

Leonard JN, Gummer CL, Dawber RP. Generalized trichorrhexis nodosa. *Br J Dermatol.* 1980;103(1):85–90. PubMed Id: 7426408.

Manzoor S, Masood C. Alopecia areata in Kashmir: a study of 200 patients. *Indian J Dermatol Venereol Leprol.* 2001;67(6):324–325.

Millikan L. Hirsutism, postpartum telogen effluvium, and male pattern alopecia. *J Cosmet Dermatol.* 2006;5(1):81–86.

Olsen EA. Female pattern hair loss. *J Am Acad Dermatol.* 2001;45:570–580.

Olsen EA. Current and novel methods for assessing efficacy of hair growth promoters in pattern hair loss. *J Am Acad Dermatol.* 2003;48:253–262.

Olsen EA, Messenger AG, Shapiro J, et al. Evaluation and treatment of male and female pattern hair loss. *J Am Acad Dermatol.* 2005;52:301–311.

Rebora A, Guarrera M, Baldari M, et al. Distinguishing androgenetic alopecia from chronic telogen effluvium when associated in the same patient: a simple noninvasive method. *Arch Dermatol.* 2005;141(10):1243–1245.

Rogers NE, Avram MR. Medical treatments for male and female pattern hair loss. *J Am Acad Dermatol.* 2008;59:547–566.

Seebacher C, Bouchara JP, Mignon B. Updates on the epidemiology of dermatophyte infections. *Mycopathologia.* 2008;166:335–352.

Sharma V, Silverberg NB, Howard R, et al. Do hair care practices affect the acquisition of tinea capitis? A case-control study. *Arch Pediatr Adolesc Med.* 2001;155(7):818–821.

Shrivastava SB. Diffuse hair loss in an adult female: approach to diagnosis and management. *Indian J Dermatol Venereol Leprol.* 2009;75(1):20–27.

Silverberg NB, Weinberg JM, DeLeo VA. Tinea capitis: focus on African American women. *J Am Acad Dermatol.* 2002;46:S120–S124.

Sinclair R. Chronic telogen effluvium: a study of 5 patients over 7 years. *J Am Acad Dermatol.* 2005;52(2 Suppl 1):12–16.

Smith RA, Ross JS, Bunker CB. Localized trichorrhexis nodosa. *Clin Exp Dermatol.* 1994;19(5):441–442. PubMed Id: 7955512.

Thomas EA, Kadyan RS. Alopecia areata and autoimmunity: a clinical study. *Indian J Dermatol.* 2008;53(2):70–74.

Trost LB, Bergfeld WF, Calogeras E. The diagnosis and treatment of iron deficiency and its potential relationship to hair loss. *J Am Acad Dermatol.* 2006;54(5):824–844.

Van den Biggelaar FJ, Smolders J, Jansen JF. Complementary and alternative medicine in alopecia areata. *Am J Clin Dermatol.* 2010;11(1):11–20.

Whiting DA. Possible mechanisms of miniaturization during androgenetic alopecia or pattern hair loss. *J Am Acad Dermatol.* 2001;45:S81–S86.

Ectodermal Dysplasias

Lynn McKinley-Grant

▪▪ Diagnosis Synopsis

Ectodermal dysplasias are a heterogeneous group of heritable disorders of the ectoderm that affect the hair, teeth, nails, eccrine (sweat) glands, or other ectodermal tissues (e.g., sebaceous glands, mucous-secreting glands of the GI and respiratory tract, lacrimal glands). There are well over 100 syndromes involving the ectoderm. X-linked ectodermal dysplasia, which primarily affects males although females have mild phenotypic expression, is described below. Another common syndrome, hidrotic epidermal dysplasia, has normal secreting, partial or complete alopecia beginning in childhood, and separation of the nail plate from the nail bed and a small and posteriorly displaced nail plate.

Anhidrotic Ectodermal Dysplasias

Anhidrotic ectodermal dysplasias (AED) are inherited disorders characterized by abnormalities of eccrine (sweat) glands, hair, teeth, nails, and other ectodermal appendages (mucous-secreting glands of the GI and respiratory tract, sebaceous glands, and lacrimal glands). The most common form of AED is X-linked (1 to 7/100,000 newborns), although rare autosomal recessive and dominant forms exist and are clinically identical. Complications can include hyperthermia due to high environmental conditions, poor growth in infancy, and recurrent respiratory infections, presumably because of abnormal mucous gland secretions. Death is rarely a complication in the neonatal period. Mentation is normal.

Other Ectodermal Dysplasias

For a complete list of syndromes, search Ectodermal Dysplasia in the Online Mendelian Inheritance in Man (OMIM) database: http://www.ncbi.nlm.nih.gov/omim.

◉ Look For

Look for hypohidrosis or anhidrosis (sweating is significantly decreased or absent), hypodontia or adontia (teeth may be absent and those present are conical or peg shaped and widely spaced; delayed eruption is the norm), hypotrichosis (fine, sparse, pale, coarse, and slow-growing scalp hair; partially or totally absent brows, lashes and body hair, and variable pubertal hair abnormalities), and distinct facies (frontal bossing, large everted lips, flat nasal bridge all becoming more obvious with age) (Fig. 4-686). Nails are usually normal but may show ridges and be brittle. The skin is extremely dry and pale; atopic dermatitis is common, and the periorbital skin is dark and wrinkled.

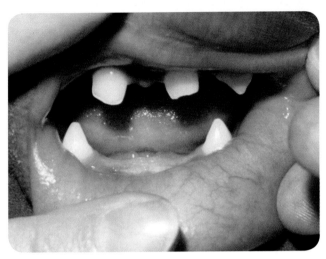

Figure 4-686 Missing teeth or malformed teeth are a clue to anhidrotic ectodermal dysplasia.

◉◉ Diagnostic Pearls

- Hypotrichosis *without* scarring.
- Consider this diagnosis in infants with fever of unknown origin and no infections and in children with recalcitrant dermatitis. Panorex jaw films can demonstrate multiple absent or malformed teeth.

?? Differential Diagnosis and Pitfalls

- Lamellar ichthyosis—if extreme scaling at birth
- Malar hypoplasia—may be mistaken for congenital syphilis
- Ectrodactyly-ectodermal dysplasia clefting syndrome (EEC)
- Hay-Wells syndrome (AEC) (Figs. 4-687 and 4-688)—with fused eyelids and often clefting of oral cavity
- Rapp-Hodgkin syndromes—all include cleft lips
- Zanier-Roubicek syndrome—normal brows and lashes
- Fried tooth and nail syndrome—normal sweating and severe nail dystrophy
- AED with hypothyroidism
- Berlin syndrome—characterized by skin pigmentation mottling, normal sweating, and developmental delay
- Rosselli-Gulienetti syndrome—includes facial clefting and popliteal pterygia as well as the skin and hair features of AED
- Hidrotic ectodermal dysplasia—is autosomal dominant, seen in ethnic groups, and has partial-to-complete non-scarring alopecia, thickened palms and soles, and small nail plates set back on the digits. Sweating is normal (Figs. 4-689 and 4-690).

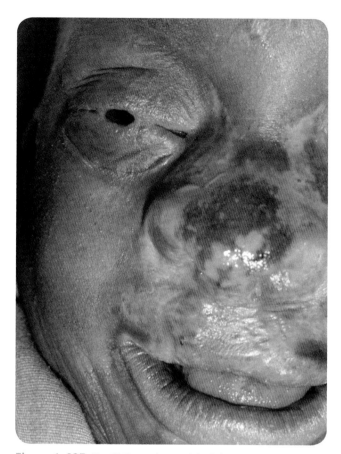

Figure 4-687 Hay-Wells syndrome with clefts and partial fusion of the eyelids.

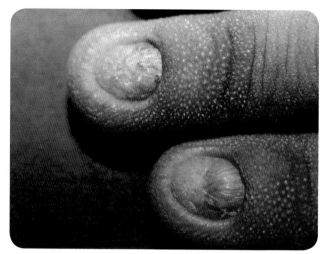

Figure 4-689 Hidrotic epidermal dysplasia with extensive proliferation of the acrosyringium.

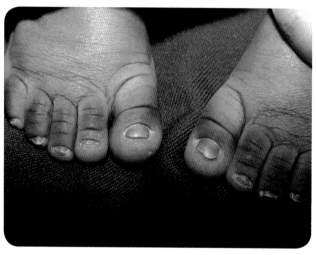

Figure 4-690 Hidrotic ectodermal dysplasia with small uplifted nail plates on the great toes and tiny remnants of nail plates on the other toes.

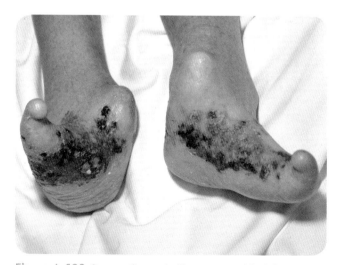

Figure 4-688 Same patient as in Figure 4-687 with clefting.

✓ Best Tests

Panorex jaw films. Genetic analysis can determine defect in ectodysplasin receptor (X-linked gene) or a second autosome coded receptor.

▲▲ Management Pearls

- Keep cool and lubricated. Hyperthermia prevention is essential. Wet shirts in high environmental temperatures help to keep cool.
- Artificial tears should be used for irritated and dry eyes.
- Humidified air and bronchodilators to keep respiratory secretions loose and to assist in keeping respiratory infections to a minimum.
- Ear drops will help to prevent cerumen impactions.
- Moisturizing lotions with sunscreen for the skin.
- Put patients in contact with the National Foundation for Ectodermal Dysplasias (http://www.nfed.org/) for pamphlets and advice.

- Because of the multiplicity of syndromes, genetic counseling can be complicated and a consultation with a medical geneticist can be very useful.

Therapy

Use an optimistic approach with parents; many of these children have been able to participate in athletics and use external water sprays for artificial heat-induced sweating.

Suggested Reading

Sybert VP. Ectodermal dysplasia. In: Wolff, K, et al., eds. *Fitzpatrick's Dermatology in General Medicine.* New York, NY: McGraw-Hill; 2008:1339–1348; chapter 143.

Scarring Alopecia

Morgana Colombo • Lynn McKinley-Grant • Mary Gail Mercurio • Ivy Lee • Alicia Ogram

■■ Diagnosis Synopsis

Central Centrifugal Cicatricial Alopecia

Central centrifugal cicatricial alopecia (CCCA) is a progressive scarring alopecia of the crown and vertex expanding symmetrically and peripherally and seen predominantly in women of African descent. CCCA now includes hot comb folliculitis, follicular degeneration syndrome, pseudopelade in African Americans, and "central elliptical pseudopelade" in whites. Onset often occurs between the second and fourth decades. The hair-grooming factors that are often attributed to CCCA are cornrow and braiding with and without extensions and weaves with sewn in or glued on hair (Fig. 4-691) resulting initially in a tender scalp.

To debunk the myths, a negative correlation between CCCA and the following practices was reported in one study: use of hair relaxers and hot combs, scalp burns from hair relaxers, frequent use of hair relaxers, and use of any of these grooming practices—including cornrows and weaves—before the age of 20. This study was based on US blacks of

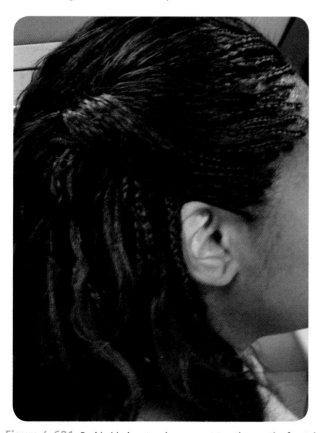

Figure 4-691 Braided hair extension can put traction on the frontal areas of the scalp and lead to hair loss.

African descent, and there are differing reports in African patients and Afro-Caribbean patients.

Traction Alopecia

Traction alopecia refers to scarring hair loss as a result of excessive and chronic tension on the hair follicles and inflammation—usually from styling. It is usually seen on the frontal and temporal margins of the scalp. The condition is more frequent in African American girls and women and less so in boys and men and is due to frequent use of tight braiding, elastic bands, tight rollers, decorative corn rowing, and excessive brushing or heat at the roots. Chemically relaxed hair with these styles is more susceptible to traction alopecia.

Traction alopecia is seen in Eskimos in Western Greenland, young Danish girls with ponytails, ballet dancers, and any ethnic group that styles hair with tension to the frontal region of the scalp. Traction alopecia also occurs with work-related gear such as helmets, hair caps, and head bands.

Folliculitis Decalvans

Folliculitis decalvans (FD) is a common form of scarring alopecia characterized by suppurative folliculitis with destruction of the hair follicle. FD can arise any time after onset of puberty but most commonly occurs in middle-aged adults of both sexes. The crown is the most frequently affected area. Although *Staphylococcus aureus* is often isolated from the follicular pustules, an abnormal host response to this pathogen has been implicated rather than a recurrent staphylococcal folliculitis.

Kerion

A kerion is an acute inflammatory reaction that accompanies cases of tinea capitis and tinea barbae caused by *Trichophyton verrucosum*, *Trichophyton tonsurans*, or *Microsporum canis*. A kerion will occur in a patient with an intact immune response who develops an intense inflammatory response to the organisms. Almost exclusively seen in children, on rare occasions, it may be seen in adolescents and young adults. Like tinea capitis, this disease is more common in patients of African descent. Fever, pain, occipital lymphadenopathy, and secondary bacterial infection may be associated. The intensity of the inflammation depends on the host immune response. If left untreated, scarring and permanent alopecia can develop.

Halo Scalp Ring

Halo scalp ring is a ring or band of alopecia that is several centimeters in width encircling or, more commonly, partially encircling the head. It is associated with caput succedaneum of the scalp in neonates and is believed to be secondary to direct pressure (sometimes with underlying necrosis) on the vertex from the cervix during difficult deliveries, often in primigravidas. Generally, the hair grows back over 6 months without scarring, but there are reported cases of scarring alopecia.

Nevus Sebaceous

Nevus sebaceous (of Jadassohn) is a common hamartomatous malformation that is usually present at birth or develops in early childhood. Its presence may be subtle, and it may not be noted until later childhood or adolescence, when it thickens because of hormonal influence. It consists of a yellow to orange oval or linear verrucous plaque, most often on the scalp or, more rarely, the forehead and neck. Most lesions are sporadic. There is no predilection for either sex or any race or ethnicity. Removal, if not cosmetically a problem, is recommended before adulthood because of the small risk of a malignancy developing within the lesion during adulthood. Risk of development of basal cell carcinoma within lesions is approximately 1%. Other benign adnexal neoplasms, including trichoblastoma and syringocystadenoma papilliferum, occur more frequently within the lesion. In very rare cases, sebaceous or apocrine carcinomas can occur within nevus sebaceous.

A small number of patients with this lesion will have nevus sebaceous syndrome, which is analogous to epidermal nevus syndrome. They may manifest neurologic, skeletal, or ocular abnormalities.

Aplasia Cutis Congenita

Aplasia cutis congenita is a congenital disorder seen in newborns, typically with an absence of the skin of the scalp (but can occur in any location). While most children have no other associated abnormalities, cleft lip and palate, tracheoesophageal fistula, double cervix and uterus, patent ductus arteriosus, coarctation of the aorta, cutis marmorata telangiectatica congenita, AV fistulas, CNS dysraphisms, and intestinal lymphangiectasia have been reported with the anomaly. There is no racial or ethnic predilection. Some reports of aplasia cutis congenita suggest it is genetically determined, and may be more prevalent in children from consanguineous parents.

The newborn can present with an open erosion or a healed, depressed scar.

◉ Look For
....

Central Centrifugal Cicatricial Alopecia

Initially starts in the crown/vertex as thinning brittle hairs with soreness and itching; progressing to shiny and scarred skin and loss of follicles (Fig. 4-692). It spreads from the center to the periphery with minimal erythema, although the histology of the peripheral lesion shows a lymphocytic infiltrate.

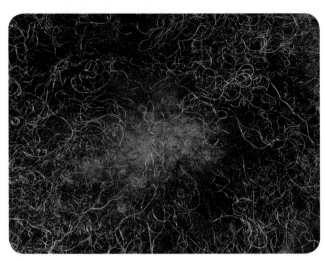

Figure 4-692 Single spot of central centrifugal cicatricial scarring alopecia.

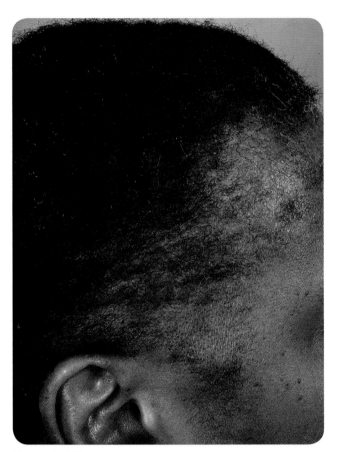

Figure 4-693 Patchy hair loss, often frontal from tight braiding.

Traction Alopecia

Hair loss corresponding to areas of braiding and pulling of the hair, usually temporal and frontal hair margins (Fig. 4-693). The scalp is nonerythematous in later-stage disease. In early disease, however, follicular erythema and hyperkeratosis, folliculitis, and broken hairs may occur. In severe cases, follicular atrophy and permanent nonscarring hair loss can be significant.

Folliculitis Decalvans

Look for crops of pustules, most commonly on the crown of the scalp. The outbreaks wax and wane periodically. Areas that are no longer involved demonstrate scarred plaques of alopecia devoid of hair follicles, and characteristic of this scarring is the occurrence of several residual hairs growing out of a single hair follicle, so-called tufting or doll's hair (Figs. 4-694 and 4-695).

Kerion

Boggy, thick, inflamed plaques or nodules on the scalp, often studded with pustules and broken hairs (Figs. 4-696 and 4-697). These lesions can suppurate. Scarring alopecia may result. Erythema associated with inflammation will appear in shades of red to purple to black in more darkly pigmented skin. Kerion formation may mimic acne keloidalis and FD. Keloidal scarring from kerions is also more common in darker skin types.

Halo Scalp Ring

Alopecia in an annular (or broken ringlike) distribution around the scalp (Fig. 4-698).

Nevus Sebaceous

A solitary yellow-orange plaque, which thickens and darkens with age, typically in early adolescence at the onset of puberty. The lesion usually occurs on the scalp and is accompanied

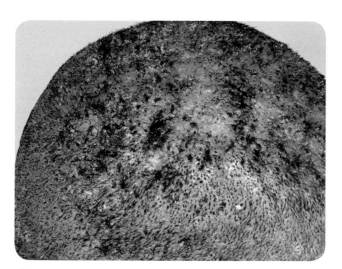

Figure 4-694 Multiple sites of scarring alopecia of folliculitis decalvans.

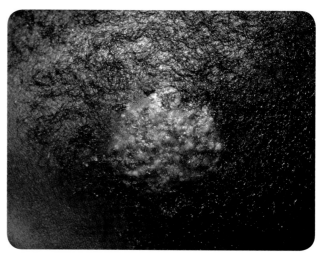

Figure 4-696 This typical kerion, due to dermatophyte, is raised, crusted, and exudative.

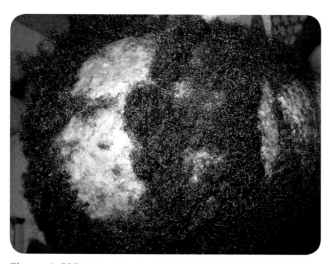

Figure 4-695 Folliculitis decalvans with characteristic tufts of hair within scarred area.

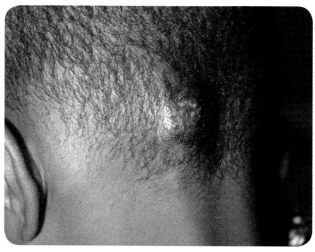

Figure 4-697 Kerion with large, deep, inflammatory component and superficial crust.

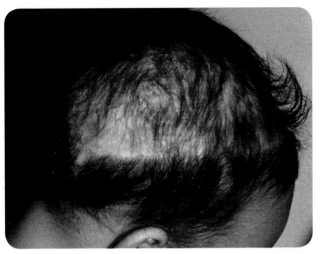

Figure 4-698 Scarring alopecia as a consequence of halo scalp ring.

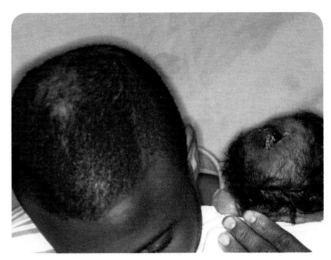

Figure 4-700 Aplasia cutis congenita in a father and child with scarring alopecia.

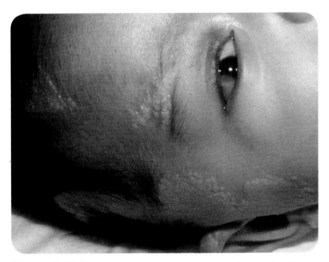

Figure 4-699 Plaquelike nevus sebaceous with peripheral papules involving scalp and face as part of the linear nevus sebaceous syndrome.

by alopecia. It often has a rubbery, verrucous quality (Fig. 4-699). In darker skin types, the plaque can appear very dark and similar in appearance to a seborrheic keratosis.

Aplasia Cutis Congenita

In neonates, aplasia cutis congenital can present as moist open erosions or healed and atrophic scars (Fig. 4-700). Bullous lesions can drain, then refill. A "hair collar sign" (presence of hypertrichosis of coarse hair circumferentially at the rim of lesion) may be associated with underlying CNS dysraphism. In older children and adults, look for noninflammatory and well-demarcated lesions on the scalp, especially along the midline, but also in other body locations. There may be a persistent area of scarring alopecia, typically seen as a depressed scar.

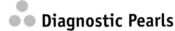

Diagnostic Pearls

Central Centrifugal Cicatricial Alopecia

History of cornrow braiding with or without extensions, of weaves with or without glue, or of central traction. There is some hair on the vertex, but the scalp is scarred.

Traction Alopecia

The location of the hair loss at the margins of the scalp, with receding hair and some broken hairs at different stages, is suggestive of the diagnosis. Look at childhood pictures to see previous hairstyles. Look at photographs of the patient's siblings to see similar styles.

Folliculitis Decalvans

The erythematous follicular pustules are often quite painful.

Kerion

The inflammatory process can lead to a false-negative fungal culture. Diagnosis is based on an index of suspicion, and clinical grounds can be used to initiate therapy.

Halo Scalp Ring

Unusual pattern of alopecia, prolonged delivery (early rupture of membranes, etc.) in a primigravida.

Nevus Sebaceous

The lesion is often flat in the neonate, but there is an absence of hair in a round or an oval shape. Large midline lesions on the forehead may be associated with convulsions and central nervous system malformations.

Aplasia Cutis Congenita

Aplasia cutis congenita may present as single or sometimes overlapping papules resembling a barbell. If the lesion is associated with lipoma or vascular stain, the likelihood of underlying CNS malformation is significantly greater. Lesions heal with scarring.

?? Differential Diagnosis and Pitfalls

- Other types of scarring alopecia, such as discoid lupus or lichen planopilaris
- Nonscarring forms of alopecia may also be considered (see "Nonscarring Alopecia")
- Sarcoidosis
- Alopecia areata usually causes round areas of nonscarring hair loss. However, the ophiasis type of alopecia areata is hard to differentiate clinically from scarring traction alopecia.
- Trichotillomania (the patient is pulling hair out)
- Frontal fibrosing alopecia
- Acne neurotic
- Dissecting cellulitis
- Pseudolymphoma
- Follicular mycosis fungoides
- Erosive pustular dermatosis
- Cicatricial pemphigoid and other scarring bullous disorders including the porphyrias
- Basal cell carcinoma and other malignancies

In Newborns and Children also Consider

- Erosions from herpes simplex virus (HSV)
- Ulceration from application of scalp electrodes or forceps
- Neonatal lupus
- Pyoderma
- Solitary mastocytoma
- Juvenile xanthogranuloma
- Nevus comedonicus
- Solitary collagenoma in tuberous sclerosis

✓ Best Tests

Central Centrifugal Cicatricial Alopecia

- A biopsy will differentiate CCCA from other causes of scarring alopecia. And although CCCA is primarily a clinical diagnosis, a biopsy will also determine whether the disease is active and requires treatment to arrest the process or whether the process is largely completed and patient will no longer benefit from therapy.
- Fungal culture
- ANA—the most frequent presentation of systemic lupus in African Americans is hair loss
- Endocrine workup—thyroid-stimulating hormone (TSH), DHEAS, LH, FSH, prolactin

Traction Alopecia

This is usually a clinical diagnosis, but a scalp biopsy is necessary to confirm. The pathology should be sent to a dermatopathologist familiar with hair and scalp pathology.

Folliculitis Decalvans

Culture of intact pustule. Scalp biopsy of an acute pustular lesion shows suppurative folliculitis, often with rupture of the hair follicle and a concomitant interstitial and perifollicular infiltrate in which neutrophils predominate. Scalp biopsy in a later stage is characterized by reparative fibrosis. Special stains or culture may demonstrate the presence of organisms, the most frequent being *S. aureus*.

Kerion

- KOH preparation of infected plucked hairs or skin scrapings. Hairs may be removed with forceps or by rubbing the area with a toothbrush or moist gauze. Firm scraping with the edge of a glass slide may dislodge small broken hairs for exam.
- *Trichophyton tonsurans*-involved hairs do not fluoresce with a Wood lamp. Animal ringworms (such as *M. canis*) fluoresce.
- Fungal culture of hairs or biopsy will provide speciation but will take several weeks. Cultures can be obtained by moistening a sterile cotton swab or toothbrush and vigorously rubbing it over affected areas of the scalp.
- Bacterial culture to evaluate for concomitant secondary bacterial infection.

Halo Scalp Ring

This is a clinical diagnosis.

Nevus Sebaceous

This is usually a clinical diagnosis. Skin biopsy is diagnostic.

Aplasia Cutis Congenita

Observation. CNS imaging if hair collar sign is present or if surgical intervention is planned. Perform a viral culture to rule out HSV if the lesion is erosive and other signs of HSV are present.

▲▲ Management Pearls

Central Centrifugal Cicatricial Alopecia

Discontinue immediately cornrows, extensions, and weaves of the hair if there is any sign of inflammation.

Early Disease
- Mid- to high-potency topical and/or intralesional steroids, with antibiotics for infection (doxycycline has anti-inflammatory properties), or more aggressive anti-inflammatory medications (see Therapy below).
- Treat any underlying conditions such as seborrheic dermatitis or tinea capitis.
- Examine the periphery of lesions for inflammation and new hair growth. Repeat biopsies can detect inflammation.

End-Stage Disease
- Surgical options.
- Patients who do not respond to therapy or who are unwilling to undergo surgical therapy can consider a hairpiece or prosthesis wig.
- Due to usual lack of visible inflammation, it may be difficult to know when CCCA is active. One clinical indicator of disease activity and need for treatment is the patient's observation that the hair loss is still spreading.

Traction Alopecia

- As the physician, you must let the patient know that you are aware of styling practices and their consequences—or, if you are not aware, have the patient explain the practice to you. If it pulls on the scalp, then it is causing mechanical damage to the hair follicle. Counsel the patient that braiding and trauma to the scalp are to be reduced.
- If traction is recognized early on—during childhood or adolescence—and hair style is loosened and practices that place tension on hair are stopped, full recovery and hair regrowth can be achieved. However, if the patient presents as an adult and reports years of hair thinning on temporal and frontal margins, most likely hair follicles have undergone years of inflammation and scar tissue has formed, making the hair loss permanent.

Folliculitis Decalvans

FD is well known for its resistance to treatment. Some benefit is afforded by antistaphylococcal antibiotics.

Kerion

- A prompt response to treatment of a kerion is critical because the patient will lose hair permanently due to the scarring. Often, the kerion occurs during the first few weeks of treatment, and you must advise patients to come back if there is increased swelling or tenderness. Such patients—adults and children—will need treatment with oral corticosteroids.
- Since fungal organisms invade the follicle, topical therapy is ineffective and oral agents are necessary. The intensity of the inflammatory reaction makes concomitant use of oral corticosteroids reasonable. Prompt and effective treatment is critical in preventing or minimizing cicatricial alopecia and scarring, which is often keloidal in darker skin types.
- Griseofulvin and terbinafine are equally effective in treating tinea capitis due to *Trichophyton* infections. Griseofulvin is fungistatic, requires an 8-week treatment duration, and is poorly absorbed; therefore, advise the patient to take it along with fatty food to enhance absorption. Terbinafine is fungicidal and requires a 4-week treatment duration. The shorter regimen may help in increasing patient compliance and decreasing resistance secondary to early termination of therapy. There is no significant difference in tolerability or adverse effects between griseofulvin and terbinafine.
- Griseofulvin is the treatment of choice in *Microsporum* infections.
- To prevent reinfection and spread of the infection—Patients with tinea capitis should not use another person's hat, comb, or brush, nor should anyone else use their hat(s) or hair-grooming utensils or pomades. Furthermore, these patients should wear a cap if sitting in high-backed chairs and should have their own pillowcase. Adjunctive use of a selenium sulfide shampoo two to three times a week may reduce the risk of spreading the infection.

Halo Scalp Ring

Avoid unnecessary workup for skin disorders.

Nevus Sebaceous

- In the adult years, both benign and rarely, malignant neoplasms can develop within a nevus sebaceous. Prophylactic excision of the entire lesion is sometimes considered for this reason.
- For larger (>1.5 cm) or facial lesions, early removal (first 3 years of life) results in overall better cosmetic outcome.

Aplasia Cutis Congenita

Scalp defects are self-limiting and heal spontaneously with scarring. In severe cases, surgery is necessary to close the defect. CNS imaging should be done prior to surgery.

Therapy

Central Centrifugal Cicatricial Alopecia

Topical treatments such as high-potency topical corticosteroids (clobetasol propionate 0.05% foam, solution or ointment twice daily), tacrolimus 0.1% ointment twice daily or pimecrolimus 1% cream twice daily, or intralesional triamcinolone acetonide, 10 mg/mL, can be used for symptom relief or if biopsy reveals dense perifollicular lymphocytic inflammation.

- Minoxidil tends not to work well but may be tried in women whose scarring is so generalized that transplantation is not practical: minoxidil 5% solution or foam twice daily.
- The combination of oral tetracycline (minocycline or doxycycline, 100 mg twice daily) or antimalarial (hydroxychloroquine, 200 mg twice daily) with either intralesional triamcinolone acetonide or potent topical corticosteroid is thought to be most helpful in active advancing cases.
- Hair transplantation may be successful if the involved area is <5 cm in diameter. It should be noted that the presence of significant scarring in the recipient may make hair transplantation more technically difficult and decrease graft survival rates.

Even if discontinuation of hot combs, relaxers, and/or excessive heat, all factors that have been identified as possibly causing this disease, has not led to cessation of progressive hair loss in most cases, it is still recommended that patients discontinue or minimize such hair treatments.

For patients unwilling to discontinue chemical relaxers, it should be recommended that chemical services be professionally done (salon), that a base (usually petrolatum derivative) be applied to the entire scalp prior to relaxer applications, and that relaxers be applied no more frequently than every 8 to 10 weeks. In addition, the chemical relaxer should never touch the scalp, and relaxers should never be applied with other straightening or coloring agents at the same time.

Traction Alopecia

First and foremost, the patient should discontinue all hair styling practices that put tension on the hair. Intralesional corticosteroid injections (5 to 10 mg/mL triamcinolone) may stimulate hair growth in patients who do not have fibrosis. If fibrosis is present, punch grafts or rotation flaps may enable hair growth. Scalp reduction or flap transplantation can be tried with a surgeon who has a lot of experience.

Folliculitis Decalvans

Antistaphylococcal antibiotics (as determined by culture sensitivities) often afford some improvement such as erythromycin, cephalosporins, trimethoprim/sulfamethoxazole, and clindamycin.

Rifampin, in combination with antistaphylococcal antibiotics, has shown additional benefits. Rapid emergence of resistance prohibits use of rifampin as monotherapy. Note that rifampin may cause secretions (such as urine, tears, saliva, etc.) to turn red-orange.

Oral corticosteroids are sometimes indicated to calm the inflammation.

Zinc sulfate has also been used successfully in a limited number of cases.

Topical antimicrobial therapy may be used as adjunctive agents.

Hair-removal lasers have recently been shown to be efficacious in management of recalcitrant cases.

Kerion

Griseofulvin ultramicrosize—375 mg daily for 4 to 8 weeks

Terbinafine—250 mg daily for 4 weeks

Itraconazole—200 mg daily for 4 to 6 weeks

For severe inflammatory lesions, add prednisone starting at 0.5 mg/kg/d and tapering to zero over 7 to 14 days.

Pediatric Patient Considerations

Griseofulvin ultramicrosize—5 to 10 mg/kg/d for 4 to 8 weeks.

Terbinafine—62.5 mg daily (weight < 20 kg), 125 mg daily (20 to 40 kg), and 250 mg daily (>40 kg).

There are limited data on the efficacy and safety of itraconazole in children.

Prednisone—starting at 0.5 mg/kg/d and tapering to zero over 7- to 14-day course.

Halo Scalp Ring

If there is scarring alopecia, hair grafting may be required.

(Continued)

Nevus Sebaceous

Both surgical excision and careful monitoring are reasonable treatments. Because the risk of malignant transformation is low, especially in children, removal can be delayed until adolescence with careful observation.

Aplasia Cutis Congenita

Standard good wound care.

Scalp defects are self-limiting and heal spontaneously with scarring. In severe cases, surgery is necessary to close the defect.

Hypertrophic lesions respond to intralesional steroid injections (10 mg/mL, 0.1 to 0.3 mL).

CNS imaging should be obtained prior to any procedure, including injections and biopsies.

Suggested Readings

Andrews M, Burns M. Common tinea infections in children. *Am Fam Physician*. 2008;77(10):1415–1420.

Borovicka JH, Thomas L, Prince C, et al. Scarring alopecia: Clinical and pathologic study of 54 African-American women. *Int J Dermatol*. 2009;48:840–845.

Fu JM, Price VH. Approach to hair loss in women of color. *Semin Cut Med Surg*. 2009;28:109–114.

Gathers CG, Jankowski M, Eide M, et al. Hair grooming practices and central centrifugal cicatricial alopecia. *J Am Acad Dermatol*. 2009;60:574–578.

Gathers RC, Lim HW. Central centrifugal cicatricial alopecia: past, present and future. *J Am Acad Dermatol*. 2009;60:660–668.

Gonzalez U, Seaton T, Bergus G, et al. Systemic antifungal therapy for tinea capitis in children (Review). *Cochrane Datab Syst Rev*. 2007;Issue 4. Art No: CD004685.

Harman RR. Traction alopecia due to 'hair extension'. *Br J Dermatol*. 1972;87:79–80.

Huang MJ, Kua KE, Teng HC, et al. Risk factors for severe hyperbilirubinemia in neonates. *Pediatric Res*. 2004;56(5):682–689.

Khumalo NP, Jessop S, Gumedze F, et al. Hairdressing and the prevalence of scalp disease in African adults. *Br J Dermatol*. 2007;157:981–988.

Khumalo NP, Jessop S, Gumedze F, et al. Hair dressing is associated with scalp disease in African schoolchildren. *Br J Dermatol*. 2007;157:106–110.

Khumalo NP, Jessop S, Gumedze F, et al. Determinants of marginal traction alopecia in African girls and women. *J Am Acad Dermatol*. 2008;59:432–434.

Mc Michael AJ. Hair and scalp disorders in ethnic populations. *Dermatol Clin*. 2003;21:629–644.

Parlette EC, Kroeger N, Ross EV. Nd: YAG laser treatments of recalcitrant folliculitis decalvans. *Dermatol Surg*. 2004;30(8):1152–1154.

Prager W, Scholz S, Rompal R. Aplasia cutis congenita in two siblings. *Eur J Dermatol*. 2002;12(3):228–230.

Ross EK, Tan E, Shapiro J. Update on primary cicatricial alopecia. *J Amer Acad Dermatol*. 2005;53:1–37.

Seebacher C, Bouchara JP, Mignon B. Updates on the epidemiology of dermatophyte infections. *Mycopathologia*. 2008;166:335–352.

Sterling JB, Sina B, Gaspari A, et al. Acne keloidalis: A novel presentation for tinea capitis. *J Am Acad Dermatol*. 2007;56(4):699–701.

Suliman TM, Quazi A. Aplasia cutis congenital of the trunk in a Saudi newborn. *Br Assoc Plast Surg*. 2004;57:582–584.

Tanzi EL, Hornung RL, Silverberg NB. Halo scalp ring: A case series and review of the literature. *Arch Pediatr Adolesc Med*. 2002;156(2):188–190.

Watchko J. Identification of neonates at risk for hazardous hyperbilirubinemia: emerging clinical insights. *Pediatr Clin North Am*. 2009;56:671–687.

Cephalohematoma

Alicia Ogram

■ Diagnosis Synopsis

Cephalohematoma is a subperiosteal hematoma caused by rupture of the diploic veins of the skull during a prolonged or difficult labor or delivery, especially one requiring vacuum assistance. Thus the incidence of cephalohematoma may be higher in populations where the vacuum extractor is more commonly used. The swelling may not become apparent for hours or days after birth. Severe lesions may be associated with underlying skull fracture. Infection of the collection has been reported. Occasionally, the hemorrhage can calcify.

Cephalohematoma can cause anemia and is a factor in causing hyperbilirubinemia. The risk of hyperbilirubinemia with cephalohematoma may be higher in neonates of Asian and African descent, given the higher prevalance of glucose-6-phosphate dehydrogenase (G6PD) deficiency and defects in the UDP glucuronosyltransferase 1A1 gene in these populations. Premature birth, more common in African Americans than European Americans, can also be a factor contributing to increased bilirubin levels, which can cause kernicterus.

◉ Look For

A large, soft mass on the scalp localized by the cranial sutures. Overlying ecchymosis or discoloration is not present (Fig. 4-701). Later stages may have alopecia.

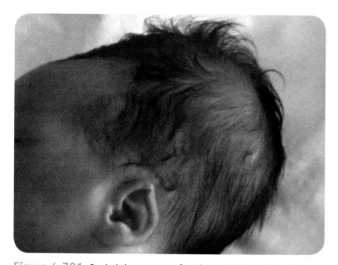

Figure 4-701 Cephalohematoma of scalp can lead to alopecia.

●● Diagnostic Pearls

Typically unilateral and over the parietal bone. Bilateral hematomas will be separated by a depression associated with the intervening suture line.

?? Differential Diagnosis and Pitfalls

- Swelling of caput succedaneum is not well demarcated.
- Encephalocele and meningocele are often associated with pulsation and an underlying bony defect.

✓ Best Tests

This is a clinical diagnosis. Culture of aspirated material can confirm infection but is rarely needed. Radiographs can detect fractures underlying massive lesions.

▲▲ Management Pearls

Treatment is rarely necessary. Spontaneous resorption occurs over weeks to months. Calcification may persist for years.

Therapy

Complications of infection, anemia, or hyperbilirubinemia may require antibiotics, transfusion, or phototherapy, respectively.

Suggested Readings

Chang HY, Chiu NC, Huang FY, et al. Infected cephalohematoma of newborns: experience in a medical center in Taiwan. *Pediatrics Int.* 2005;47:274–277.

Dahl KM, Barry J, DeBiasi RL. Escherichia hermannii infection of a cephalohematoma: case report, review of the literature, and description of a novel invasive pathogen. *Clin Infect Dis.* 2002;35(9):e96–e98.

Huang MJ, Kua KE, Teng HC, et al. Risk factors for severe hyperbilirubinemia in neonates. *Pediatric Res.* 2004;56(5):682–689.

Kaplan M, Herschel M, Hammerman C, et al. Hyperbilirubinemia among African American, glucose-6-phosphate dehydrogenase-deficient neonates. *Pediatrics.* 2004;114(2):e231–e219.

Okpere EE, Itabor AI. The use of the vacuum extractor in a Nigerian Hospital. *Int J Gynaecol Obstet.* 1982;20:29–33.

Watchko J. Identification of neonates at risk for hazardous hyperbilirubinemia: emerging clinical insights. *Pediatr Clin North Am.* 2009;56:671–687.

Pediculosis Capitis

Morgana Colombo

■■ Diagnosis Synopsis

Pediculosis capitis, also known as head lice, is caused by *Pediculous humanus capitis* (head lice). Pediculosis typically affects children of all socioeconomic groups between ages 3 and 11. Transmission is by close contact (direct head-to-head contact) and possibly via fomites (e.g., via clothes, brushes, linens, combs, and hats). Lice live approximately 30 days on the host and 1 to 3 days off the host. Eggs (nits) hatch within 7 to 10 days.

The incidence in hair with a tighter curl, as seen in African hair, is lower than in naturally straight or processed straight hair. Contributing to this lower incidence are several factors: the frequent use of hair pomades and heat to straighten hair and the elliptical shape of African American hair shaft, which makes it harder for the lice to grasp on. However, with current grooming practices such as relaxers, weaves, and permanents, there is an increase of lice in African American children. Also, hair that is imported from India and used in weaves can have lice and will infect a person who uses that hair.

◉ Look For

Lice and nits in the scalp and hair.

Lice—the adult lice are small, wingless ectoparasites. They are 1 to 3 mm long with elongated bodies and three pairs of claw-like legs.

Nits—nits appear as 0.5- to 1-mm gray-white specks that are firmly attached to individual hair shafts (Figs. 4-702 and 4-703). Microscopy will reveal an oblong structure attached to the hair at an acute angle with a lobular breath-

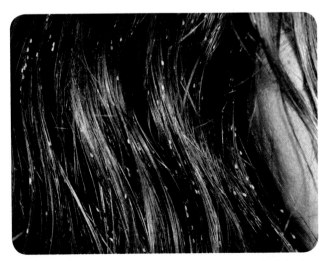

Figure 4-702 Multiple nits from head lice on multiple hairs in a patient in South America.

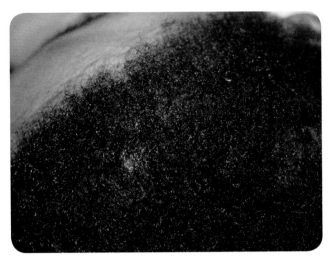

Figure 4-703 Scattered nits in an African American child.

ing apparatus at its superior end. Nits are often present in the occipital and the retroauricular portions of the scalp.

Pruritus is common. Bite reactions, excoriations, cervical lymphadenopathy, and conjunctivitis are also frequently seen.

●● Diagnostic Pearls

- Pyodermas in the scalp along with occipital and cervical lymphadenopathy suggest possible pediculosis infestation.
- Identification of lice may be easiest by combing hair.
- Nits alone are not diagnostic of active infection, but if nits are within ¼ inch of the scalp, active infestation is likely. Nits farther away are not viable except in warmer climates, where viable nits can be seen 8 or more inches from the scalp.

?? Differential Diagnosis and Pitfalls

- Nits can be mistaken for hair casts, debris on hair shaft left by hair spray, and accumulated flakes of seborrheic dermatitis.
- Unlike nits, hair casts—seen in other scalp disorders—freely move along the hair shaft. Microscopic examination allows easy distinction between the opaque amorphous hair cast seen on both sides of the hair shaft and the transparent flask-shaped nit firmly attached to one side of the hair shaft.
- The scales of seborrheic dermatitis are greasy, yellow, and irregular in shape and are easily removable.
- Tinea capitis has similar pruritus and lymphadenopathy but is associated with alopecia. Nits are not found on close examination of the hair.

✓ Best Tests

Demonstration of lice or nits on hair visually or under microscope.

▲▲ Management Pearls

- Although fomite transmission of head lice has not been proven, lice and ova have been found in common household objects, and it is best to eradicate them from these environments. On the day of treatment, clothing worn that day and bed linens can be machine washed or dry cleaned to decrease the risk of fomite transmission. Vacuuming may also be of benefit.
- Many "resistant" infestations are due to improper use of pediculicides, misdiagnosis of active infestations, or reinfestation. After treatment, only individuals found to have living lice (move extremities when stimulated) should be considered to have an active infestation. Patients should carefully read all product labels for over-the-counter topical pediculicides and use exactly as directed by the manufacturer. All household contacts should be examined and treated concurrently.
- Therapeutic failure may also result from resistance of lice and ova to the agent used or insensitivity of the ova to the agent used. There is evidence of increasing resistance of lice to treatment with permethrin. If there is no response with permethrin, use an alternative therapy. Use of a higher-strength permethrin formulation (5% instead of 1%) may be tried first to overcome relative resistance to the lower-strength formulation. Resistance to permethrin may extend to pyrethrins and other pyrethroids.

Therapy

Multiple topical and oral therapies are available for pediculosis. There are worldwide reports of resistance of the lice to some of the current treatments. Prescription products should be reserved for patients with proven infestations that do not respond to proper application of over-the-counter pediculicides. Manual nit removal must be used as an adjuvant to topical therapy. Most herbal and home remedies are unproven in effectiveness and safety.

Over-the-Counter Pediculicides
- Permethrin 1%—Apply to dry hair and rinse after 10 minutes. Repeat in 1 to 2 weeks.
- Pyrethrins with piperonyl butoxide—Apply to dry hair and rinse after 10 minutes. Repeat in 1 to 2 weeks.

Prescription Products
- Malathion 0.5% lotion—Apply to dry hair and rinse after 8 to 12 hours. A repeat application is recommended after 1 to 2 weeks. Not indicated in children aged younger than 6 years.
- Permethrin 5%—Apply to dry hair and rinse after 8 to 12 hours. Repeat in 1 to 2 weeks. Not indicated in infants younger than 2 months.
- Oral ivermectin—200 µg/kg in one oral dose. Repeat in 7 to 10 days. Not indicated in children younger than 5 years or weighing <15 kg.
- Lindane, DDT, and carbaryl—Use of these products is rarely recommended due to potential systemic toxicity and limited effectiveness.
- An oral sulfa antibiotic when added to topical permethrin has been shown to be superior to monotherapy with permethrin.

Physical Nit Removal
Although chemical modalities of treatment are the mainstay of therapy, they do not reliably kill all louse ova; therefore, physical removal of nits is still widely used as an addition to chemical modalities.

Shaving of scalp hair eradicates head lice and ova; however, it is usually not cosmetically acceptable.

Traditional nit and louse removal involves nit picking or combing with a fine-tooth comb. One way of doing this is with wet combing (combing wet hair with a designated comb every 3 to 4 days); however, the rate of nit removal with this technique is quite low. Application of diluted vinegar or 8% formic acid may aid in the removal of nits and improve compliance by making combing easier.

Suggested Readings

Burkhart CN, Burkhart CG. Head lice: scientific assessment of the nit sheath with clinical ramifications and therapeutic options. *J Am Acad Dermatol.* 2005;53:129–133.

Burkhart CG, Burkhart CN, Burkhart KM. An assessment of topical and oral prescription and over-the-counter treatments for head lice. *J Am Acad Dermatol.* 1998;38:979–982.

Elewski BE. Clinical diagnosis of common scalp disorders. *J Investig Dermatol Symp Proc.* 2005;10:190–193.

Elston DM. Controversies concerning the treatment of lice and scabies. *J Am Acad Dermatol.* 2002;46:794–796.

Heymann WR. Head lice treatments: Searching for the path of least resistance. *J Am Acad Dermatol.* 2009;61:323–324.

Ko CJ, Elston DM. Pediculosis. *J Am Acad Dermatol.* 2004;50:1–12.

CHAPTER 5

Medical, Surgical, and Cosmetic Dermatologic Therapies

Dermatologic care makes extensive use of topical and systemic agents, and this chapter emphasizes important practical points for the safe and optimal use of these medications. Surgical therapies and cosmetic treatments should be approached realizing some of the special challenges of certain therapies in pigmented skin. Patients with pigmented skin are most bothered by uneven skin tones or any changes in their appearance that are not received positively by other people of their culture. Physicians should be sensitive to therapies that cause pigment change, either hypopigmentation or hyperpigmentation, as it may not be well accepted. Many patients come from cultural considerations where specific folk medicines are commonly used. These may interact with many of the physician-initiated therapies, and the physician should be sensitive to the use of these unprescribed folk medicines in patients being treated. Details of drug use for specific diseases are covered when specific diseases are considered in Chapter 4.

Topical Medications

Percutaneous Absorption of Topical Medications

The total systemic absorption of topical medicines is related to the concentrations of the medication, the vehicle in which the medication is compounded, intactness of the epidermis, the maturity of the epidermis, and the percentage of the body to which the medication is applied.

General Considerations

Body Surface Area and Topical Medications

Percentage of body surface area (BSA) is useful in determining the extent of dermatologic disease and in roughly estimating the amount of topical medication to be prescribed. Obesity is a major health issue in the United States with a higher prevalence in African Americans and Hispanics and should be considered, since it increases the BSA as well as weight. If the BSA of a patient is known, one can utilize percentages found in the Lund-Browder chart to calculate the amount of topical medication required for a patient to treat his or her dermatosis (Table 5-1).

Vehicle Recommendations

Vehicles, or bases, are major determinants of medication stability, tolerability, absorption, efficacy, ease of application, and patient acceptance. The fundamental ingredients of vehicles are liquids, powders, and lipids. For most dermatologic conditions, vehicles with higher lipid content are preferred (i.e., ointments and oils) because of their increased moisturizing properties, decreased burning on application, and ability to increase percutaneous absorption of most medications. There is a difference in preference for vehicles in men and women and among ethnic groups. For example, men prefer

TABLE 5-1 Amount of Topical Ointment Required to Cover Each Area Twice Daily for a Month (in Grams)

Area	Birth–1 year	1–4 years	5–9 years	10–14 years	15 years	Adult
Entire body	250	500	1,000	1,250	2,000	2,250
Head (back or front)	25	50	60	75	85	85
Upper leg	15	35	70	115	150	215
Lower leg	15	30	50	70	125	150
Trunk (back or front)	35	75	115	150	250	300
Upper arm	10	20	35	45	80	90
Lower arm	10	15	30	35	60	65

no cream or nongreasy creams. African Americans prefer ointment on moist skin. Asians prefer no oils. For locations of the body where the skin is thin or naturally occluded (intertriginous areas) or for dermatoses that are weeping or oozing, vehicles with higher liquid content should be considered (i.e., creams, lotions, gels, and solutions). These enhance spreadability and are better tolerated in moist areas of the body and for "wet" dermatoses. Vehicles with powder added (i.e., pastes and shake lotions) are also useful in intertriginous areas, where they can be used to decrease friction and absorb excess moisture. Recently, foams—which have a more cosmetically elegant presentation—have been developed to improve compliance.

Special Therapeutic Agents

Topical Corticosteroids

Topical corticosteroids are anti-inflammatory and antiproliferative agents that are used extensively in dermatology. Multiple assays have been developed to rank the clinical efficacy of topical steroids, and potency ratings may vary slightly depending on the reference utilized. The Stoughton vasoconstriction assay, in which steroids are classed based on their vasoconstrictive activity, is the most commonly used rating system for the potency of steroids. For most topical corticosteroids, clinical efficacy is well correlated with their position on this ladder (Table 5-2). This is a numerical scale, not a linear ladder, and patients are often confused when they look at the concentration of a steroid and try to correlate that with its potency. Stronger steroids have lower class numbers. It is also important to remember that corticosteroids of the same strength will be of higher potency in lipophilic vehicles (ointments) than in aqueous (lotion) vehicles. Understanding this relationship is imperative to choosing the correct topical corticosteroid in the most appropriate vehicle. Attention to these factors will optimize treatment while avoiding undesired corticosteroid side effects.

When using topical corticosteroids in children, it is important to recognize that many corticosteroids are approved only above a certain age and for a limited period of time.

Potential Adverse Effects of Topical Steroids

The risk for adverse effects from topical corticosteroids is increased in areas of the body where skin is thinnest (eyelids, face, or intertriginous areas where skin touches skin). Although rare in adults, suppression of the hypothalamic-pituitary-adrenal axis may result within a week of exposure to small amounts of superpotent topical steroids (class 1) or extensive and prolonged exposure to medium-potency topical steroids (classes 3 and 4). Serious adverse effects, however, have been reported only after gross misuse over years of topical corticosteroid application.[1–3] Local atrophy can occur with repeated exposure of normal skin to superpotent topical corticosteroids.

Potential Systemic Adverse Effects

- Suppression of the hypothalamic-pituitary-adrenal axis
- Iatrogenic Cushing syndrome

TABLE 5-2 Steroid Potency Ladder: From Most Potent (Class 1) to Least Potent (Class 7)

Ointments and Creams

Class 1

Clobetasol propionate 0.05% ointment and cream

Halobetasol propionate 0.05% ointment and cream

Class 2

Betamethasone dipropionate 0.05% ointment and cream

Amcinonide 0.1% ointment

Mometasone furoate 0.1% ointment

Fluocinonide 0.05% ointment and cream

Diflorasone diacetate 0.05% ointment and cream

Desoximetasone 0.25% ointment and cream

Halcinonide 0.1% cream

Class 3

Triamcinolone acetonide 0.1% ointment

Triamcinolone acetonide 0.5% cream

Betamethasone valerate 0.1% ointment

Fluticasone propionate 0.005% ointment

Halcinonide 0.1% ointment

Amcinonide 0.1% cream

Desoximetasone 0.05% cream

Class 4

Flurandrenolide 0.05% ointment

Fluocinolone acetonide 0.025% ointment

Hydrocortisone valerate 0.2% ointment

Triamcinolone acetonide 0.1% cream

Mometasone furoate 0.1% cream

Class 5

Flurandrenolide 0.025% ointment

Prednicarbate 0.1% ointment and cream

Hydrocortisone butyrate 0.1% ointment and cream

Betamethasone valerate 0.1% cream

Clocortolone pivalate 0.1% cream

Flurandrenolide 0.05% cream

Fluocinolone acetonide 0.025% cream

Hydrocortisone probutate 0.1% cream

Fluocinolone acetonide 0.01% cream

Hydrocortisone valerate 0.2% cream

Fluocinolone acetonide 0.01% oil

Class 6

Alclometasone dipropionate 0.05% ointment and cream

Desonide 0.05% ointment and cream

Triamcinolone acetonide 0.025% cream

Flurandrenolide 0.025% cream

Class 7

Hydrocortisone 2.5% ointment and cream

TABLE 5-3 Suggested Therapeutic Ladder

Potency (Example)	Dermatosis	Thickness	Skin Location	Length of Continuous Use
Superpotent (Clobetasol propionate 0.05% ointment)	Resistant and chronic	Very thick or lichenified	Avoid face and skin folds Caution on torso	Monitor closely if >2–3 wk
High (Fluocinonide 0.05% ointment)	Severe and chronic	Very thick or lichenified	Peripheral extremities Avoid face and skin folds Caution on torso	Monitor closely if >2–3 wk
Intermediate (Triamcinolone acetonide 0.1% ointment)	Moderate acute or chronic	Moderately thick Mildly lichenified	Torso and extremities Caution on face and skin folds	Monitor closely if >2–3 wk on face or skin folds or >3 mo on body
Low (Desonide 0.05% ointment)	Mild and acute	Minimal thickness No lichenification	Face and skin folds	Monitor regularly if >4 wk on face or skin folds
Very low (Hydrocortisone 2.5% ointment)	Very mild and acute	No thickening No lichenification	Face, skin folds occluded areas	Monitor regularly if >4 wk on face

Potential Local Adverse Effects

All of the adverse effects below will appear worse in pigmented skin and leave severe postinflammatory hyperpigmentation.

- Epidermal atrophy
- Striae
- Purpura
- Hypopigmentation
- Glaucoma (from absorption around the eyes)
- Cataracts (from absorption around the eyes)
- Hypertrichosis
- Folliculitis or steroid-induced acne
- Perioral dermatitis
- Delayed wound healing

Guidelines and Tips for the Use of Topical Steroids
- Familiarize yourself with a small group of generic topical corticosteroid ointments to use as a practical therapeutic ladder (Table 5-3) (Micromedex).[4] Build upon this ladder as you gain experience with topical corticosteroids. In the United States, 1% hydrocortisone is available without a prescription.
- Utilize the lowest-strength corticosteroid that will clear dermatitis in a short amount of time (i.e., fewer than 7 days).
- If long-term chronic therapy is required (e.g., for atopic dermatitis), intermittent therapy is recommended over continuous therapy. An ideal topical corticosteroid will clear the patient's dermatitis within 3 days and maintain clearance for a week before more topical corticosteroid is required.
- Use only very mild topical corticosteroids on eyelids or intertriginous areas.
- Recognize that ointments are usually stronger than other formulations when changing vehicles (e.g., changing from an ointment to a solution to treat a dermatosis of the scalp).

Antiparasitic Agents

Most cases of lice and scabies are treatable with topical agents and sometimes systemic agents. Those agents and their usage are listed in Table 5-4.

TABLE 5-4 Common Antiparasitic Agents and Their Uses

Name	Available Formulations	Use
Pyrethrins with piperonyl butoxide	0.3% shampoo or lotion 0.18% lotion	Pediculosis
Permethrin	1% and 5% cream	Pediculosis and scabies
Ivermectin (200 μg/kg)	3 or 6 mg tablets	Pediculosis and scabies
Lindane	1% shampoo or lotion	Pediculosis and scabies
Crotamiton	10% cream or lotion	Scabies
Malathion	0.5% lotion	Pediculosis
Benzyl benzoate	20%–25% solution	Scabies
Thiabendazole (1.5 g p.o. b.i.d. × 2 d)	500 mg tablets	Cutaneous larva migrans
Precipitated sulfur	6% ointment	Scabies

TABLE 5-5 Onset of Action for Topical Anesthetics

Brand	Active Ingredients	Onset of Action
EMLA	2.5% lidocaine and 2.5% prilocaine	60–120 min
LMX-4	4% lidocaine	30–60 min
LMX-5	5% lidocaine	30–60 min
Topicaine	4% lidocaine	30–60 min

TABLE 5-7 Onset of Action for Local Anesthetics

Name	Onset of Action	Duration
Lidocaine	<1 min	30–120 min
Lidocaine with epinephrine	<1 min	60–400 min
Bupivacaine	2–10 min	120–240 min
Bupivacaine with epinephrine	2–10 min	240–480 min
Mepivacaine	3–20 min	30–120 min

Topical Anesthetics

Topical anesthetics are useful for minor procedures on intact skin (needle or laser procedures). More invasive procedures, such as excisions, require the addition of local anesthetics or general anesthesia. Contraindications to topical anesthetics include allergy to amide anesthetics, nonintact skin, and for lidocaine/prilocaine, recent sulfonamide antibiotic use and methemoglobinemia. Dosing and proper application of topical anesthetics are described in Tables 5-5 and 5-6 (Drugdex [Thomson Micromedex Healthcare Series]).[5,6]

Local Anesthetics

Local anesthetics are required for invasive dermatologic procedures (e.g., biopsies and excisions).[7] Onset-of-action information for local anesthetics can be found in Table 5-7. Table 5-8 shows the maximum doses of local anesthetics in children and neonates.

Topical Antifungal Agents

Many topical antifungal agents are available for the treatment of superficial dermatophyte and yeast infections (Table 5-9). They are usually applied twice daily, but more frequent application may be required if agents are removed by bathing or perspiration. Several agents, such as clotrimazole, miconazole, and terbinafine, are available as over-the-counter medications and are good first-line agents. Undecylenic acid and tolnaftate are usually less effective than prescription medications. The use of combination products containing corticosteroids is not recommended.

Acne Medications

The basic principle in treating acne is to utilize the simplest regimen possible that adequately controls the disease. Patients with pigmented skin are more bothered by the postinflammatory changes than the acne. The physician needs to encourage the patient to treat acne quickly to avoid these changes. Once a treatment regimen is begun, medications should be titrated regularly to optimize clinical response and minimize irritation, but allow at least 8 weeks before alterations are made for lack of efficacy.

As retinoids affect all acne lesions, they should be included as first-line agents in every acne regimen. Topical retinoids are ranked by the efficacy of their anti-acne action in increasing strength from azelaic acid as the weakest retinoid to adapalene, to tretinoin, and to tazarotene as the strongest agent in the retinoid class (Table 5-10). Irritancy parallels efficacy, such that tazarotene—the strongest retinoid—is also the most irritating. Many physicians start with a topical tretinoin product (e.g., tretinoin 0.05% cream) and titrate up or down the retinoid ladder based on clinical response and level of irritation.

Other medications may be used in addition to topical retinoids to reduce specific acne lesions. Topical antibiotics are most useful in decreasing inflammatory (erythematous or pustular) acne lesions. Oral antibiotics are most useful in decreasing deep acne nodules. Hormonal therapies are especially useful in women who have acne flares around their periods. Combination products are used to simplify a patient's acne regimen. Systemic retinoids are used when the above regimens fail.

TABLE 5-6 Maximum Dose of Lidocaine Cream

Weight (kg)	Maximum Application Area (cm²)
<10	100
10–20	200

Source: Drugdex (Thomson Micromedex Healthcare Series).

TABLE 5-8 Maximum Dose for Local Anesthetics in Children and Neonates

Name	Max Neonatal Dose	Max Pediatric Dose
Lidocaine	4 mg/kg	5 mg/kg
Lidocaine with epinephrine	5 mg/kg	7 mg/kg
Bupivacaine	2 mg/kg	2.5 mg/kg
Bupivacaine with epinephrine	2 mg/kg	4 mg/kg
Mepivacaine	4 mg/kg	5 mg/kg

TABLE 5-9 Topical Antifungal Agents

Name	Spectrum	Formulation
Ciclopirox	Dermatophytes, yeast	Cream, gel, lotion, solution, nail lacquer
Clotrimazole	Dermatophytes, yeast	Cream, lotion, spray
Miconazole nitrate	Dermatophytes, yeast	Cream
Econazole nitrate	Dermatophytes, yeast	Cream
Sulconazole	Dermatophytes, yeast	Cream, solution
Ketoconazole	Dermatophytes, *Candida* *Pityrosporum*	Shampoo Cream
Oxiconazole	Dermatophytes, yeast, *Pityrosporum*	Cream, lotion
Naftifine	Dermatophytes, *Candida*, *Pityrosporum*	Cream, gel
Terbinafine	Dermatophytes *Pityrosporum*	Cream, solution, spray
Butenafine	Dermatophytes, *Candida*, *Pityrosporum*	Cream
Nystatin	*Candida*	Cream, ointment, powder
Undecylenic acid	Dermatophytes, *Candida*	Cream, foam, spray, powder, ointment
Tolnaftate	Dermatophytes	Cream, gel, spray, powder

TABLE 5-10 Dosage of Acne Medications

Class	Name	Dosage/Application
Topical Retinoids—prevent formation of precursor lesions and decrease comedones and inflammatory lesions		
	Tazarotene	0.05%–0.1% gel or cream qhs
	Tretinoin	0.025%–0.1% cream, gel, or solution qhs
	Adapalene	0.1%, 0.3% cream, gel, lotion qhs
	Azelaic acid	15%–20% cream or gel qhs
Topical Antibiotics—decrease inflammatory lesions		
	Clindamycin phosphate	1% solution, lotion, pad, foam, or gel q.d. to b.i.d.
	Erythromycin	2% ointment, solution, or pad b.i.d.
	Benzoyl peroxide	2.5%–10% cream, gel, lotion, liquid, pad, soap, or solution q.d. to b.i.d.
	Sulfur	1%–10% lotion, ointment, cream, or soap q.d. to t.i.d.
	Sodium sulfacetamide	10% lotion, pad, cream, or soap b.i.d.
Combination Products—combined effects of 2 topical therapies in 1 formulation		
	Benzoyl peroxide/erythromycin	3%/5% cream b.i.d.
	Benzoyl peroxide/clindamycin	1%/5% cream q.d.
	Clindamycin phosphate/benzoyl peroxide	1.2%/2.5%
	Clindamycin/tretinoin	1.2%/0.025% gel qhs
	Adapalene/benzoyl peroxide	0.1%/2.5% gel qhs
Systemic Antibiotics—decrease superficial and deep inflammatory lesions		
	Tetracycline	500 mg b.i.d.
	Doxycycline	100 mg b.i.d.
	Minocycline	100 mg b.i.d.
Systemic Retinoids—decrease comedones and superficial and deep inflammatory lesions		
	Isotretinoin	Up to 2 mg/kg daily or divided b.i.d.
Hormonal Therapies—decrease comedones and superficial and deep inflammatory lesions in women		
	Spironolactone	50–100 mg b.i.d.
	Oral contraceptives	Various

Over-the-Counter Medications

Sunscreens

The American Academy of Dermatology recommends use of broad-spectrum sunscreens with sunburn protection factor (SPF) 15 and above that are water resistant.

Sunscreen Labeling
- SPF—time to produce erythema (redness) on protected skin divided by time to produce erythema on unprotected skin
- Broad-spectrum protection—protection over UVA and UVB spectra
- Water resistant—maintains SPF after 40 minutes of water immersion
- Very water resistant/waterproof—maintains SPF after 80 minutes of water immersion

Insect Repellants

Products containing *N,N*-diethyl-m-toluamide (DEET) or picaridin are formulated for use directly on the skin.[8] Repellants containing permethrin are formulated for use on clothing. DEET is sold over the counter in concentrations ranging up to 100% DEET. The higher the concentration, the longer the protection will last. The CDC recommends 30% to 50% DEET formulations to repel most insects.

Systemic Toxicity from Topical Agents

Serious systemic toxicity has been reported in neonates and children from topical agents. The toxicity is more prone to happen in those with impaired epidermis and those with a lower weight (and hence a high surface area or volume area). Some of those agents are listed in Table 5-11.

Systemic Medications

Systemic Corticosteroids

The use of systemic corticosteroids is limited to specific severe disorders in dermatology, including lupus erythematosus, autoimmune disease, bullous dermatoses, acute allergic reactions, and severe drug reactions. Systemic steroids are very rarely indicated for psoriasis or atopic dermatitis. The most commonly used steroids are prednisone and prednisolone, typically at doses between 0.5 and 2 mg/kg/d (Table 5-12). While on long-term therapy (longer than 2 to 4 weeks), patients should be closely monitored for adverse effects (see below); have their blood pressure followed; and be started on vitamin D, calcium, and a bisphosphonate to prevent osteoporosis. Peptic ulcer prophylaxis can be achieved with proton pump inhibitors.

TABLE 5-11 Potential Toxicities in Children and Infants from Commonly Used Topical Agents

Compound	Use	Toxicity	Risk Factors/Comments
Alcohols	Antiseptic	Hemorrhagic necrosis	Occlusion Preterm infants
Topical corticosteroids	Anti-inflammatory agent	Adrenal suppression	Occlusion (diaper area) Superpotent corticosteroids Use over extensive body Surface area
Calcipotriol	Vitamin D analogue	Hypercalcemia	Regular monitoring of serum calcium recommended in children and infants
Diphenhydramine	Topical antipruritic	Central anticholinergic Syndrome	Not recommended in infants Apply to affected area no more than 4× daily
Lidocaine	Topical anesthetic	Petechiae, seizures	Children <2 y Use over recommended amount (see lidocaine dosing chart)
Lindane	Scabicide	Neurotoxicity	Children <50 kg Other skin conditions (atopic dermatitis) Seizure disorder Use over 2 ounces
DEET	Insect repellant	Neurotoxicity	Infants <2 mo Use over 30% concentration Reapplication more than recommended by manufacturer
Neomycin	Topical antibiotic	Ototoxicity	Premature infants
Povidone-iodine	Antiseptic	Hypothyroidism	Premature infants
Prilocaine	Topical anesthetic	Methemoglobinemia	Use over recommended amount (see EMLA dosing chart)
Salicylic acid	Keratolytic agent	Salicylism, encephalopathy Metabolic acidosis	Use >20% BSA
Silver sulfadiazine	Topical antibiotic	Kernicterus, agranulocytosis	Infants <2 mo

Source: Micromedex.

TABLE 5-12 Systemic Corticosteroid Equivalent Dosing (mg)

Cortisone	25
Hydrocortisone	20
Prednisone	5
Prednisolone	5
Methylprednisolone	4
Triamcinolone	4
Dexamethasone	0.75
Betamethasone	0.75

Before prescribing systemic steroids, patients should have a PPD and control test. Also review history of infectious disease, particularly tuberculosis. The physician must be aware of the higher incidence of hypertension, diabetes, and glaucoma in many patients with pigmented skin. These conditions can affect the decision to use systemic steroids.

Potential Adverse Effects of Systemic Steroids

- Suppression of the hypothalamic-pituitary-adrenal axis
- Adrenal crisis
- Hyperglycemia
- Hypertension
- Congestive heart failure
- Hyperlipidemia
- Cushingoid changes
- Osteoporosis
- Osteonecrosis
- Peptic ulcer disease
- Bowel perforation
- Cataracts
- Agitation
- Immunosuppression
- Myopathy
- Delayed wound healing
- Pseudotumor cerebri
- Perioral dermatitis
- Steroid acne
- Striae

Commonly Used Oral Antibiotics

Some of the antibiotics commonly used for cutaneous infections are outlined in Table 5-13.[9,10] The choice for specific antibiotics is discussed in the section for each disease in Chapter 4.

TABLE 5-13 Commonly Used Oral Antibiotics

Name	Formulations	Dose	Max Dose
Amoxicillin	Drops: 50 mg/mL Suspension: 125, 200, 250, or 400 mg/5 mL Caps: 250, 500 mg Tabs: 500, 875 mg Chewable tabs: 125, 200, 250, 400 mg Tabs for oral suspension: 200, 400, 600 mg	250–500 mg/dose t.i.d.	2–3 g/24 h
Amoxicillin-clavulanic acid	Tabs: 250, 500, 875 mg amoxicillin Extended release tabs: 1 g amoxicillin Chewable tabs: 125, 200, 250, 400 mg amoxicillin Suspension 125, 200, 250, 400 mg amoxicillin/5 mL	250–500 mg/dose t.i.d.	2–3 g/24 h
Ampicillin	Suspension: 125, 250 mg/5 mL Caps: 250, 500 mg	250–500 mg q6h	2–3 g/24 h
Azithromycin	Tabs: 250, 500 mg Suspension: 100, 200 mg/5 mL	500 mg on day 1 followed by 250 mg × 4 d	Multiple-day regimens: 500 mg/24 h 1-d regimen: 1,500 mg/24 h
Cefaclor	Caps: 250, 500 mg Suspension: 125, 187, 250, 375 mg/5 mL	250–500 mg/dose q8h	4 g/24 h
Cephalexin	Tabs: 250, 500 mg Caps: 250, 500 mg Suspension: 125, 250 mg/5 mL	1–4 g/24 h divided b.i.d. to q.i.d.	4 g/24 h
Clarithromycin	Film tablets: 250, 500 mg Extended-release tabs: 500 mg Granules for suspension: 125, 250 mg/5 mL	250–500 mg/dose b.i.d.	1 g/24 h

(Continued)

TABLE 5-13 Commonly Used Oral Antibiotics (*Continued*)

Name	Formulations	Dose	Max Dose
Ciprofloxacin	Tabs: 100, 250, 500, 750 mg Extended-release tabs: 500, 1,000 mg Suspension: 250, 500 mg/5 mL	250–750 mg/dose b.i.d.	2 g/24 h
Clindamycin	Caps: 75, 150, 300 mg Oral solution: 75 mg/5 mL	150–450 mg/dose q6–8h	1.8 g/24 h
Dicloxacillin sodium	Caps: 250, 500 mg	125–500 mg/dose q6h	4 g/24 h
Doxycycline	Caps: 20, 50, 75, 100 mg Tabs: 20, 40 SR, 50, 100 mg Syrup: 50 mg/5 mL Suspension: 25 mg/5 mL	100–200 mg/24 h divided q.d. to b.i.d.	200 mg/24 h

Erythromycin	Estolate:
	  Suspension: 125, 250 mg/5 mL
	Ethyl succinate:
	  Suspension: 200, 400 mg/5 mL
	  Oral drops: 100 mg/2.5 mL
	  Chewable tabs: 200 mg
	  Tabs: 400 mg
	Base:
	  Tabs: 250, 333, 500 mg
		1–4 g/24 h divided q6h	4 g/24 h

Minocycline	Tabs: 50, 75, 100 mg Caps: 50, 75, 100 mg Caps (pellet filled): 50, 100 mg Oral suspension: 50 mg/5 mL	50–100 mg/dose q.d. to t.i.d.	200 mg/24 h
Nafcillin	Caps: 250 mg	250–1,000 mg q4–6h	12 g/24 h
Oxacillin	Oral solution: 250 mg/5 mL	500–1,000 mg/dose q4–6h	12 g/24 h
Penicillin V potassium	Tabs: 250, 500 mg Oral solution: 125, 250 mg/5 mL	250–500 mg/dose divided q6–8h	3 g/24 h
Tetracycline	Caps: 250, 500 mg Suspension: 125 mg/5 mL	1–2 g/24 h divided q6–12h	3 g/24 h

Trimethoprim-
  sulfamethoxazole
	Tabs (regular strength): 80 mg
	  TMP/400 mg SMX
	Tabs (double strength): 160 mg
	  TMP/800 mg SMX
	Suspension: 40 mg TMP/200 mg
	  SMX/5 mL
		160 mg TMP/dose b.i.d.	320 mg TMP/24 h

TABLE 5-14 H1-Antihistamines

Name	Antihistamine Effect	Anticholinergic Effect	Sedative Effect
Chlorpheniramine	Moderate	Moderate	Mild
Cyproheptadine	Moderate	Moderate	Mild
Diphenhydramine	Mild	Strong	Strong
Hydroxyzine HCL	Strong	Moderate	Strong
Loratadine	Strong	Weak	Rare
Fexofenadine	Strong	Weak	Rare
Cetirizine HCL	Strong	Weak	Occasional
Promethazine	Very strong	Strong	Strong

TABLE 5-15 Dosing of Commonly Used H1-Antihistamines

First-Generation H1-Antihistmines

Diphenhydramine	25–50 mg every 4–6 h; maximum 300 mg/d
Hydroxyzine	2 mg/kg/24 h divided q6–8h

Second-Generation H1-Antihistamines

Cetirizine	10 mg daily
Levocetirizine	5 mg daily
Loratadine	10 mg daily
Desloratadine	5 mg daily
Fexofenadine	60 mg b.i.d. or 180 mg daily

Source: Modified from Milgrom H, Leung DY. Allergic rhinitis. In: Kliegman R, Nelson WE, eds. *Nelson Textbook of Pediatrics*. 18th Ed. Philadelphia, PA: Saunders; 2007:951.

H1-Antihistamines

Antihistamines can be very useful for pruritus. Specific dosing is important to prevent adverse effects (Tables 5-14 and 5-15).[11,12]

Immunomodulators

Systemic immunomodulators are important agents for patients with significant cutaneous and systemic disorders and should be used by those with experience with these agents and their side effects (Table 5-16).

TABLE 5-17 Commonly Used Systemic Retinoids

Name	Indication	Dose
Acitretin	Psoriasis	0.5 mg/kg/d
Isotretinoin	Acne	0.5–1 mg/kg/d

Systemic Retinoids

Systemic retinoids are used to treat acne when standard therapies fail. Treatment for acne with isotretinoin usually lasts approximately 5 to 6 months, after which patients are either "cured" of their acne or have residual acne that is much more sensitive to standard therapies. The use of isotretinoin is highly regulated and requires close monitoring. Proper training in the regulatory system and treatment guidelines is required for prescribers through the iPLEDGE program (www.ipledgeprogram.com/PrescriberInformation.aspx). Both systemic retinoids have the potential for causing birth defects in women of childbearing potential, and established guidelines for their use *must* be followed (Table 5-17).

Cosmetic Consideration of Therapies

General Considerations

The concept of beauty has evolved, and now celebrities and models with pigmented skin are more commonly seen and

TABLE 5-16 Dosage of Commonly Used Immunomodulators

Name	Dermatologic Indications	Dosage Range
Methotrexate	Psoriasis Morphea Immunobullous disease	5–25 mg weekly
Azathioprine	Atopic dermatitis Immunobullous disease Lupus erythematosus	3–5 mg/kg/d[a]
Mycophenolate mofetil	Atopic dermatitis Psoriasis Immunobullous disease	2–3 g/d divided b.i.d.
Cyclosporine	Psoriasis Atopic dermatitis	2.5–5 mg/kg/d
Hydroxychloroquine	Lupus erythematosus Polymorphous light eruption	200–400 mg q.d.
Dapsone	Immunobullous disease Pyoderma gangrenosum Pustular psoriasis	50–100 mg q.d.

[a]Initial dosing based on TMPT level.

admired. Hispanics like Jennifer Lopez, African Americans like Beyoncé, and Bollywood actresses like Preity Zinta are commonly depicted in the media and contribute to popular cultural concepts of beauty. Those with deeply pigmented skin account for an increasing proportion of the cosmetic market and are often looking for treatment of conditions such as acne, keloid, dyschromia, and alopecia[13]; however, many cosmetic preparations are a two-edged sword and can aggravate conditions such as acne.

Surgical procedures should always be performed by those with specific training and experience. Some common cosmetic procedures are listed below, with considerations to keep in mind when treating a patient with more deeply pigmented skin.

Fillers

Darker-skinned patients develop more volume loss in the lower face (compared with the deep furrows and rhytides of the lower face seen in whites),[14] so injectable soft tissue fillers are an increasingly used procedure.

Studies have shown that patients with pigmented skin can receive the same benefits of filler injections without experiencing dyspigmentation sequelae, making this a safe procedure for patients with darker skin.[15]

Laser Treatment

Patients with pigmented skin are at a greater risk of developing pigment-related complications after laser treatment, so extreme care and planning as well as knowledge of different lasers is necessary before performing these procedures in darker-skinned patients.

The most common side effect seen after laser treatment is postinflammatory hyperpigmentation.[16] It is more commonly seen with ablative lasers (CO_2, erbium:YAG) and fractional laser treatments. For skin rejuvenation, nonablative lasers such as 1064 nm, 1450 nm, and 1540 nm should be considered because of the lower risk of postinflammatory hyperpigmentation.

Skin tightening with infrared devices has been used for treatment of cutaneous laxity with good results and minimal side effects.

Ethnic patients often request hair removal procedures, especially for hirsutism and pseudofolliculitis barbae. The diode and Nd:YAG lasers are the most effective wavelengths to treat darker skin types,[17] with the long-pulsed Nd:YAG being the treatment of choice for these conditions in African Americans with Fitzpatrick skin types V and VI.[14]

Chemical Peels

Dyspigmentation, lentigines, seborrheic keratosis, and dermatosis papulosa nigra are common concerns in patients with more deeply pigmented skin and may be a cultural concern in some populations such as in Asians and Hispanics. The decision to perform a chemical peeling in pigmented skin should be individualized. Postinflammatory hyperpigmentation is the most common complication in patients with darker skin and occurs with most types of peels, especially deep ones.[18] Glycolic acid peels in lower concentrations may be the safest, but these procedures should only be done by an experienced dermatologist.

Botox

Botox for dynamic rhytides has been used in patients with more deeply pigmented skin with similar results as in light skin. This is considered a safe procedure in this population.[17]

Hair Transplantation

Hair transplantation is performed rarely in African Americans. If considered, caution must be taken because of the possibility of keloidal scarring in the donor site.[18]

References

1. Katz HI, Prawer SE, Mooney JJ, et al. Preatrophy: covert sign of thinned skin. *J Am Acad Dermatol.* 1989;20(5 Pt 1):731–735.
2. Gilbertson EO, Spellman MC, Piacquadio DJ, et al. Super potent topical corticosteroid use associated with adrenal suppression: clinical considerations. *J Am Acad Dermatol.* 1998;38(2 Pt 2):318–321.
3. Warner MR, Camisa C. Topical corticosteroids. In: Wolverton SE, ed. *Comprehensive Dermatologic Drug Therapy.* 2nd Ed. Philadelphia, PA: Saunders Elsevier; 2007:595–624.
4. Drake LA, Dinehart SM, Farmer ER, et al. Guidelines of care for the use of topical glucocorticosteroids. American Academy of Dermatology. *J Am Acad Dermatol.* 1996;35(4):615–619.
5. Soriano TT, Lask GP, Dinehart SM. Anesthesia and analgesia. In: Robinson JK, Hanke WC, Sengelmann R, Siegel D, eds. *Surgery of the Skin: Procedural Dermatology.* Philadelphia, PA: Elsevier Mosby; 2005:39–58.
6. *Physicians' Desk Reference: PDR 2003.* 57th Ed. Montvale, NJ: Thomson PDR; 2003.
7. Lubenow TR, Ivankovich AD, Barkin RL. Management of acute postoperative pain. In: Barash PG, Cullen BF, Stoelting RK, eds. *Clinical Anesthesia.* 5th Ed. Philadelphia, PA: Lippincott Williams & Wilkins; 2006:1405–1440.
8. Katz TM, Miller JH, Herbert AA. Insect repellents: historical perspectives and new developments. *J Am Acad Dermatol.* 2008;58:865–871.
9. Lee C, Robertson J, Shilkofski N. Drug doses. In: Robertson J, Shilkofski N, eds. *Johns Hopkins: The Harriet Lane Handbook: A Manual for Pediatric House Officers.* 17th Ed. Philadelphia, PA: Elsevier Mosby; 2005: chap 27.
10. Schleiss MR. Principles of antibacterial therapy. In: Kliegman RM, Behrman RE, Jenson HB, Stanton BF, eds. *Nelson Textbook of Pediatrics.* 18th Ed. Philadelphia, PA: Saunders; 2007:1110–1122.
11. Scheman AJ, Severson DL, eds. *Pocket Guide to Medications Used in Dermatology.* Philadelphia, PA: Lippincott Williams & Wilkins; 2003.
12. Milgrom H, Leung DY. Allergic rhinitis. In: Kliegman R, Nelson WE, eds. *Nelson Textbook of Pediatrics.* 18th Ed. Philadelphia, PA: Saunders; 2007:951.
13. Taylor Sc. Epidemiology of skin diseases in ethnic populations. *Dermatol Clin.* 2003;21:601–607.

14. Burgess CM. Soft tissue augmentation in skin of color: market growth, available fillers, and successful techniques. *J Drugs Dermatol.* 2007; 6(1):51–55.

15. Odunze M, Cohn A, Few JW. Restylane and people of color. *Plast Reconstr Surg.* 2007;120:2011–2016.

16. Carniol PJ, Woolery-Lloyd H, Zhao AS, et al. Laser treatment for ethnic skin. *Facial Plast Surg Clin N Am.* 2010;18:105–110.

17. Ross EV, Cooke LM, Timko AL, et al. Treatment of pseudofolliculitis barbae in skin types IV, V, and VI with a long-pulsed neodymium:yttrium aluminum garnet laser. *J Am Acad Dermatol.* 2002;47(2):263–270.

18. Rullan P, Karam AM. Chemical peels for darker skin types. *Facial Plast Surg Clin N Am.* 2010;18:111–131.

Suggested Readings

Grimes PE, ed. *Aesthetics and Cosmetic Surgery for Darker Skin Types.* Philadelphia, PA: Lippincott Williams & Wilkins; 2008.

Talakoub L, Wesley NO. Differences in perceptions of beauty and cosmetic procedures performed in ethnic patients. *Sem Cut Med Surg.* 2009;28:115–129.

Index

Note: Page numbers followed by "f" denote figures and those followed by "t" denote tables.